HUMAN ANATOMY & Physiology I

3rd EDITION

Mark F. Taylor, Ph.D.

Baylor University

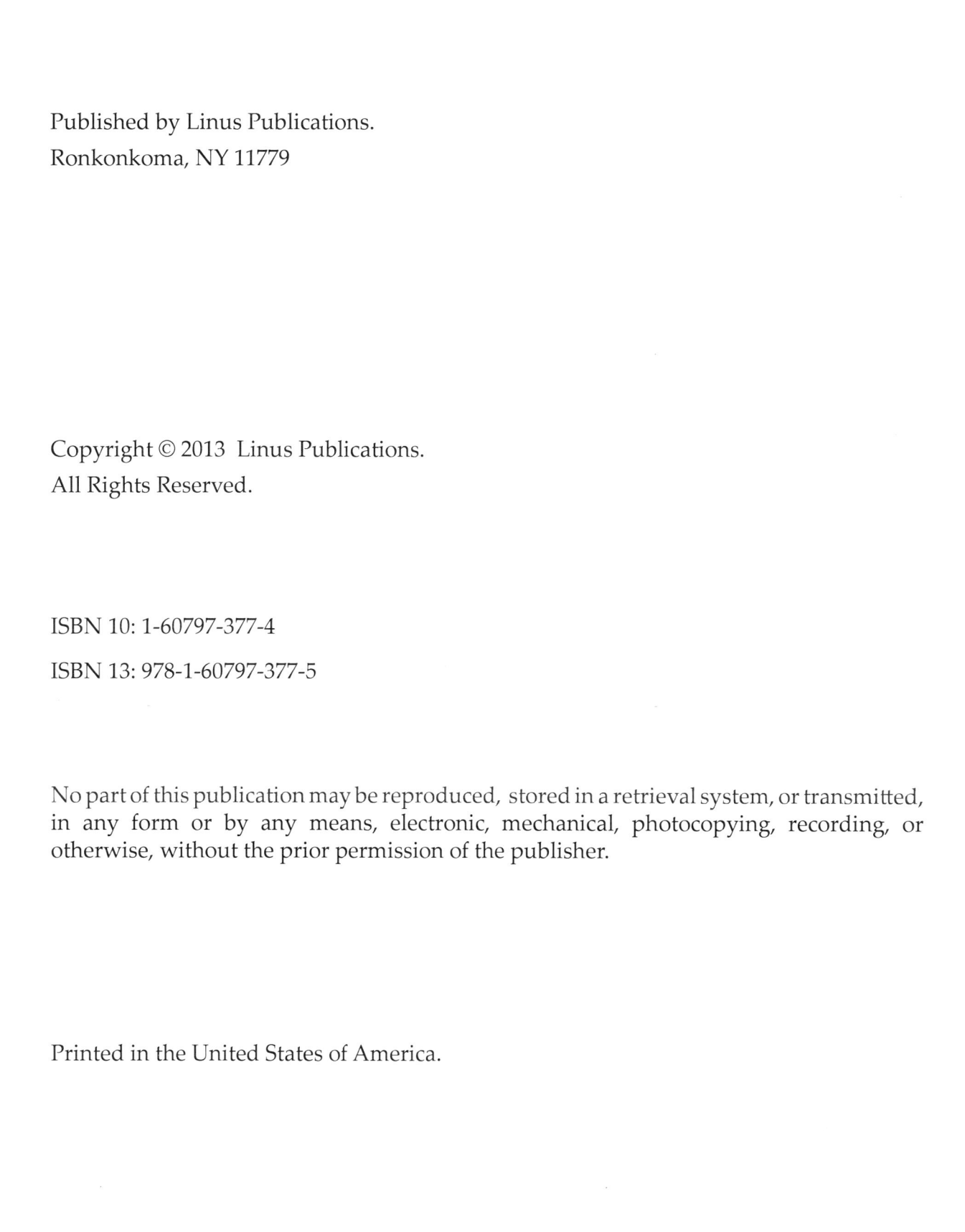

Published by Linus Publications.
Ronkonkoma, NY 11779

Copyright © 2013 Linus Publications.
All Rights Reserved.

ISBN 10: 1-60797-377-4

ISBN 13: 978-1-60797-377-5

No part of this publication may be reproduced, stored in a retrieval system, or transmitted, in any form or by any means, electronic, mechanical, photocopying, recording, or otherwise, without the prior permission of the publisher.

Printed in the United States of America.

Print Numbers   5   4   3   2   1

Acknowledgements

I would like to express my sincere appreciation to Linus Learning, for its willingness to publish this text. Specifically, I would like to thank Jay Herarth for his unending support of this work and his frequent encouragement along the way. I would also like to thank the editors who worked diligently on putting together the artwork and formatting the text. I want to thank Ekerd and Nash for your efforts as well. Last, but not least, I want to thank my wife, Linda, for her undying support of me through this and all the other time-intensive endeavors I have undertaken.

Preface

Human anatomy and physiology (A&P) is a course about the characteristics of the human body: its multitude of structures and their functions. Most students who enroll in an A&P course may be planning for a career in a health profession, such as nursing, nutrition science, physical or occupation therapy, or medicine. However, a student does not need to be headed toward any specific career in order to derive benefits from taking an A&P course. This text is designed to enlighten the reader with up-to-date information about basic human form and function, but it is not an exhaustive assemblage of every A&P fact. Nevertheless, it presents to the reader more detail than might be found in a book designed to highlight only the most basic facts about the human body. Indeed, scientific information is ever changing, and even facts about anatomy, or the shape of things, can change over time. In the future, it will likely be necessary to change the way we view or explain various aspects of the human body, but for now our current information will have to suffice. So, even if you have had an A&P course in the past, read this text with an expectation to learn something new. Even looking at "old" facts can be enlightening when viewed from a different perspective.

Table of Contents

Chapter 1:
Introduction to Human Anatomy & Physiology ... 1

    Anatomy & Physiology ... 2
    The Science of Anatomy ... 2
    The Science of Physiology ... 3
    Organization of the Body ... 3
    The Characteristics of Life ... 5
    Environmental Requirements for Life ... 7
    Homeostasis ... 8
    Homeostatic Control Systems ... 8
    Feedback Mechanisms in Homeostasis ... 9
    Relationships among Variables ... 11
    Homeostasis and Disease ... 12
    Review ... 12
    Topics to Know in Chapter 1 ... 13

Chapter 2:
Body Organization ... 15

    The Axial Region ... 15
    The Appendicular Region ... 15
    Directional Terms ... 15
    Planes and Sections ... 19
    Body Cavities ... 20
    Serous Membranes ... 21
    Mucous Membranes ... 22
    Abdominopelvic Quadrants and Regions ... 23
    Topics to Know in Chapter 2 ... 24

Chapter 3:
Chemistry Overview 27

    Atoms, Molecules, and Compounds 27

    Mixtures 28

    Chemical Bonds 29

    Isotopes 30

    Energy 30

    Chemical Reactions 31

    Water 33

    Acids, Bases, and Salts 33

    Buffers 35

    Inorganic and Organic Compounds 35

    Enzymes 35

    Carbohydrates 38

    Lipids 39

    Protein 41

    Nucleic Acids 43

    Topics to Know for Chapter 3 45

Chapter 4:
Overview of the Cell 47

    Overview of a Typical Cell 47

    The Cytosol and Inclusions 47

    The Cytoskeleton 49

    The Projections of a Body Cell 52

    Cytoplasmic Organelles 53

    Topics to Know in Chapter 4 61

Chapter 5:
The Nucleus, DNA Expression, and the Cell Cycle ... 63

- Function of the Nucleus ... 63
- Structure of the Nucleus ... 64
- Organization of the Genetic Material ... 64
- DNA Expression ... 66
- Transcription ... 66
- Translation ... 70
- Cellular Differentiation ... 73
- The Cell Cycle ... 73
- Interphase ... 74
- Mitosis ... 75
- Cytokinesis ... 76
- Closer look at DNA Replication ... 77
- Mutations ... 78
- Control of the Cell Cycle ... 79
- Predetermined Limits on Cell Division ... 80
- Topics to Know for Chapter 5 ... 81

Chapter 6:
Membrane Structure and Function ... 83

- Membrane Lipids ... 83
- Membrane Carbohydrates ... 85
- Membrane Proteins ... 86
- Membrane Transport ... 87
- Membrane Permeability ... 87
- Gradients Across A Membrane ... 87
- Diffusion ... 88
- Osmosis: A Special Case of Diffusion ... 90
- Factors Affecting Diffusion ... 93

    Carrier-Mediated Transport..94

    Vesicular Transport 98

    Topics to Know for Chapter 6 101

Chapter 7:
Tissues 103

    Cell Connections 103

    Epithelial Tissue 104

    Classification of Membranous Epithelium 105

    Specific Membranous Epithelia 106

    Connective Tissue 108

    Cells In Connective Tissues 109

    Connective Tissue Proper 109

    Cartilage 111

    Osseous Tissue 112

    Blood 112

    Tissue Healing 113

    Tissue Necrosis 113

    Topics to Know for Chapter 7 114

Chapter 8:
The Integumentary System 115

    Integumentary System Overview...115

    The Skin as an Organ 116

    Layers of the Skin 116

    Types of Skin 117

    Functions of the Skin 118

    Topical Features of the Skin 119

    The Epidermis 120

    The Dermis 124

The Hypodermis 126

Cutaneous Sensation 126

Skin Color 127

Skin Derivatives 129

Skin Repair 135

Topics to Know for Chapter 8 137

Chapter 9:
Osseous Tissue 139

Overview of the Skeletal System 139

Accessory Parts of the Skeletal System 140

Functions of the Skeletal System 141

Classification of Bones 142

Anatomy of a Long Bone 143

Anatomy of Short Bones, Flat Bones, and Irregular Bones 146

Osseous Tissue 146

Bone Deposition by Osteoblasts 148

Bone Resorption by Osteoclasts 149

Development and Growth of Bones 149

Patterns of Bone Growth 152

Factors Affecting Bone Development 154

Bone Remodeling 155

Bone Remodeling and Bone Density 155

Bone Remodeling and Ca^{2+} Homeostasis 156

Repair of Fractures 156

Topics to Know for Chapter 9 158

Chapter 10:
The Axial Skeleton 159

Overview of the Skeleton 159

The Skull	161
Frontal Bone	165
Parietal Bones	166
Temporal Bones	166
Occipital Bone	167
Sphenoid Bone	167
Ethmoid Bone	168
Maxillae	169
Palatine Bones	171
Mandible	171
Nasal Bones	172
Vomer	172
Inferior Nasal Conchae	172
Zygomatic Bones	172
Lacrimal Bones	172
The Orbits and Nasal Cavity	173
Paranasal Sinuses	173
Fontanels	173
The Hyoid Bone	175
General Structure of the Spine	175
Cervical Vertebrae	178
Thoracic Vertebrae	179
Lumbar Vertebrae	180
The Sacrum	180
The Thoracic Cage	182
Sternum	182
Topics to Know for Chapter 10	183

Chapter 11:
The Appendicular Skeleton 185

The Pectoral Girdle	185
Clavicles	186

Scapulae	186
The Upper Limb	187
Humerus	187
Ulna	188
Radius	189
Carpals	189
Metacarpals	191
Phalanges	191
The Pelvis and Pelvic Girdle	191
Ilium	192
Ischium	192
Pubis	193
True Pelvis and False Pelvis	193
The Lower Limb	193
Femur	194
Patella	196
Tibia	196
Fibula	197
Tarsals	198
Phalanges	199
Arches of the Foot	199
Topics to Know for Chapter 11	200

Chapter 12:
Joints 201

Naming and Classifying Joints	201
Classification of Joints by Movement	202
Anatomy of Fibrous Joints	203
Anatomy of Cartilaginous Joints	204
Anatomy of Synovial Joints	205
Joint Stability and Range of Motion	208

Classification of Synovial Joints 208

Body Movements at Synovial Joints 209

Characteristics of Selected Joints 213

The Shoulder Joint 213

The Elbow Joint 214

The Wrist Joint 215

The Hip Joint 216

The Knee Joint 217

The Ankle Joint 218

What Makes Synovial Joints "POP"? 218

Topics to Know for Chapter 12 223

Chapter 13:
Membrane Potentials 225

Membrane Potential 225

Factors Affecting Ion Movement.. 226

Major Ions Affecting Potentials.. 226

Development of a Membrane Potential... 227

Graded Potential.. 228

Action Potentials.. 228

Topics to Know for Chapter 13 231

Chapter 14:
Muscle Tissue 233

Overview of Muscle Tissues... 233

Types of Muscle Tissues 234

Functions of Muscle Tissue 234

Characteristics of Muscle Tissue.. 235

Anatomy of a Skeletal Muscle 236

Anatomy of a Skeletal Muscle Fiber.. 239

Myofilaments 241
Contraction and Relaxation of Skeletal Muscle Fibers 243
Regulation of Muscle Contraction 246
Excitation-Contraction Coupling..249
Tension in Skeletal Muscle Fibers 250
Energy for Contraction..254
Muscle Fatigue 257
Types of Skeletal Muscle Fibers...258
Distribution of Muscle Fibers 260
Regeneration of Muscle Fibers 260
Contraction of Whole Skeletal Muscles..261
Cardiac Muscle Cells...266
Smooth Muscle Tissue..267
Topics to Know for Chapter 14 273

Chapter 15:
The Muscular System...275

Introduction to the Skeleltal Muscles 275
Muscle Interactions 275
Skeletal Muscle Names 276
Learning Skeletal Muscles 277
Muscles of the Head 277
Muscles of the Neck And Spine 283
Muscles of the Torso 285
Muscles of the Arm 290
Muscles of the Forearm 290
Intrinsic Hand Muscles..294
Muscles of the Iliac And Gluteal Regions 295
Muscles of the Lower Limb...297
Intrinsic Foot Muscles 302
Topics to Know for Chapter 15 303

Chapter 16:
Introduction to the Nervous System 305

Regulatory Systems 305

Overview of the Nervous System 305

Glial Cells 306

Neurons 308

Myelination of Axons 309

Unmyelinated Axons 311

Gray Matter and White Matter 311

Classification of Neurons 312

Repair of Damaged Axons 312

Neurotransmitters 313

Action Potentials in Neurons 314

Signal Summation 316

Signal Integration 316

Methods of Impulse Conduction 316

Factors Affecting Impulse Conduction 317

Classification of Axons 318

Topics to Know for Chapter 16 318

Chapter 17:
Central Nervous System 321

Overview of the CNS 321

Overview of the Brain 321

The Cerebrum 321

The Diencephalon 325

The Brain Stem 327

Mesencephalon 327

Cerebellum	328
Brain Ventricles	328
Functional Systems of the Brain	329
Brain Waves	329
Sleep	330
Protection of the Brain	331
The Spinal Cord	332
Topics to Know for Chapter 17	335

Chapter 18:
Peripheral Nervous System (Part 1): Nerves and Somatic Reflexes 337

Peripheral Nervous System	337
Overview of Nerves	337
Spinal Roots	340
Spinal Nerves	341
Rami, Plexuses, and Peripheral Nerves	341
Reflexes	343
Somatic Reflexes	345
Topics to Know for Chapter 18	347

Chapter 19:
Peripheral Nervous System (Part 2): The Autonomic Nervous System 349

Autonomic Nervous System	349
Sympathetic Division	350
Parasympathetic Division	351
Receptors for ANS Neurotransmitters	352
Control of the ANS	353
Visceral (Autonomic) Reflexes	353
Topics to Know for Chapter 19	355

Chapter 20:
The Senses..357

    Sensation and Perception..357

    Sensory Receptors 357

    Receptor Adaptation...357

    Classification of Receptors 358

    Spatial Discrimination 359

    Pain Sensations..359

    Taste 360

    Smell 361

    The Eye and Vision 362

    Anatomy of the Eye...362

    Fibrous Tunic 362

    Vascular Tunic 362

    Nervous Tunic 363

    Photoreceptors..364

    Other Cells in the Retina 364

    Lens 365

    Chambers of the Eye...365

    Accessory Structures of the Eye..365

    Light Refraction in the Eye 367

    Eye Movement..367

    Stimulation of Photoreceptors 368

    Retinal Processing...368

    Perception of Color 369

    Light Adaptation 369

    Visual Pathway 370

    Visual Field and 3-D Vision..370

    Visual Acuity 370

    The Ear and Hearing 370

External Ear 371
Middle Ear 371
Inner Ear (Labyrinth) 371
Perception of Sound 373
Physiology of Hearing 373
Equilibrium 373
Topics to Know for Chapter 20 375

Appendix 1: Keys for Chapter Figures 377
Appendix 2: Eponyms in Anatomy & Physiology 393
Index 397

CHAPTER 1

Introduction to Human Anatomy & Physiology

Imagine driving along in your car when you hear an awful clatter under the hood. Your first thought, "What's wrong?" Most people do not think much about how a car works until something goes wrong with it. In this situation, it would be beneficial to know something about the car's design and the function of its parts in order to narrow down the possible problems. In the same way, most people do not think about how their body works as long as everything is working properly. However, as soon as they feel ill or have an injury, parts of the body and how they work become first and foremost in their minds.

A human body is something we all live with, and increasing your knowledge about its parts can help you understand and appreciate ways to keep it in working condition. However, just like a fine-tuned car that can sometimes break down, even the most health-conscious individual can become sick or experience "body" damage. This book can teach you about the human body in much the same way that a service manual can teach a mechanic about an automobile.

It identifies the parts of the body and describes how each part works. For those seeking a career in the healthcare profession, this in-depth knowledge of the body is essential to understanding how drugs and medical procedures can help correct problems brought about by disease and injury.

This first chapter provides a foundation on which to build your knowledge of the human body. First, we introduce the scientific disciplines that study human form and function. Then we describe the body's levels of organization so you can understand how both large and small parts of the body operate. Next, we describe what makes your body "living" and what the body needs to stay alive. Finally, we introduce vocabulary that will help you locate various body parts. To help you learn this vocabulary, we provide a pronunciation key next to most scientific terms when we first define them. We may also show the term's literal meaning alongside an italicized root word or surrounded by quotation marks. **Etymology** (et-a-MOL-ō-jē; *etymo*, true meaning) is the study of word origins, and it can help you remember difficult terms. Knowing the etymology of a structure's name may reveal something about the structure's shape, location, or function. Another word, *etiology* (et-ē-OL-ō-jē; *etio*, cause) sounds like etymology but is the study of the causes of diseases.

ANATOMY & PHYSIOLOGY

Anatomy and physiology (A&P) are two branches of **biology** (bī-OL-ō-jē; *bio*, life; *logos*, words), which is the study of living things. Thus, A&P provides insight into understanding how the living human body works.

Anatomy (a-NA-tō-mē) is the study of form and structure, and it describes how different structures in the body relate to one another. Anatomy also refers to the actual structure of a body part; for example, someone may ask you to describe the anatomy of the heart. The etymology of *anatomy* (*ana*, apart; *tome*, to cut) reminds us that much of our knowledge of the human body arose from *dissection* (dis-EK-shun; "cutting apart") of dead bodies. A dead body is a *cadaver* (ka-DAV-er; "to fall"). During medieval times, much knowledge of anatomy was gained through dissecting condemned prisoners while they were still alive. The cutting up of living things is called *vivisection* (VIV-i-sek-shun; *vivi*, living).

Physiology (fiz-ē-OL-ō-jē; *physio*, nature of) is the study of how structures function, but it also refers to the actual function of a body part. After describing the anatomy of the heart, someone may ask you to explain the physiology of the heart.

The ordering of the words *anatomy & physiology* in this book's title is no accident. Before we can explain how a structure performs a particular function, we must first describe the structure's anatomy. Imagine how vaguely a person would understand vision or hearing if he or she knew nothing about the anatomy of the eyeball or the ear.

THE SCIENCE OF ANATOMY

Anatomy includes the study of *gross* and *microscopic* structures of the body. There are many ways to study the structure of the human body, but all aspects of anatomy fall into two major subdivisions: gross anatomy and microscopic anatomy.

Gross Anatomy

While vivisecting prisoners might seem gross or grotesque, anatomists use the word gross in a different way. **Gross anatomy** (grōs; "obvious"), also called **macroscopic anatomy** (*macro*, large; *scope*, to view), is the study of structures that are large enough to see with the naked eye. There are three major approaches to learning gross anatomy: *regional*, *systemic*, and *surface anatomy*.

- **Regional anatomy** focuses on describing all structures within a certain region of the body before moving on to another region. For example, a regional approach might expect you to learn all the muscles, bones, blood vessels, nerves, and other structures in the arm before moving on to learn the various structures in the leg. Most medical schools use this approach because it integrates a vast amount of information that medical students have learned from undergraduate courses.

- **Systemic** (sis-TEM-ik) **anatomy** deals with one *system* in the body at a time before moving on to study another system. A *system* includes specialized structures called *organs* that work together to perform a particular function. An example of an organ system is the digestive system, which includes organs such as the stomach, intestines, and liver. The digestive system processes food so the body can obtain nutrients for maintaining good health.

- **Surface anatomy** relates the position of internal structures to anatomical features that are visible on the body's external surface. For example, a *phlebotomist* (flē-BOT-ō-mist; *phleb*, vein; *tomy*, to cut) uses surface anatomy to locate and puncture blood vessels with a needle to obtain a blood sample. Physicians and nurses rely on knowledge of surface anatomy when placing a stethoscope on the chest to hear the heart or lungs, or on the arm to measure blood pressure.

Microscopic Anatomy

In contrast to gross anatomy, **microscopic anatomy** (*micro*, small) is the study of structures that are so small that we cannot see them with the naked eye. Therefore,

INTRODUCTION

we must magnify them with the aid of a *microscope* (MĪ-krō-skōp; *micro*, small; *scop*, to view). There are two major subdivisions of microscopic anatomy.

- **Cytology** (sī-TOL-ō-jē; *cyto*, cell) is the study of cells, which are the smallest "living" components of the body.
- **Histology** (his-TOL-ō-jē) is the study of *tissues*, which are groups of cells that work together to perform a particular function.

Developmental anatomy

Incorporating aspects of microscopic and gross anatomy is **developmental anatomy**, which focuses on structural changes that occur in the body from conception to adulthood. Developmental anatomy has three subdivisions:

- **Embryology** is the study of the *embryo*, or the first two months of development in the womb.
- **Fetology** (fē-TOL-ō-jē) is the study of the *fetus*, or the stages of development from the embryo to birth.
- **Postnatal development** is the study of the stages between birth and adulthood.

THE SCIENCE OF PHYSIOLOGY

Physiology relates microscopic anatomy to the function of gross anatomical structures. Like anatomy, physiology has a number of subdivisions ranging from studies of microscopic structures such as individual cells to studies of entire systems in the body.

- **Cell physiology** is the study of how individual cells carry out their activities. Obviously, this is the study of physiology at the cellular level.
- **Renal physiology** is the study of how the kidneys filter the blood and produce urine; this is an example of physiology at the "organ" level.
- **Neurophysiology** is the study of how different parts of the nervous system (brain, spinal cord, and nerves) work; this is an example of physiology at the "system" level.

In addition to studies that deal with the normal functioning of different parts of the body, some studies deal with what can go wrong with body parts.

- **Pathophysiology** (PATH-ō-fiz-ē-OL-ō-jē; *patho*, suffering) is the study of how disease disrupts body parts.
- **Pathology** deals with all aspects of disease, including its cause and the anatomical and physiological changes that occur in the affected structures. Pathophysiology is a subdivision of pathology.

ORGANIZATION OF THE BODY

Thus far, we have hinted that the human body is not as simple as it might seem when viewed from a surface anatomy perspective. There are many levels of organization in the body, much like there are different levels of organization in this book, from letters to words, to sentences, and so on. We will use this analogy to gain a better understanding of the body's organization. Like this book, the human body consists of many smaller components that function together as a whole. From microscopic to macroscopic, the human body includes chemical, cellular, tissue, organ, organ system, and organismal levels of organization.

1. **Chemical level:** The chemical level of organization deals with *matter*, which is anything in the universe that occupies space; therefore, the body is made of **matter**. The building blocks of matter are **elements**, so-named because they represent the "elementary" (lowest or simplest) form of matter. Examples of elements in the body are carbon (C), hydrogen (H), and oxygen (O). The smallest stable form of an element is an **atom**, which can bind with other atoms to form **molecules**. Atoms and molecules, which we collectively call **chemicals**, represent the lowest level of organization in the body. In our book analogy, the chemical level of organization would be the ink used for letters in words.

2. **Cellular level:** The cellular level of organization deals with *cells*. A **cell** is the basic unit of life; that is, it is the smallest thing in the body that can be "living." The word "cell" literally means "small room," and was applied because the first cells viewed under a microscope looked like tiny rooms occupied by monks in a monastery. Molecules come together to form **organelles**, which

are specialized structures that perform specific functions inside cells. Examples of cells include liver cells, skin cells, and pancreas cells. An average adult body may contain 100 trillion cells and there are about 200 different kinds of cells in the body. Cells would be like the letters on this page, with each letter consisting of ink ("chemicals").

3. **Tissue level: A tissue** (TISH-ū; "woven") is a group of cells working together to perform a similar function. A tissue would be like a word in this paragraph, since most words contain two or more letters ("cells") functioning together to form a meaningful term. The body contains four general types of tissues: *epithelial*, *connective*, *muscle*, and *nervous*. A specific type of epithelial tissue functions as a membrane to cover a surface. The visible part of your skin is a type of epithelium.

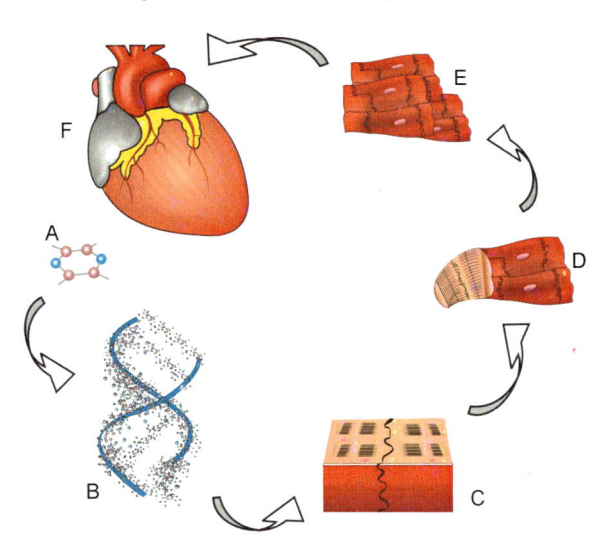

Figure 1-1. Organization in an organ. Label each level.

4. **Organ level:** An **organ** ("instrument") is a well-defined, anatomical structure consisting of two or more tissues working together to perform one or more functions for the body. We could compare an organ to this sentence, which has multiple words ("tissues") functioning together to make a meaningful statement. An example of an organ is the heart, which contains muscle tissue, epithelial tissue, connective tissue, and nervous tissue. The levels of organization in an organ are shown in Figure 1-1.

5. **System level**: An **organ system** ("organized whole") is a group of organs working together to perform a specific task. In our analogy, this paragraph is like a system because it contains multiple sentences ("organs") that function together to elaborate on a particular thought. The stomach, intestines, pancreas, and liver are examples of organs that are part of the *digestive system*. Some organs play important roles in several systems. For example, the pancreas makes chemicals that break down food in the intestine, making it part of the digestive system. It also produces hormones, chemicals that affect other cells in the body, making it part of the endocrine system. The body's eleven organ systems include the following and are shown in Figure 1-2:

- *Integumentary*: skin, hair and nails.
- *Skeletal*: bones, cartilage, ligaments, tendons
- *Muscular*: muscles attaches to skeletal components
- *Nervous*: brain, spinal cord, nerves, sensory organs
- *Endocrine*: endocrine glands
- *Cardiovascular*: heart, blood vessels
- *Lymphatic*: lymphatic vessels, lymph nodes, spleen, thymus gland
- *Respiratory*: nasal cavity, larynx (voice box), trachea (windpipe), lungs
- *Digestive*: mouth, teeth, tongue, salivary glands, throat, esophagus, stomach, small intestines, large intestines, liver, gall bladder, pancreas
- *Urinary*: kidneys, ureters, urinary bladder, urethra
- *Reproductive (Female)*: ovaries, oviducts, uterus, vagina, accessory glands; *(Male)*: testes, vas deferens, seminal vesicles, prostate and bulbourethral glands, and penis

6. **Organismal level:** The organismal level includes all organ systems working together to form the human body, which we call an *organism*. An **organism** (OR-gan-izm) is any living thing, and as the name might imply, living things are highly organized. A human body is a *multicellular* organism, meaning

INTRODUCTION 5

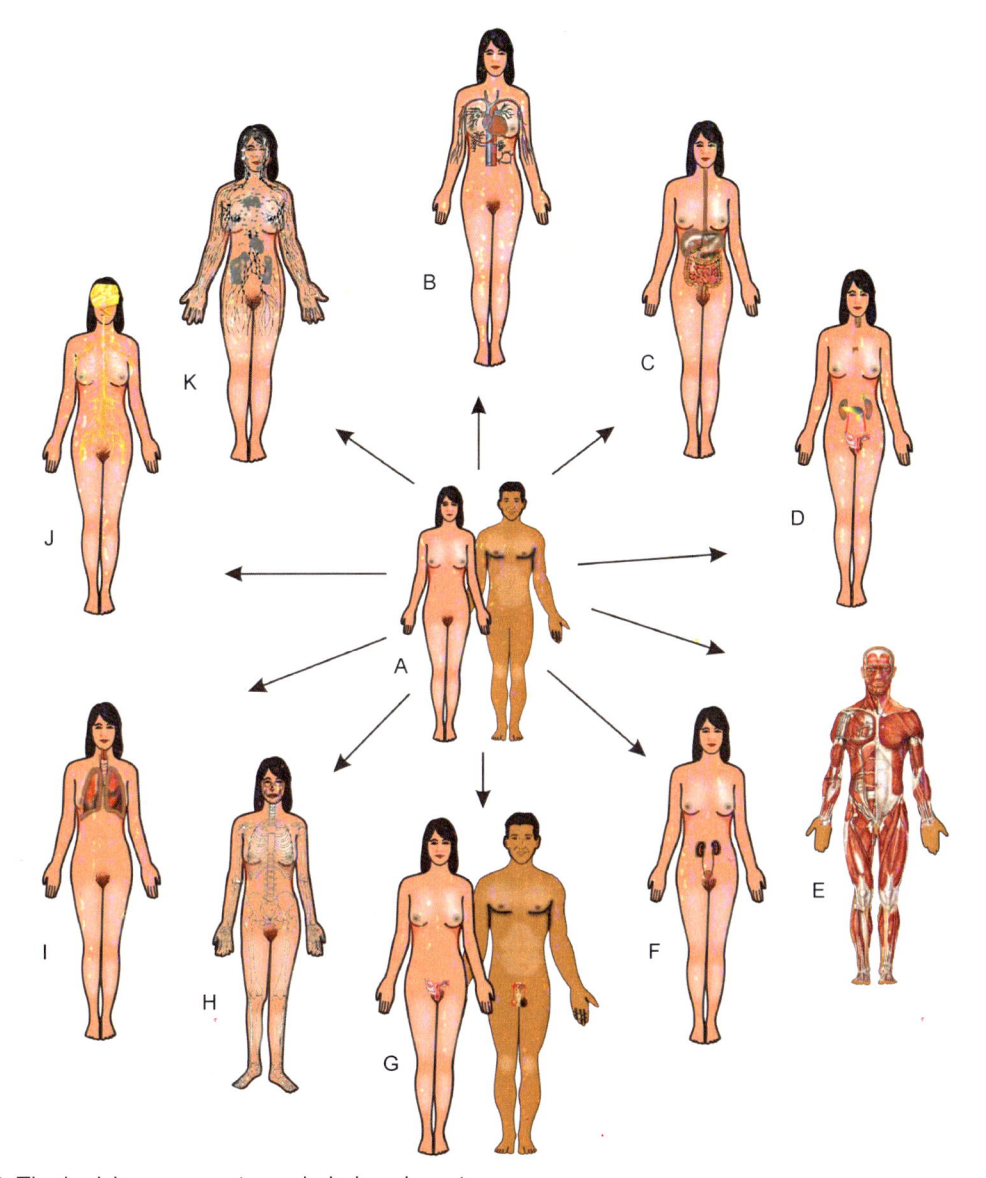

Figure 1-2. The body's organ systems. Label each system.

it has numerous cells (*multi*, many). Some organisms, such as bacteria and yeast, consist of only one cell, which makes them *unicellular* (*uni*, one). To finish our analogy, we could say this page is like an organism because it consists of multiple paragraphs ("organ systems"). There are still more subdivisions in biology, and the next two would include a *population*, two or more similar organisms living in the same area, and a *community*, two or more populations living in the same area. This chapter would be like a population and the entire book would be like a community. But how can you tell that your body is "alive" and this book is not? You will find the answer in the next section.

THE CHARACTERISTICS OF LIFE

The fact that you are reading this sentence means you are alive, but what is life? Answering this question requires more than a simple one-line response; instead, it requires describing a number of "life" characteristics. In this section, we describe the characteristics that distinguish humans from nonliving objects. Humans exhibit cellularity, metabolism, excretion, growth, reproduction, organization, adaptability, irritability, movement, homeostasis, and inheritance.

> **Note:** The following mnemonic (ne-MON-ik; "memory") may help you remember the traits of life; each letter represents one trait: C-ME-GRO-AIM-HI (Pronounced "See Me Grow Aim High").

Earlier, we stated that a cell is the smallest thing that can be alive, but in your body, a single cell does not function independently of other cells. Amazingly, the trillions of cells that comprise your body work together as a single, living unit. In a biological sense, the following eleven characteristics help validate that your body is alive:

- **Cellularity** (sell-ū-LAR-i-tē) implies that the body is made of tiny functional units called **cells** ("little room"). *The cell theory* in biology states that the cell is the basic unit of life, so all organisms exhibit cellularity and contain at least one cell. You have trillions of cells in your body. The "C" could also stand for "carbon." All living things consisting of matter contain organic compounds, which are those that contain carbon. Examples of carbon compounds include proteins, carbohydrates, and lipids.

- **Metabolism** (me-TAB-ō-lizm; *metabol*, change) refers to the countless chemical reactions, or interactions between two or more chemicals, that occur in the body continuously. Simply, metabolism includes all the chemical reactions in the body and includes *anabolism* and *catabolism*. **Anabolism** (a-NAB-ō-lizm; *anabol*, raise up) includes reactions that produce larger, more complex molecules. **Catabolism** (ka-TAB-ō-lizm; catabol, cast down) includes reactions that break down large, complex molecules into smaller, simpler ones.

- **Excretion** (eks-KRĒ-shun; to separate) refers to the elimination of wastes from the body. Catabolism always generates certain waste molecules, and allowing these wastes to accumulate would poison the body and eventually cause death. Four organ systems perform excretion, or have *excretory* (EKS-krē-tor-ē) functions. The urinary (ŪR-i-nar-ē) system excretes liquid waste in the form of urine; the digestive system excretes solid waste called feces (FĒ-sēz); the respiratory (RES-pir-a-tor-ē) system excretes gaseous waste—primarily carbon dioxide; and the integumentary (in-teg-ū-MEN-ta-rē) system excretes certain wastes in sweat and oil.

- **Growth**, the process of getting larger, is a feature of the body as a whole and a characteristic of its cells at some time in their life. You began life as a single cell that was smaller than the head of a pin, but look at you now! Your body grew as that original cell divided repeatedly to form additional cells. However, simply dividing one cell again and again does not cause growth, since that process might simply produce smaller and smaller cells. The body can grow only if its newly formed cells grow too. Seeing yourself in the mirror without the aid of a microscope validates the notion that your cells grew after they formed, although they remain microscopic.

- **Reproduction**, or producing "copies" of oneself, can occur at different levels of organization. It occurs at the cellular level, which is how you became multicellular, and it occurs at the organismal level when a person produces a child. Many of your cells reproduce throughout your lifetime, with the newly formed cells replacing worn-out or damaged ones. In addition, special cells called *gametes* (GAM-ēts) from a male and female can unite to form a single-celled *zygote* (ZĪ-gōt; "yoked"), which divides repeatedly to form a new human body.

- **Organization**, or the ordered arrangement of structures, implies that the body is not simply a collection of matter arranged in a haphazard fashion. Recall that organization is the basis for why we call living things *organisms*. This is also the basis of the term *organic*, which refers to the carbon-based compounds made within organisms.

- **Adaptability** is the ability to change over time in response to a change in lifestyle or a change in the external environment; *adapt* means "to adjust." If an inactive, sedentary person began a vigorous exercise regimen that included lifting weights and running, the body would *adapt* to this new lifestyle.

INTRODUCTION

Changes would include stronger and larger skeletal muscles, thicker bones, and a stronger heart able to pump blood through blood vessels more effectively. *Acclimation* (ak-li-MĀ-shun), also called *acclimatization* (a-clī-ma-ti-ZĀ-shun), refers to the adaptation of an individual to a different climate or altitude, and this type of adjustment may take several days or longer.

- **Irritability** (ir-i-ta-BIL-i-tē) is the ability to change quickly in response to a change that occurred inside or outside the body. To be *irritable* means to be excitable. Whereas adaptability is a relatively slow change, irritability is a more immediate reaction to a sudden environmental change. For instance, you demonstrate irritability when you flinch at the sound of a firecracker or jerk your hand away from a hot stove.

- **Movement** may not seem applicable to all living organisms, such as a tree, but movement occurs, albeit not necessarily at all levels of organization. Fluids and various microscopic structures move around inside cells, blood moves within blood vessels, and food moves through your digestive system. Moreover, most people can move their body from one place to another and can move items in their surrounding environment.

- **Homeostasis** (hō-mē-ō-STĀ-sis; *homeo*, same; *stasis*, stand still) refers to the maintenance of relatively stable internal conditions. For example, you can maintain a core body temperature (that is, deep inside the body) near 37°C (98.6°F) even if the room temperature is 0°C (32°F). The roles that various cells, tissues, organs, and organ systems play in maintaining homeostasis will be a recurring theme in this book.

- **Inheritance** refers to passing on chemical information from one generation to the next, whether at the cellular or the organismal level of organization. You inherited chemicals from your parents that influenced your anatomy and physiology. *Inheritance* comes from a word meaning "heir." Even for people who never produce a child, each time one of their cells divides, it passes chemical information to the newly formed cells.

Nonliving things may exhibit some of the "life" characteristics described above, but only in a limited way. For instance, mineral crystals grow and exhibit organization, while a virus reproduces and demonstrates inheritance, but neither crystals nor viruses exhibit cellularity, metabolism, irritability, or any other "life" characteristic. Although they are nonliving, viruses can cause certain diseases, including the cold, the flu, and acquired immune deficiency syndrome (AIDS).

ENVIRONMENTAL REQUIREMENTS FOR LIFE

In this final section, we point out certain factors that humans need from their external environment in order to stay alive. While some factors in our external environment could harm us, we can identify four factors that are necessary for our survival: *water, nutrients, oxygen,* and a *suitable temperature*.

Water is the most vital substance that you obtain from the external environment. It makes up about 70% of your body's weight and is important to your survival in the following ways: (1) it provides the medium in which all metabolic reactions occur; (2) it transports nutrients and cellular wastes in the blood; and (3) it is an effective heat absorber, preventing dramatic fluctuation of body temperature.

Nutrients are chemicals found in food that cells can use for energy, building cellular components, or maintaining normal metabolism. Nutrients include *carbohydrates, lipids, proteins, vitamins,* and *minerals*. Carbohydrates are the body's major energy source and lipids provide energy and form the boundaries of cells. Proteins are the major building blocks for cells and their products, while vitamins help maintain normal chemical reactions within cells. Minerals are common in the earth's crust and examples include calcium, sodium, and phosphorus. Minerals provide structural support to bones, function in transmitting nerve signals, play a role in certain chemical reactions, and serve in many other capacities.

Oxygen is a gaseous element that enables most cells in the body to obtain more useable energy from certain nutrients. Some cells, such as many of those in the brain, are so dependent on oxygen that experiencing an oxygen-deficit for more than a few minutes can cause irreversible cell damage and even death. Oxygen from the atmosphere enters the blood in the lungs and then the blood transports it to cells throughout the body.

Temperature around the body must remain within tolerable limits to allow the body to maintain normal metabolism. If a high outside temperature causes the body's core temperature to rise to 41°C (106°F), certain proteins and other molecules begin to lose their ability to function properly. A core temperature of 42°C (109°F) is usually fatal. If a low outside temperature causes the body's core temperature to drop to near 27°C (82°F), most metabolic reactions cease. In the next section, we will describe several mechanisms that enable the body to maintain its core temperature at or near optimum (37°C).

HOMEOSTASIS

Now that you know about certain factors in the external environment that are necessary for life, we will elaborate on mechanisms the body uses to deal with changes in its internal environment. Rephrasing from the previous section, **homeostasis** (*homeo*, same; *stasis*, standing still) is a relatively stable internal environment in which cells can live. The internal environment is the fluid surrounding the body's cells. This fluid has several general names: **extracellular fluid** (**ECF**; *extra*, outside), **intercellular fluid** (*inter*, between), and **interstitial fluid** (in-ter-STI-shul; "between spaces"). The ECF that flows within blood vessels is called **plasma** (PLAZ-ma), while the ECF that flows within lymph vessels is called **lymph** (pronounced "limpf").

Although *homeostasis* translates "to stay the same," many aspects of the ECF fluctuate continuously above or below a desired value. For example, the temperature and the amounts of water, nutrients, and oxygen in the ECF are always changing. However, the key to homeostasis, or the key to maintaining good health, is to make sure these fluctuations stay within tolerable limits. Any aspect of the environment that can change is a *variable* ("to vary"), but a variable that the body has some control over is a *regulated variable*.

Minor fluctuations in regulated variables are normal and unpreventable, but sometimes these minor fluctuations can quickly lead to major disruptions to homeostasis and pose a threat to life if not corrected quickly. Fortunately, the body has a number of regulatory mechanisms that can counter minor disruptions in homeostasis before they develop into life-threatening situations. One of these mechanisms involves homeostatic control systems.

HOMEOSTATIC CONTROL SYSTEMS

Control systems monitor variables and help regulate homeostatic activities of other systems. The nervous system and endocrine system play important roles as *homeostatic control systems*, because they direct many of the homeostatic activities of other systems.

We can compare a control system to a person riding a bicycle along a thin line in the middle of a sidewalk (see Figure 1-3). The thin line running along the center of the sidewalk represents a desired value for some regulated variable, while the bike's tire path

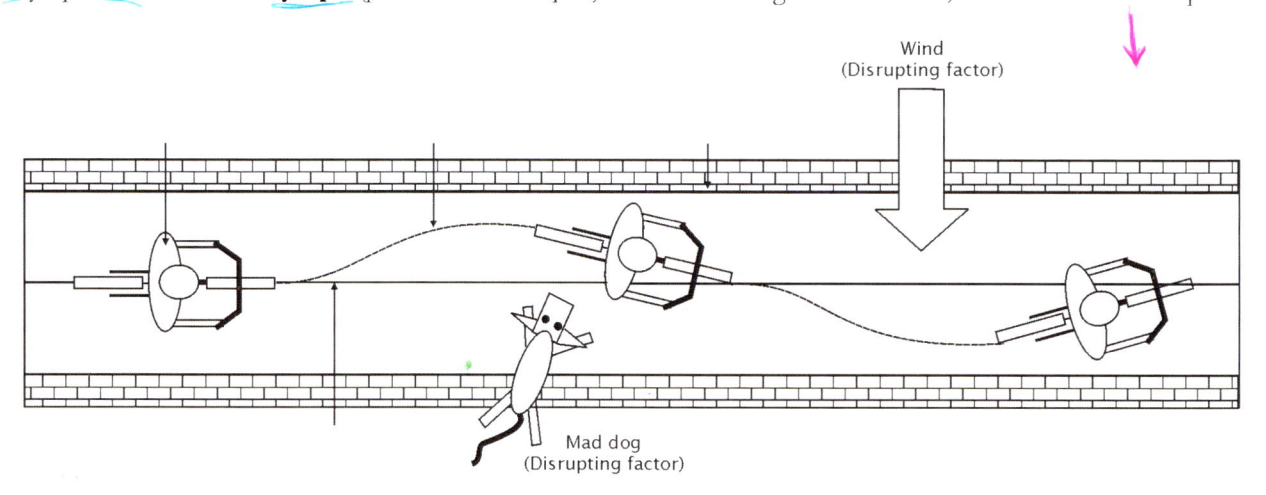

Figure 1-3. Example of negative feedback. See text for explanation.

INTRODUCTION

denotes the actual value for the variable. The edges of the sidewalk symbolize the tolerable limits within which values of the variable can fluctuate before the body "crashes" (suffers ill effects). Finally, because ferocious dogs and strong winds cause the bike to veer off the line, they correspond to factors that disrupt homeostasis. In the case of the dog's effect, the rider may actually cause the bike to veer off course, and this is a temporary disruption in the control system itself.

While it would be virtually impossible to prevent the bike from veering off the line from time to time, even without dogs or strong winds present, the rider's corrective steering may at least keep the bike near the middle of the sidewalk. Similarly, a homeostatic control system cannot prevent regulated variables from fluctuating, but can help keep them within tolerable limits. To elaborate further, the rider integrates the actions of three anatomical features to keep the bike on the line: the *eyes*, which inform the brain about the bike's position; the *brain*, which decides when the arms should move; and the *arms*, which turn the handlebars to guide the bike back on course. In a similar way, a homeostatic control system integrates the actions of three components: *sensors, integrating center,* and *effectors*.

A sensor (also called a **receptor**) is a structure that monitors a particular regulated variable and sends information about it to an integrating center. Examples of sensors in the body include *chemoreceptors* (KĒ-mō-rē-sep-terz), which detect changes in the amounts of various chemicals in the blood, and *thermoreceptors* (THUR-mō-rē-sep-terz) which detect changes in body temperature (*thermo*, heat). Any factor that causes a sensor to respond in some way is a stimulus (STIM-ū-lus, "to provoke"), and exposing a sensor or other structure to a stimulus is *stimulation*.

The **integrating** (or **control**) **center** receives information about a regulated variable from a sensor, compares it to a desired value, called the **set point**, and then sends information to a structure called the *effector* that helps return the variable to its set point. In other words, the integrating center "knows" what to do when the variable's value moves away from the set point. Since information sent from a receptor comes into the control center, we call it *input*, or *afferent* information (AF-er-ent, "bring in"). Information that leaves the control center is *output*, or *efferent* information (EF-er-ent, "bring out"). The brain and certain endocrine glands determine the set point for various chemicals in the blood, while the brain alone determines the set point for body temperature.

An **effector** (ē-FEK-tor) is a structure that receives efferent information from a control center and produces a reaction (an effect) that brings the value of a regulated variable back to its set point. Hence, we say the control center *stimulates* the effector to produce a certain effect. Most organs in the body act as effectors for either the nervous system or endocrine system, and some organs are effectors for both systems. To avoid confusion over the words "affect" and "effect," you could say, "The control center's output *affects* the effector," or "The control center's output has an *effect* on the effector."

FEEDBACK MECHANISMS IN HOMEOSTASIS

Feedback involves reacting to a stimulus in a way that either counteracts or intensifies the stimulus. After stimulating an effector that helps adjust the value of a regulated variable, the control center must re-evaluate the variable's status to determine whether stimulation of the effector must continue or cease. For re-evaluation to occur, a homeostatic control system relies on a process called *feedback*, in which the sensor "feeds back" information about the variable to the control center. In some situations, feedback does not involve a homeostatic control system; however, feedback always includes a stimulus and a reaction that either counteracts or intensifies the stimulus.

Negative Feedback

If the body's reaction to a stimulus *negates* (opposes or counteracts) the stimulus, the process is **negative feedback**. In other words, when a stimulus changes the value of a regulated variable in one direction, negative feedback moves the value in the *opposite* direction. In this sense, being "negative" is a good thing because negative feedback prevents dramatic fluctuations in the values of regulated variables. If we plot the actual values for a regulated variable over time, negative feedback produces an oscillating pattern that might look something like the tire path in our bicycle analogy. In that figure, the rider demonstrates negative feedback control when trying to keep the bike on the line. When the bike veers left, the rider negates that movement by turning the handlebars to the right; when the bike veers right, the rider negates that movement by turning the handlebars to the left.

An example of negative feedback is *thermoregulation*, in which a homeostatic control system counteracts fluctuations in body temperature. First, thermoreceptors in the skin and brain respond to changes in body temperature by sending afferent signals to the *thermoregulatory center* (TRC) located in the brain. The TRC then compares the afferent signals to the brain's temperature set point. If the temperature is higher than the set point, the TRC initiates *heat-loss mechanisms*. This includes sending efferent signals to sweat glands, causing them to release sweat onto the skin's surface. As the sweat evaporates, the body cools. In addition, the brain causes blood vessels in the skin to dilate (DĪ-lāt, "open up"), allowing more warm blood to come near the body's surface where it can radiate heat into the surrounding environment.

If body temperature is lower than the set point, the TRC initiates *heat-producing mechanisms*. This includes causing efferent signals to be sent to skeletal muscles, which "shiver" in response. Shivering generates heat and causing the body temperature to rise. Additionally, the brain causes blood vessels in the skin constrict (become narrower) so that less warm blood is brought near the body's surface, thus, preventing excessive heat loss. While the TRC cannot prevent fluctuations in body temperature, it attempts to minimize those fluctuations. See Figure 1-4 for a depiction of thermoregulation.

Positive Feedback

If the body's reaction to a stimulus intensifies the stimulus, the process is **positive feedback**. Defined another way, when a stimulus moves the value of a regulated variable in one direction, positive feedback moves the value farther along in the *same* direction. Positive feedback has been called "a vicious cycle" because it involves a cycle of recurring events that reinforce each other. When we plot these events on a circle, each complete cycle or *positive feedback loop*, occurs faster than the previous cycle. Although it seems that positive feedback could quickly cause the variable's value to get out of control, several events prevent that from happening: (1) some factor eliminates the stimulus; or (2) the body lacks the resources or energy to continue reacting to the stimulus.

Since positive feedback causes the value of a regulated variable to move quickly *away from* homeostatic conditions, how can this process ever be beneficial to one's health? The answer is that sometimes the body must amplify or intensify the effect of a stimulus in order to remove the stimulus as quickly as possible. It might help to think of positive feedback as the body's way of "fighting fire with fire." Firefighters often fight forest fires by *starting* fires ahead of the main fire in order to burn up potential fuel; as a result, the forest fire burns out more quickly. Childbirth and blood clotting are two examples that incorporate positive feedback loops as a way of reducing the amount of time that the body is under stress. We will describe childbirth in a later chapter but will provide a brief overview of blood clotting here.

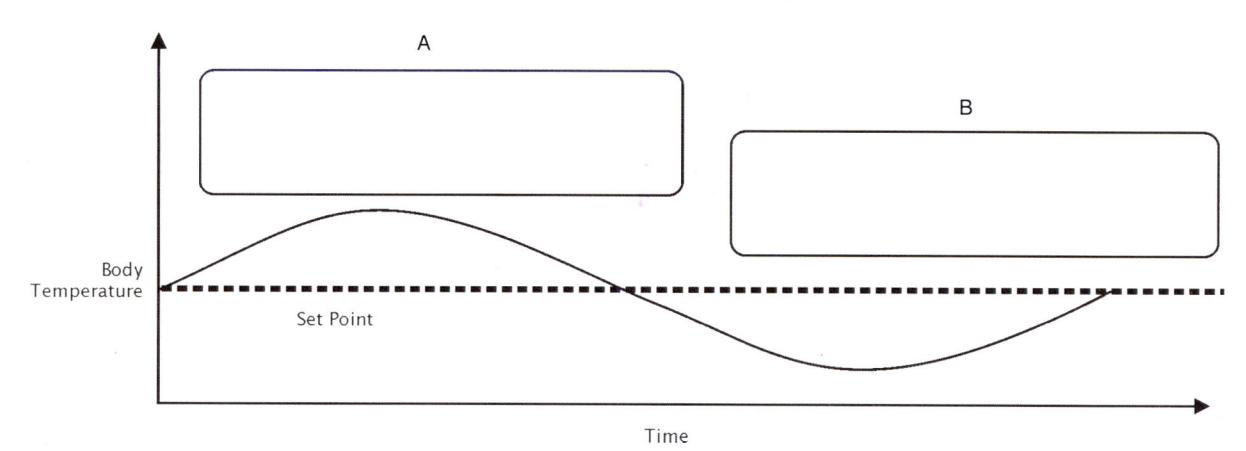

Figure 1-4. Thermoregulation is an example of negative feedback.

INTRODUCTION

Blood clotting (formation of a blood clot) is an example of how a self-amplifying positive feedback loop can counter a potentially life-threatening loss of blood. A blood clot is a jelly-like mass that plugs a tear or cut in a blood vessel's wall. First, tearing a blood vessel disrupts homeostasis by causing bleeding, which reduces the amount of cell-nourishing blood circulating through the body. The tear in the vessel acts as a stimulus, causing platelets (tiny particles in the blood) to attach to the damaged tissue and then release a variety of chemicals. Some of these chemicals cause the platelets at the damaged site to become "sticky," and some of the chemicals initiate reactions necessary for forming a blood clot. A positive feedback loop begins as more platelets arrive on the scene, stick to the platelets already there, and release their chemicals like the platelets that arrived earlier. As a result, the newly arrived platelets become sticky and their added chemicals speed up the clotting process. This positive feedback loop continues until the clot seals the tear in the vessel wall and bleeding stops.

RELATIONSHIPS AMONG VARIABLES

When discussing feedback and describing how a change in one variable affects a change in some other variable, it is often helpful to show the relationship between the two variables on a graph. The variable we place on the X-axis (*abscissa*—ab–SIS–uh, or horizontal line at the bottom of the graph) is the **independent variable**, so-named because we assume that its value is not dependent on the value of the other variable of interest. In contrast, the variable we place on the Y-axis (*ordinate*—ORD–nat, or vertical line forming the left side of the graph) is the **dependent variable**, so-named because we assume its value depends on the value of the independent variable. We sometimes call the dependent variable the *response variable* because its value changes in response to changes in the independent variable. See Figure 1-5 for a depiction of a *relational graph*.

We can illustrate the usefulness of a graph by showing the relationship between two regulated variables, body temperature and sweating. First, we might ask, "How does body temperature affect sweating," or "How does sweating respond to a change

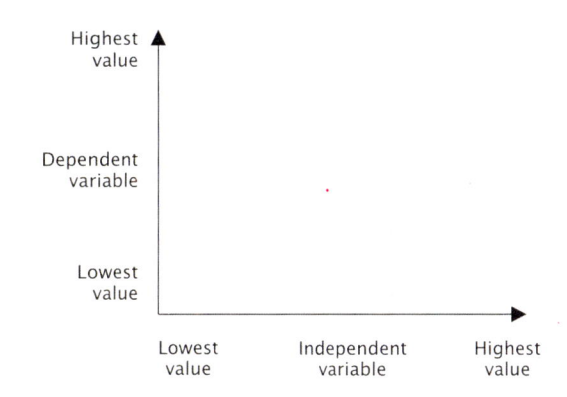

Figure 1-5. Relational graph.

in body temperature?" In this case, body temperature is the independent variable and the amount of sweating is the dependent variable. If body temperature rises only slightly above the set point, the body responds by producing a small amount of sweat in a given time. To show this, we first find the measured temperature on the X-axis then move upward to plot a point at a level corresponding to a "small" amount of sweat on the Y-axis. At higher and higher temperatures, the body sweats more and more. For each measured temperature value, there is a corresponding point that represents the amount of sweat produced at that temperature.

So, what do the points on our graph tell us about the relationship between body temperature and sweating? If we draw a straight line among the dots, we see that it slants upward and to the right. (The procedure for determining the exact slope of this line is based on a statistical formula and is beyond the scope of this book, so the line we will draw here is simply an educated guess.) A line with this type of slope indicates a **positive relationship** between the variables (see Figure 1-6a).

Recall in positive feedback, the body's response to a stimulus moves in the same direction as the stimulus. In a positive relationship, the response variable (Y) changes in the same direction as the X variable. In our example of thermoregulation, if body temperature increases, then the amount of sweating increases too, whereas if body temperature decreases, then the amount of sweating decreases. Now you can say, "The amount of sweating is *positively* related to body temperature," or "Body temperature has a *positive* effect on the amount of sweating."

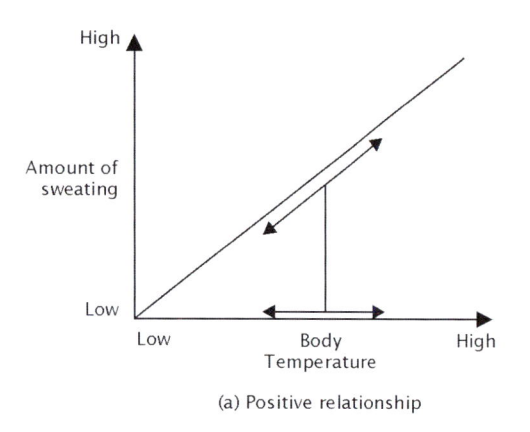

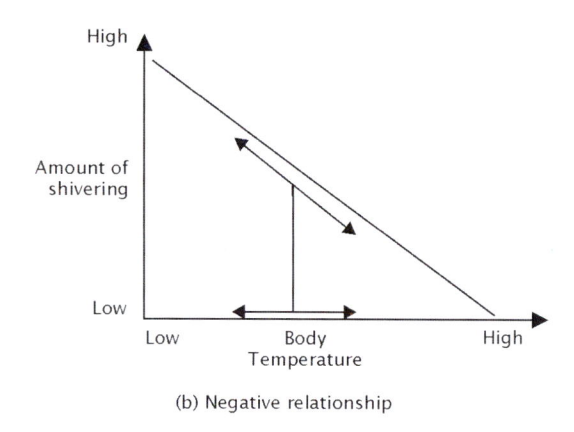

Figure 1-6. Positive and negative relationships

A negative (or **inverse**) **relationship** exists if the value of variable Y changes in the *opposite* direction to that of variable X. That is, if the value of X increases, then the value of Y decreases, or if the value of X decreases, then the value of Y increases. This would be the case if we ask, "How does body temperature affect the amount of shivering?" Since shivering generates body heat, it tends to increase when body temperature decreases. In contrast, shivering decreases as body temperature increases. Thus, we can say, "The amount of shivering is negatively related to body temperature," or "Body temperature has a *negative* effect on the amount of shivering" (see Figure 1-6b).

HOMEOSTASIS AND DISEASE

While the body may be able to prevent dramatic fluctuations in regulated variables through negative feedback, and it may be able to cope quickly with certain stimuli through positive feedback, there are limitations to its ability to maintain homeostasis. Sometimes the body may face stimuli that push the value of a regulated variable beyond tolerable limits, at which time we say the body experiences a *homeostatic imbalance*. We can compare a homeostatic imbalance to our bike rider losing his/her balance and suffering injury because the bike swerves too far and gets off the sidewalk. The body's reaction to any stimulus that causes a homeostatic imbalance is stress. If the body's homeostatic control systems are able to reestablish homeostasis through negative feedback, we can now define negative feedback in the body simply as "reaction negates stress."

When a homeostatic imbalance causes an interruption or cessation of some bodily function, we say the person is ill or experiences **illness**. A **disease** (*dis-*, not + *ease*) is an illness that produces certain recognizable *signs* and *symptoms* that usually have a known cause. **A sign** is some aspect of a disease that is visible or measurable, such as redness, swelling, fever, vomiting, bleeding, etc. A **symptom** is a "feeling" or subjective description of the way a person feels and includes nausea, fatigue, headache, pain, etc. A **syndrome** (*sym-*, together; *drom-*, running) is a combination of signs and symptoms for a particular disease; two examples are respiratory distress syndrome (RDS) and acquired immune deficiency syndrome (AIDS).

REVIEW

Before moving on to the next chapter, take some time to review the *Topics to Know in Chapter 1* that follow.

INTRODUCTION

TOPICS TO KNOW IN CHAPTER 1 (INTRODUCTION TO ANATOMY & PHYSIOLOGY)

- acclimation
- acclimatization
- adaptability
- afferent information
- AIDS
- anabolism
- anatomy
- atom
- cadaver
- carbohydrates
- carbon
- catabolism
- cell
- cell physiology
- cellularity
- chemical
- chemoreceptor
- C-ME-GRO-AIM-HI
- connective tissue
- cytology
- dependent variable
- developmental anatomy
- disease
- dissection
- ECF
- effector
- efferent
- elements
- embryo
- embryology
- epithelial tissue
- etiology
- etymology
- examples of feedback
- excretion
- excretory systems
- extracellular fluid
- feedback mechanisms in homeostasis
- fetology
- fetus
- gametes
- gross anatomy
- growth
- histology
- homeostasis
- homeostasis and disease
- homeostatic control systems
- homeostatic imbalance
- illness
- independent variable
- inheritance
- input
- integrating (control) center
- intercellular fluid
- internal environment
- interpreting graphs
- interstitial fluid
- inverse correlation
- irritability
- life
- lipids
- lymph
- macroscopic anatomy
- matter
- metabolism
- minerals
- mnemonic
- molecules
- multicellular organism
- muscle tissue
- negative correlation
- negative feedback
- nervous tissue
- neurophysiology
- nutrients
- organ
- organ system
- organelles
- organic
- organism
- organization
- organization in the body
- output
- oxygen
- pathology
- pathophysiology
- physiology
- plasma
- positive correlation
- positive feedback
- positive feedback loop
- postnatal development
- proteins
- receptor
- regional anatomy
- regulated variable
- renal physiology
- reproduction
- requirements for life
- response variable
- sensor
- set point
- sign
- stimulation
- stimulus
- stress
- surface anatomy
- symptom
- syndrome
- system
- systemic anatomy
- thermoreceptors
- thermoregulation
- thermoregulatory center
- tissue
- variable

CHAPTER 2

Body Organization

To prevent misunderstanding when reading and discussing anatomy, it is necessary to understand and use universally accepted terminology. You can begin building your anatomy vocabulary by learning the major surface regions of the body. We can identify these regions most effectively by looking at a body that is in anatomical position. In **anatomical position**, the person is standing erect with the head, palms, and feet facing forward, the feet slightly apart, and the arms by the sides. We will first highlight the basic layout of the body and the boundaries of selected regions. At the most basic level of gross anatomy, we can divide the body into two major regions: the *axial* and *appendicular* regions.

THE AXIAL REGION

The **axial region** (AK-sē-ul), so-named because it forms the body's *axis* or central "core," includes the head, neck, and trunk. Table 2-1 provides an alphabetized list of the axial regions and their sub-regions.

THE APPENDICULAR REGION

The **appendicular region** (ap-en-DIK-ū-lar), so-named because its parts *append* (attach) to different parts of the axial region, includes the *upper limbs* and *lower limbs*. Table 2-2 provides an alphabetized list of the appendicular regions and their sub-regions.

After learning the names and locations of the axial and appendicular regions, your expanded vocabulary will provide a basis for locating numerous structures *inside* the body. For instance, the femoral region, or thigh, contains the *femur* (thighbone), *femoral* artery, *femoral* vein, and *femoral* nerve. The fibular region contains the *fibula*, a long bone. Where would you expect to find the *occipital artery* and the *popliteal vein*? If you said the back of the head and the back of the knee then you are correct. Now that you have read about the major surface regions of the body, label those regions in Figure 2-1.

DIRECTIONAL TERMS

Now that you are familiar with the body's surface landmarks, it's time to learn the directional terms

Table 2-1. Axial Regions

	Pronunciation	Literal meaning	Common Name
HEAD			
Buccal	BUK-ul	Cheek	Cheek
Cephalic	se-FAL-ik	Head	Entire head (cranial and face regions)
Cranial	KRĀ-nē-ul	Skull	Skull (frontal, occipital, otic regions)
Face	fās	Face	Face (mental, nasal, buccal, oral, orbital regions)
Frontal	FRUN-tul	Forehead	Forehead
Mental	MEN-tul	Chin	Chin
Nasal	NĀ-sul	Nose	Nose
Occipital	ok-SIP-i-tul	Back of head	Back of head
Oral	OR-ul	Mouth	Mouth
Orbital	OR-bi-tul	Circle	Eye socket
Otic	Ō-tik	Ear	Ear region
NECK			
Cervical	SER-vi-kul	Neck	Neck (connects head to trunk)
Nuchal	NŪ-kul	Nape	Back of neck
TRUNK			
Abdominal	ab-DOM-i-nul	Belly	Abdomen (includes umbilical region)
Acromial	a-KRŌ-mē-ul	Point of shoulder	Tip of shoulder
Axillary	AK-sil-ār-ē	Axle	Armpit; joins trunk to upper limb
Coxal	COK-sul	Hip	Hip; joins trunk to lower limb
Gluteal	GLŪ-tē-ul	Buttock	Buttocks (separated by natal cleft)
Inguinal	ĒNG-gwi-nul	Groin	Groin; joins trunk to lower limbs
Lumbar	LUM-bar	Loin	Lower back
Mammary	MAM-a-rē	Breast	Breast
Natal cleft	NĀ-tul	Birth	Groove separating buttocks
Pelvic	PEL-vik	Basin (bowl)	Pelvis
Perineal	Payr-i-NĒ-ul	Between thighs	Triangle region from anus to genitalia
Pubic	PŪ-bik	Grown up*	Front of pelvis
Sacral	SĀ-krul	Sacred**	Between the hips
Scapular	SKAP-ū-lar	Shoulder blade	Shoulder blade
Shoulder	SHŌL-der	Shoulder	Shoulder (joins trunk and arm)
Spinal	SPĪ-nul	Thorn	Backbone
Sternal	STER-nul	Chest	Breastbone
Thoracic	THŌ-ras-ik	Chest	Chest (mammary and sternal regions)
Umbilical	um-BIL-i-kul	Navel	Navel
Vertebral	VER-tuh-brul	Turning joint	Spinal column

* Named for the coarse hairs, or pubes (PŪ-bēz), that appear in the pubic region when a person becomes sexually mature (reaches puberty).

** Some ancient cultures thought this part of the skeleton was sacred and would rise from the dead.

BODY ORGANIZATION

Table 2-2. Appendicular Regions

	Pronunciation	Literal meaning	Common name
UPPER LIMBS			
Antebrachial	an-tē-BRĀ-kē-ul	Forearm	Forearm (from elbow to wrist)
Antecubital	An-tē-KŪ-bi-tul	Front of elbow	Front of elbow
Brachial	BRĀ-kē-ul	Arm	Arm (from shoulder to elbow)
Carpal	KAR-pul	Wrist	Wrist (junction of forearm and hand)
Cubital	KŪ-bi-tul	Elbow	Elbow region
Digital	DIJ-i-tul	Fingers	Fingers (same as phalangeal)
Manual	MAN-ū-ul	Hand	Hand
Olecranal	ō-LEK-ra-nul	Point of elbow	Back of elbow
Palmar	PAL-mar	Palm	Palm (same as volar)
Phalangeal	Fa-LAN-jē-ul	Line of soldiers	Fingers (same as digital)
Pollex	POL-eks	Thumb	Thumb
Volar	VŌ-lar	Palm	Palm (same as palmar)
LOWER LIMBS			
Calcaneal	kal-KĀ-nē-ul	Heel	Heel
Crural	KROO-rul	Leg (anterior portion)	Leg
Digital	DIJ-i-tul	Digit	Toes
Femoral	FEM-o-rul	Thigh	Thigh (hip to knee)
Fibular	FIB-ū-lar	Outer side of leg	Side of leg (knee to ankle)
Gluteal	GLŪ-tē-ul	Buttock	Buttock (common site of injections)
Hallux	HAL-uks	Great toe	Big toe
Leg	leg	From knee to foot	Leg
Patellar	Pa-TEL-er	Kneecap	Kneecap
Pedal	PED-al	Foot	Foot
Peroneal	payr-ō-NĒ-ul	Fibular	Side of leg (same as fibular)
Phalangeal	fa-LAN-jē-ul	Line of soldiers	Toes
Plantar	PLAN-tar	Sole of foot	Sole
Popliteal	Pop-LIT-ē-ul	Back of the knee	Back of knee
Sole	sōl	Bottom of foot	Bottom of foot
Sural	SOO-rul	Calf	Back of leg
Tarsal	TAR-sul	Ankle	Ankle (joins leg to foot)
Thigh	thī	Thigh	Thigh
Volar	VŌ-lar	Sole	Sole of foot

18   CHAPTER 2

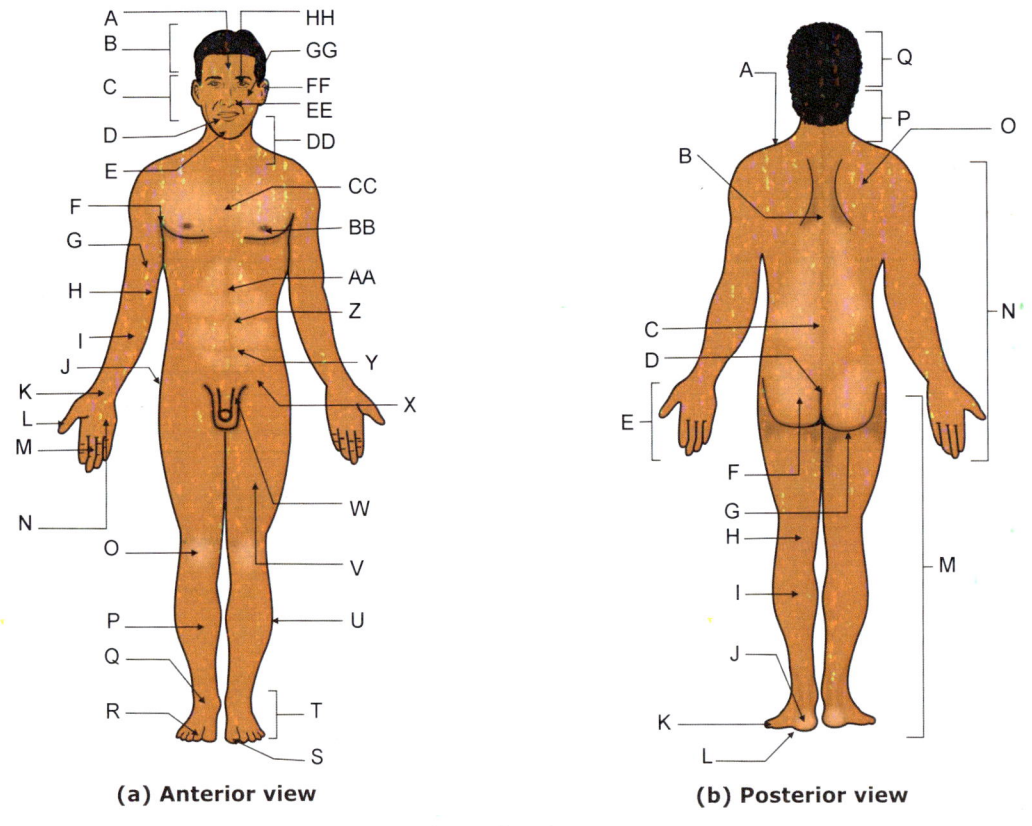

(a) Anterior view

(b) Posterior view

Figure 2-1. Anatomical position and the body's major surface features

that relate the location of one body part to another. Using these directional terms can allow you to avoid prolonged explanations and misunderstanding when describing a particular location on or inside the body. Without this terminology, someone could interpret the statement, "The buccal region is next to the eye region," to mean the forehead, nose, side of the head, or the cheek. However, saying, "The buccal region is *inferior* to the eye," eliminates the forehead, nose, and side of the head as possibilities.

To ensure consistency when using anatomy-related directional terms, we always assume the body we are describing is in anatomical position. In this way, a given term can always relate the location of one body part relative to another, even when the body changes its position. For example, *superior* means "above," so we can always say your cephalic region is superior to your trunk, even if you "stand on your head." Also, keep in mind that in anatomy, *right* and *left* means the right and left sides of the body you are viewing, not your own right and left sides. Become familiar with the directional terms in Table 2-3 and then label them in Figure 2-2.

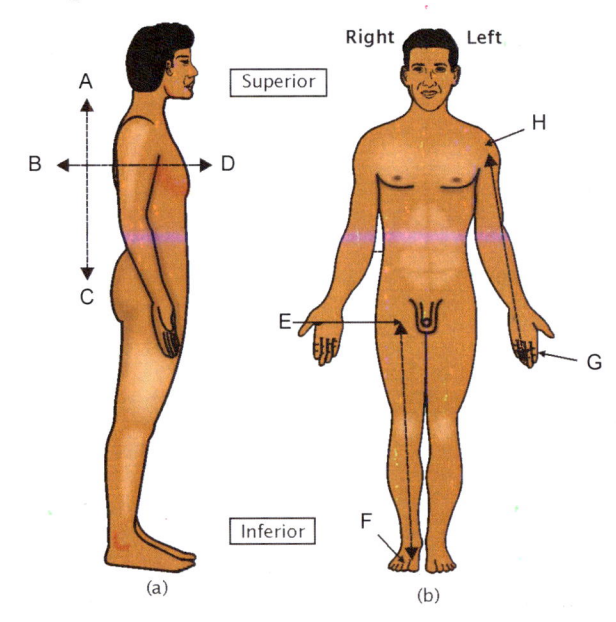

Figure 2-2. Directional Terms

BODY ORGANIZATION

Table 2-3. Directional Terms

Term	Description	Example
Anterior	Toward the front or in front of a structure	The toes are anterior to the heel.
Posterior	Toward the back or behind a structure	The heel is posterior to the toes.
Caudal	Toward the tail or coccyx (inferior end of spine)	The lumbar region is caudal to the thoracic region.
Contralateral	On opposite sides of the midline	The right lung and left kidney are contralateral.
Ipsilateral	On the same side of the midline	The left lung and left kidney are ipsilateral.
Deep	Away from the body's surface or body part	Muscles are deep to the skin.
Superficial	Toward or on the body's surface or body part	The skin is superficial to the muscles.
Distal	Away from the point of origin of a body part	The elbow is distal to the shoulder.
Proximal	Closer to the point of origin of a body part	The shoulder is proximal to the elbow.
Dorsal	Back or toward the back	The olecranon is dorsal to the antecubital region.
Ventral	Toward the front	The antecubital region is ventral to the olecranon.
Inferior	Toward the feet or lower part of a structure	The elbow is inferior to the shoulder.
Superior	Toward the head or upper part of a structure	The shoulder is superior to the elbow.
Intermediate	Between two structures	The heart is intermediate to the lungs.
Lateral	Away from a midline or toward the outer side	The thumb is lateral to the little finger.
Medial	Toward a midline or toward the inner side	The little finger is medial to the thumb.

PLANES AND SECTIONS

Now that you are familiar with the body's surface anatomy, let's take a look at some of the body's internal features. To do this, we must consider the angles at which anatomists cut the body they want to study. This is important because many images in this text show flat cut surfaces within three-dimensional body parts. In anatomy, a *section* is a cut that follows a straight path along an imaginary flat surface called a *plane*. Most anatomical studies utilize sections made along three planes that intersect the body at right angles; these include the *sagittal, frontal,* and *transverse* planes. A section made along a given plane has the same name as that plane; for example, to make a sagittal section, one cuts along a sagittal plane.

A **sagittal** (SAJ-i-tul) **plane** runs **vertically** and divides the body into right and left sides. We can be more specific when considering a sagittal plane's location relative to the body's *midline* (an imaginary vertical line running along the exact center of the body). A **midsagittal plane** lies on the midline to divide the body into two *equal* sides. **A parasagittal plane** runs alongside (*para-*, beside) the midline to divide the body into two *unequal* sides. Most images showing sagittal sections of the body or one of its parts are actually midsagittal sections.

A **transverse**, or **horizontal, plane** runs perpendicular (at right angles) to the sagittal and frontal planes and, for this reason, we sometimes call a transverse section a **cross section**. Any section made between the transverse plane and either a sagittal or a frontal plane is an **oblique section** (*oblique*, slanting).

A **frontal**, or **coronal, plane** (kō-RŌ-nul) runs vertically and divides the body into anterior and posterior parts. The word *corona* means "crown," so imagine you are placing a crown on your head and look at the orientation of your thumbs. Since they point toward your head from each side, they can remind you of a coronal plane's orientation. There are many frontal planes, but most images of frontal sections show the body or an organ divided into nearly equal anterior and posterior parts.

All of the sections just described can provide useful information about the anatomy of a particular body part, but each section produces a unique-looking image. Thus, to help you understand sectional views, we will provide small *orientation diagrams* that show the sectioned body part and the particular plane along which the cut occurred. You may have to make cuts along each of these planes on models provided in lab. Label the planes in Figure 2-3.

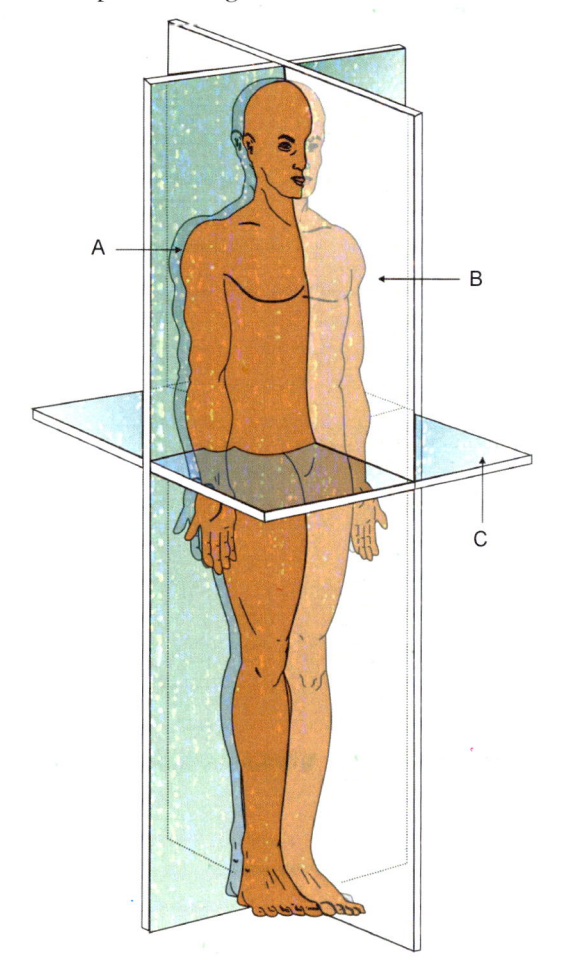

Figure 2-3. Planes of the body.

BODY CAVITIES

Making either a midsagittal or a frontal section through the axial region reveals two major body cavities, the *dorsal* and *ventral* cavities. These cavities have no connections with the outside of the body and serve three major functions: (1) to provide a location to hold vital organs; (2) to protect vital organs from the external environment; and (3) to allow room for certain internal organs, such as the heart and lungs, to expand without compressing adjacent organs.

Dorsal Body Cavity

The **dorsal body cavity** is the more posterior of the body's two major cavities and it contains a *cranial cavity* and a *vertebral cavity*. The **cranial cavity**, located inside the cranium of the cephalic region, is the more superior cavity and holds the brain. **The vertebral (spinal) cavity** is in the vertebral region and holds the spinal cord. The cranial and vertebral cavities are continuous with one another; that is, there is no barrier between them. Thick bones and tough connective tissue surround the dorsal cavity and protect the brain and spinal cord against external blows. In addition, the dorsal cavity contains a watery fluid that cushions the vital organs against the jarring effects of walking and running. The fluid also helps maintain a stable temperature within the cavity.

Ventral Body Cavity

The **ventral body cavity** is much larger than the dorsal cavity and is anterior to it. The ventral cavity has two major subdivisions: a *thoracic cavity* and the *abdominopelvic cavity*, separated from one another by a dome-shaped muscle called the *diaphragm* (DĪ-a-fram; "partition"). In general, anatomists refer to all organs within the ventral body cavity collectively as **visceral organs** (VIS-er-ul) or the **viscera** (VIS-er-a; "internal organ").

The **thoracic cavity** is superior to the diaphragm and contains four smaller cavities. Two of these, the right and left **pleural cavities** (PLOO-rul), each hold a lung and are so-named because they occupy the lateral portions (*pleura*, side) of the thoracic cavity. Located intermediate to the right and left pleural cavities is the **mediastinum** (mē-dē-a-STĪ-num; "middle"). It contains the trachea (windpipe), esophagus, thymus gland, major blood vessels, and the **pericardial cavity** (per-i-KAR-dē-ul), which encloses the heart (*peri*, around; *cardia*-, heart). To review the organization of the thoracic cavity, you could say, "The heart is in the pericardial cavity, which is in the mediastinum, which is in the thoracic cavity, which is in the ventral cavity," or "The ventral cavity contains the thoracic cavity, which contains the left pleural cavity, which contains the left lung."

The **abdominopelvic cavity** is inferior to the diaphragm and has two major parts: the *abdominal cavity* and the *pelvic cavity*, although these cavities are

BODY ORGANIZATION

Table 2-4. Major cavities of the body

Body Cavity	Location	Major organs within cavity
Abdominopelvic	Inferior to diaphragm	Stomach, intestines, liver, gall bladder, spleen, pancreas, kidneys, reproductive organs, urinary bladder
Abdominal	Inferior to diaphragm and superior to pelvis	Stomach, small intestine, large intestine, liver, gall bladder, spleen, pancreas, and kidneys *(no reproductive organs or urinary bladder)*
Cranial	Within skull	Brain
Dorsal	Cranial and vertebral cavities	Brain and spinal cord
Mediastinum	Between pleural cavities	Esophagus, trachea, thymus gland, and heart
Middle ear	Temporal bones	Ear ossicles
Nasal	Superior to oral cavity	Nasal septum, conchae
Oral	Inferior to nasal cavity	Tongue and teeth
Orbital	Anterior-superior skull	Eyeballs
Pelvic	Within pelvis	Reproductive organs, urinary bladder, and rectum
Pericardial	Mediastinum	Heart
Peritoneal	Inferior to diaphragm	Same as in abdominopelvic cavity
Pleural	Lateral to mediastinum	Lungs
Spinal	Within vertebrae	Spinal cord
Synovial	Around movable joints	Synovial fluid to reduce friction
Thoracic	Superior to diaphragm	Esophagus, trachea, lungs, and heart
Ventral	Thoracic and abdominopelvic	Abdominal and thoracic organs
Vertebral	Same as spinal cavity	Spinal cord
Visceral	Same as ventral cavity	Same as in ventral cavity

continuous with one another. The **abdominal cavity** extends from the diaphragm to the pelvic region and contains the stomach, liver, pancreas, and other organs, including most of the intestines. The **pelvic cavity** is inferior and slightly posterior to the abdominal cavity. The pelvic cavity lies within the bony pelvis and contains the urinary bladder, internal reproductive organs, and the rectum (inferior part of the large intestine).

To reinforce your knowledge of different body cavities, practice describing the location of various internal organs, beginning with the most general cavity and ending with the most specific cavity and vice versa. For example, you could say, "The brain is within the cranial cavity, which is within the dorsal cavity," or "The dorsal cavity contains the vertebral cavity, which contains the spinal cord. Use Table 2-4 to review the body's major cavities and then label those cavities in Figure 2-4.

SEROUS MEMBRANES

A thin membrane, called a **serous membrane** (SĒR-us) protects the walls of the ventral cavity and the surfaces of visceral organs as these organs carry out their normal functions. Some visceral organs, such as the heart and lungs, change shape constantly, while other organs, including the stomach, intestines, and urinary bladder, change shape on a regular basis. These movements generate friction between adjacent visceral organs and between these organs and the walls of the ventral cavity. The serous membranes produce a slippery **serous fluid** that reduces this friction. The word *serous* relates to "whey," or the watery part of curdled milk. (The "curd" is the solid part of curdled milk used to make cheese.)

There are several serous membranes in the ventral cavity, and each has two layers: the *parietal* (pa-RĪ-e-tul)

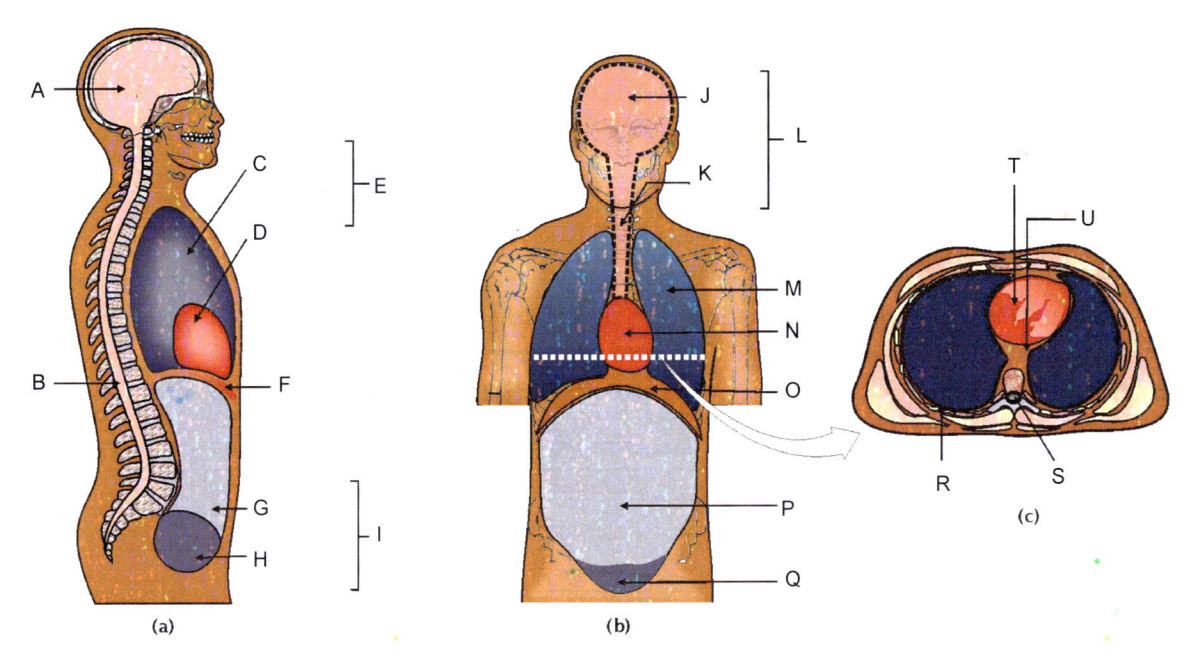

Figure 2-4. Major cavities and serous membranes of the body.

layer attaches to the wall of the cavity (*paries*, wall), and the *visceral* layer surrounds individual visceral organs. Serous fluid is between the parietal and visceral layers of each serous membrane. You can make a model of a serous membrane by inserting your fist into a sealed balloon filled with water. The outer part of the balloon represents the parietal layer and the inner part represents the visceral layer. Your fist represents a visceral organ and the fluid in the balloon represents serous fluid.

Two serous membranes, the *pleura* and *pericardium*, lie within the thoracic cavity. The serous membrane associated with the lungs is the **pleura** (PLOO-ra). The two layers of the pleura include the **parietal pleura**, located on the walls of the thoracic cavity, and the **visceral pleura** on the surface of the lungs. The pleural cavity lies between the parietal and viscera pleura. The serous membrane associated with the heart is the *pericardium* (per-i-KAR-dē-um). The **parietal pericardium** lines the inner wall of the *pericardial sac*, a bag-like structure that holds encloses the heart. The **visceral pericardium** covers the surface of the heart. The pericardial cavity lies between the parietal and visceral pericardium.

The most extensive serous membrane, the *peritoneum* (per-i-tō-NĒ-um; "stretched around"), lies within the abdominal cavity. The **parietal peritoneum** lines the walls of the abdominal cavity and the **visceral peritoneum** surrounds most of the visceral organs within the cavity. A few organs, such as the kidneys, adrenal glands, pancreas, and parts of the small and large intestine lie posterior to the parietal peritoneum. For this reason, we say these organs are *retroperitoneal* (*retro*, behind). The inferior portion of the parietal peritoneum extends into much of the pelvic cavity to cover portions of certain reproductive organs and the urinary bladder. The space between the parietal and visceral peritoneum is the *peritoneal cavity*. In much of the abdominopelvic cavity, the peritoneal cavity is only a "virtual" space because the peritoneal membranes lie next to one another. Review the body's serous membranes and then label those membranes in Figure 2-4.

MUCOUS MEMBRANES

If an internal body cavity ultimately has connection with the outside of the body, the inner lining of that cavity is a **mucous membrane** (MŪ-kus). These membranes usually contain a thin coat of material called **mucus** (note the spelling). Mucus is a viscous (thick) material most often secreted by specialized *goblet cells* that are part of the mucous membrane. Mucous membranes include the inner linings of organs in the digestive, respiratory, urinary and reproductive systems.

BODY ORGANIZATION

ABDOMINOPELVIC QUADRANTS AND REGIONS

Just as a grid on a city map can help you locate a particular street, an imaginary grid on the abdominopelvic cavity can help you locate a particular visceral organ. The simplest grid, and the one used mostly by healthcare professionals, has one vertical line and one horizontal line intersecting at the *umbilicus* (navel). This simple grid forms four **abdominopelvic quadrants** (*quad-*, four). The names of the quadrants refer to their location relative to the subject's right and left sides and include the *upper right, upper left, lower right, and lower left*.

Some anatomists may prefer a more elaborate grid to compartmentalize the abdominopelvic cavity. This grid resembles a tic-tac-toe grid with two parallel vertical lines intersecting two parallel horizontal lines, thereby dividing the abdominopelvic cavity into nine **abdominopelvic regions**.

- The two **hypochondriac regions** (hī-pō-KON-drē-ak; *hypo*, below; *chondr-*, cartilage) are the most superior, lateral regions. *Hypochondriac* denotes a region below cartilage (a type of connective tissue) on the anterior, inferior portion of the rib cage.
- The **epigastric** region (ep-ē-GAS-trik) is intermediate to the right and left hypochondriac regions and is so-named because it contains most of the stomach (*epi-*, above; *gastr-*, stomach).
- The two **lumbar** regions are immediately inferior to the right and left hypochondriac regions.
- The **umbilical** region is in the center of the grid (in the vicinity of the *umbilicus*, or navel), which is immediately inferior to the epigastric region and medial to the right and left lumbar regions.
- The two **inguinal (iliac)** regions are the most inferior, lateral regions and are immediately inferior to the right and left lumbar regions.
- The **hypogastric (pubic) region** is intermediate to the inguinal regions.

Table 2-6 lists the abdominopelvic quadrants and the nine abdominopelvic regions with their associated structures. After you become familiar with these items, label them in Figure 2-5.

Table 2-6. Divisions of the abdominopelvic cavity and their associated structures.

ABDOMINOPELVIC QUADRANTS	
Lower left	Small intestine, colon (parts), urinary bladder, reproductive organs
Lower right	Small intestine, colon (parts), urinary bladder, reproductive organs
Upper left	Spleen, stomach, pancreas, small intestine, colon (parts), left kidney
Upper right	Liver, gall bladder, stomach, small intestine, colon (parts), right kidney
ABDOMINOPELVIC REGIONS	
Epigastric	Liver, stomach, pancreas, colon (part)
Hypogastric (Pubic)	Small intestine, colon (part), urinary bladder, reproductive organs
Left hypochondriac	Spleen, stomach, pancreas, small intestine (part), left kidney, colon (parts)
Left Inguinal	Colon (parts)
Left Lumbar	Small intestine, colon (part), left kidney
Right Hypochondriac	Liver, gall bladder, small intestine (part), colon (parts), right kidney
Right inguinal	Small intestine, colon (parts)
Right lumbar	Small intestine, colon (part), right kidney
Umbilical	Small intestine, both kidneys

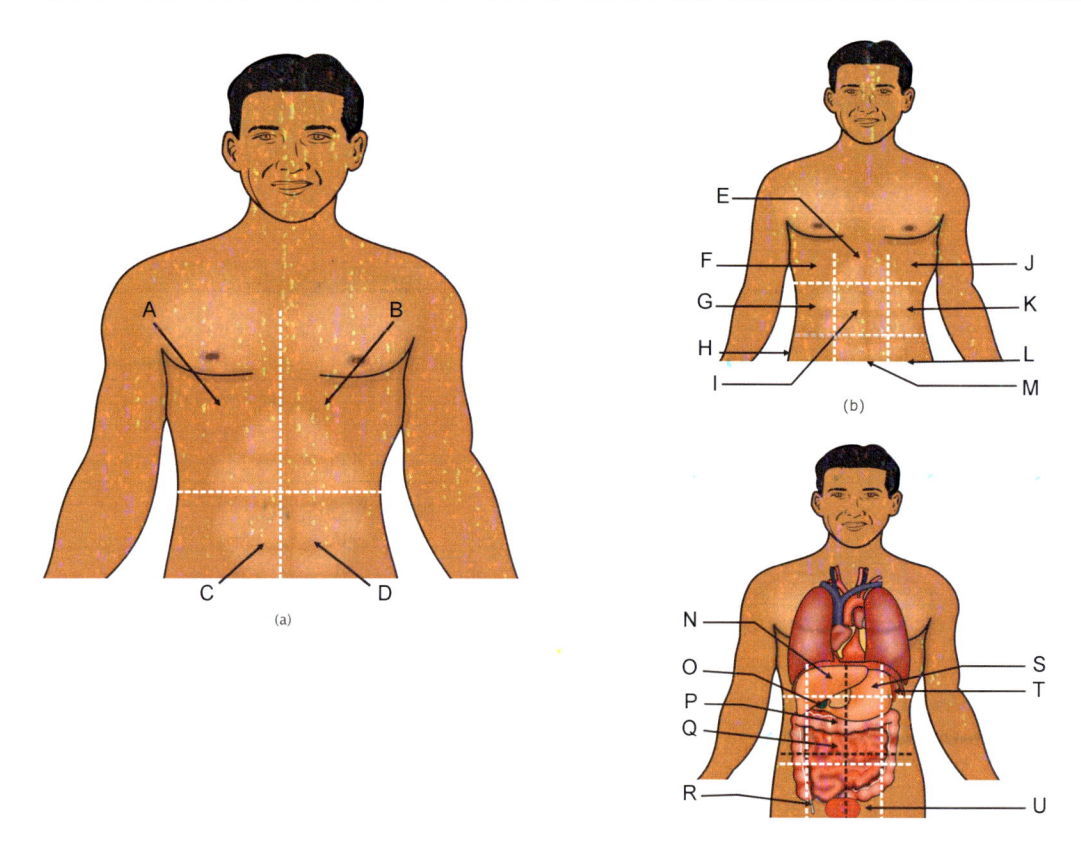

Figure 2-5. Abdominopelvic quadrants and regions.

TOPICS TO KNOW IN CHAPTER 2 (BODY ORGANIZATION)

abdominal cavity
abdominal region
abdominopelvic region
acromial region
anatomical position
antebrachial region
antecubital region
anterior
appendicular regions
axial regions
axillary region
brachial region
buccal region
calcaneal region
carpal region
caudal
cephalic
cervical region
contralateral
coronal plane
coxal region
cranial region
cross section
crural region

cubital region
deep
digital region
distal
dorsal
dorsal cavity
epigastric region
face
femoral region
fibular region
frontal region
frontal plane
gluteal region
hallux region
hypochondriac region
hypogastric region
iliac region
inferior
inguinal region
intermediate
ipsilateral
lateral
leg region
lower limb

lumbar region
mammary region
manual
medial
mediastinum
midsagittal plane
mucous membrane
mucus
natal cleft
neck
nuchal region
oblique section
occipital region
olecranal region
oral
orbital region
otic region
palmar region
parasagittal plane
parietal pericardium
parietal peritoneum
parietal pleura
patellar region
pedal

BODY ORGANIZATION

pelvic region
pericardial cavity
perineal region
peritoneal region
peroneal region
phalangeal
plantar region
pleura
pleural cavity
pollex region
popliteal region
posterior
proximal
pubic region
quadrant

sacral region
sagittal plane
scapular region
serous fluid
serous membrane
shoulder
skull
sole
spinal region
sternal region
superficial
superior
sural region
tarsal region
thigh

thoracic cavity
thoracic region
transverse plane
umbilical region
upper limb
ventral
ventral cavity
vertebral cavity
vertebral region
viscera
visceral pericardium
visceral peritoneum
visceral pleura
volar region

CHAPTER 3

Chemistry Overview

The study of human anatomy and physiology is really a study of chemicals, and to understand the makeup and function of these **chemicals** requires a basic knowledge of chemistry. Chemistry is the study of the material that comprises all physical objects; i.e., chemistry is the study of *matter*. **Matter** is anything in the universe that occupies space or has mass, and it consists of basic building blocks called **elements**. An element is so-named because it is the most *elementary* ("beginning") level of organization in matter. There are 92 naturally occurring elements. Six of these—carbon (C), hydrogen (H), nitrogen (N), oxygen (O), phosphorus (P), and sulfur (S)—make up most of the matter when considering all living things on Earth. However, the six most abundant elements in humans are C, H, N, O, P, and Ca (calcium).

> **Note**: Remember CHNOPS ("Shnops") for the most common elements in most organisms, and CHNOPCa ("Shnop-kuh") for the most common elements in the human body.

The body contains chemicals at several different levels of complexity, including *atoms, molecules,* and *compounds*.

ATOMS, MOLECULES, AND COMPOUNDS

To understand the chemical makeup of your body, you must begin with an understanding of atoms. An **atom** (literally, "indivisible") is the smallest subunit of an element that has characteristics associated with that element. An atom contains one or more subatomic particles, including protons, neutrons, and electrons. Figure 3-1 shows examples of atoms.

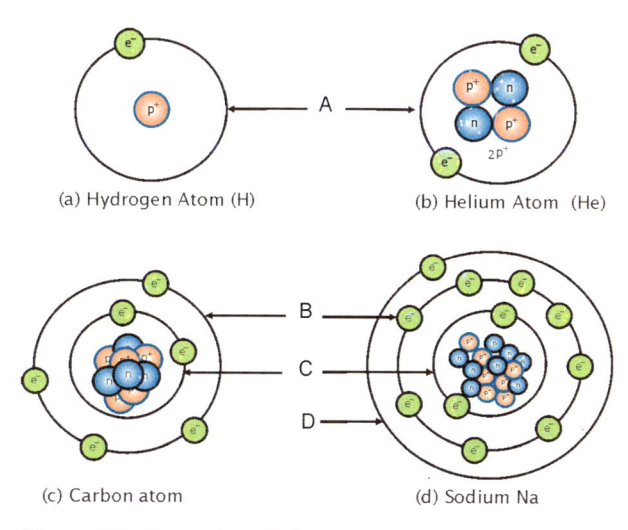

(a) Hydrogen Atom (H)   (b) Helium Atom (He)

(c) Carbon atom   (d) Sodium Na

Figure 3-1. Examples of atoms

A **proton** has a positive charge, whereas a **neutron** does not have a charge. These two types of subatomic particles exist in the nucleus ("nut" or "kernel"), located at the center of the atom. An **electron** has a negative charge and orbits the nucleus. An element's **atomic number** is the number of protons that exist within the nucleus of one of the element's atoms. The **atomic weight** (or **atomic mass**) is the weight of all protons and neutrons within the nucleus, and it is approximately equal to the number of protons and neutrons present. An atom is neutral (lack a charge) when its number of protons equals its number of electrons.

The human body is more than just a collection of individual atoms clumped together. Instead, it consists of atoms interacting with one another in complex ways. Atoms can interact with one another in a process called a **chemical reaction**, which involves the formation of **chemical bonds**. Chemical reactions can form complex levels of matter, including *molecules* and *compounds*. A **molecule** is a combination of any two or more atoms. Examples of small molecules include hydrogen gas (H_2), oxygen gas (O_2), water (H_2O), and methane (CH_4). A **macromolecule** is a large chain-like molecule such as DNA. A **compound** is a combination of two or more different elements, and includes water (H_2O), methane (CH_4), glucose ($C_6H_{12}O_6$), and DNA.

> Note: All compounds are molecules but not all molecules are compounds. For example, O_2 is a molecule but not a compound, while H_2O is both a molecule and a compound

Since physiology involves the study of various chemicals reacting in different ways, it is necessary to understand how physiologists measure chemicals. The customary unit of measurement for molecules is the *mole*. A **mole** is equal to the compound's molecular weight expressed in grams; whereas, a **millimole** (mmole) is equal to its molecular weight measured in milligrams (mg). One mole of any element contains the same number of atoms as one mole of any other element, and this number is 6.023×10^{23} (called *Avogadro's number*), or 602.3 billion trillion atoms. For practice, calculate the number of milligrams in one mmole of *glucose* ($C_6H_{12}O_6$) and one mmole of *sodium chloride* (NaCl; table salt). (These compounds have important medical importance that you will learn about later.) First, we must first know the atomic weight of each element in these compounds: C=12, H=1, O=16, Na=23 and Cl=35. Therefore, one mmole of glucose is:

$$(C=6\times12) + (H=12\times1) + (O=6\times16) = 180 \text{ mg}$$

One mmole of NaCl (table salt) is:

$$(Na=1\times23) + (Cl^-1\times35) = 58 \text{ mg}$$

Before describing chemical bonds, you must have an understanding of *mixtures*, which are combinations of matter that do not share chemical bonds.

MIXTURES

The body contains a variety of *mixtures*, which are combinations of substances in which each substance retains its own chemical properties. A *homogeneous* mixture (hō-mō-JĒ-nē-us; *homo*, same) has particles distributed evenly throughout and cannot be separated by filtration. Although a homogeneous mixture may absorb light, the particles are so small that light rays are not scattered (deflected or refracted). In contrast, a *heterogeneous* mixture (het-er-ō-JĒN-ē-us; *hetero*, different) has particles large enough to scatter light rays. There are three types of mixtures: *solutions, colloids,* and *suspensions*.

A **solution** is a homogeneous mixture in which one substance, called the **solute**, is scattered evenly throughout another substance called the **solvent**. A solute will not settle out of a solution; i.e., it will not separate from the solvent. The solute's **concentration** is the amount of solute divided by the total amount of solution:

$$\text{Concentration} = \frac{\text{Amount of Solute}}{\text{Amount of Solution}}$$

In this book, brackets around a term denote a concentration. For example, we will write the concentration of glucose as [glucose]. A one-millimolar (1 mM) glucose solution contains 1 mmole of glucose (180 mg) dissolved in 100 ml of solution, where the solvent is pure water. Other common units of measure for a substance's concentration include parts per million (ppm), milligrams per liter (mg/L—the same as ppm), and micrograms per deciliter (μg/dl).

CHEMISTRY OVERVIEW

A **colloid** (KOL-oyd; *coll*, glue; *oid*, appearance) is a heterogeneous mixture in which particles are large enough to scatter light, yet they are too small to settle out of the mixture. Common colloids are gelatin and milk.

A **suspension** is a heterogeneous mixture that contains particles large enough to settle out of the mixture. An example of a suspension is muddy water in a flask. If allowed to stand undisturbed for some time, the suspended dirt and clay particles will settle to the bottom of the flask.

CHEMICAL BONDS

Your body holds together because atoms have the ability to form chemical unions, or *bonds*, between one another. A **chemical bond** is an attraction or force that holds atoms together. Electrons are the subatomic particles responsible for this attractive force. Electrons orbit the atom's nucleus at different distances called **electron shells** (or **energy shells**). The actual flight path for electrons within an electron shell is an **orbital**. Each orbital can contain no more than two electrons. The energy shell closest to the nucleus has the lowest energy and contains only one orbital; therefore, it can hold a maximum of two electrons. Shells farther away from the nucleus have more energy and may contain many orbitals. Most outer electron shells contain four orbitals, and thus can hold a maximum of eight electrons.

An atom interacts with other atoms in a way that either completely fills or completely empties its *outermost* electron shell. Since most atoms have outer electron shells that can hold a maximum of eight electrons, chemists refer to this tendency of interaction as the **octet rule** (*oct-*, eight). Exceptions to this rule are hydrogen and helium atoms, which have only one orbital and, therefore, can have only two electrons in their outer electron shell. If the outer shell of a neutral atom is full, that atom will not react with another atom and the element is *inert* (literally means "sluggish"). Helium (He) is an inert element. Three major types of chemical bonds that can hold molecules together include *ionic*, *covalent*, and *hydrogen* bonds.

Ionic Bonds

An **ionic** (ī-ON-ik) **bond** is the force of attraction between oppositely charged particles of matter called ions. Since ions in a solution are able to conduct an electrical current, chemists call them **electrolytes** (ē-LEK-trō-lītz). An **ion** (Ī-on) is an atom or molecule that has more or fewer electrons than protons. A positively charged ion is a **cation** (KAT-ī-on), which results when a neutral atom or molecule loses one or more electrons. An example of a cation is a hydrogen ion (H^+). Whereas, a hydrogen atom is neutral when it has one electron and one proton, losing the electron makes the atom become a hydrogen ion. Other examples of cations include the sodium ion (Na^+) and calcium ion (Ca^{2+}). A negatively charged ion is an **anion** (AN-ī-on), which results when a neutral atom or molecule gains one or more electrons. One way that an anion can form is when one atom "steals" one or more electrons from another atom. In this process, the atom that loses the electron becomes a cation. For example, when a neutral chlorine atom steals an electron from a sodium atom, the chlorine atom becomes a chloride ion and the sodium atom becomes a sodium ion. Since these ions have opposite charges, they attract one another and form an ionic compound called NaCl, or table salt. The reaction is as follows:

$$Na + Cl \rightarrow Na^+ + Cl^- \rightarrow NaCl$$

Covalent Bonds

A **covalent bond** (kō-VĀ-lent; *co-*, together; *valence*, power) forms when two atoms share one or more outer electrons. Covalent bonds are found within a single water molecule, in which one oxygen atom shares electrons with two hydrogen atoms:

$$2H + O \rightarrow H_2O$$

Covalently bonded molecules are either *nonpolar* or *polar*. **Nonpolar** molecules share electrons *equally*; that is, a shared electron spends about the same amount of time orbiting both atoms. **Polar** molecules share electrons *unequally*, in which an electron orbits one of the atoms longer than it orbits the other atom. Overall, a polar compound is neutral because its number of electrons equals its number of protons. However, due to the unequal sharing of electrons, a polar compound has a *positive* and a *negative* region. Think of a polar molecule as being like a battery. Although the battery has a positive end and negative end (these oppositely charged ends are called *poles*), the battery as a whole is electrically neutral because the total number of positive charges equals the total number of negative charges. Water is a polar compound, but carbon dioxide (CO_2) is nonpolar.

Sometimes two atoms share two or more electrons. In these cases, double or triple lines drawn between the atoms indicate the number of electrons shared. Hydrogen atoms can form only one covalent bond, while oxygen atoms can form two. Carbon atoms, which exist in all organic molecules, can form four covalent bonds.

Hydrogen Bonds

A hydrogen bond (H-bond) is an attraction between a hydrogen atom located within one polar molecule and an oxygen or nitrogen atom located within another molecule. If the H-bond exists within one large macromolecule, it is an *intra*molecular H-bond (*intra*, within). Intramolecular H-bonds allow the macromolecule to coil and bend to form unique 3-dimensional shapes. If the H-bond exists between molecules that are not part of a macromolecule, it is an *inter*molecular H-bond (*inter*, between). Intermolecular hydrogen bonds hold adjacent water molecules together in a process called **cohesion** (cō-HĒ-shun; *cohes*, stick together). Intermolecular hydrogen bonds also allow water molecules to stick to non-water molecules in a process called **adhesion** (ad-HĒ-shun; *adhes*, stick to).

ISOTOPES

Sometimes different atoms of the same element have different molecular weights, and these unique atoms are called isotopes. An **isotope** (Ī-sō-tōp; *iso*, same; *-tope*, part) is an element with an atomic weight that is different from that of the most common form of the element. For example, most hydrogen atoms have one proton (p^+) and no neutrons (n^o). On the other hand, one type of hydrogen isotope is *deuterium* (^2H; dū-TĒR-ē-um), which has one p^+ and one n^o (*deuter* means "second," referring to the second particle present in the nucleus). Another hydrogen isotope, called *tritium* (^3H; TRIT-ē-um), has one p^+ and two n^o (*tri* means "three," referring to the three particles in the nucleus). Some isotopes are **radioactive**, meaning they are unstable and lose nuclear particles and energy over time. This decomposition of an isotope is **radioactive decay**.

Medical technology makes use of a variety of radioisotopes and utilizes special instruments to detect radioactive decay. Clinicians sometimes inject small amounts of radioisotope into a patient and trace it through the body to locate obstructions, tumors, and to map out metabolic pathways. In other cases, clinicians deliberately concentrate radioactive isotopes inside cancerous tumors, allowing the release of nuclear particles and energy from the radioisotopes to destroy the tumor cells.

ENERGY

Energy is the force that moves matter, and **work** is the movement of matter; therefore, energy is the force responsible for work. Stored energy, or the energy of "position," is **potential energy**, so named because while it is not moving matter at that moment, it can perform work later. Potential energy exists in a car battery because it can start the car's engine when you turn on the ignition switch. In your cells, certain molecules (such as glucose) have potential energy in their chemical bonds, and a cell can release this energy to do work.

Energy in motion is **kinetic energy** (ki-NE-tik; *kinesis*, movement), and includes the following:

- **Chemical energy**: energy released when a chemical bond is broken, or the energy required to form a chemical bond
- **Electrical energy**: movement of electrons along a wire, through a liquid, or in the atmosphere
- **Electrochemical energy**: movement of *ions*
- **Radiant** (also called **electromagnetic**) **energy**: energy that travels in waves or rays; examples are visible light, ultraviolet (U-V) radiation, and X-rays
- **Mechanical energy**: energy existing in matter as it moves; this energy can be transferred directly to other matter. When a moving object transfers mechanical energy to a second object, the second object may (1) move, (2) change shape, or (3) change its direction of movement if it is already moving. Golf involves transferring mechanical energy from a moving golf club to a stationary ball in order to move the ball.

CHEMISTRY OVERVIEW

Heat relates to the relative speed of particles in motion, but it is unavailable to do work. Heat is released when one form of energy transforms into another form. **Temperature** is a measure of heat and relates directly (is positively related) to the speed of the particles in motion. The faster the particles are moving, the higher the temperature.

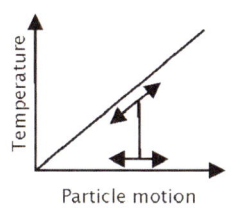

Moreover, when the temperature of particles increases, so does the speed at which those particles move.

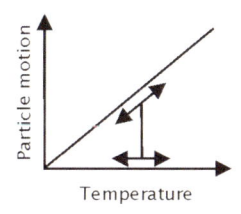

Looking back and forth at these two graphs suggests that a positive feedback mechanism is possible. This is what happens during either *hypothermia* or *hyperthermia*. In hypothermia (hī-pō-THER-mē-a; *hypo*, low; *therm*, heat), a person's body temperature is decreasing, which causes metabolic reactions to slow down. The slower metabolism generates less heat, which causes the body temperature to decrease even more, which in turn causes the metabolic processes to slow down even more, and so on. In hyperthermia (*hyper*, high), the reactions are the opposite of that in hypothermia: an increasing body temperature causes an increase in metabolism, which generates more heat to cause an increase in body temperature and a subsequent increase in metabolism, and so on. Unless counteracted in some way, hypothermia and hyperthermia are life-threatening conditions.

The generation of heat indicates that the transfer of energy from one form to another form is not 100% efficient. Heat released when a gallon of gasoline burns cannot propel a car. Likewise, when a cell "burns" food molecules, some of the energy can perform work inside the cell, but the remaining energy is released as heat.

CHEMICAL REACTIONS

A **chemical reaction** is an interaction between atoms or ions and involves the breaking or forming of chemical bonds. Particles that interact with one another are **reactants**, while the substance formed during a reaction is the **product**. In some cases, several reactants interact to form a larger product. In other cases, a single reactant breaks down into smaller products.

Depending on whether energy is absorbed or released during the process, a chemical reaction is either *endergonic* or *exergonic*. Reactions that *absorb* energy are **endergonic** (en-der-GON-ik; *ender*, inside; *gonic*, work). Thus, the product contains more stored energy than all the reactants combined. An example of an endergonic reaction is photosynthesis, in which plants use light energy to produce glucose and oxygen from carbon dioxide and water:

$$6CO_2 + 6H_2O + \text{light energy} \rightarrow C_6H_{12}O_6 + 6O_2$$

Reactions that *release* energy are **exergonic** (eks-er-GON-ik; *exer*, outside). Consequently, the product of an exergonic reaction contains less stored energy than all the reactants combined. An example of an exergonic reaction is the breakdown of glucose. The complete breakdown of glucose inside a cell involves a series of reactions known collectively as *cellular respiration*, so-named because it proceeds only when oxygen molecules are available, and humans take in oxygen molecules through the *respiratory* system. Cellular respiration is summarized as follows:

$$C_6H_{12}O_6 + O_2 \rightarrow CO_2 + H_2O + \text{energy}$$

A cell can utilize the energy released during cellular respiration to drive various cellular activities, which is to say that the cell uses the released energy to do work.

Classification of Chemical Reactions

Chemical reactions are classified in a number of ways, but the major types include *synthesis, decomposition, reversible,* and *oxidation-reduction* reactions.

Recall from chapter 1 that all chemical reactions in the body account for **metabolism**. One aspect of metabolism is **anabolism**, in which reactants combine to form a larger compound. Anabolic reactions are **synthesis** reactions (SIN-the-sis; *syn*, together; *thesis*, arranging) and we can summarize them as follows:

X + Y → XY

The opposite of anabolism is **catabolism**, which involves the breakdown of compounds. Catabolic reactions are decomposition reactions:

XY → X + Y

A **reversible** reaction is one in which the reactants generate a product that readily breaks apart, or *dissociates* (diss-Ō-sē-ātz; to separate), to form the original reactants. Chemists denote these reactions with double arrows (← →). An example of a reversible reaction is the formation and breakdown of carbonic acid (H_2CO_3). Following the reaction to the right, carbon dioxide and water combine to form carbonic acid, which then dissociates to form hydrogen ions (H^+) and bicarbonate ions (HCO_3^-). Then following the reaction to the left, some of the H^+ and HCO_3^- may combine to form H_2CO_3, which dissociates to form CO_2 and H_2O:

$$CO_2 + H_2O \leftrightarrow H_2CO_3 \leftrightarrow H^+ + HCO_3^-$$

Carbonated beverages are made by bubbling CO_2 into the beverage under high pressure. The added CO_2 binds with water and forces the above reactions to the *right*. As a result, more H^+ ions form and these ions can "burn" your throat when you drink the beverage. If you leave the carbonated drink uncovered, CO_2 diffuses into the atmosphere. To replace the CO_2 that is lost, the above reactions move to the *left*; therefore, more H^+ ions react with HCO_3^- to form H_2CO_3, which dissociates to form CO_2 and H_2O. When sufficient H^+ ions leave the solution, the drink no longer produces that burning sensation when you drink it, and we say the drink is "flat."

Oxidation-reduction (redox) reactions involve synthesis and decomposition. The *loss of an electron is* **oxidation**. In most biological reactions, when an electron leaves a compound, a proton (hydrogen ion) goes with it. Since one proton and one electron together make up a hydrogen atom, we can also say oxidation is a *loss of a hydrogen atom*. An oxidizing agent is one that readily "steals" electrons from other atoms. Oxygen atoms are strong oxidizing agents because they each have two vacant spots in their outer electron shell, which causes them to react in a way to fill those spots with electrons. Oxygen atoms can readily oxidize iron (Fe) atoms in a shiny, new nail exposed to moisture and air. The result is iron oxide (Fe_2O_3, or rust). Since oxygen interacts with many different chemicals, we can also say oxidation is the *addition of an oxygen atom* to a substance.

The opposite of oxidation is **reduction**, and we can define it as the *gain of an electron*, the *gain of a hydrogen atom*, or the *loss of an oxygen atom*. A sodium atom experiences oxidation when it loses an electron to a chlorine atom; in turn, the chlorine atom becomes reduced. In photosynthesis, a plant reduces CO_2 by adding hydrogen atoms to form glucose ($C_6H_{12}O_6$). Since glucose is a highly reduced compound, you could think of it as being *RED*-hot with energy ("RED" standing for REDuced.) Certain chemical reactions oxidize glucose by removing some of its hydrogen atoms. The oxidized form of a compound has fewer carbon-hydrogen (C-H) bonds and, therefore, has less stored energy than its reduced form. In the above example, CO_2 has less stored energy than $C_6H_{12}O_6$.

> Note: Ways to remember redox reactions: (1) "OIL RIG": **O**xidation **I**s **L**oss, **R**eduction **I**s **G**ain, or (2) "LEO GER", the GER is the growl of LEO the Lion: **L**oss of **E**lectrons is **O**xidation; **G**ain of **E**lectrons is **R**eduction.

Some chemical reactions produce molecules called free **radicals**, which are molecules that have unpaired electrons in their outer electron shell. An example of an important free radical formed in the human body is the superoxide ion (O_2^-). This free radical reacts violently with other atoms, stealing electrons from them, because the radical has a strong tendency to pair all of its electrons. Reacting with a free radical causes oxidation of a compound, and this may cause the compound to change its 3-dimensional shape. In turn, the change in shape could adversely affect the function of the oxidized compound. **Antioxidants** are chemicals that react with free radicals and prevent their reaction with vital cellular compounds. Certain vitamins, such as A, C, and E are important antioxidants.

Factors Affecting Reaction Rate

Several variables can affect the rate at which a chemical reaction occurs:

CHEMISTRY OVERVIEW

(1) *Size of reactants*: Reaction rate correlates *negatively* with the size of the reactants because smaller particles move faster and, thus, react faster than larger particles. *smaller = faster*

(2) *Concentration of reactants*: Concentration of reactants has a positive effect on reaction rate; i.e., the more reactants present, the more likely they will interact.

(3) *Temperature*: Reaction rate is positively affected by temperature. Heated molecules move faster, and this increases the likelihood that they will react. *Hotter = faster*

(4) *Concentration of catalysts*: **A catalyst** is a substance that speeds up a reaction without becoming part of any product; thus, the greater the concentration of catalysts, the greater the reaction rate.

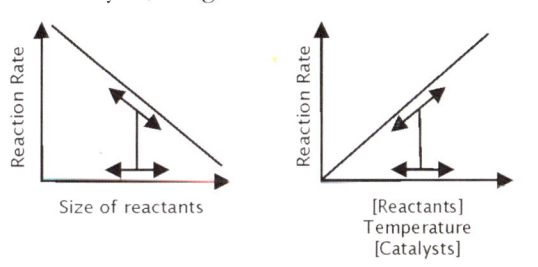

WATER

Since water makes up 50-60% of our bodies, we should take a moment to consider its importance to life. Water is a *polar* compound that has many important functions in the body:

(1) It is the medium in which chemical reactions occur.

(2) It can act as a chemical reactant.

(3) It acts as a lubricant to reduce friction.

(4) It absorbs and dissipates heat.

(5) It acts as a shock absorber.

Related to the first function, water has the ability to dissolve many substances. The ability of a substance to disperse evenly in a fluid is **dissolution**, which is why we say a substance can *dissolve* in a particular fluid. Additionally, if a compound can dissolve in a fluid, we say it is *soluble* in that fluid. Since water can dissolve so many things, it has been called the "universal solvent." So, what gives water this special ability?

Water's polarity allows it to form **hydration shells** around ions and polar molecules. The positive (hydrogen) end of a water molecule attracts anions and the negative regions of polar compounds, while the negative (oxygen) end of a water molecule attracts cations and the positive regions of polar compounds. Hydration shells keep ions and polar molecules dispersed (dissolved). Figure 3-2 shows hydration shells around solute particles.

ACIDS, BASES, AND SALTS

A number of different compounds dissociate in solution to form ions, and these substances play vital roles in homeostasis. Examples of compounds that dissociate in this way include *water, acids, bases,* and *salts*. While it might seem logical that ionic bonds would be found in all these compounds, ionic bonds are found only in salts. In contrast, water, acid, and base molecules are held together by covalent bonds. Water dissociates

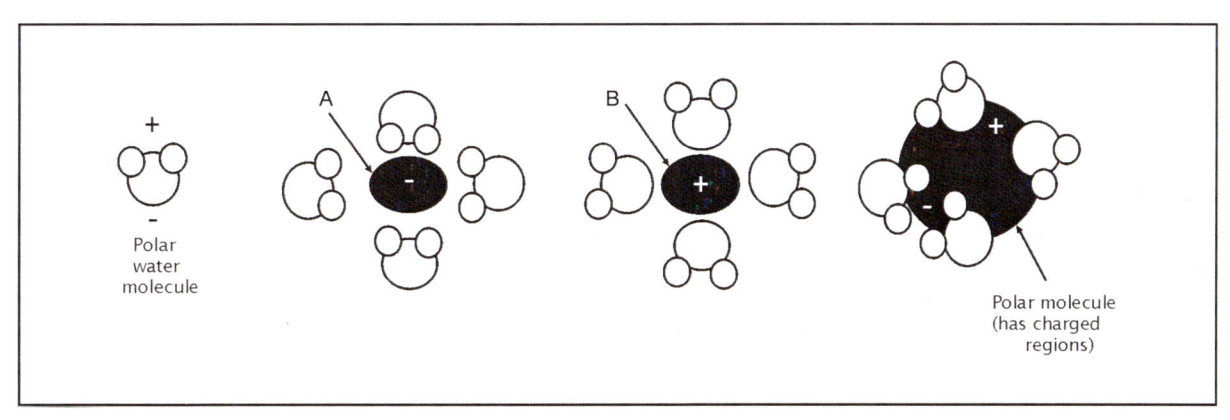

Figure 3-2. Hydration shells around ions and a polar molecule

into hydrogen ions and hydroxide ions (OH⁻), which can then come together again to form water as follows:

$$H_2O \leftarrow\rightarrow H^+ + OH^-$$

An **acid** is a compound that dissociates to yield H⁺ ions in a solution. An example is *hydrochloric acid* (HCl), which dissociates to yield hydrogen ions and chloride ions:

$$HCl \rightarrow H^+ + Cl^-$$

A *strong acid*, such as HCl, dissociates completely and irreversibly; thus, we show the reaction with a single arrow. On the other hand, a *weak acid* dissociates incompletely and the reaction is reversible. This means that some undissociated acid molecules are always in the solution along with the H⁺ ions and anions yielded when some of the acid molecules dissociated. *Carbonic acid* (H_2CO_3) is a weak acid and its dissociation is shown with a double arrow:

$$H_2CO_3 \leftarrow\rightarrow H^+ + HCO_3^-$$

Acids taste sour, and some of the more common acids that you have probably tasted include *ascorbic acid* (vitamin C), *citric acid* (abundant in fruits such as oranges and grapefruits), and acetic acid (vinegar).

A **base** is a substance that removes H⁺ ions from a solution. *Sodium hydroxide* (NaOH), also known as lye and found in drain cleaners, is an example of a *strong base*. Like strong acids, strong bases dissociate completely and irreversibly. Furthermore, dissociation of a strong base always yields a hydroxide ion, and this anion readily reacts with H⁺ ions to form water. The dissociation of NaOH and its ability to remove H⁺ from a solution is shown below:

$$NaOH + H^+ \rightarrow Na^+ + OH^- + H^+ \rightarrow Na^+ + H_2O$$

Minerals that dissociate to form base compounds are referred to as alkaline (AL-ka-līn) compounds.

A *weak base* dissociates incompletely and the reactions are reversible. Sodium bicarbonate ($NaHCO_3$), which is used as baking soda, is a weak base; thus, we show its dissociation with a double arrow:

$$NaHCO_3 \leftarrow\rightarrow Na^+ + HCO_3^-$$

The bicarbonate ion (HCO_3^-) is the base component that can bind with H⁺; when this happens, H_2CO_3 (carbonic acid) forms. However, HCO_3^- ions do not react with H⁺ as readily as do the OH⁻ ions released from strong bases. The ability of bicarbonate released from $NaHCO_3$ to act as a base is shown below:

$$NaHCO_3 + H^+ \rightarrow Na^+ + HCO_3^- + H^+ \leftarrow\rightarrow Na^+ + H_2CO_3$$

A **salt** is an ionic compound that dissociates to yield cations other than H⁺ and anions other than OH⁻. An example is sodium chloride (NaCl), commonly called table salt:

$$NaCl \rightarrow Na^+ + Cl^-$$

When a strong acid and a strong base mix, the reaction forms salt and water. The following shows the reaction between hydrochloric acid and sodium hydroxide:

$$HCl + NaOH \rightarrow NaCl + H_2O$$

The pH scale and measurements of [H⁺]

Chemists use a mathematical formula to calculate the *pH* of a solution, and this formula relates to the amount of H⁺ in that solution. The calculation for pH is as follows:

$$pH = -\log_{10}[H^+]$$

The [H⁺] is the concentration of H⁺ reported as moles of H⁺ per liter of solution. The $\log_{10}$ of a number is the power to which 10 is raised to equal that number. For example, the $\log_{10}$ of 100 is 2, since 10^2 equals 100. However, when dealing with numbers less than 1, the exponent will be a negative number. For instance, the $\log_{10}$ of 0.001 is -3 (obtained from 10^{-3}). Since the [H⁺] expressed in grams per liter is extremely small, the logarithm of the [H⁺] will always be negative. Therefore, by adding a negative sign to the equation, pH values become positive.

The pH scale ranges from 0-14, with acids having a pH below 7 and bases having a pH above 7. Since a mole of H⁺ weighs approximately one gram, a solution at pH 7 has 0.0000001 g of H⁺ in every liter (notice the number 1 is in the *seventh* place to the right of the decimal). A solution at pH 2 has 0.01 g H⁺ per liter of

CHEMISTRY OVERVIEW

solution. At pH 7, the [H⁺] = [OH⁻] and the solution is said to be *neutral*. Pure water is neutral although it acts like an acid and a base at the same time by dissociating into H⁺ and OH⁻ ions. To get a better feel for the logarithmic nature of the pH scale, consider the following:

Solution at pH 7 has 100 times <u>more</u> H⁺ than at pH 9
Solution at pH 8 has 10,000 times <u>fewer</u> H⁺ than at pH 4
Solution at pH 7 has 10,000 times <u>more</u> OH⁻ than at pH 3

The normal range of pH in the body is 7.35 to 7.45. When the tissue fluids have a pH below 7.35, the person is experiencing *acidosis* (as-i-DŌ-sis; *osis*, condition). When the tissues have a pH above 7.45, the person is experiencing *alkalosis* (al-ka-LŌ-sis).

BUFFERS

While dramatic fluctuations in blood or tissue fluid pH can be life threatening, the body contains certain chemicals that help maintain pH levels within tolerable limits. A **buffer** is a substance that prevents dramatic pH changes in a solution by reacting with either H⁺ or OH⁻ that enter the solution. The word "buffer" relates to how a soft body reacts when struck; that is, it absorbs the punch. A *buffer system* consists of several related chemicals that react to the addition of either an acid or a base. One important buffer system in the body is the **carbonic acid-bicarbonate (H_2CO_3-HCO_3^-) buffer system**. The basis of this buffer system involves the reaction of carbon dioxide with water to form carbonic acid. The carbonic acid-bicarbonate buffer system is as follows:

(1) $CO_2 + H_2O \longleftrightarrow H_2CO_3 \longleftrightarrow H^+ + HCO_3^-$
        (Weak acid)   (Weak base)

(2) Added acid (H⁺) reacts with HCO_3^- to form a weak acid, which does not readily give up H⁺ ions; thus, the decrease in pH is minimized:

   $HCO_3^- + $ Added $H^+ \rightarrow H_2CO_3$ (Weak acid)

(3) Added base (OH⁻) reacts with H_2CO_3 to form a weak base, which does not readily remove H⁺ ions; thus, the increase in pH is minimized:

   $H_2CO_3 + $ Added $OH^- \rightarrow HCO_3^-$ (Weak base) $+ H_2O$

INORGANIC AND ORGANIC COMPOUNDS

Compounds are either *inorganic* or *organic*. All organic compounds contain carbon, while those that lack carbon are inorganic. Originally, scientists thought that only *organisms* could make organic compounds (hence, the name). However, scientists can now synthesize various organic compounds in the lab. Although all organic compounds contain carbon, some carbon compounds traditionally have been considered inorganic because they can form naturally without an organism being involved. Three examples of "inorganic" carbon compounds include carbon monoxide (CO), carbon dioxide (CO_2), and bicarbonate (HCO_3^-). Many major organic compounds in the body contain numerous carbon atoms arranged in either chains or rings.

When organic compounds react with one another, only a small portion of each molecule actually interacts with the other molecule. The "reactant" part of an organic compound is a **functional group**. Think of a functional group as being responsible for an organic molecule's reactivity in the same way that the outer electrons are responsible for a single atom's reactivity. Examples of functional groups found in various organic compounds of the body include the **hydroxyl** (OH), **amino** (NH_2), **carboxyl** (COOH), **carbonyl** (C=O), **sulfhydryl** (SH), **methyl** (CH_3), and **phosphate** (PO_4) groups. These major functional groups are highlighted in Figure 3-3.

The most abundant organic compounds in the body are *carbohydrates*, *lipids*, *proteins*, and *nucleic acids*. Vitamins are also organic, but their concentrations are extremely low compared to the four listed above. Some organic compounds are **macromolecules**, also called *polymers*. A **polymer** (POL-i-mer; *poly*, many; *mer*, part) is a long chain of smaller, repeating subunits called **monomers** (MON-ō-merz; *mono*, one). Each monomer may exist freely by itself, apart from the polymer. Examples of polymers include protein, consisting of amino acid monomers, and starch, consisting of glucose monomers. If a polymer is like a train, then monomers are like the boxcars.

ENZYMES

Major organic compounds in the body are built and broken down by special chemicals called *enzymes*. An

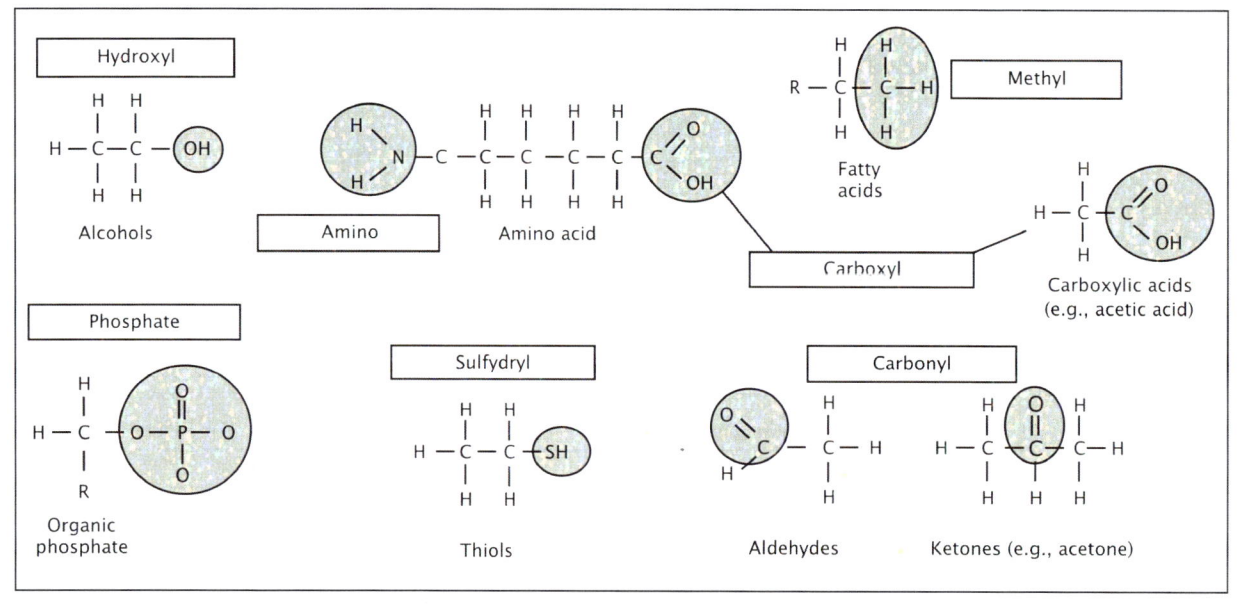

Figure 3.3. Major functional groups

enzyme (EN-zīm) is a protein that functions as a *catalyst*, or chemical that speeds up a chemical reaction without becoming part of the product. As a result, a single enzyme can do its job repeatedly without being used up. However, enzyme molecules eventually "wear out" and must be replaced. Enzyme means "yeast," and just as yeast can cause a change in bread dough, making it rise, so an enzyme can cause a change in other compounds. A *coenzyme* is not an enzyme, but is a non-protein that helps an enzyme in some way. The coenzyme may form part of the enzyme's substrate-binding site, supply a reactant to the enzyme, and/or remove by-products of a reaction. Most coenzymes are derived from vitamins. Figure 3-4 shows the basic functioning of an enzyme and coenzyme.

Enzymes speed up chemical reactions by lowering the **activation energy**, which is the energy required to initiate a reaction. Enzymes do not necessarily cause reactions that could not occur otherwise, but they cause them to occur much quicker than would be possible without the enzyme. In order to speed up a reaction enough to sustain life without an enzyme being present would require so much energy that the cell could not survive the heat.

The body contains thousands of different enzymes and each enzyme is very specific in regard to the type of chemical on which it works. A **substrate (reactant)** is the chemical worked on by an enzyme. The exact way in which an enzyme fits together with its specific substrate is not fully understood, but the substrate must first attach to the enzyme at a site called the **substrate-binding site.** Early on, scientists assumed that substrates fit into enzymes rigidly, much like a key fits into a lock. This idea was known as the *lock-and-key model* of enzyme action. However, recent research suggests that when the substrate binds to the

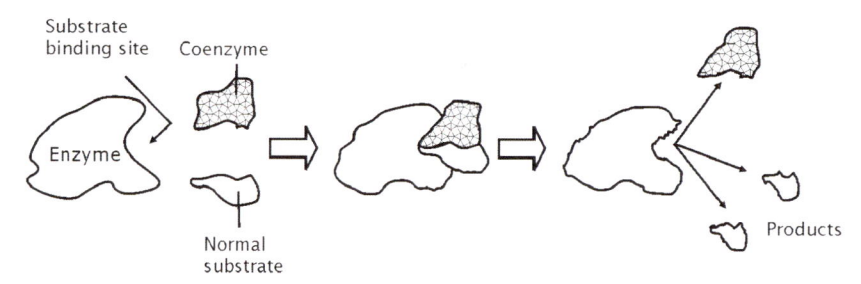

Figure 3-4. Function of an enzyme and coenzyme

CHEMISTRY OVERVIEW

enzyme, the binding site changes shape and conforms more to the shape of the substrate. This idea, called the *induced-fit model*, is probably a more accurate explanation of how enzymes and their substrates interact. The common way of visualizing this is thinking about how a sock conforms to the shape of a foot that is inserted into it. High temperature or varying the pH can alter the shape of the substrate-binding site and prevent the enzyme from functioning properly. Any change in an enzyme's shape that adversely affects its normal functioning is called **denaturation** (dē-nā-chur-Ā-shun; de, take away; *nature*, function).

Enzymes in Dehydration Synthesis and Hydrolysis

Enzymes are responsible for synthesizing and decomposing organic compounds in the body. The formation of most organic compounds occurs through a process called **dehydration synthesis**. In this process, an enzyme forms a covalent bond between two compounds after it removes a hydrogen atom (H) from one of the compounds and a hydroxyl group (OH) from the other compound. The removed H and OH then combine to form a water molecule. Since the enzyme removes components from the reactants that combine to form water while the enzyme synthesizes a new organic molecule, the process is aptly called *dehydration* synthesis (*hydra*, water). We can summarize the process as follows:

$$A\text{-}H + B\text{-}OH \rightarrow AB + H_2O$$

Most decomposition of organic compounds occurs through a process called **hydrolysis** (hī-DROL-i-sis; *hydro-*, water; *lysis*, breaking), in which an enzyme breaks the compound into two smaller products and breaks a water molecule into H and OH. The enzyme then attaches the H to one of the products and attaches the OH to the other product. At first glance, hydrolysis may seem like dissolution in that both processes utilize water to break apart a substance. However, hydrolysis involves breaking a covalent bond within an organic compound and this process requires an enzyme. In contrast, dissolution does not involve breaking a covalent bond, and thus it does not require an enzyme. We summarize hydrolysis as follows:

$$AB + H_2O \rightarrow A\text{-}H + B\text{-}OH$$

It is important to distinguish hydrolysis from dissolution, which you read about earlier. While dissolution involves the formation of hydration shells around ions or polar molecules, it does not break covalent bonds. For example, a crystal of table sugar (called *sucrose*; SŪ-krōs) can dissolve in water and this dissolution involves the liberation of many individual sucrose molecules from the crystal, but individual sucrose molecules are not hydrolyzed. However, if an enzyme called *sucrase* (SŪ-krās) is added to the solution then it will hydrolyze the sucrose, breaking it into two smaller molecules: glucose and fructose (see Figure 3-5).

Regulation of Enzyme Activity

It is important to regulate enzyme activity in the body so that products vital to good health will remain in optimum concentrations. The regulation of enzyme activity occurs through various negative feedback mechanisms. An example is **end-product inhibition**, in which products of a reaction bind to an enzyme and prevent it from working. Thus, the number of product molecules formed over time remains relatively constant (see flowchart).

Two ways to inhibit enzymes without causing permanent denaturation are through *competitive inhibition* and *allosteric inhibition*. In **competitive inhibition**, a "foreign" substrate competes with the normal substrate for the substrate-binding site. If the foreign substrate binds to the site, the normal substrate cannot attach to the enzyme. Heavy metals, such as lead, can inhibit

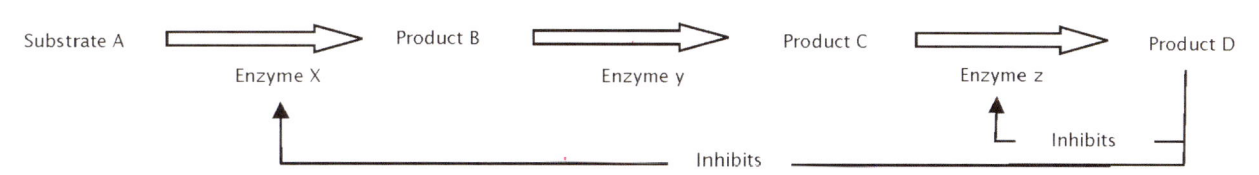

Substrate A → (Enzyme X) → Product B → (Enzyme y) → Product C → (Enzyme z) → Product D

Inhibits (Enzyme X) ←
Inhibits (Enzyme z) ← Product D

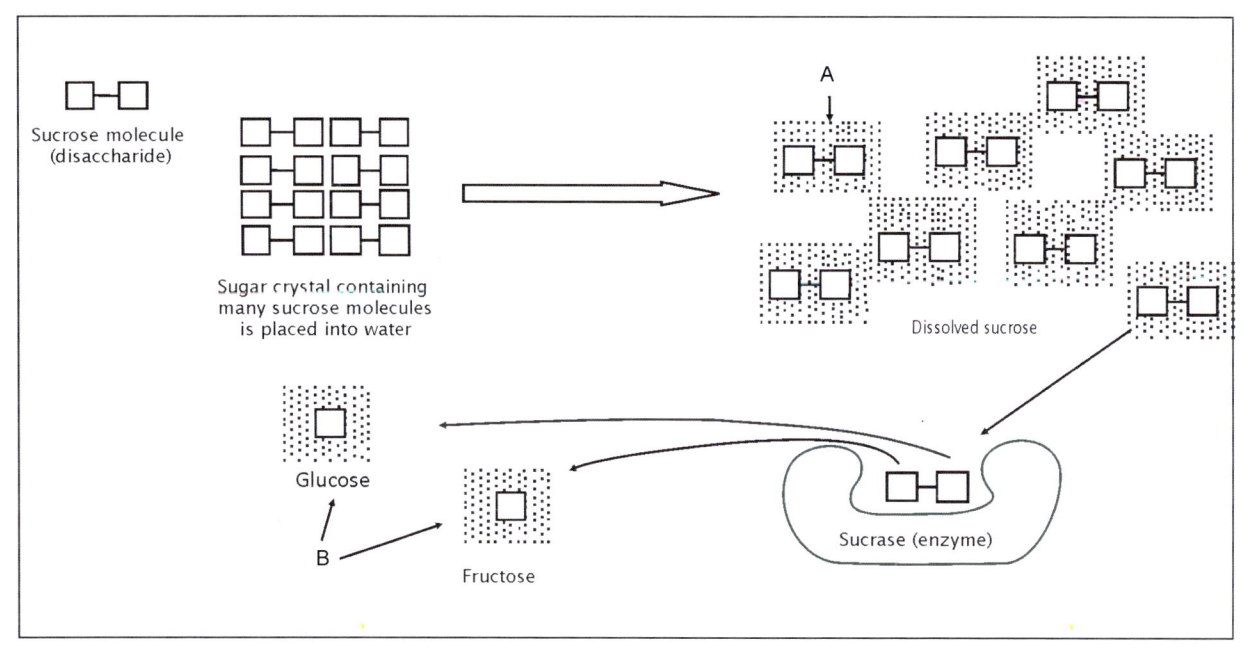

Figure 3-5. Dissolution and hydrolysis of sucrose sugar

cellular metabolism in this manner. In **allosteric** (al-ō-STER-ik; allo, other), or **noncompetitive inhibition**, a foreign substance binds to a part of the enzyme other than the substrate-binding site. This causes the enzyme, including its substrate-binding site, to change shape, and this prevents the normal substrate from attaching to the enzyme. Sulfanilamide (sul-fa-NIL-a-mīd) and other *sulfa* drugs act in this way to inhibit certain enzymes inside bacteria, which in turn inhibits bacterial growth. Figure 3.6 shows the regulation of enzymes in different ways.

CARBOHYDRATES

Carbohydrates, also called **saccharides** (SAK-ar-īdz; *sacchar*, sugar), serve as the primary source of energy for the body's cells, but they also function as cell markers and are part of nucleic acids (DNA and RNA). Carbohydrates contain carbon, hydrogen, and oxygen, and exist at different levels of complexity.

- **Monosaccharides** (mon-ō-SAK-ar-īdz; *mono*, one), also called simple sugars, are the simplest carbohydrates and include *pentoses* (with 5 carbons; *pent*, five) and *hexoses* (with 6 carbons; *hex*, six). Important pentoses include **ribose** (RĪ-bōs) in RNA and **deoxyribose** (dē-oks-sē-RĪ-bōs) in DNA. Common hexoses include **glucose** (also called **dextrose**; DEKS-trōs), **fructose** (FRŪK-tōs), and **galactose** (ga-LAK-tōs). These three hexoses have the chemical makeup ($C_6H_{12}O_6$), but their 3-dimensional shapes differ; therefore, they

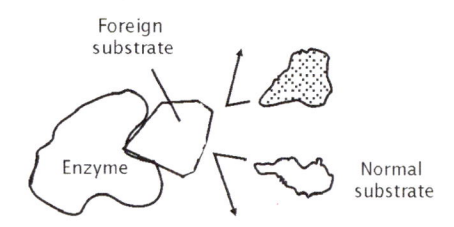

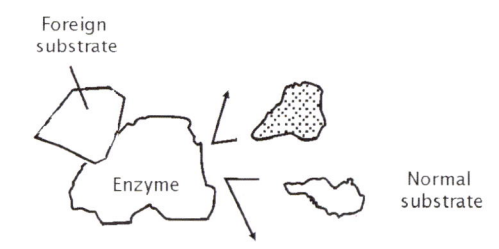

(a) Competitive inhibition

(b) Noncompetitive (allosteric) inhibition

Figure 3-6. Methods of enzyme inhibition

CHEMISTRY OVERVIEW

are considered *isomers* (Ī-sō-merz; *iso*, same; *-mer*, part). Glucose is the most common carbohydrate circulating in your blood.

- **Oligosaccharides** (ol-i-gō-SAK-ar-īdz; *oligo*, few) contain up to 20 simple sugars bonded together by an enzyme during dehydration synthesis reactions. The most common oligosaccharides are **disaccharides** (*di*, two), which contain two simple sugars. Examples of disaccharides include **sucrose** (SŪ-krōs), or table sugar consisting of glucose and fructose, **maltose** (MAL-tōs), or malt sugar consisting of two glucoses, and **lactose** (LAK-tōs), or milk sugar consisting of glucose and galactose. **Dextrin**, or starch gum, is an oligosaccharide consisting of 3-20 glucose molecules and is derived from polysaccharides such as starch.

- **Polysaccharides** (pol-ē-SAK-ar-īdz) are polymers consisting of simple sugars (usually glucose). The presence or absence of specific polysaccharides on the plasma membrane of red blood cells determines your blood type. Examples of polysaccharides include *glycogen*, *starch*, and *cellulose*.
    - **Glycogen** (GLĪ-kō-jen; *glycol*, sugar; *gen*, generating) is a highly branched compound made of glucose molecules. The liver and muscle cells store glycogen as a source of glucose molecules, which can be broken down for energy.
    - **Starch** is similar to glycogen except it is not highly branched. Plant cells store glucose molecules as starch. *Complex carbohydrates* in the diet consist of starches found in potatoes, beans, etc.
    - **Cellulose** is the most abundant organic molecule in the world and forms the walls of plant cells. Like starch, cellulose consists entirely of glucose molecules. Humans cannot utilize cellulose as an energy source because they lack the enzyme *cellulase* needed to hydrolyze cellulose. Any cellulose you eat passes through your body undigested, but it is important in the diet as "fiber," which can help push other materials through the digestive system. On the other hand, cows and horses have cellulase-producing bacteria in their intestines, meaning these animals can eat grass and release glucose from the plants' cellulose walls. The released glucose molecules can then serve as a source of energy.

Cells use most of the energy extracted from carbohydrates to synthesize molecules called *ATP*, which in turn is used to perform work in the cells. The amount of energy released during the complete oxidation of glucose is approximately four kilocalories (Kcal) per gram (g) of glucose, written 4 Kcal/g. A kilocalorie is the amount of heat needed to raise the temperature of one kg (or 1 liter) of pure water 1° C. A cell can use about half of the energy released from glucose to synthesize ATP; the other half escapes as heat.

LIPIDS

Like carbohydrates, lipids contain C, H, and O, and they are an important source of energy in the body. However, unlike many carbohydrates, lipids are insoluble in water. Since lipids have many more C-H bonds than simple sugars, they contain much more stored energy. Animals usually have more stored energy in the form of lipids than in carbohydrates. Chemists classify lipids according to their chemical composition and structure, and include *fatty acids, glycerides, phospholipids, glycolipids, eicosanoids*, and *steroids*.

Fatty acids consist of carbon chains with hydrogen atoms attached along the sides and at one end and a carboxyl group (COOH) attached at the other end. A *saturated* fatty acid has no double bonds between any of the carbon atoms in the carbon chain and, therefore, has the maximum number of hydrogen atoms attached along the sides of the chain. In other words, we say the carbon chain is "saturated" with hydrogen atoms. An *unsaturated* fatty acid has one or more double bonds within the carbon chain. If there is only one double bond in the chain, the fatty acid is *monounsaturated*; if there are two or more, the fatty acid is *polyunsaturated*.

It is possible to convert an unsaturated fatty acid into a saturated fatty acid by breaking double bonds in the carbon chain and adding H atoms at these sites. This process, called *hydrogenation* (hī-DRAH-jen-Ā-shun),

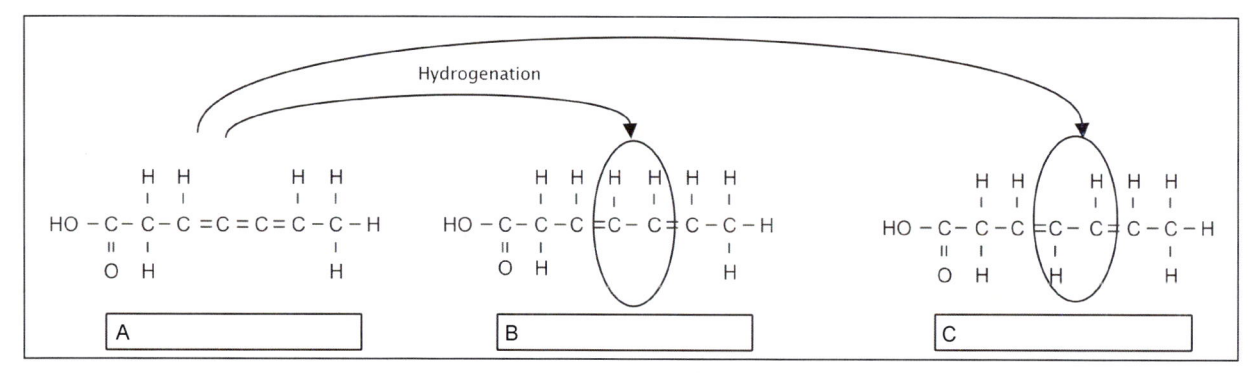

Figure 3-7. Hydrogenation process

can result in the formation of either cis fatty acids, if the added H bind to the same side of the carbon chain, or trans fats, if the added H bind to opposite sides of the carbon chain (*trans* means "across") (see Figure 3-7). *Trans* fatty acids, like saturated fatty acids, do not bend readily and tend to be solid at room temperature. They are not found naturally, but may be present in margarines and other foods that have been *partially hydrogenated*. *Trans* fats have been implicated in the clogging of blood vessels in the heart, the most common form of heart disease.

Glycerides (GLIS-er-īdz) consist of a glycerol (GLIH-ser-ol) molecule attached to one or more fatty acids. A *monoglyceride* (MON-ō-glih-ser-īd) contains one fatty acid; a *diglyceride* (DĪ-glih-ser-īd) contains two fatty acids; and a *triglyceride* (TRĪ-glih-ser-īd) contains three fatty acids. **Oils** are triglycerides containing unsaturated fatty acids. The double bonds in unsaturated fatty acids create "kinks" that prevent the fatty acid from lying flat or forming a straight line; this causes the triglyceride to remain liquid at room temperature. **Fats** are triglycerides containing saturated fatty acids. The solid nature of fats at room temperature results when adjacent, non-kinked, saturated fatty acids pack together tightly. Fats are important as a source of stored energy and for insulation and protection of underlying tissues.

Phospholipids (FOS-fō-lih-pidz) contain a glycerol molecule covalently bonded to a phosphate molecule and two fatty acids. The phosphate group is polar, and therefore water-soluble or *hydrophilic* (hi-drō-FIL-ik; "water-loving"). The fatty acids are nonpolar, and therefore non-water soluble or *hydrophobic* (hī-drō-FŌ-bik; "water-fearing"). Any molecule that has both hydrophobic and hydrophilic regions is **amphipathic** (am-fē-PATH-ik; *amphi*, both; *pathic*, feeling). When phospholipids containing relatively short fatty acids mix with water, they spontaneously form a **micelle** (MĪ-sel; "small morsel"), a tiny sphere with the fatty acid "tails" pointing inward away from the surrounding water. Micelles transport lipid-soluble nutrients in the intestines. When phospholipids containing relatively long fatty acids mix with water, they form a **bilayer** (BĪ-lā-er; *bi*, two), two layers of phospholipids with the fatty acid tails pointing inward. Phospholipid bilayers comprise all membranes that are part of a cell.

Glycolipids (glī-kō-LIP-idz) are diglycerides attached to carbohydrates and function in the cell membrane that separates a cell from its surrounding environment.

Eicosanoids (ī-KŌS-i-noyds; *eicos*, twenty; *oid*, form) are lipids derived from *arachidonic acid* (a-RAK-i-don-ik), a 20-carbon fatty acid. Two major groups of eicosanoids include *leukotrienes* (lū-kō-TRĪ-ēnz) and *prostaglandins* (pros-ta-GLAN-denz). White blood cells (*leuko* means "white") release leukotrienes in response to tissue damage and disease. Virtually all cells produce prostaglandins, especially when the cells are damaged, and these compounds can influence various cellular activities.

Steroids (STĒR-oydz) consist of carbon rings but do not have fatty acids. Steroids are hydrophobic

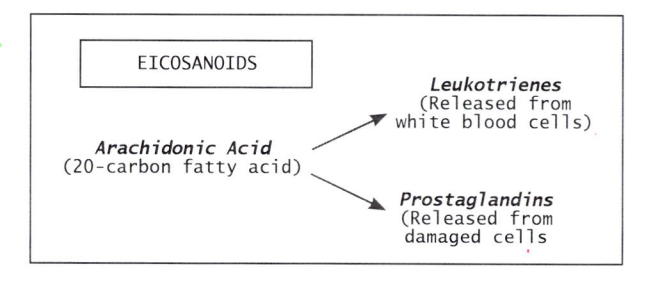

CHEMISTRY OVERVIEW

and include *cholesterol, vitamin D, hydrocortisone,* and sex hormones (*testosterone, progesterone,* and *estrogen*).

PROTEIN

Proteins are the most important structural component in the body, and compared to other organic compounds they have the widest range of functions in the body. A **protein** (PRŌ-tēn) is a polymer of *amino acids*. All amino acids contain C, H, O, and N, but a few also contain sulfur. In addition, all amino acids contain an amino group (NH$_2$) and a carboxyl (COOH) group. During protein synthesis, an enzyme removes a hydrogen atom from one amino acid's amino group and removes a hydroxyl group from an adjacent amino acid. The H and OH combine to form water and a covalent bond forms between the two amino acids. The covalent bond that holds two amino acids together is called a **peptide** (PEP-tīd) **bond**.

There are 20 different structural designs for amino acids in the body. The body can make twelve of these types but cannot make the other eight, which are called *essential* amino acids, so-named because it is essential that a person obtain them in their final form through the diet. A complete protein contains all essential amino acids and likely contains all or most of the other ones as well. Varying numbers of amino acids can bond together to make different sized molecules. Two amino acids bonded together form a **dipeptide** (DĪ-pep-tīd); three amino acids form a **tripeptide** (TRĪ-pep-tīd); 4-20 amino acids form an **oligopeptide** (OL-i-gō-pep-tīd; oligo, few); and >20 amino acids form a **polypeptide**. Some books reserve the name protein for polypeptides containing more than 50 amino acids.

Levels of Complexity in Proteins

The structure of a protein can exist at four different levels of complexity (see Figure 3-8):

(1) **The primary level** (*prima*, first) refers to the protein's amino acid sequence; i.e., the specific order of different amino acids within the protein. The primary structure ultimately determines a protein's shape and function.

(2) The **secondary level** results from coiling or creasing the amino acid chain to form a 3-dimensional shape.

(3) A **tertiary level** (TER-shē-ār-rē; "third") results when a secondary-level protein bends back on itself to form a more globe-like shape.

(4) A **quaternary level** (kwah-TER-na-rē; quarter, four) exists when two or more tertiary proteins unite.

Denaturing a protein alters its 3-dimensional shape, which then alters the protein's function. In some cases, denaturation is permanent (irreversible). You can witness permanent denaturation of a protein when you fry an egg. *Albumin* (al-BŪ-men) is the protein found in the clear part of an egg that turns white when heated (*albu* means "white"). Exposure to different pH levels or various chemicals can also denature proteins. See the levels of protein complexity in Figure 3-8.

Classification by Shape

Physiologists classify proteins by shape and by function. Based on shape, proteins are either *globular* or *filamentous*.

- **Globular** (GLOB-ū-lar; *glob*, sphere) **proteins** resemble a sphere and may exist at the tertiary or quaternary level of complexity. Examples of globular proteins are *enzymes, antibodies* (which protect you from many disease-causing agents), and *hemoglobin* (HĒ-mō-glō-bin), which is responsible for the red color of red blood cells.

- **Filamentous proteins** (fil-a-MEN-tus; *filament*, thread), also called **fibrous proteins**, are thread-like fibers consisting of secondary-level proteins intertwined like a rope. Examples of filamentous proteins are *keratin* (KAIR-a-tin; found in skin, hair, and nails), *collagen* (KOL-a-jen; helps hold organs together and is the most abundant protein in the body), and elastin (ē-LAS-tin; makes tissues elastic or stretchy).

Classification by Function

Any protein in the body can be classified into one of six groups of proteins based by function, and these groups include *transport, regulatory, immunological, contractile, catalytic,* and *structural* proteins. The acronym, TRICCS, can help you remember this classification.

42

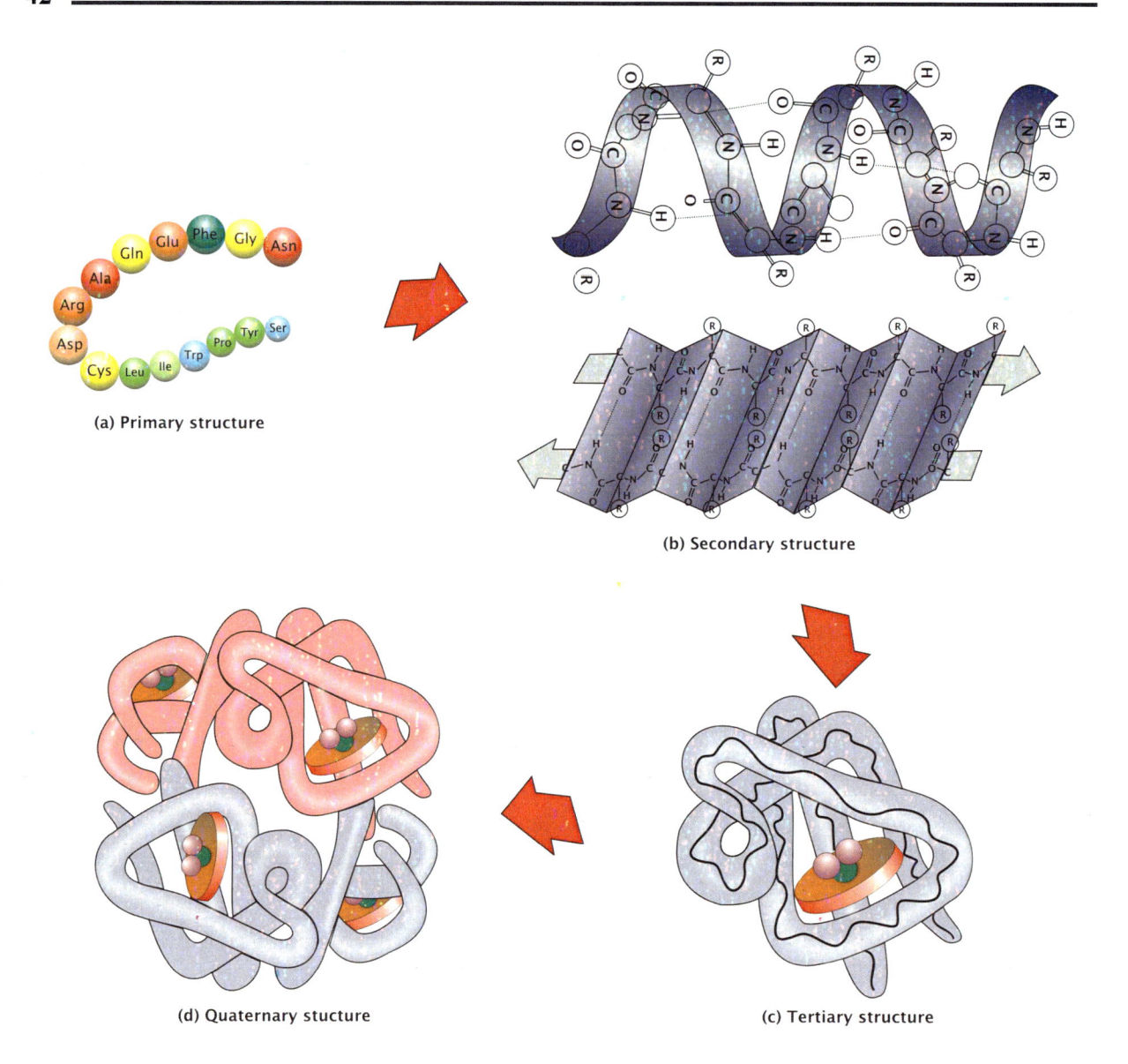

(a) Primary structure

(b) Secondary structure

(c) Tertiary structure

(d) Quaternary stucture

Figure 3-8. Levels of complexity in a protein.

- **Transport proteins** carry substances from one place to another. *Hemoglobin* is an example and transports gases throughout the body. In addition, certain proteins inside the membranes of cells can transport substances from one side of the membrane to the other.

- **Regulatory proteins** control the activity of a cell. For example, *insulin* (IN-su-lin) is a protein hormone that regulates the rate at which cells remove glucose from the blood.

- **Immunological proteins** (im-ū-nō-LOJ-i-kal) protect the body from potentially harmful, foreign particles. *Antibodies* (AN-ti-bod-ēz; anti, against) are immunological proteins that bind to bacteria and viruses to help prevent them from harming the body.

- **Contractile proteins** can shorten the length of a cell or cause the cell's shape to change in other ways. *Actin* (AK-tin) and *myosin* (MĪ-ō-sin) are contractile proteins that interact to shorten muscle cells when you contract your muscles.

CHEMISTRY OVERVIEW

Table 3-1. Major Groups of Enzymes and their general functions.

General Name for Certain Enzyme	Function
Catalase (KAT-a-lās)	Breaks hydrogen peroxide (H_2O_2) into water and oxygen molecules
Dehydrogenase (dē-hī-DROJ-en-ās)	Removes H from a molecule
Hydrolase (HĪ-dro-lās)	Hydrolyzes (breaks up) a larger compound to form smaller compounds
Kinase (KĪ-nās)	Adds a phosphate group to a compound; i.e., it phosphorylates other compounds
Ligase (LĪ-gās)	Joins two molecules using energy supplied from an ATP molecule
Phosphatase (FOS-fa-tās)	Removes a phosphate from a compound; i.e., it dephosphorylates a compound
Phosphorylase (fos-FOR-i-lās)	Adds a phosphate group to a compound
Polymerase (po-LIM-er-ās)	Combines monomers to form a polymer
Synthetase (SEN-the-tās)	Synthesizes a compound
Transferase (TRANS-fer-ās)	Transfers items from one compound to another compound

- **Catalytic proteins** (kat-a-LIT-ik) are enzymes, which increase the rate of chemical reactions. The names of most enzymes end with the suffix "ase". For example, *sucrase* (SŪ-krās) hydrolyzes sucrose to form glucose and fructose molecules; *maltase* splits maltose into two glucose molecules, and *lactase* splits lactose into glucose and galactose. Thus, the name of an enzyme may suggest the enzyme's action. Enzymes with names not ending in "ase" are usually secreted in an inactive form and then activated later. For example, pepsin is an enzyme that hydrolyzes proteins in the stomach, but it is secreted as an inactive compound called *pepsinogen*. The pepsinogen becomes active only after exposure to acid in the stomach. Table 3-1 summarizes the major groups of enzymes.

- **Structural** proteins strengthen and support a structure. Examples include *collagen* and *elastin* fibers in the skin and tendons, and *keratin* in the skin, hair, and nails.

NUCLEIC ACIDS

The last major group of organic compounds we will describe is **nucleic acids** (nū-KLĀ-ik), so-named because they are abundant in a cell's nucleus. Nucleic acids are polymers consisting of monomers called *nucleotides*. A **nucleotide** (NŪ-klē-ō-tīd) contains a simple, pentose sugar (either *ribose* or *deoxyribose*), a nitrogenous (nitrogen-containing) base, and a phosphate group. The nitrogenous base within a nucleotide is either a *purine* or a *pyrimidine*. **Purines** (PŪR-ēnz) have two carbon rings, and include **adenine** (AD-e-nēn) and **guanine** (GWA-nēn), abbreviated **A** and **G**, respectively. **Pyrimidines** (pī-RIM-i-dēnz) have only one carbon ring and include **cytosine** (SĪ-tō-sēn), **thymine** (THĪ-mēn), and **uracil** (YUR-ō-sil), or **C, T,** and **U,** respectively.

Nucleotides can connect to one another by covalent bonds and by hydrogen bonds. Covalent bonds form between the phosphate group of one nucleotide and the sugar of another nucleotide, whereas hydrogen bonds can form between a purine and pyrimidine. The nitrogenous bases always pair up in the following way: A with T, A with U, and G with C. These specific pairings are called **complementary base pairing**.

Due to *covalent* bonding, nucleotides can form a *single-stranded* polymer called a nucleic acid. A polymerase enzyme is responsible for bonding nucleotides together to form the nucleic acid. Note that the polymerase enzyme is a protein; therefore, it is also a polymer. One end of the nucleic acid or chain of nucleotides has a sugar molecule exposed and is called the 3' (three-prime) end. The other end of the chain has a phosphate group exposed and is called the 5' (five-prime) end. Remembering this will help you understand how polymerases construct nucleic acids.

Due to *hydrogen* bonding between complementary base pairs, a single-stranded nucleic acid can either (1) fold back on itself to take on a more 3-dimensional shape, or (2) bond to another single-stranded nucleic acid to form a *double-stranded* nucleic acid (see Figure).

DNA, or deoxyribonucleic acid (dē-OK-sē-RĪ-bō-nū-KLĀ-ik), consists of nucleotides containing a deoxyribose sugar, a phosphate group, and either A, T, C, or G; there are no uracils in DNA nucleotides. The DNA of living cells is always a double-stranded polymer with two parallel polymers of nucleotides held together by hydrogen bonds between complementary base pairs. This double-stranded DNA molecule coils into a form known as a *double helix* (helix means "coil"). Within viruses, which are not classified as organisms, the DNA may exist as either a single-stranded polymer (abbreviated ssDNA) or a double-stranded helix (abbreviated dsDNA).

RNA, or ribonucleic acid (RĪ-bō-nū-KLĀ-ik) consists of nucleotides containing a ribose sugar, a phosphate group, and either A, U, C, or G (there are no thymines in RNA nucleotides). In living cells, RNA is always a single-stranded polymer instead of a double helix. Viruses may contain RNA that is either single-stranded (ssRNA) or double stranded (dsRNA). The well-known human immunodeficiency virus (HIV), which causes acquired immune deficiency syndrome (AIDS), contains dsRNA.

ATP and GTP

Two important standalone nucleotides are **adenosine triphosphate** (**ATP**; a-DEN-ō-sēn trī-FOS-fāt) and **guanosine triphosphate** (**GTP**; GWAN-ō-sēn). ATP contains adenine, ribose, and three phosphates, whereas, GTP contains guanine, ribose, and three phosphates. ATP is the major "fuel" molecule that cells hydrolyze to release energy for work. Additionally, certain enzymes may use ATP or GTP as a source of phosphate in order to phosphorylate (add a phosphate ion to) other compounds. After being phosphorylated, a compound may change shape and become either activated or inactivated. Removing one phosphate from ATP or GTP produces **ADP** (adenosine diphosphate) and **GDP**, respectively. Removing two phosphates from ATP or GTP produces **AMP** (adenosine monophosphate) and **GMP**, respectively. Uses of ATP energy include the transfer of materials across cell membranes, dehydration synthesis, hydrolysis, and muscle movement. In Figure 3-9, the third phosphate group on ATP or GTP is transferred to molecule X. In this process, the ATP or GTP is dephosphorylated and molecule X is phosphorylated. Phosphorylating molecule X causes the molecule to change shape.

CHEMISTRY OVERVIEW

ATP and GTP

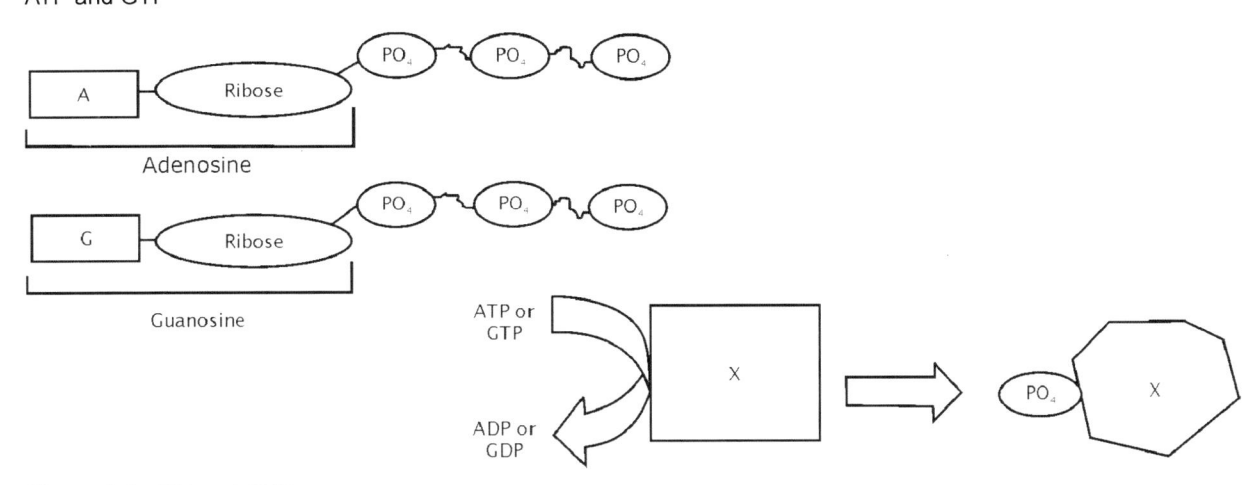

Figure 3-9. ATP and GTP

TOPICS TO KNOW FOR CHAPTER 3 (CHEMISTRY OVERVIEW)

3' end
5' end
acid
acid solutions
acidosis
actin
activation energy
adenine
adhesion
ADP
albumin
alkaline compounds
alkalosis
allosteric inhibition
amino acid
amino group
AMP
amphipathic
anabolism
anion
antibodies
antioxidant
-ase
atom
atomic mass
atomic number
atomic weight
ATP
base
basic solutions
bilayer
buffers
carbohydrates
carbonic acid reactions

carbonic acid-bicarbonate buffer
carbonyl group
carboxyl group
catabolism
catalase
catalyst
catalytic proteins
cation
cellular respiration
cellulase
cellulose
chemical bond
chemical energy
chemical reaction
chemistry
CHNOPCa
CHNOPS
cholesterol
cis fatty acid
classification of proteins by function
classification of proteins by shape
coenzyme
cohesion
collagen
colloids
competitive inhibition
complete protein
complex carbohydrate
complementary base pairing
compound
concentration
contractile proteins
covalent bond
cytosine

decomposition reaction
dehydration synthesis
dehydrogenase
denaturation
deoxyribose
deuterium
dextrin
dextrose
diglyceride
dipeptide
disaccharides
dissociation
dissolution
DNA
double helix
dsDNA
dsRNA
eicosanoids
elastin
electrical energy
electrochemical energy
electrolytes
electromagnetic energy
electron shells
electrons
elements
endergonic
end-product inhibition
energy
energy shells
enzyme
essential amino acid
estrogen
exergonic

factors affecting reactions
fats
fatty acids
fibrous proteins
filamentous proteins
free radical
fructose
functional group
functions of water
galactose
globular proteins
glucose
glycerides
glycogen
glycolipids
GTP
guanine
heat
hemoglobin
heterogeneous mixture
hexoses
homogeneous mixture
hydration shells
hydrocortisone
hydrogen bond
hydrogenation
hydrolase
hydrolysis
hydrophilic region
hydrophobic region
hydroxyl group
immunological proteins
induced-fit model
inorganic compound
insulin
intermolecular H-bond
intramolecular H-bond
ion
ionic bond
isomers
isotope
keratin
kilocalorie
kinase
kinetic energy
lactase
lactase
lactose
leukotriene
levels of complexity in proteins
ligase
lipid soluble
lipids
lock-and-key model
macromolecule
maltase
maltose
matter

mechanical energy
metabolism
methyl group
micelle
millimole
mixtures
mole
molecule
monoglyceride
monomer
monosaccharides
monounsaturated fatty acid
myosin
neutrons
noncompetitive inhibition
nonpolar molecules
nucleic acids
nucleotides
octet rule
oils
oligopeptide
oligosaccharides
orbital
organic compound
-ose
oxidation
oxidation-reduction reaction
pentoses
pepsin
pepsinogen
peptide bond
pH
ph scale
phosphatase
phosphate group
phospholipids
phosphorylase
polar compound
polymer
polymerase
polypeptide
polysaccharides
polyunsaturated fatty acid
potential energy
primary level
product
progesterone
prostaglandin
protein
protons
purines
pyrimidines
quaternary level
radiant energy
radioactive decay
radioactivity
reactant
redox reaction

reduction
regulation of enzymes
regulatory proteins
reversible reaction
ribose
RNA
saccharides
salt
saturated fatty acid
secondary level
simple sugars
single-stranded polymer
sodium bicarbonate
sodium chloride
solute
solutions
solvent
ssDNA
ssRNA
starch
starch gum
steroid
strong acid
strong base
structural proteins
subatomic particles
substrate
substrate-binding site
sucrase
sucrose
sulfhydryl group
superoxide ion
suspension
synthesis reaction
synthetase
temperature
template
tertiary level
testosterone
thymine
trans fatty acid
transcription
transferase
transport proteins
TRICCS
triglyceride
tripeptide
tritium
unsaturated fatty
uracil
vitamin D
water
water-soluble
weak acid
weak base
work

CHAPTER 4

Overview of the Cell

OVERVIEW OF A TYPICAL CELL

The body of an average sized adult consists of between 50 and 100 trillion cells, including over 200 different cell types. With regard to their general characteristics, human cells fall into two groups: *somatic cells* and *sex cells*. **Somatic cells** (sō-MA-tik; *soma*, body), also called *body cells*, include all cells in the body except gametes. **Gametes** (GAM-ēts; "spouse"), or **sex cells**, function only in sexual reproduction and include *sperm* in the male and *ova* (Ō-vuh; "eggs") in the female. Considering the variety of cells in the body, it is difficult to portray a "typical" body cell exactly. However, all body cells share certain structural features. This section describes these features, along with a few other characteristics that are present only in certain types of cells (see Figure 4-1).

A typical somatic cell consists of three major parts: the *plasma membrane*, the *cytoplasm*, and the *nucleus*. The **plasma membrane** (also called the **cell membrane**) forms the cell's outer surface and holds the cell's inner contents intact. The **cytoplasm** (SĪ-tō-plazm; *cyto*, cell; *plasm*, something formed) includes all parts of the cell between the plasma membrane and the nucleus. The nucleus is an example of an *organelle*, a specialized structure or compartment that performs a particular function inside the cell.

THE CYTOSOL AND INCLUSIONS

Almost two-thirds of the human body consists of fluids, and about 70 percent of this fluid volume is *intracellular* (inside cells). The **cytosol** (SĪ-to-sol) is the intracellular fluid between the plasma membrane and the nucleus. In most body cells, the cytosol consists mostly of water and accounts for more than half of the cell's volume. Since water has a high specific heat (that is, it takes a relatively high amount of heat energy to change its temperature), the watery cytosol helps protect the cell against sudden temperature changes. More importantly, because it is a "universal solvent," water is a favorable medium for holding the reactants and products of the millions of chemical reactions that occur every second in the cell.

Proteins are abundant in the cytosol and cause it to behave like a colloid. For this reason, the consistency of the cytosol is more like liquid gelatin or raw egg white. The cytosol's relatively high viscosity (thickness), along with a network of filamentous (thread-like) proteins supports the organelles. Without this support, organelles would tend to "sink" to the bottom of the cell or bounce around when the body moves. With the help of its plasma membrane, a cell maintains concentrations of proteins and other chemicals in its

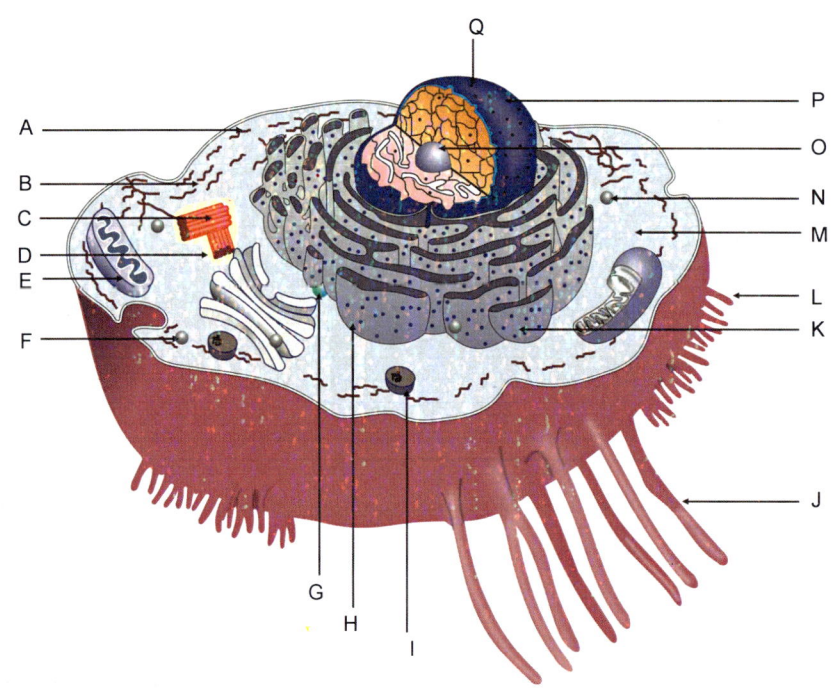

Figure 4-1. A generalized cell

cytosol that differ substantially from the extracellular fluid. The relative concentrations of major ions and groups of organic compounds in the cytosol and extracellular fluids are shown in Table 4-1.

In addition to cushioning the organelles, the cytosol is a storage depot. Cellular products may collect in the cytosol into variable-sized clumps called inclusions (in-KLŪ-shunz). The **inclusions** in most body cells consist of metabolic products or substances that the cells can quickly convert to energy. The four most common inclusions are:

- **Fat droplets**: consist mainly of triglycerides and may occupy up to 95% of the cytosol in the fat-storing cells called *adipocytes* (AD-i-pō-sīts; *adipo*, fat). These cells are abundant just beneath the skin where they cushion and help insulate the body. Between meals, the adipocytes release their energy-rich triglyceride molecules into the blood so other cells can use them as a source of energy.

- **Glycogen**: a polymer (long chain) of glucose molecules and is the body's principal carbohydrate reserve. Liver and muscle cells in particular store large amounts of glycogen as inclusions called *glycogen granules*. During strenuous physical activity, liver cells release the glucose molecules into the blood for other cells to use as an energy source.

Table 4-1. Relative concentrations of major substances in the cytosol and extracellular fluid

Substance	Intracellular Fluid	Extracellular Fluid
Bicarbonate ions (HCO_3^-)		Higher
Calcium ions (Ca^{2+})		Higher
Chloride ions (Cl^-)		Higher
Glucose		Higher
Oxygen gas (O_2)		Higher
Sodium ions (Na^+)		Higher
Amino Acids	Higher	
Carbon dioxide (CO_2)	Higher	
Lipids	Higher	
Magnesium ions (Mg^{2+})	Higher	
Phosphate ions (PO_4^{3-})	Higher	
Potassium ions (K^+)	Higher	
Proteins	Higher	
Sulfate ions (SO_4^{2-})	Higher	

- **Melanin** (MEL-a-nin; *melan*, black): the dark pigment (coloring agent) that is responsible for most variations in skin and hair color. Its synthesis oc-

OVERVIEW OF THE CELL

curs inside cells called *melanocytes* (MEL-a-nō-sīts or mel-AN-ō-sīts) which are abundant in the skin, hair roots, and the light-sensitive parts of the eyeball. Melanin absorbs ultraviolet light, protecting deeper tissues from these potentially harmful rays.

- **Hemoglobin** (HĒ-mō-glō-bin; *hemo*, blood): the oxygen-carrying compound that is responsible for the color of red blood cells (RBCs). In fact, mature RBCs have no organelles, leaving hemoglobin as the main organic ingredient in their cytosol. Hemoglobin binds to oxygen molecules (O_2) as RBCs flow through the lungs and releases O_2 as RBCs flow through other tissues.

THE CYTOSKELETON

In addition to inclusions, the cytosol contains a vast network of interlocking filamentous proteins that forms the cell's **cytoskeleton**. Similar to the way in which an internal, bony skeleton supports your body, an internal cytoskeleton supports each of your cells. Additionally, the cytoskeleton can change the location or position of organelles in the cytosol, enable certain kinds of cells to move about within the body, and help a cell to divide. In fact, some cell biologists assert that the cytoskeleton's indispensable role in directing motion is what allows a cell to "do" rather than merely to "be." The cytoskeleton consists of three types of protein filaments: *microfilaments, microtubules, and intermediate filaments* (see Figure 4-2).

Microfilaments

Extending everywhere in the cytosol, **microfilaments** are the **smallest**, but **most numerous**, components of the cytoskeleton. Microfilaments consist of **actin** molecules (AK-tin; beam), the most common free protein in the cytosol. Numerous globular (G) actin molecules join to form a thin, flexible, helical (coiled) strand that resembles a pearl necklace. What is more, the G-actin molecules line up so regularly that they give the microfilament "endedness," in which G actin molecules on opposite ends of the filament display different parts of their chemical structure. For this reason, cell biologists refer to one end of the filament as the "plus" end and the other end as the "minus" end. Keep this fact in mind, because endedness is one of the keys to understanding how a cell moves things around in its interior. Some microfilaments form stable and long-lasting structures in the cytosol, but more often a cell repeatedly builds and then dismantles microfilaments as it goes about its business. The most important roles of microfilaments include:

1. **Shaping and Supporting the Plasma Membrane:** Most microfilaments pack densely near the plasma membrane in a region called the **cell cortex** (KOR-teks, "bark"). Here, the microfilaments crisscross on top of one another and bond to projections of proteins in the plasma membrane to form a web-like pattern. This web of microfilaments gives each type of body cell its characteristic shape, and it helps prevent the plasma membrane from splitting open if stretched.

2. **Facilitating Cell Crawling**: Some body cells use a process called **cell crawling** to move. The cell thrusts out its plasma membrane in the direction of travel and, at the same time, "reels in" the membrane behind it. To accomplish this feat, the cell adds actin monomers to microfilaments

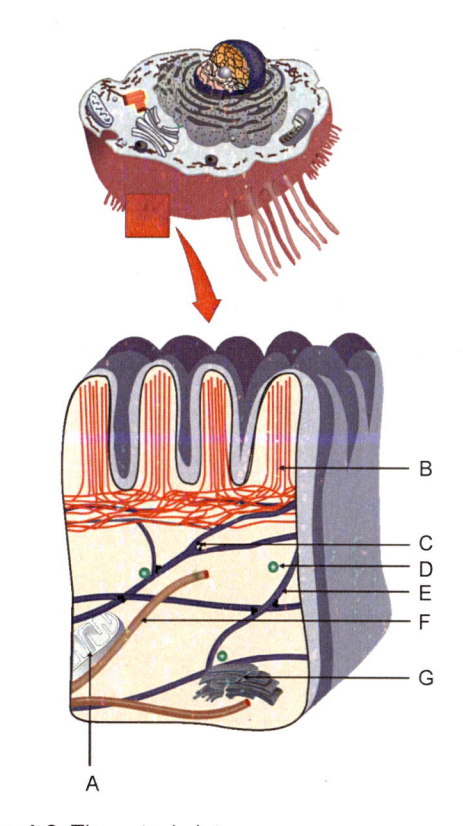

Figure 4-2. The cytoskeleton

aimed at the plasma membrane. The growing microfilaments act like battering rams that push the plasma membrane forward in little streamers called **pseudopodia** (sū-dō-PŌ-dē-a; *pseudo*, false; *podia*, feet). At the cell's "tail end," **motor molecules** made of the protein **myosin** (MĪ-ō-sin) form bridges between the plasma membrane and nearby microfilaments. Using energy from ATP, the motor molecules change shape repeatedly, "walking" towards the plus end of the microfilament. As a result, the motor molecules tug the microfilaments toward the interior of the cell, dragging the plasma membrane along. Some white blood cells employ cell crawling to search for invading microorganisms or dead cells to ingest. Then again, truly spectacular examples of cell crawling occur during fetal life, when cells migrate in vast swarms as they form the tissues and organs.

> **Note**: Some biologists have estimated that neurocytes, the earliest forms of brain cells, crawl a collective one million miles before reaching their final destinations in the brain.

3. **Moving cell vesicles**: A cell's actin microfilaments also serve as an intracellular railroad. Large substances drawn into a cell, and many of a cell's products, don't float about randomly in the cytosol. Instead, a cell packages them in membrane-enclosed sacs, called *vesicles*. One end of a myosin motor molecule attaches to a vesicle while the other end attaches to a microfilament. By regularly changing its shape, the motor molecule "walks" the cargo-containing vesicle through the cytosol to its destination inside or outside the cell, but this movement is always toward the "plus" end of the microfilament (Figure 4-3).

4. **Completing cell division**: When a cell divides, microfilaments in the cell cortex gather in parallel bands around the cell's "midsection" and cleave the cell in two. During this process, myosin motor molecules attach between adjacent microfilaments in the band and "walk" both filaments past each other. Like slowly tightening a belt around the waist, the microfilaments pull the plasma membrane in towards the interior of the cell. This process continues until the cell pinches in two, forming independent cells.

Microtubules

Now, let's consider the structure and functions of the largest threads in the cytoskeleton. A cell's **microtubules** are large-diameter filaments that extend from an "organizing center" out toward the plasma membrane. Each microtubule consists of a hollow coil of **tubulin** (TŪ-byoo-lin) molecules. Each tubulin molecule is a globular protein that resembles a pearl in a necklace. The regular arrangement of its molecules gives microtubules "endedness," just like microfilaments. The cell changes the length of its microtubules by adding or removing tubulin molecules from the "plus" end. Microtubules play three distinct roles in a body cell:

1. **Positioning cytoplasmic organelles**: Your first glimpse at a generalized cell might give you the impression that the cytoplasm is like a "tossed salad" in which organelles are scattered haphazardly. Nothing could be further from the truth! The cell uses microtubules to position its organelles precisely where they are needed most and where they function best. Just as important, the shape and integrity of some of the cell's most important organelles solely depend on microtubules. If these large cytoskeletal filaments were to disappear, some organelles would collapse like puppets with cut strings. Still others would come apart and drift uselessly within the cytosol. The microtubule-based movement of organelles occurs when tubulin joins forces with two motor molecules of its own: **kinesins** (ki-NĒ-sinz) and **dyneins** (DĪ-nēnz). The motor molecules work by sensing the "endedness" of the microtubule strand: kinesins "walk" their load toward the

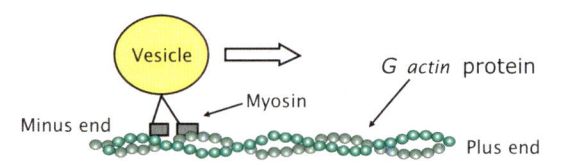

Figure 4-3. Microfilament

plus end, while dyneins "walk" theirs toward the *minus* end (Figure 4-4). A cell needs many motor molecules of both varieties to position its largest organelles. The net effect is like moving a large curtain along a curtain rod: the cell can bunch up the "curtain" (organelle), spread it out, or move it away from or toward the cell's interior.

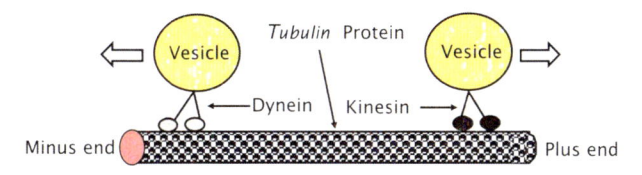

Figure 4-4. Microtubule

2. **Moving motile cell extensions:** Some body cells have relatively long finger-like or tail-like extensions. Columns of microtubules linked by dynein motor molecules cause these extensions to beat back and forth like tiny whips. Rhythmic beating starts as dynein molecules form crossbridges between microtubules on one side of an extension. The dynein molecules "walk" the adjacent microtubules past one another causing the extension to bend. After a moment, dynein molecules on the opposite side of the extension perform the same walking routine, causing the extension to bend in the reverse direction.

3. **Facilitating cell reproduction:** Before a dividing cell pinches in two, it replicates (makes copies of) its chromosomes. A chromosome is a dense package of DNA and proteins that holds a portion of a cell's genetic code. After the replication process is complete, each chromosome consists of two "sister" strands of DNA called *chromatids* (KRŌ-ma-tidz), held together at a site called the *centromere* (SEN-trō-mēr). Clusters of microtubules called **spindle fibers** grow towards and attach to the chromatids. One spindle fiber attaches to one chromatid at a site called the **kinetochore** (ki-NE-tō-kor). Just before the cell divides, each kinetochore begins to dismantle the plus ends of their attached microtubules. In a process that can be compared to a firefighter sliding down the pole at the fire station, the chromosomes aren't so much "pulled apart" but rather slide away from one another by unraveling the spiral ends of the microtubules that hold them together.

Like a bicycle wheel, microtubules fan out through a body cell in a hub-and-spoke pattern. The hub is the cell's **centrosome** (SEN-tro-sōm; *centro*, center; *some*, body), the production center for microtubules. A hazy-looking sphere with an indefinite border, a centrosome huddles close to the nucleus in non-dividing cells. A centrosome consists of hundreds of tiny rings of a special type of tubulin protein. The "minus" end of a microtubule emerges from but stays "plugged in" to one of the centrosome's tubulin rings. In this way, a centrosome controls the number, orientation, and location of all the microtubules that extend into the cytosol.

A centrosome is not an organelle, but it encloses two cylindrical organelles called **centrioles** (SEN-trē-olz), which align perpendicularly to one another inside a centrosome. Each centriole consists of nine bundles of microtubules, with three microtubules per bundle. Cell biologists still don't know what centrioles do. They once thought that centrioles made spindle fibers, but this is unlikely, since plant cells lack centrioles but make plenty of spindle fibers. Also, when biologists experimentally plucked out the centrioles from a centrosome, the cell still made spindle fibers at the right time and divided with ease. You might say that centrioles are organelles in search of a job!

Intermediate Filaments

Finally, let's turn our attention to the third—and toughest—component of the cytoskeleton. As their name implies, **intermediate filaments** are thicker than microfilaments but thinner than microtubules. These filaments are the strongest parts of the cytoskeleton and their strength helps cells endure mechanical stress. Many cells have intermediate filaments made of **keratins** (KAIR-i-tinz), a diverse family of proteins. These cells weave their intermediate filaments from small keratin subunits, rather like a rope-maker weaves a braided rope. Two pairs of keratin filaments bundle into a four-filament subunit, then eight subunits twist together to form a finished intermediate filament. Since they lack the "strand-of-beads" design like microfilaments and microtubules, intermediate filaments lack "endedness," which means they can't guide cell movement. However, intermediate filaments are exceptionally durable. Your hair and nails are the fused remnants of intermediate filaments that originated inside special skin cells.

Intermediate filaments are a part of most body cells, but they predominate in cells that need strong internal support. Some nerve cells, for example, have long slender extensions called *axons* that pass electrical-like signals to distant parts of the body. Numerous intermediate filaments within the axons prevent them from snapping like overstretched rubber bands whenever you move your body. Intermediate filaments are also abundant in sheets of cells that form the *epidermis*, or outer portion of the skin. Intermediate filaments span the cytoplasm from protein plugs called *cell junctions* that "weld" together the plasma membranes of neighboring cells. If external force stretches tissue cells, the intermediate filaments snap tight like ropes to prevent the cells from rupturing or pulling apart from their neighbors. Table 4-2 provides a summary of the cytoskeletal structures.

THE PROJECTIONS OF A BODY CELL

In addition to the host of proteins and carbohydrates that protrude from the plasma membrane, a body cell may have larger organelle-like projections that serve to (1) increase the cell's surface area, (2) sweep extracellular substances along the plasma membrane, or (3) propel the cell from place to place. The most important projections of a body cell include its *microvilli*, *cilia*, and a *flagellum*.

Microvilli

The tiniest projections found on certain body cells are **microvilli** (mī-krō-VIL-ī; *villi*, shaggy hair). Each of these stubby little cylinders is so small (measured in nanometers or billionths of a meter) that you would need to use a powerful electron microscope to see them clearly. An internal scaffolding of actin microfilaments supports each microvillus, and the entire mass of microvilli gather into a dense patch extending from only one side of a body cell. A patch of microvilli gives a cell a soft, peach-fuzz texture when viewed under a light microscope, a feature that biologists call the cell's **brush border**.

Microvilli are useful because they dramatically increase a cell's surface area. A demonstration you can try at home suggests why a large surface matters. Take a shower and dry off with your favorite towel. After your next shower, dry off using a bed sheet trimmed

Table 4-2. Cytoskeleton of a Body Cell

Filament Type	Composition	Distribution	Functions	Motor Molecules
Microfilaments	G-actin monomers	Concentrated along cell cortex, but present throughout cytosol	• Support and shape cell membrane • Transport cytoplasmic vesicles • Cell crawling (amoeboid movement) • Pinch cell in two to form daughter cells during cell division	Myosins
Microtubules	Tubulin subunits	Hub-and-spoke pattern extending from centrioles to plasma membrane	• Distribute organelles in cytoplasm • Movement of large cell projections • Enable duplicate chromosomes to separate during cell division	Kinesins Dyneins
Intermediate filaments	Varies; usually keratin protein	Hub-and-spoke pattern extending from nucleus to cell junctions	• Reinforce cell junctions • Prevent cells from pulling apart • Major component in hair and nails	None

OVERVIEW OF THE CELL

to match the size of a towel. Which drying device do you think would be more effective? Although the towel and sheet are the same size, the long fiber loops projecting from the towel vastly increase the towel's surface area, speeding its absorption of water. Similarly, cells that need to take up substances from the extracellular fluid fast usually bear microvilli. Examples of such "absorbent" cells include those lining your intestines. Keep in mind that an individual microvillus is a temporary structure, one that can form and fade away in as little as 15 minutes. Compare this to a snail's eyes that extend out but can retract quickly whenever the snail senses danger. The short "cycling time" of microfilaments allows a cell to adjust the topography of its plasma membrane quickly to cope with changes in the surrounding environment.

Cilia and Flagella

Although on the surface they resemble microvilli, **cilia** (SIL-ē-a; small hair) and **flagella** (fla-JEL-a; whip) are much larger. And, unlike microvilli, which are specialized for absorption, cilia and flagella devote themselves solely to pushing extracellular fluids. A cilium and a flagellum have the same basic design and operate the same way. Both are cylinders made of a circle formed by nine pairs of microtubules, called *doublets*, with an additional microtubule pair running down the center; this arrangement of microtubules is referred to as a "9 + 2" array (Figure 4-5).

A **basal body** anchors a cilium or flagellum to the cell cortex and directs the assembly of microtubules. Basal bodies and centrioles are identical organelles. Cell biologists still haven't figured out how a basal body's microtubule "triplets" give rise to the microtubule "doublets" in a cilium or flagellum. Recall that dynein motor molecules can form cross-bridges between microtubule pairs and "walk" one pair past the other. This repeated process generates the force that makes a cilium or flagellum alternately bend and straighten.

Although they work the same way, cilia and flagella behave differently and have different functional roles. Cilia project from the surface of tissue cells that face a body cavity, and a patch of ciliated cells work in unison. In an initial thrust called the *power stroke*, all the cilia sweep against the extracellular fluid in the same direction. During a subsequent *recovery stroke*, the cilia coil back into a "question-mark like" shape before extending to full length. Both movements in succession generate a forceful ciliary "wave" that can propel fluids and small particles across a tissue surface in a single direction, even against the force of gravity. Think of how spectators at a sports event do "the wave" in the stands, with whole blocks of people standing and throwing their hands in the air then sitting down, to produce a rhythmic wave that "rolls" across the stands. Ciliary movement pushes debris up and out of the respiratory tract, and it is a critical process for moving an ovum (female reproductive cell) through the female reproductive system.

Cilia wave back and forth to push extracellular fluids past a stationary cell, but a flagellum pushes a motile cell through the extracellular fluid. The focus of a flagellum's purpose in humans is in reproduction. A flagellum forms the tail of a sperm cell, a free-floating male reproductive cell. The flagellum whips about far more forcefully and rapidly than a cilium. And, since a sperm cell is able to move from one place to another, the beating flagellum can propel the sperm through the female reproductive system. The structure of a centriole, basal body, and cilium is shown in Figure 4-5.

CYTOPLASMIC ORGANELLES

You've been reading to this point about a body cell's "infrastructure;" that is, the cellular structures that maintain the cell's physical integrity, act as a biochemical barrier, and move substances from place to place. Earlier you read that a body cell is a kind of biochemical factory; therefore, let's consider the cytoplasmic subunits that conduct most of the chemical reactions in the cytoplasm—the **cytoplasmic organelles**. Back when cell biologists and biochemists started "unpacking" the parts of cells, they assigned the newly discovered organelles to one of two categories. **Membranous organelles** come wrapped in a double-layered membrane of phospholipids, also known as a *phospholipid bilayer* (*bi*, two); **non-membranous organelles** do not have this lipid wrapper.

Why do some organelles need a membrane? Recall that one trademark of a cell is its ability to maintain the unique chemical balance of its cytosol. Membranous organelles are a further refinement of this strategy. Just as the cytosol differs chemically from the extracellular

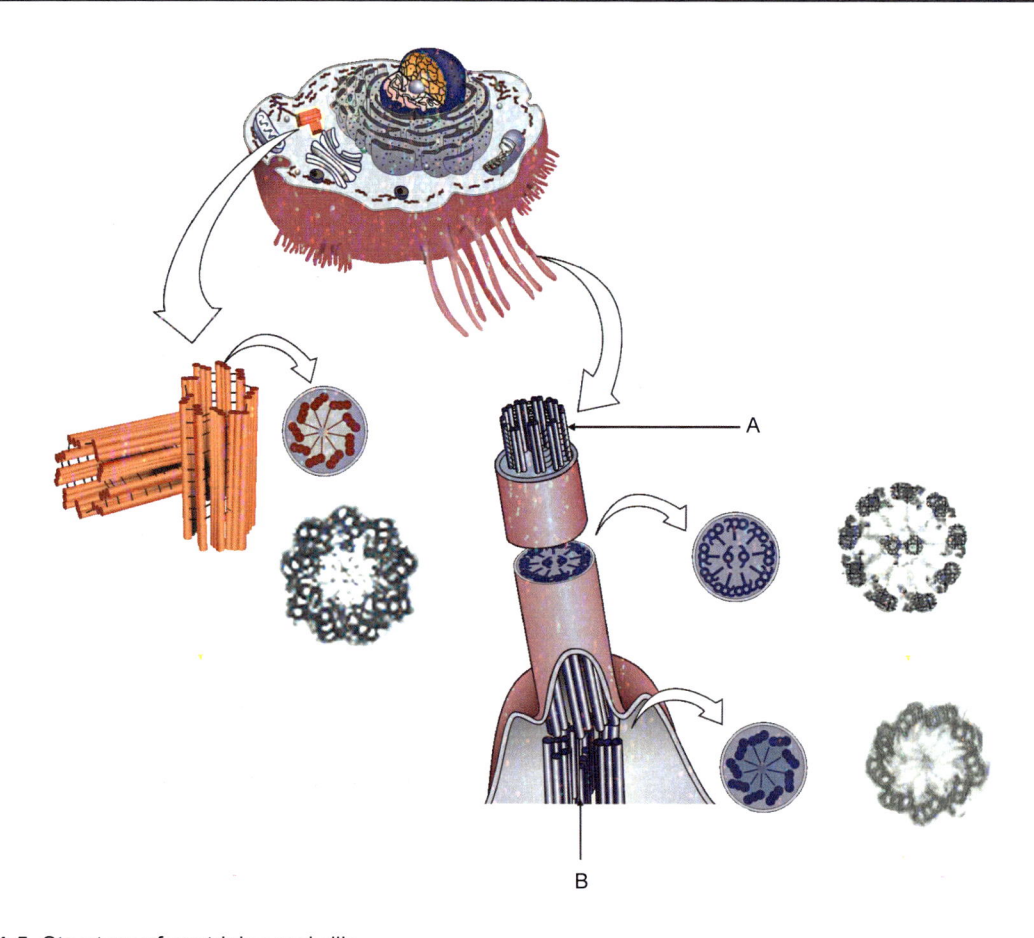

Figure 4-5. Structure of centrioles and cilia

fluid, the chemical environment inside a membranous organelle can differ substantially from that of the cytosol. In fact, some of the chemical reactions that take place within some organelles are so toxic that if leaked into the cytosol they would kill the cell in an instant. Apart from its role as a chemical barrier, the lipid bilayer surrounding membranous organelles serves as a kind of "universal mailing envelope" for *intracellular* transport. Vesicles that pinch off from the membrane of one organelle move along the cytoskeleton to neighboring organelles or to the plasma membrane.

Nevertheless, as most cell biologists would admit, knowing that a particular organelle has (or lacks) a membrane doesn't tell us much about what that organelle does for the cell. For this reason, we will conclude the tour of the cell's cytoplasm by grouping cellular organelles into two broad (but still imperfect) functional categories: (1) organelles that synthesize, modify, or package essential molecules, and (2) organelles that transport or digest organic molecules.

Organelles that Produce, Modify, or Package Molecules In Chapter 3, you read that synthesis reactions unite smaller molecules to make larger molecules, consuming energy in the process. Synthesis reactions occur constantly in a cell in order for it to:

- Build and maintain its organelles, membranes, and cytoskeleton
- Make the molecular products it exports to other cells
- Replace the macromolecules it consumes as part of cellular metabolism

Like goods rolling down a factory assembly line, some of a cell's newly synthesized products require customizing, sorting, and packaging before they are ready for delivery and use elsewhere. The first functional category of organelles, which synthesize, modify, sort, or package a cell's molecular products, includes ribosomes, mitochondria, endoplasmic reticula, and Golgi complexes.

OVERVIEW OF THE CELL

Ribosomes

Ranked among the cell's smallest components, **ribosomes** (RĪ-bō-sōmz) are non-membranous organelles that serve as construction sites for synthesizing proteins. A functional ribosome consists of one large and one small subunit, each of which forms from the union of *ribosomal proteins* and *ribosomal RNA* (rRNA) molecules. (Note: even the proteins that make up part of a ribosome are made at ribosomes.) Ribosomal subunits are given numbers based on their size, which determines their "sedimentation" rate in a liquid. Since the larger subunits sink faster, they are assigned a larger number than the small subunit. The large and small ribosomal subunits in bacteria (also known as *prokaryotic cells*; prō-kair-ē-OT-ik) are numbered 50s and 30s, respectively, whereas, in cells that have a nucleus (also known as *eukaryotic* cells; ū-kair-ē-OT-ik) they are 60s and 40s. The "s" relates to sedimentation rate. Figure 4-6 shows a basic ribosome.

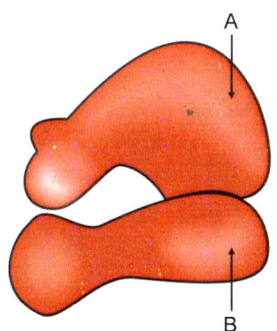

Figure 4-6. Ribosome

The destination of proteins made at a ribosome depends on the location of the ribosome in the cell. Some ribosomes attach to the surfaces of other organelles, becoming **bound ribosomes**, while other ribosomes move about in the cytosol as **free ribosomes**. Most proteins made at bound ribosomes leave the cell and function elsewhere in the body. For example, certain cells in the pancreas use bound ribosomes to make the protein insulin, an indispensable hormone that helps most other cells in the body take in glucose from the blood. Most proteins made at free ribosomes remain inside the cell and carry out various cellular functions.

Mitochondria

A cell needs a constant supply of ATP to carry out its normal metabolic activities. Adenosine triphosphate (ATP) is a molecular "fuel" that a body cell uses to drive nearly all of its endergonic reactions. Most of this fuel is produced inside **mitochondria** (mīt-ō-KON-drē-a) which under a microscope look like tiny packets filled with threads and grains of sand (*mito*, thread; *chondria*, granules). A typical body cell may have between 1000 and 2000 mitochondria, but this number can rise or fall depending on a cell's need for ATP. In fact, cell biologists sometimes figure out a body cell's level of physiological activity by counting the number of mitochondria in its cytoplasm. Cells that engage in unusually rapid or complex chemical reactions (e.g., cells in the brain, muscles, and liver) typically are jam-packed with mitochondria.

Mitochondria are exceptional organelles because they possess two phospholipid bilayers, one inside the other. The outer membrane is smooth, but the inner membrane has many folds called **cristae** (KRIS-tē; "crests"). The cristae project into an inner compartment that contains an enzyme-rich gel called the **matrix** (MĀ-triks; "womb"). A narrow **intermembrane space** separates the inner and outer membranes. This configuration is important because most ATP synthesis occurs along the inner membrane, and the cristae increase the surface area of the membrane that is responsible for ATP synthesis (see Figure 4-7).

Mitochondria have some curious features that have lead biologists to speculate that these organelles once lead an independent life. Mitochondria have one double helix DNA molecule that is "circular" (without an end—like a rubber band), which is similar to the DNA molecules found in bacteria. What is more, a mitochondrion's protein-synthesizing ribosomes resemble bacterial ribosomes, and a mitochondrion divides inside a cell through *binary fission*, the same method bacteria use to divide. Hence, biologists suspect that mitochondria were once free-living bacteria that survived after they entered a larger cell. The theory of their origin is known as the *endosymbiotic theory* (en-dō-sim-bī-OT-ik; *endo*, inside; *bio*, life). If so, both entities came to benefit from this event--the mitochondrion lives sheltered inside the cell's stable chemical environment, and in exchange for lodging, it

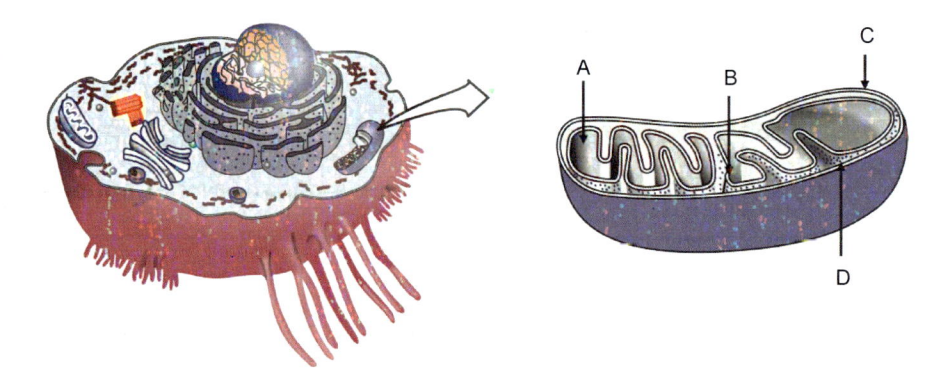

Figure 4-7. Mitochondrion

exports astounding numbers of ATP molecules every second into its "host's" cytoplasm. Figure 4-8 illustrates the endosymbiotic theory.

Mitochondria obtain energy for ATP synthesis by breaking the chemical bonds in molecules derived from glucose and fatty acids. This type of ATP synthesis involves a string of chemical reactions that are collectively known as **aerobic (cellular) respiration**, a process that requires oxygen. In the absence of oxygen, mitochondria stop producing ATP.

Endoplasmic reticulum

A body cell's largest membranous organelle is its **endoplasmic reticulum**, or **ER** (en-dō-PLAZ-mik re-TIK-ū-lum). In fact, the ER's membrane has a greater surface area than the plasma membrane. As the second part of its name suggests (*reticul-*, net), the ER is a membranous network that extends from the surface of the nuclear membrane like a pleated curtain. While the endoplasmic reticulum may look haphazardly unfurled in the cytoplasm, microtubules precisely arrange the ER into functionally advantageous shapes. The ER has many roles, but its chief role is being a site for the synthesis of proteins and lipids. Closer inspection of the ER reveals that it has two quite visually distinct parts: (1) the wavy *rough ER* and, (2) the more tube-like *smooth ER*.

The **rough endoplasmic reticulum** is continuous with, and remains positioned close to the cell's nuclear membrane. The wavy layers of the rough ER's lipid bilayer enclose **cisternae** (sis-TER-nā; "reservoirs"), fluid-filled chambers that modify and store newly formed proteins. The rough ER is so-named because of its grainy appearance, which is due to the numerous ribosomes that dot its face like sesame seeds on a bun (Figure 4-9).

The ribosomes don't permanently fasten to the membrane, but attach and release as they start and finish synthesizing a protein. Actually, the newly emerging protein helps to "thumbtack" its ribosome to the rough ER's outer membrane. In addition, the rough ER often

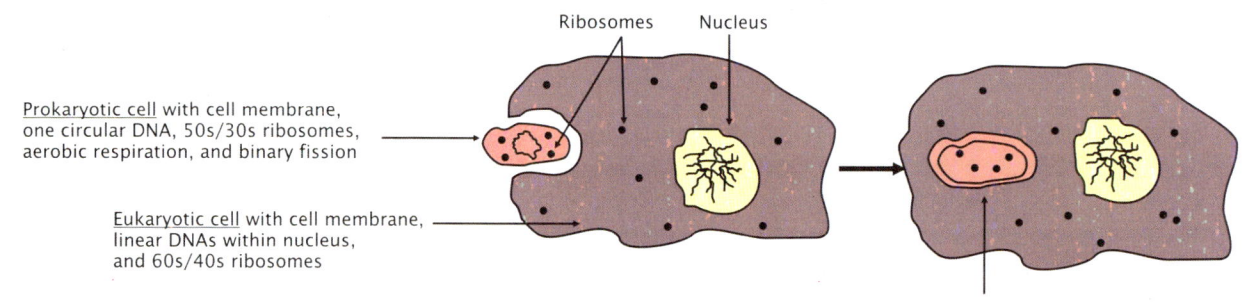

Prokaryotic cell with cell membrane, one circular DNA, 50s/30s ribosomes, aerobic respiration, and binary fission

Eukaryotic cell with cell membrane, linear DNAs within nucleus, and 60s/40s ribosomes

Mitochondrion with two membranes, circular DNA, 50s/30s ribosomes, aerobic respiration, and binary fission

Figure 4-8. Endosymbiotic theory

OVERVIEW OF THE CELL

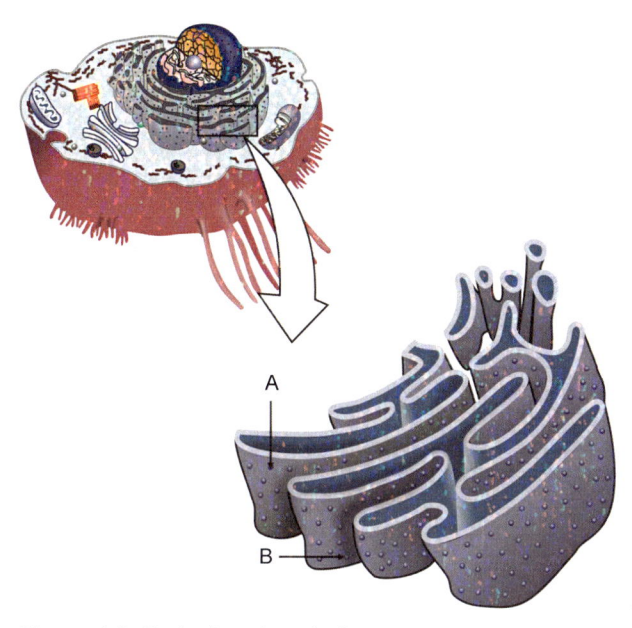

Figure 4-9. Endoplasmic reticulum

attaches carbohydrates to proteins in a process called **glycosylation** (glī-kos-i-LĀ-shun), transforming them into *glycoproteins*. All proteins that a cell exports to the rest of the body originate at the rough ER. Thus, cells that specialize in secreting substances tend to have exceptionally large rough ERs.

Moving out from the nucleus, the folds of the rough ER eventually break into the networks of tubules and sacs known as the **smooth endoplasmic reticulum**, so named because its surface lacks ribosomes. The smooth ER is the principle construction site for phospholipids and cholesterol. In some specialized cells, however, the smooth ER takes on equally specialized roles. For example, in muscle cells the smooth ER stores vast amounts of calcium ions, which it releases on cue to stimulate muscle contraction. In other cells, the smooth ER is heavily coated with enzymes that can transform substances as they enter or leave the cell. The unusually large smooth ER of liver cells, for example, holds enzymes that detoxify harmful substances in the blood such as drugs, alcohol, or various environmental toxins. After synthesizing and processing proteins and lipids, the ER packages these products into vesicles for transport to other organelles. Most of these vesicles, called *transport vesicles*, move to the Golgi complex.

Golgi complex

Newly synthesized proteins do not linger in the cisternae of the rough ER for very long. Within minutes, vesicles engulf these proteins, pinch off from the ER, and travel along microtubule railroads toward a **Golgi complex** (GŌL-jē), also called a **Golgi body** or **Golgi apparatus**. Perhaps the most curious-looking of all the membranous organelles, the Golgi complex consists of a stack of plate-like sacs. The wide *cis* face of a Golgi complex points at the rough ER, while its narrower *trans* face points at the plasma membrane (Figure 4-10).

Transport vesicles arriving from the ER enter the cis face and pass from plate-to-plate in the direction of the trans face. Ultimately, the Golgi complex packages these substances into large vesicles that move to and fuse with the plasma membrane, or they unite with smaller vesicles that travel to other organelles.

> **Note**: Since vesicles from the ER enter the *cis* face of the Golgi complex, think of *cis* as the "come in site."

The Golgi complexes are a cell's protein modifiers, sorters, and packagers. Just as an automobile maker customizes vehicles on an assembly line to meet the preferences of individual buyers, each plate in a Golgi complex sequentially modifies proteins until they reach their "ready-to-use" form. How a Golgi complex does this is a complex story that cell biologists are still unraveling. As vesicles arrive at each plate, they display membrane markers that serve as biochemical "order tickets" that tell enzymes in the plate what to do to the incoming proteins. The Golgi complex modifies individual proteins in a step-by-step fashion, just as a car on an assembly line may have a stick shift installed earlier on the line, and red leather seats installed further along. What is more, the Golgi complex "reads" the membrane markers and markers on the proteins it modifies, in order to sort out and package proteins that are bound for different destinations.

The major kind of "customizing" that the plates of a Golgi complex do is adding carbohydrates (glycosylation) and lipid molecules to proteins. For example, the Golgi complex synthesizes and attaches

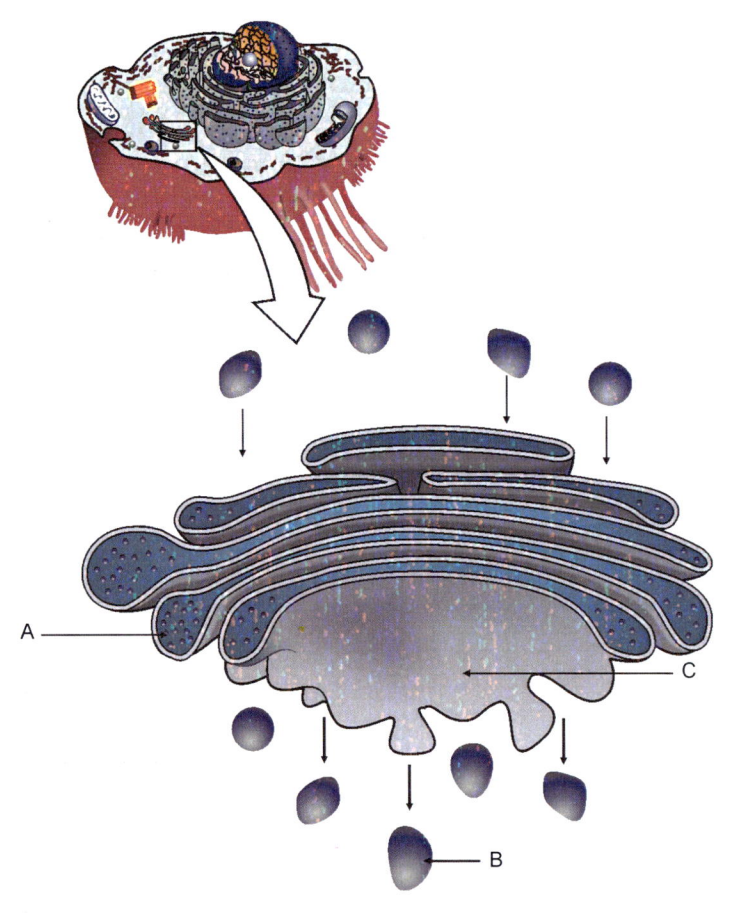

Figure 4-10. Golgi complex

very large polysaccharides to proteins to form *proteoglycans* (prō-tē-ō-GLĪ-kanz), substances that give connective tissues such as ligaments and tendons their flexibility and strength. The Golgi complex also attaches carbohydrates to lipid molecules, forming many of the *glycolipids* that become part of the plasma membrane.

Organelles that Transport and Digest Products

If the organelles just described function as the cell's "factories," then vesicles, lysosomes, and peroxisomes function as shipping containers, recycling centers, and decontamination sites. Simply put, vesicles are containers for hauling molecules on their membranous surfaces or within their fluid-filled interiors. On the other hand, you can distinguish lysosomes and peroxisomes by something unique that happens *inside* these spherical organelles, which both function as chemical reaction chambers.

Vesicles

You have likely noticed that previous sections mentioned vesicles time and again to this point in our tour of a body cell. That's to be expected, since vesicles interact directly with a number of membranous organelles and with the plasma membrane. **Vesicles** (VES-i-klz, "bags") are small, spherical organelles that transport substances through the cytoplasm, and they originate at certain membranous organelles and at the plasma membrane. Several organelles, including the ER, Golgi complex, and lysosomes, interact with one another through vesicles. Because all of these organelles are "membranous," and because they work together as a coordinated system to perform vital functions for the cell, cell biologists refer to them collectively as the cell's **endomembrane system**. Vesicles function as the "pick-up and delivery trucks" between the endomembrane system and the plasma membrane; coincidentally, cell biologists refer to the movement of vesicles within a cell as *vesicular traffic*.

OVERVIEW OF THE CELL

Just as a steady flow of truck traffic moving products and supplies within a city keeps the city operational, a steady flow of vesicular traffic moving molecular products and supplies within a cell keeps the cell functioning properly. Vesicular traffic runs along two major routes within a cell:

(1) An outbound *secretory pathway* (SĒ-kre-tor-ē) moves materials from parts of the endomembrane system to the plasma membrane

(2) An inbound *endocytic pathway* moves materials from the plasma membrane to the endomembrane system

In brief, the secretory pathway involves synthesizing molecular products at the endomembrane system and exporting them from the cell at the plasma membrane. The endocytic pathway involves taking in substances from the extracellular environment at the plasma membrane and transporting them to the endomembrane system for processing. Based on their particular roles in these pathways, cell biologists classify vesicles as *transport, secretory, or endocytic*.

Transport vesicles carry organic molecules from the ER to the Golgi complex and from the Golgi complex to other organelles and the plasma membrane. Watching transport vesicles develop on the surface of the ER and Golgi complex is sort of like watching someone blow bubbles with bubblegum. After synthesizing proteins on its outer surface and modifying them in its interior, the ER packages its molecular products inside budding transport vesicles. After pinching off of the ER, the transport vesicles latch onto motor molecules that pull them along the cytoskeleton to the cis face of the Golgi complex. After fusing with the cis face membrane, the vesicle releases it contents into the Golgi complex for further processing. After modification, the organic molecules enter transport vesicles that bud off of the *trans* face of the Golgi complex. Some of the Golgi-generated vesicles fuse with endocytic vesicles, while others fuse with the plasma membrane.

When a transport vesicle fuses with the plasma membrane, some of the vesicle's contents may spill into the extracellular fluid in a process called **secretion** (sē-KRĒ-shun). But what prevents a transport vesicle containing contents destined for secretion from fusing with a mitochondrion or some other organelle instead of the plasma membrane? The answer is membrane proteins. Certain proteins that project from the vesicle's surface function as receptors that recognize specific proteins or other compounds in the plasma membrane. Therefore, vesicles that bump into membranes other than the plasma membrane will not fuse with them because they lack the appropriate protein receptors. On the other hand, transport vesicles that bind with other organelles have receptors that recognize specific proteins on the other organelle's surface.

> **Note:** The word *secretion* can refer to the process by which a vesicle releases a substance into the ECF, or it can refer to the actual substance released from a vesicle into the ECF.

Secretory vesicles (SĒ-kre-tor-ē) are specialized transport vesicles that bud off of the Golgi complex and congregate near the plasma membrane, but secrete their contents only when prompted by a chemical cue in the ECF. (Recall that transport vesicles reaching the plasma membrane do not require such a cue before they can secrete their contents.) This chemical signal is a specific molecule that binds to a receptor molecule on the outer face of the plasma membrane and initiates chemical reactions inside the cell. These chemical reactions cause the secretory vesicles to fuse with the plasma membrane and secrete their contents. Since the body carefully controls the concentrations of the extracellular chemical signals, the release of substances from secretory vesicles is *regulated* secretion. Only certain kinds of cells, called *secretory cells*, produce secretory vesicles and release large amounts of one type of secretion. For example, following a meal, secretory cells in your pancreas secrete large amounts of digestive enzymes that help break down the food molecules in your intestine.

In addition to expelling cellular products into the ECF, transport and secretory vesicles supply new lipids and proteins to the plasma membrane. This is important for two reasons. First, molecules in the plasma membrane eventually "wear out" and the cell must replace them. When a vesicle fuses with the plasma membrane, any molecules that are part of the vesicle's membrane become part of the plasma membrane. Since the transport vesicle folds inside out during the fusion process, any molecules (including glycoproteins and glycolipids) adhering to the *inner* surface of the vesicle will end up facing the ECF. Conversely, any molecules adhering to the outer surface of the vesicle will end up facing the cytoplasm. Second, the plasma membrane must grow as a cell grows. Before dividing, a cell must grow larger; to grow also, the plasma membrane incorporates membranes of transport vesicles.

Endocytic vesicles (en-dō-SIT-ik) pinch off of the plasma membrane and deliver substances from the ECF *into* the cell. These vesicles form in a process called *endocytosis* (en-dō-sī-TŌ-sis), during which a portion of the plasma membrane pinches inward while enclosing substances from the ECF. After moving into the cytoplasm, endocytic vesicles eventually fuse with lysosomes (described next). Endocytic vesicles are common in certain types of white blood cells that ingest and destroy bacteria and viruses.

Lysosomes

Lysosomes (LĪ-sō-sōmz) are highly specialized vesicles that pinch off of the Golgi complex, remain inside the cell, and decompose food molecules and worn-out organelles. Lysosomes contain enzymes called *hydrolases* (HĪ-drō-lā-sez) that digest large organic molecules, breaking them into smaller molecules by hydrolysis. Since certain byproducts of hydrolysis are reusable, lysosomes function like recycling centers for the cell. Hydrolases work only in an acid environment (about pH 5), which is the case inside of the lysosome. The cytosol's pH is around 7; therefore, if a few hydrolase molecules leak into the cytosol, they cease to function and usually do not harm the cell.

One of the most important functions of lysosomes is to digest the contents of endocytic vesicles. Some of the large molecules that a cell takes in from the ECF and packages into endocytic vesicles can serve as a source of energy or building blocks for cellular components. However, in order to release this energy or make the building blocks available, the cell must first digest or break down the large molecules. After forming at the plasma membrane, an endocytic vesicle moves through the cytosol and fuses with a lysosome. The lysosome's hydrolase enzymes mix with the contents of the vesicle, quickly digesting them. Some of the chemical byproducts of this digestion enter the cytosol for use in various metabolic activities, while the unusable materials remain inside the vesicle. Finally, motor molecules attach to the vesicle and transport it to the plasma membrane where the "waste" molecules enter the ECF.

Lysosomes also perform "housekeeping" chores by removing worn-out organelles from the cytoplasm and recycling their reusable molecules. When a cell digests one of its own organelles, the process is called **autophagia** (aw-tō-FĀ-jē-a; *auto*, self; *phag*, eating). Cell biologists have not yet determined how lysosomes identify worn-out organelles and mark them for destruction. However, prior to autophagia, a vesicle derived from the ER envelops the worn-out organelle. Motor molecules then transport the vesicle along the cytoskeleton where it can unite with a lysosome. Just as a salvage yard strips out all the "good stuff" from worn-out automobiles, lysosome enzymes strip out usable molecules from worn-out organelles. Lastly, lysosomes are responsible for **autolysis** (aw-TOL-i-sis; "self-breaking") of certain cells. When these cells reach the end of their life span, numerous lysosomes rupture allowing the hydrolase enzymes to spill into the cytosol. As mentioned earlier, a small amount of hydrolase leaking into the cytosol would likely be neutralized by the higher-pH cytosolic liquid; however, having numerous lysosomes rupture can overwhelm the buffering capacity of the cytosol, resulting in the cell being digested from the inside out. Thus, lysosomes have the nickname "suicide bags."

Peroxisomes

Peroxisomes (per-OX-i-sōmz) are tiny organelles that break down a variety of compounds, including fatty acids, amino acids, and various toxins. In the process, the peroxisome makes **hydrogen peroxide** (H_2O_2), which is responsible for the organelle's name. Although peroxisomes may seem similar to lysosomes, there are several key differences between these organelles. First, lysosomes bud off the Golgi complex, while peroxisomes reproduce by simply pinching in two. Second, peroxisomes contain different enzymes than those found in lysosomes. Free ribosomes synthesize these enzymes, which then enter a peroxisome through carrier proteins located in the peroxisome's membrane.

The two enzymes that allow peroxisomes to play a unique role inside cells are *oxidase* and *catalase*. **Oxidase** (OKS-si-dās) removes electrons from (oxidizes) fatty acids and other molecules, causing these molecules to break apart. By-products of fatty acid oxidation leave the peroxisome and can enter the smooth ER, which converts them to cholesterol or other lipids. Oxidase also detoxifies harmful molecules, such as free radicals. Recall that free radicals are molecules that have unpaired electrons, a condition that causes them to steal electrons from other compounds. This action can damage DNA and other vital molecules. Oxidase converts the free radicals to H_2O_2, but H_2O_2 is also detrimental to the cell. Fortunately, the peroxisome contains **catalase** (KAT-a-lās), an enzyme that converts the H_2O_2 into water and oxygen: $2H_2O_2 \rightarrow 2H_2O + O_2$. Like oxidase, catalase can detoxify certain harmful compounds, such as formic acid (found in the venom of insect stingers) and alcohol. Hydrogen peroxide in an open wound forms bubbles containing O_2 liberated when catalase from damaged cells converts the peroxide into oxygen and water.

Table 4-3 summarizes the cytoplasmic organelles.

Peroxisomes

Table 4-3. Membranous vs. non-membranous organelles and their relationship to their functional categories

Membranous organelles	*Functional category**	*General Function*
Mitochondria	1	Aerobic ATP production
Endoplasmic reticulum	1	Lipid synthesis, forms transport vesicles
Golgi complex	1	Sorting and packaging of molecules for export
Vesicles	2	Storage, digestion, transport
Lysosomes	2	Digestion
Peroxisomes	2	Neutralize toxic substances
Non-membranous organelles		
Centrioles	1	Unknown, but associated with centrosome, which synthesizes microtubules
Ribosomes	1	Protein synthesis

*1 = Synthesize and/or sort; 2 = Transport and/or digest

TOPICS TO KNOW IN CHAPTER 4 (OVERVIEW OF THE CELL)

"9 + 2" array of microtubules
50s and 30s ribosomal units
60s and 40s ribosomal units
actin
adipocytes
aerobic (cellular) respiration
autolysis
autophagia
basal body
binary fission
biochemists
bound ribosomes
brush border

catalase
cell
cell biologists
cell cortex
cell crawling
cell junctions
cell theory
centrioles
centrosome
cilia
circular DNA
cis face
cisternae

cytoplasm
cytoplasmic organelles
cytoskeleton
cytosol
direction of motor molecule movement
dyneins
endocytic pathway
endocytic vesicles
endocytosis
endomembrane system
endoplasmic reticulum
endosymbiotic theory
fat droplets

flagella
free ribosomes
gametes
glycogen
glycogen granules
glycolipids
glycosylation
Golgi complex
hemoglobin
hydrogen peroxide
hydrolases
inclusions
intermediate filaments
keratins
kinesins
kinetochore
lysosomes
melanin
melanocytes
membranous organelles
microfilament "endedness"
microfilaments
microtubules
microvilli
minus end
mitochondria
mitochondrial cristae
mitochondrial matrix
mitochondrial ribosomes
molecular biologists
motor molecules
myosin
non-membranous organelles
organelle
organelles that produce, modify, or package molecules
organelles that transport and digest products
overview of cells
oxidase
peroxisomes
plus end
proteoglycans
pseudopodia
regulated secretion
ribosomal proteins
ribosomal RNA
ribosomes
roles of microfilaments
rough endoplasmic reticulum
secretion
secretory cells
secretory pathway
secretory vesicles
smooth endoplasmic reticulum
somatic cells
spindle fibers
trans face
transport vesicles
tubulin
vesicles
vesicular traffic

CHAPTER 5

The Nucleus, DNA Expression, and the Cell Cycle

In order for an organization to sustain itself and grow, it must have an effective leader and the same holds true for the highly organized cell. In this chapter, we complete our tour of a typical body cell with a look at the cell's "chief supervisor," the nucleus. After describing its form and chemical makeup, we will explain how the nucleus controls the cell's day-to-day activities through the action of its genetic material, DNA. Finally, as a logical connection to an upcoming chapter, the study of groups of cells called tissues, we will conclude this chapter by explaining how cells reproduce.

FUNCTION OF THE NUCLEUS

The most recognizable organelle in most cells is the nucleus, and its enormous size compared to other organelles suggests that it plays a major role in the normal functioning of the cell. The nucleus is the largest organelle in our typical cell, and is so-named because it resembles a round seed (*nucleus*, nut). It serves as a storehouse and library for genetic material, which, in the form of DNA molecules, provides the chemical "blueprints" for constructing the cell's proteins. Because the nucleus directs protein synthesis, and because proteins (notably enzymes) control most of the cell's metabolic activities, the nucleus is nicknamed the cell's "control center."

The number of nuclei within a cell relates directly to the amount of protein the cell must synthesize to maintain its structure and metabolic activity. Most cells in the body are **uninucleate** (oo-ni-NŪ-klē-āt; *uni*, single) having only one nucleus, but a few types of cells are **multinucleate**, having more than one nucleus. Examples of multinucleate cells that synthesize large amounts of protein include skeletal muscle cells and certain cells in bones and liver. Red blood cells are unique in that they develop as uninucleate cells inside bones but become **anucleate** (ā-NŪ-klē-āt) when they eject their nucleus prior to entering the blood (the prefix *a-* means "without"). This seemingly bizarre act enables red blood cells to carry more oxygen, but it also leaves the cells without any genetic material. Consequently, red blood cells can't replace worn-out proteins and live only three or four months.

STRUCTURE OF THE NUCLEUS

The most noticeable features of the nucleus are the *nuclear envelope*, *nucleoplasm*, and *nucleolus* (Figure 5-1). The **nuclear envelope** encloses the nucleus and consists of an outer and inner membrane. The outer membrane is continuous with the rough endoplasmic reticulum, and like the rough ER, has numerous ribosomes on its surface. Large, circular openings, called **nuclear pores**, exist where the inner and outer membranes fuse and allow the nucleus to exchange materials with the cytosol. Nuclear pores are large enough to allow ions and small molecules (including nucleotides) to move freely into and out of the nucleus. However, macromolecules such as proteins and RNA can move into or out of the nucleus only with the help of proteins that line the nuclear pores. The exact mechanism by which this transport occurs is unknown, but it is a process that requires the cell to expend energy.

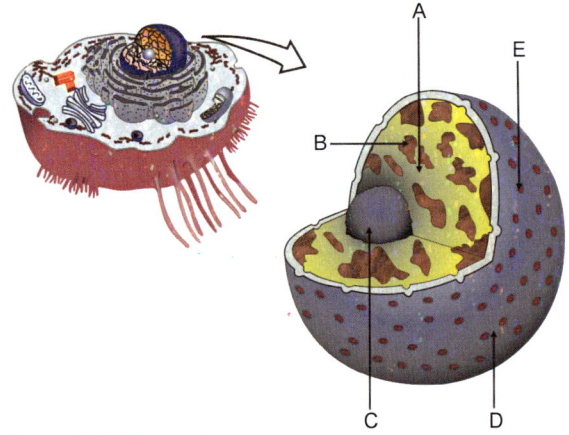

Figure 5-1. The nucleus

The inner membrane of the nuclear envelope surrounds the **nucleoplasm** (NŪ-klē-ō-plazm), the fluid inside the nucleus. Nucleoplasm has a consistency similar to cytosol and its major organic components include DNA, RNA, ribosomal proteins, enzymes, and nucleotides. A **nucleolus** (nū-KLĒ-ō-lus) is a dark-staining region inside the nucleoplasm where RNA molecules and proteins come together to form large or small ribosomal subunits. The ribosomal subunits eventually exit the nucleus through the nuclear pores and come together in the cytosol to form functional ribosomes. Although it appears to have a well-defined border, a nucleolus does not have a membrane. What is more, the size of a nucleolus is ever changing, growing when new ribosomal subunits become part of it and shrinking when subunits leave it to enter the cytoplasm. Cells that synthesize large amounts of protein need many ribosomes and, therefore, usually have more than one nucleolus inside the nucleus.

ORGANIZATION OF THE GENETIC MATERIAL

Genetic material consists of DNA and protein bound together in a way that allows it to exist either as fine, entangled threads during cell growth or as highly condensed, well-defined packages during cell division. The genetic material exists in the nucleus of a non-dividing cell as fine, intertwining threads called **chromosomes** (KRŌ-mō-somz; *chromo*, color; *somes*, bodies). The structural material that comprises a chromosome is **chromatin** (KRŌ-ma-tin), so-named because it appears dark when stained with certain dyes. A closer look at chromatin reveals that it is a complex union between DNA and a group of globular proteins called **histones** (HIS-tōnz). Histone proteins look like small marbles and bunch together in groups of eight. A short segment of a double helix DNA molecule wraps around these clusters of histones, much like a thread wraps around a spool. The entire DNA-histone complex resembles a beaded necklace, in which each "bead" is a **nucleosome** (NŪ-klē-ō-sōm). Figure 5-2 shows the structure of a nuclear chromosome.

Chromosome Number

The number of chromosomes in the nucleus of a human gamete (sex cell—egg or a sperm) is 23, referred to as the human's **haploid number (n)**. Each of these chromosomes is *different*; that is, each one contains genetic information for different inheritable traits. One of the 23 different chromosomes is called the **sex chromosome**, because it plays a role in determining the sex of the person. The other 22 chromosomes in the gamete are called **autosomes**.

Within the nucleus of a human somatic cell, the 23 different chromosomes exist in *pairs*; therefore, the number of chromosomes in the nucleus of a typical body cell is 46, referred to as the human's **diploid number** (2n; DIP-loyd). The two chromosomes within

THE NUCLEUS, DNA EXPRESSION, AND THE CELL CYCLE

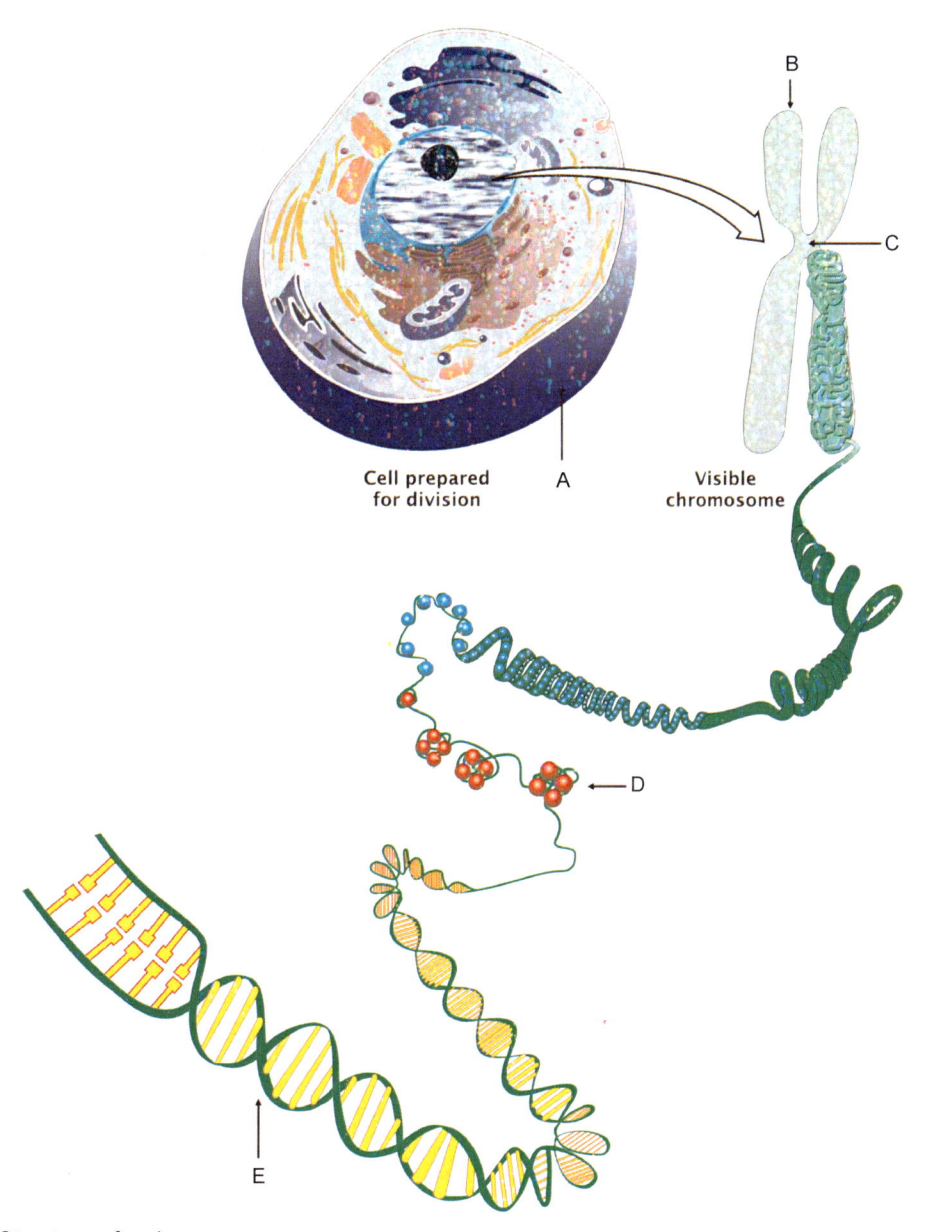

Figure 5-2. Structure of a chromosome

a given pair are said to be *homologous* (hō-MOL-o-gus), because they contain genetic information for the same inheritable traits (*homo*, same; *logo*, words). One member of each homologous pair of chromosomes comes from the mother and the other member of the pair comes from the father. Chromosomes derived from the mother are **maternal chromosomes** (muh-TER-nal; *mater*, mother), while those derived from the father are **paternal chromosomes** (puh-TER-nal; *pater*, father).

To make sure you understand the numbers and terms just described, let's recap what you just read. The haploid number (n) refers to the number of *different kinds* of chromosomes in an organism. For humans, n=23. The diploid number is the number of chromosomes present when there are two copies (one maternal and one paternal) for each kind of chromosome. For humans, 2n=46. Human gametes are haploid (n), containing only 23 chromosomes (22 autosomes and 1 sex chromosome). Human somatic cells are diploid (2n), containing 46 chromosomes (22 pairs of autosomes and 1 pair of sex chromosomes).

DNA EXPRESSION

Each DNA molecule in the nucleus consists of functional segments called **genes** (jēnz) that provide a chemical code specifying the number, type, and arrangement (sequence) of amino acids in proteins. The word *gene* implies that information within these segments of DNA can be used to generate proteins. Recall that two or more amino acids linked together comprise a *peptide*; therefore, since proteins consist of *many* amino acids, biochemists refer to them as *polypeptides*. Biochemists have determined that genes contain chemical instructions necessary to synthesize polypeptides, and this concept became the **one gene-one polypeptide theory**. All the genes on all the different types of chromosomes in your cells make up your **genome** (je-NŌM). An example of how genes might align on a chromosome is shown in Figure 5-3. The small segments that have no labels represent "promoters" and other regions not encoded directly onto RNA molecules. The names of actual genes would be written in italics using lowercase letters; e.g., genes that code for the enzymes sucrase and lactase might be written *suc* and *lac*, respectively. The Human Genome Project is attempting to identify every gene on every chromosome in the human species. Identifying gene location would allow researchers and clinicians to know which genes are "linked" (located on the same chromosome) and might allow defective genes to be replaced.

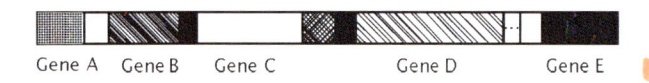

Figure 5-3. Genes on a chromosome

The Genetic Code

What exactly is the genetic information inside a gene that helps direct the sequencing of amino acids in a protein? First, recall the DNA of living organisms is a double helix molecule, comprised of two polymers of nucleotides held together by hydrogen bonds. Each nucleotide consists of a sugar (deoxyribose), a phosphate ion, and one of four nitrogenous bases: adenine (A), thymine (T), cytosine (C), or guanine (G).

Think of the letters A, T, C, and G as the alphabet for the cell's genetic language (code), which consists of 3-letter "words" called **triplets**. With four letters available to arrange in groups of three, there are 4^3 or 64 triplets possible. Sixty triplets specify amino acids that can become part of a protein; three triplets function as "stop" signals for protein synthesis; and the remaining triplet functions as a "start" signal for protein synthesis. Since the body contains only 20 different kinds of amino acids, more than one DNA triplet can specify the same amino acid. For example, the triplets CAT, CAG, CAC, and CAA all specify the amino acid valine.

The genes in a non-dividing cell remain inside the nucleus and do not guide protein synthesis directly, but instead employ RNA molecules to carry genetic information to ribosomes in the cytoplasm. Biochemists refer to the phenomenon whereby genetic information passes from a DNA molecule to an RNA molecule and ultimately to protein as the **central dogma of molecular biology** (*dogma*, opinion). We can summarize the central dogma as follows:

DNA→RNA→Protein

However, DNA does not become RNA, and RNA does not become protein. Instead, genetic information in DNA guides the synthesis of RNA, and then the information in RNA guides the synthesis of a protein. The central dogma involves two major processes: *transcription* and *translation*.

TRANSCRIPTION

Transcription, or RNA synthesis, represents the first step in the central dogma whereby genetic information passes from one type of nucleic acid to another type (*trans*, across; *script*, writing). The normal pathway is to transfer information from DNA into a molecule of RNA. To grasp the significance of this process, consider the following analogy. Let's say that you want to build a certain type of house (which we will say is comparable to a protein). You can find a blueprint (gene) for this house in a special book (chromosome) located in the library (the cell's nucleus). The book cannot leave the library, however, but you can copy (transcribe) the blueprint and take the copied version (RNA) to the construction site (ribosome). Although the blueprint copy is not the same kind of paper

THE NUCLEUS, DNA EXPRESSION, AND THE CELL CYCLE

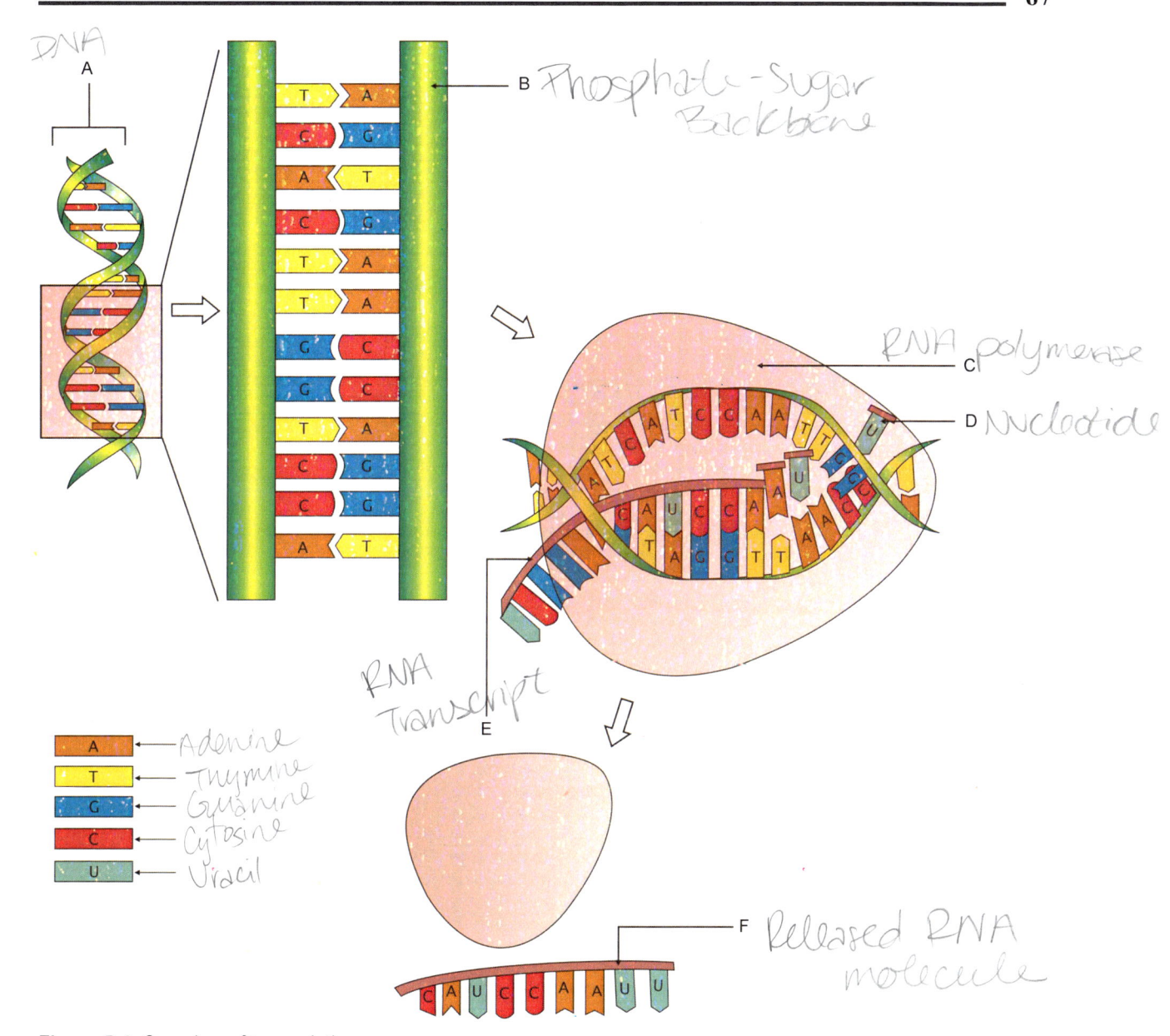

Figure 5-4. Overview of transcription

(nucleic acid) as the original blueprint, it contains the appropriate information for building the specific house (synthesizing the specific protein). Figure 5-4 provides an overview of transcription.

How does a cell determine which genes to transcribe? Before transcription can begin, gene activation must occur, which means a special chemical must "turn on" the gene, making it ready for transcription. Identifying gene-activating chemicals, called *transcription factors*, and learning how they work is a major goal of modern biochemistry research. Suffice it to say, negative feedback regulates the concentrations of transcription factors within the nucleus. For example, a deficiency of a particular cellular protein causes increased production of transcription factors that activate the gene responsible for generating that protein. Just before transcription begins, transcription factors uncoil the chromatin and expose a portion of the DNA molecule called a **promoter** (prō-MŌ-ter), located next to the gene of interest. The gene is now ready to be transcribed.

Transcription, like other synthesis reactions in a cell, requires an enzyme. In this case, the enzyme is **RNA polymerase** (puh-LIM-er-ās), so-named because it constructs a polymer called RNA. After binding to the promoter located on the DNA, the RNA polymerase breaks the hydrogen bonds between the parallel strands of the DNA's double helix, effectively "unzipping" the DNA molecule in that region. Separating the double helix is necessary to expose the DNA triplets that specify the amino acids in a protein. This initial phase in transcription is comparable to opening a book of blueprints to the page showing the blueprint that you want to copy. Furthermore, let's say that this blueprint exists on only *one* page in the open book. Similarly, RNA polymerase binds to only *one* strand of the DNA double helix; this strand is the **DNA template** and it contains the base sequence used to direct the synthesis of an RNA molecule.

In the second phase of transcription, RNA polymerase moves along the DNA template toward the template's 5' end. While doing this, the RNA polymerase pulls in RNA nucleotides from the nucleoplasm and aligns their bases (A, U, C, or G) alongside complementary bases on the DNA template. (Recall from Chapter 2, RNA substitutes uracil for thymine; thus, uracil is complementary to adenine.) Hydrogen bonds form between the complementary bases, temporarily holding them together. When the RNA polymerase positions two RNA nucleotides side by side, it forms a covalent bond between them. In this way, RNA polymerase constructs an RNA molecule having a base sequence that is complementary to the base sequence on the DNA template. Since the polymerase moves along the template in a 3' to 5' direction, it constructs the RNA molecule in a 5' to 3' direction. In other words, it always adds new RNA nucleotides to the 3' end. The portion of the RNA trailing behind the RNA polymerase detaches from the template, allowing the separated DNA strands in that region to come back together, much like re-zipping a zipper, to form a double helix (see Figure 5-5).

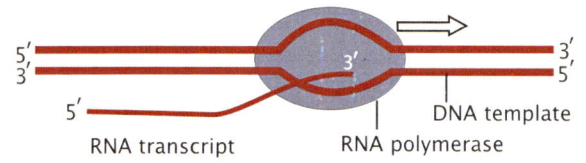

Figure 5-5. Direction of transcription

Transcription stops when the RNA polymerase comes to a region of the gene called the **terminator**. Reaching the terminator causes RNA polymerase to detach from the DNA template and release the newly formed RNA molecule, called an **RNA transcript**. Let's now look at the three types of RNA generated by transcription.

Types of RNA

Transcription of various genes is responsible for producing all RNA molecules used by a cell for protein synthesis, but not all RNAs have the same function in protein synthesis. RNA comes in three different functional forms: *ribosomal RNA*, *messenger RNA*, and *transfer RNA*.

Ribosomal RNA. Ribosomal RNA (rRNA) helps structurally reinforce a ribosome and may play a role in linking amino acids together during protein synthesis. Soon after their synthesis, rRNA molecules bind to special proteins inside the nucleus to form large and small ribosomal subunits. When needed for protein synthesis, these ribosomal subunits pass through nuclear pores and come together in the cytoplasm to form functional ribosomes. Biochemists have identified five different chromosomes in the nucleus of a human cell that generate rRNA molecules during transcription.

Messenger RNA. Carrying a copy of the DNA's genetic message for protein synthesis from the nucleus to a ribosome is the function of **messenger (mRNA)** molecules. Each "word" in the mRNA's message consists of three nucleotide bases called **codons** (KŌ-donz), so-named because they represent the codes for specific amino acids. Codons are complementary to triplets in DNA. For example, transcribing the DNA triplet CAT results in the codon GUA. Since there are 64 possible DNA triplets, there are 64 possible codons. While a single codon can specify only one of the 20 different kinds of amino acids in the body, more than one codon can specify the same amino acid. Redundancy in the genetic coding system means that changing one of the bases in a triplet or codon may not necessarily change the amino acid specified originally. Table 5-1 lists all possible codons and the amino acids they specify. (Note the three "stop" codons do not

THE NUCLEUS, DNA EXPRESSION, AND THE CELL CYCLE

Table 5-1. The Genetic Code – A list of codons on mRNA and the corresponding amino acids for which they code

Adenine as first base	Cytosine as first base	Guanine as first base	Uracil as first base
AAA Lysine	CAA Glutamine	GAA Glutamine	**UAA (Stop)**
AAC Asparagine	CAC Histidine	GAC Asparagine	UAC Tyrosine
AAG Lysine	CAG Glycine	GAG Glutamine	**UAG (Stop)**
AAU Asparagine	CAU Histidine	GAU Asparagine	UAU Tyrosine
ACA Threonine	CCA Proline	GCA Alanine	UCA Serine
ACC Threonine	CCC Proline	GCC Alanine	UCC Serine
ACG Threonine	CCG Proline	GCG Alanine	UCG Serine
ACU Threonine	CCU Proline	GCU Alanine	UCU Serine
AGA Arginine	CGA Arginine	GGA Glycine	**UGA (Stop)**
AGC Serine	CGC Arginine	GGC Glycine	UGC Cystine
AGG Arginine	CGG Arginine	GGG Glycine	UGG Tryptophan
AGU Serine	CGU Arginine	GGU Glycine	UGU Cystine
AUA Isoleucine	CUA Leucine	GUA Valine	UUA Leucine
AUC Isoleucine	CUC Leucine	GUC Valine	UUC Phenylalanine
AUG Methionine (Start)	CUG Leucine	GUG Valine	UUG Leucine
AUU Isoleucine	CUU Leucine	GUU Valine	UUU Phenylalanine

code for amino acids.) You do not need to memorize this table, but you do need to know the "start" codon (AUG) and its corresponding amino acid (methionine; meth-Ī-ō-nēn).

Before an mRNA molecule carries the DNA's genetic message to a ribosome, it undergoes a process called **mRNA processing**. Before processing occurs, the mRNA, known as *pre-mRNA*, contains nonfunctional segments called **introns** (EN-tronz) that do not properly code for segments of a protein. Special enzymes in the nucleus remove the introns and splice together the remaining functional segments called **exons** (EKS-onz). Introns are so-named because they remain *inside* the nucleus after mRNA processing. Exons are so-named because they bond together and exit the nucleus. As a result, the functional mRNA that ends up at a ribosome may be considerably shorter than the original pre-mRNA (see Figure 5-6).

In addition to cleaning up a pre-mRNA molecule by removing introns, mRNA processing offers another advantage. By splicing exons together in different

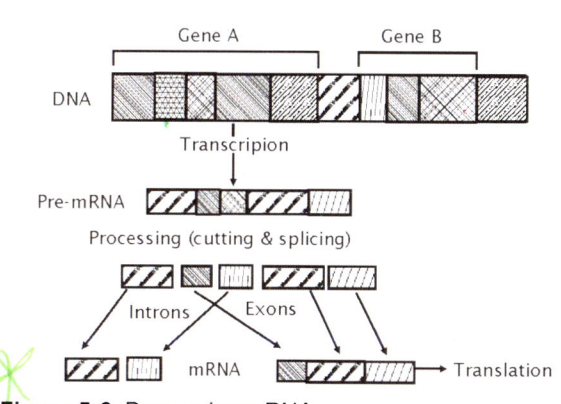

Figure 5-6. Processing mRNA

sequences, a single gene can generate more than one functional mRNA molecule. This explains how the human genome's approximately 30,000 functional genes can give rise to more than 100,000 different proteins in the body.

Transfer RNA. Bringing amino acids to a ribosome so they can come together to form a protein is the function of **transfer RNA (tRNA)**. This relatively small, clover-shaped molecule consists of less than 100 nucleotides. Hydrogen bonds between complementary bases in certain regions of the molecule are responsible for a tRNA's unique shape. One end of the tRNA displays three nitrogenous bases, called an **anticodon**, which can form hydrogen bonds with complementary codons on mRNA. For example, a tRNA with the anticodon CAU will bind only to the mRNA codon GUA. At the other end of the tRNA, an enzyme in the cytoplasm attaches a specific amino acid. The tRNA then carries its amino acid passenger to the ribosome to become part of a protein. In this respect, tRNA is like a delivery truck that carries house-building materials to a construction site. Let's now look at how tRNA and mRNA interact at a ribosome to build a protein.

TRANSLATION

Translation is the process by which a cell uses the sequence of codons on an mRNA molecule to determine the sequence of particular amino acids in a protein. To grasp the relevance of the word *translation*, think of mRNA as a translator that converts words (triplets) of one language (DNA) into appropriate words (amino acids) of another language (protein). In our blueprint analogy, the RNA polymerase is like the carpenter who "translates" the information on a photocopied house blueprint (mRNA) in order to build an actual house (protein).

Translation occurs in the cytoplasm and involves the collective efforts of mRNA, tRNA, and small and large ribosomal subunits. Before translation begins, mRNA molecules and the ribosomal subunits exit the nucleus through nuclear pores in the nuclear membrane. In the cytoplasm, the ribosomal subunits come together around the mRNA to form a functional ribosome. The mRNA then shifts through the ribosome one codon at a time. Each time the mRNA shifts, a tRNA molecule brings in the next amino acid specified by the codon occupying a precise location within the ribosome. Within the ribosome-mRNA complex, a covalent bond forms between two adjacent amino acids so that the ribosome builds a protein one amino acid at a time. Translation involves five major steps (see Figure 5-7 and the description of each step that follows).

1. Binding mRNA with small ribosomal subunit: After entering the cytoplasm, mRNA binds to an mRNA-*binding site* located on the small ribosomal subunit. The region of the mRNA that binds first with the small ribosomal subunit displays the "start" codon having the base sequence AUG. Then a tRNA with the complimentary anticodon UAC binds with the start codon. This "first" tRNA, called the *initiator tRNA* because it initiates the translation of the genetic code, always carries the amino acid methionine.

2. Formation of ribosome and entry of next tRNA: After binding with the mRNA, the small ribosomal subunit locks together with a large ribosomal subunit to form a functional ribosome. The initiator tRNA and its methionine amino acid now fit into a region called the **P site** located on the large ribosomal subunit. The P, or *peptidyl* (PEP-ti-dil) site is so-named because it will hold the growing polypeptide (protein) when another amino acid arrives at the ribosome. The next tRNA that can enter the ribosome has an anticodon that is complementary to the next codon on the mRNA. After entering the ribosome, the tRNA binds to the complementary codon and occupies a site in the large ribosomal subunit called the **A site**. The "A" stands for *aminoacyl* (a-mē-nō-AS-il), implying that this site receives the incoming amino acids, which the ribosome will add to the growing polypeptide, held in the P site.

3. Formation of a peptide bond: With tRNA molecules occupying the P and A sites in the ribosome, an enzyme in the large ribosomal subunit forms a peptide (covalent) bond between the two adjacent amino acids resting atop their respective tRNAs. At this point, the two amino acids together comprise a *dipeptide*, which is held by the tRNA in the A site.

4. Translocation: After a peptide bond forms, the P site releases its tRNA, which no longer holds an amino acid. At the same time, the ribosome shifts the mRNA so that the third codon enters the ribosome. During this shifting process, called **translocation**, the tRNA located in the A site moves to the P site, leaving the A site empty. The next tRNA, which has an anticodon that is complementary to the third codon, enters the

THE NUCLEUS, DNA EXPRESSION, AND THE CELL CYCLE

71

- A — Amino Acid (methionine)
- B — tRNA
- C — Large Ribosomal Subunit
- D — mRNA
- E — Amino Acid
- F — Small Ribosomal Subunit
- G — Amino Acids
- H — Large Ribosomal Subunit

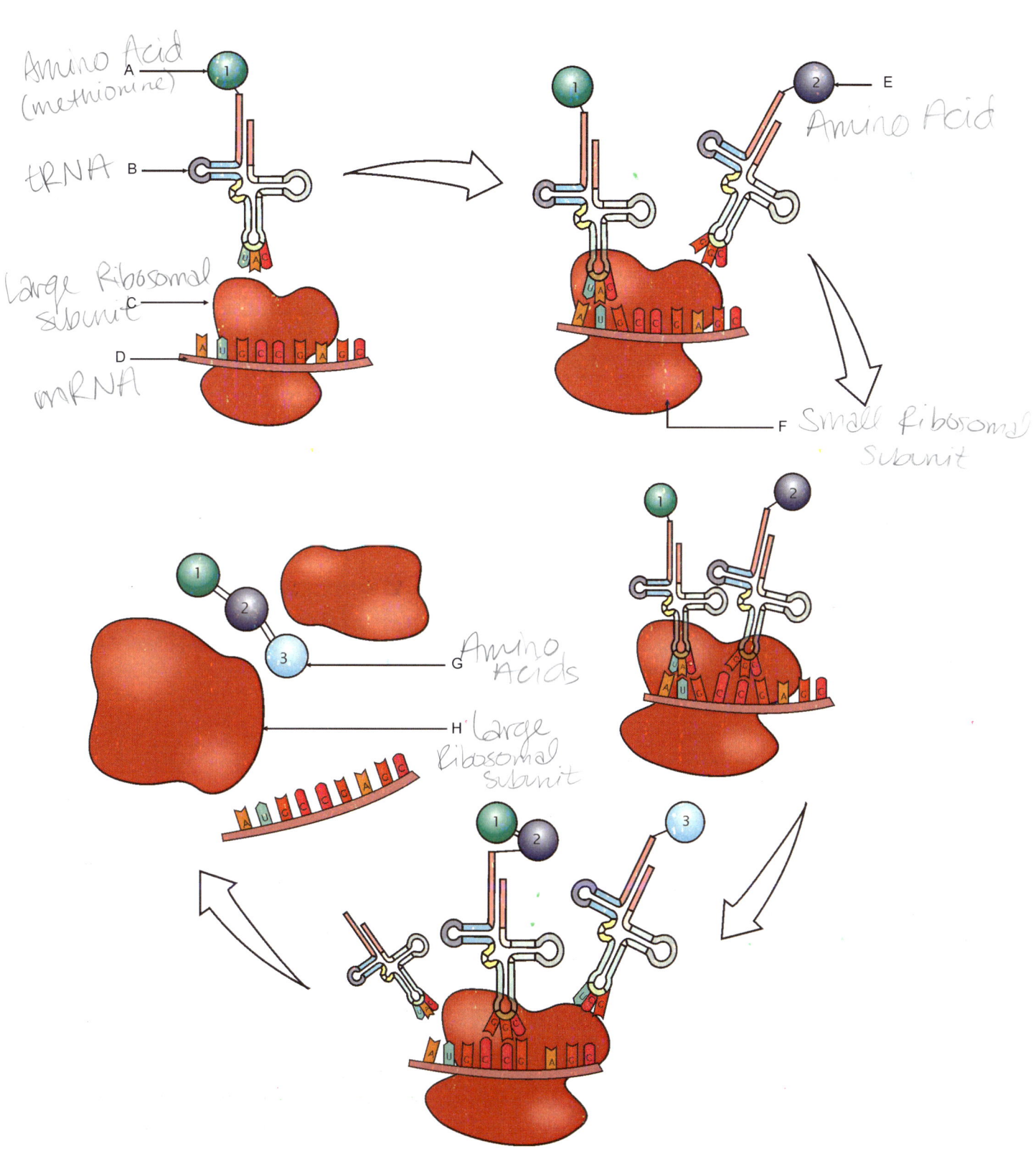

Figure 5-7. Translation

ribosome and binds to the A site. A peptide bond then forms between the second and third amino acids so that the dipeptide becomes a tripeptide, containing three amino acids. Translocation and peptide bond formation occur again and again resulting in an oligopeptide, and finally a polypeptide.

5. **The stop codon ends translation.** Translation ends when translocation pulls a "stop" codon (UGA, UAG, or UAA) into the A site of the ribosome. At that moment, the tRNA molecule located in the P site releases the polypeptide and detaches from the P site. The large and small ribosomal subunits then disconnect from one another and release the mRNA. The released polypeptide twists and coils to develop different levels of complexity and may perform a specific duty as one of the TRICCS proteins.

> **Note:** On average, a ribosome can form about 15 peptide bonds per second; therefore, it takes about 20 seconds for a ribosome to synthesize a typical protein consisting of 300 amino acids.

Each ribosomal subunit and RNA molecule mentioned above may participate in translation over one thousand times before finally wearing out. After detaching from mRNA, the ribosomal subunits are free to bind again to the same mRNA or they can bind to a different mRNA. Likewise, after detaching from a ribosome's P site, a tRNA is free to pick up another amino acid (specific for that tRNA) and bring it to either the same ribosome or a different ribosome. Furthermore, a single mRNA molecule can undergo translation by more than one ribosome at a time. When two or more ribosomes translate the same mRNA at the same time, the ribosomes collectively make up a **polyribosome**. A polyribosome enables a cell to generate large amounts of a specific protein in a relatively short amount of time with relatively few mRNA molecules.

Like all other compounds within a cell, the chemical components of translation have a limited life span. While some mRNA molecules may endure repeated translation for several hours or even a day or two before degrading, other mRNAs degrade and break apart after only a few minutes. The mechanisms responsible for this degradation are somewhat complicated, so let's just think of mRNA as being like a cotton thread that eventually wears out and breaks because we have been pulling it repeatedly through a bead (ribosome) or a series of beads (polyribosome). Of course, even the bead would wear out eventually. When needed, a cell can call upon its nucleus to synthesize new RNA molecules through transcription to replace the worn-out strands. Translation of specific mRNAs generates new ribosomal proteins, which enter the nucleus to become part of new ribosomal subunits.

Site of Protein Synthesis

What determines whether a cell synthesizes a particular protein in the cytosol (on a free ribosome) or on the rough ER? Interestingly, the synthesis of all proteins begins at free ribosomes, and then the ribosome either remains free in the cytosol to complete translation or attaches itself to the rough ER (becoming a bound ribosome) where it completes translation. If completion of translation is to occur at the rough ER, the first few amino acids to become part of the growing polypeptide function as a **leader sequence**. While the ribosome continues with translation, the leader sequence of the growing polypeptide attaches to a **signal recognition particle (SRP)** in the cytosol. The SRP then enables the ribosome to attach to a receptor site on the rough ER. As translation continues, the growing polypeptide chain enters the ER through a tiny pore at the receptor site. Proteins made in this way are modified inside the ER and Golgi complex. After incorporation into a vesicle that pinches off the Golgi complex, the new protein may be: (1) inside a lysosome; (2) inserted into the cell membrane, or (3) secreted into the extracellular fluid.

If completion of translation is to occur in the cytosol, the polypeptide may or may not have a leader sequence. (If a leader sequence is present, it has a different amino acid sequence than the one found on proteins completed at the rough ER.) If there is no leader sequence, the polypeptide will be completed at the free ribosome and remain in the cytosol. If a leader sequence is present, it will specify that the new polypeptide will enter the nucleus, a mitochondrion, or a peroxisome. In summary, the destination of proteins completed at free ribosomes depends on the presence or absence of a leader sequence. Moreover, the type of organelle into which some of these proteins enter depends on the specific type of leader sequence present on the polypeptide.

CELLULAR DIFFERENTIATION

Since the trillions of cells in a human body arise from a single cell (fertilized egg) and have virtually the same genes, how does the body come to possess more than 200 *different* kinds of cells? The answer relates primarily to how different cells utilize their genetic material. While all nucleated cells in the body have virtually the same genes, some kinds of cells transcribe certain genes that other types of cells do not transcribe. Consequently, some cells make certain types of proteins that other cells do not make. In other words, although cells may have the same kind of library (nucleus) with the same kinds of books (chromosomes), not every cell utilizes the same pages (genes) from those books. **Cellular differentiation** is the process by which similar cells become different from one another through the expression of different genes.

Cellular differentiation occurs primarily due to a cell's interaction with its extracellular environment. Let's consider how this happens. When a cell divides, the resulting daughter cells are genetically identical to the dividing (parent) cell. After repeated cell divisions, the cells cluster in masses so that some cells exist completely surrounded by other cells. Due in part to the accumulation of various cellular products in the extracellular fluid, cells in the middle of the cluster live surrounded by a slightly different chemical environment than cells along the edge of the cluster. Consequently, various chemicals may either activate or deactivate certain genes in some cells, while the same genes in other cells remain unaffected. In turn, cells that produce different types of proteins become structurally and functionally different from one another.

THE CELL CYCLE

A human body can grow, replace damaged and worn-out cells, and experience cellular differentiation only because many of its cells can reproduce themselves. **Cell division**, or cellular reproduction, results when a cell splits to form two new cells called **daughter cells**.

The series of events that occur in the life of a typical cell from the moment it forms until it divides comprise the **cell cycle**. The word "cycle" implies a return to a beginning point; in the cell cycle, daughter cells grow and divide producing more daughter cells, which in turn, grow and divide, and so on. A few types of cells, including neurons and skeletal muscle cells, do not divide; therefore, they do not go through a cell cycle.

In addition to body growth, cell replacement, and cellular differentiation, cell division is important because it maintains a high surface area to volume (SA/V) ratio for cells. Understanding this fact will help you understand why cells are so small. First, the plasma membrane represents the cell's surface area through which exchange of nutrients and wastes can occur. Second, as a cell grows larger, its volume and surface area both increase, but the surface area increases at a slower rate. Consequently, the SA/V for a large cell is *lower* than that of a smaller cell. This means that the larger cell has a smaller proportion of its mass (volume) exposed to the extracellular fluid than does the smaller cell. The larger cell may not have enough surface area through which to absorb nutrients or expel wastes in order to survive. By dividing in two, a cell can produce two daughter cells, each with a higher SA/V ratio than the dividing cell. In the following examples, you can see the effect of increasing size on the SA/V ratio of a cube-shaped cell.

1. A *small* cell is 1 unit long on each side and has a SA/V ratio of 6; i.e., it has 6 square units of SA for each cubic unit of volume.

$$\frac{\text{Surface area}}{\text{Volume}} = \frac{1 \times 1 \times 6 \text{ sides}}{1 \times 1 \times 1} = \frac{6 \text{ units}^2}{1 \text{ unit}^3}$$

2. A *medium*-sized cell is 2 units long on each side and has a SA/V ratio of 3; i.e, it has 3 square units of SA for each unit of volume.

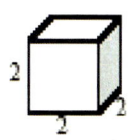

$$\frac{\text{Surface area}}{\text{Volume}} = \frac{2 \times 2 \times 6 \text{ sides}}{2 \times 2 \times 2} = \frac{24 \text{ units}^2}{8 \text{ unit}^3} = \frac{3 \text{ units}^2}{1 \text{ unit}^3}$$

The shape of a cell also influences it SA/V ratio. Consider a cell that is long and cylindrical. Notice that this cell has the same volume as the medium-sized cube-shaped cell, but has a larger SA/V ratio.

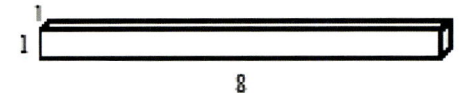

$$\frac{\text{Surface area} = (1\times8\times4\text{sides})+(1\times1\times2\text{ ends}) = 34 \text{ units}^2 = 4.3 \text{ units}^2}{\text{Volume} = 1\times1\times8 = 8 \text{ unit}^3 = 1 \text{ unit}^3}$$

In the lab you will calculate the SA/V ratios for cells of different size and shape, and also determine how the ratio affects a cell's ability to obtain nutrients and expel wastes.

The cell cycle involves three major phases: *interphase*, when the cell is growing and preparing for cell division; *mitosis*, when the cell's genetic material divides to form two nuclei; and *cytokinesis*, when the cell's cytoplasm divides to form two daughter cells. The length of time that a cell spends in each stage varies, but interphase is always the longest. Rapidly dividing epithelial cells in the intestine may spend 10-12 hours in interphase, but only an hour in mitosis and cytokinesis. At the other extreme, liver cells may spend a year or longer in interphase before they enter mitosis. We will now describe the major events that occur in a typical cell with a life cycle lasting about 24 hours. Figure 5-8 illustrates this typical cell cycle.

INTERPHASE

A typical cell spends most of its time in the cell cycle carrying out normal metabolic activities and preparing to divide. Because this part of the cell cycle includes cellular activities that occur between cell divisions, cell biologists refer to it as **interphase** (*inter-*, between). In our typical cell, interphase lasts 15-20 hours and includes three sub-phases: G_1, S, and G_2. The S stands for "synthesis," and denotes the time when the cell is synthesizing DNA molecules prior to mitosis. The G's stand for "gaps," which refer to the times before and after DNA replication but not does not include mitosis. To say that a cell is in G_1 phase suggests that the cell will eventually enter the S and G_2 phase. For this reason, cells that will not divide are in a **G_0 phase** (G zero).

G_1 phase

The **G_1 phase (1st gap phase)** lasts 8-10 hours and is the period between when the cell forms and the time it begins replicating DNA. During G_1 the chromatin inside the nucleus is uncoiled, allowing RNA polymerases to transcribe genes. The newly formed RNAs then leave the nucleus to participate in protein synthesis (translation) at ribosomes. Throughout G_1 phase, the cell grows and reproduces its organelles, ensuring that after cell division the daughter cells will have all the necessary cellular components they need to survive. Near the end of G_1, the cell replicates its centrosomes for use in mitosis.

S phase

The **S phase** (or DNA synthesis phase), which usually lasts 6-8 hours, is the period when the cell replicates each of the DNA molecules within the nucleus. During this phase, additional histone proteins generated at ribosomes enter the nucleus and bind with the newly synthesized DNA molecules to form new strands of chromatin. The nucleus of a human somatic cell entering the S phase contains 46 strands of chromatin; after S phase, the nucleus contains 92 strands of chromatin. Replicating the DNA molecules ensures that the future daughter cells will each have 46 strands of chromatin containing the same genetic information as that in the parent cell. This is crucial, since the daughter cells will need to synthesize different types of proteins to build cellular components and perform normal metabolic activities.

G_2 phase

The **G_2 phase** is the time after DNA replication when the cell makes final preparations for mitosis. Protein synthesis continues and the cell is still growing. The centrioles complete their replication and the nuclear membrane is still intact. The genetic material is still in the form of chromatin, but not yet visible with a light microscope. (Recall that each strand of chromatin consists of a double helix DNA molecule wrapped around clusters of histone proteins to form a chain of nucleosomes.) However, due to DNA replication in S phase, the 46 strands of chromatin from G_1 phase

THE NUCLEUS, DNA EXPRESSION, AND THE CELL CYCLE

have become 92 strands of chromatin. The G_2 phase lasts 4-6 hours.

MITOSIS

During **mitosis** (mī-TŌ-sis) the replicated genetic material condenses and separates so that a copy of each original DNA molecule moves to opposite ends of the cell, yielding two identical nuclei. This process ensures that each daughter cell, formed later during cytokinesis, will have the same genetic material as its parent cell. Mitosis lasts about 2 hours in a typical cell and involves *prophase*, *metaphase*, *anaphase*, and *telophase*.

Prophase

Mitosis begins with **prophase**, when replicated strands of chromatin condense, centrosomes migrate, the mitotic spindle develops, and the nuclear membrane dismantles. During early prophase, the strands of chromatin undergo *condensation*, during which the nucleosomes coil repeatedly to form tighter and larger loops that eventually become visible under the light microscope. By the end of prophase, each strand of chromatin is fully condensed and called a **chromatid**. The two identical chromatids (called *sister* chromatids) resulting from the replication of a single strand of chromatin remain attached to one another at a region called the **centromere** (SEN-tro-mēr). Two sister chromatids held together by a centromere make up a **replicated chromosome**.

Why is it important to condense the DNA during prophase? Condensing the chromatin in prophase makes it easier for a cell to organize and separate its genetic material prior to cytokinesis. However, when tightly packed into chromosomes, the DNA's genetic information is inaccessible to the cell to use for protein synthesis. In contrast, when a cell is not preparing to divide, the DNA molecule remains uncoiled and only loosely associated with the histone proteins, making the genetic information available for use in protein synthesis. Condensing 92 strands of chromatin into 46 replicated chromosomes is like coiling 92 long cotton threads around 46 spools to make them easier to manage until you need them later for sewing.

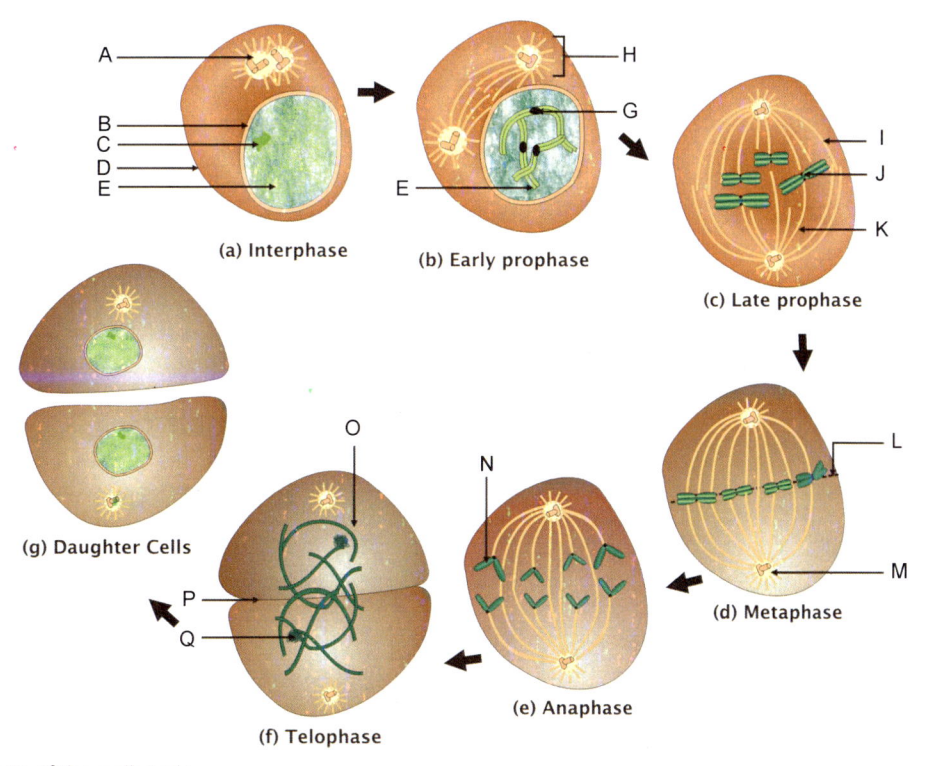

Figure 5-8. Parts of the cell cycle

While chromatin condenses to form chromosomes, the other events that occur during prophase prepare the way for separating the sister chromatids from one another. First, the two centrosomes (replicated from a single centrosome during G₁ phase) begin assembling microtubules. Some of these microtubules, called *polar fibers*, connect the two centrosomes to each other. As the polar fibers lengthen, they push the two centrosomes to opposite ends (poles) of the cell. Other microtubules, called *kinetochore fibers*, extend from both centrosomes and bind to each chromosome. The polar and kinetochore fibers together constitute the **mitotic spindle**. The two sister chromatids of each chromosome face different poles; thus, each sister chromatid normally binds only to kinetochore fibers originating from the centrosome they face. The **kinetochore** (ki-NE-tō-kor) is a protein-rich site on each chromatid that anchors a kinetochore fiber, and it is located in the centromere region of the chromosome. Near the end of prophase, the nuclear membrane dismantles, leaving the chromosomes suspended in the cytoplasm. This event will allow the sister chromatids to separate in a later phase of mitosis.

Metaphase

During **metaphase**, the replicated chromosomes align themselves along the equator or middle of the mitotic spindle. While aligned in this manner, the chromosomes occupy a region called the *metaphase plate*. During metaphase, the chromosomes jerk back and forth along the metaphase plate. This movement suggests that the kinetochores are attempting to pull the chromatids toward opposite poles.

Anaphase

During **anaphase**, the sister chromatids pull apart and move toward opposite poles. To separate sister chromatids from one another, special enzymes must break the connection at the centromere. After this happens, motor molecules located in the kinetochores pull the sister chromatids, now called *sister chromosomes*, along the kinetochore fibers toward their respective poles. As the chromosomes move, the kinetochore fibers become shorter by losing tubulin subunits in the region of the kinetochore. A chromosome moving toward a centromere appears V-shaped, with its kinetochore at the "point" leading the way. At the same time, other motor molecules interacting with the polar fibers cause the centrosomes to move farther apart, which also helps pull the sister chromosomes apart. This action also lengthens the cell as it prepares to pinch in two.

Telophase

Telophase (TĒ-lō-fāz; *telo*, end), the last phase of mitosis, begins when all sister chromosomes stop moving having reached their respective poles around the centrosomes. The cell now has two identical sets of 46 chromosomes at opposite ends of the cell. During telophase, the mitotic spindle disassembles and vesicles in the cytoplasm collect around the masses of chromosomes and fuse to form nuclear envelopes; the cell now has two nuclei. Shortly thereafter, proteins enter the nuclei through newly constructed nuclear pores and bind with rRNA molecules to form nucleoli. In addition, the chromosomes uncoil to become fine strands of chromatin that RNA polymerases can transcribe for protein synthesis. The only thing left to do to complete the cell cycle is to divide the cytoplasm to form two cells.

> **Note**: A fully condensed chromosome during mitosis is about 10,000 times shorter than it is when existing as an uncoiled strand of chromatin during G₁ phase of interphase.

CYTOKINESIS

Cytokinesis (sī-tō-kin-Ē-sis) is the last part of the cell cycle and involves division of the cytoplasm into two cells. Usually beginning in late anaphase, cytokinesis begins when a **cleavage furrow** or indentation forms around the cell's midsection perpendicular to the mitotic spindle. The cleavage furrow develops when a *contraction ring*, consisting of actin microfilaments with associated myosin motor molecules, squeezes inward on the cytoplasm as if someone were tightening a belt around the cell. As the contraction ring tightens, the cleavage furrow deepens and eventually pinches the cell in two, forming two daughter cells. Because the

THE NUCLEUS, DNA EXPRESSION, AND THE CELL CYCLE

contraction ring is perpendicular to the mitotic spindle, each daughter cell contains a nucleus. The daughter cells are genetically identical to each other and the parent cell, although they are smaller than the parent cell. After cytokinesis, each daughter cell is in G$_1$ phase.

> **Note**: Remember that mitosis is nuclear division and cytokinesis is *cytoplasmic* division.

CLOSER LOOK AT DNA REPLICATION

To understand how daughter cells produced during cell division will be genetically identical to one another, we need take a closer look at how DNA replicates itself. To some extent, DNA replication resembles gene transcription in which an enzyme uses the DNA molecule as a template when forming an RNA molecule. However, unlike transcription, which utilizes only one strand of the DNA's double helix as a template, DNA replication utilizes both strands.

DNA replication is a very precise process, producing two identical DNA molecules that are exact replicas of the original DNA molecule. However, after replication, the original (copied) DNA molecule no longer exists, but its two strands of DNA nucleotides form half of the new DNA molecules. Since this method of replication preserves half of the original DNA molecule in each new DNA molecule, biochemists refer to it as **semiconservative replication** (see Figure 5-9).

Before replication can begin, the parallel strands of the original DNA molecule must separate so that enzymes can "read" their nitrogenous bases while building new complimentary DNA strands. An enzyme called **helicase** (HĒ-li-kās) "unzips" the DNA molecule by breaking hydrogen bonds between complimentary base pairs holding the double helix together. The Y-shaped region where a helicase is unzipping the DNA is *a replication fork*. More than one helicase can work on a DNA molecule at one time, resulting in numerous replication forks. This allows other enzymes responsible for replication to attach to different regions of the same DNA molecule, thus speeding up the replication process.

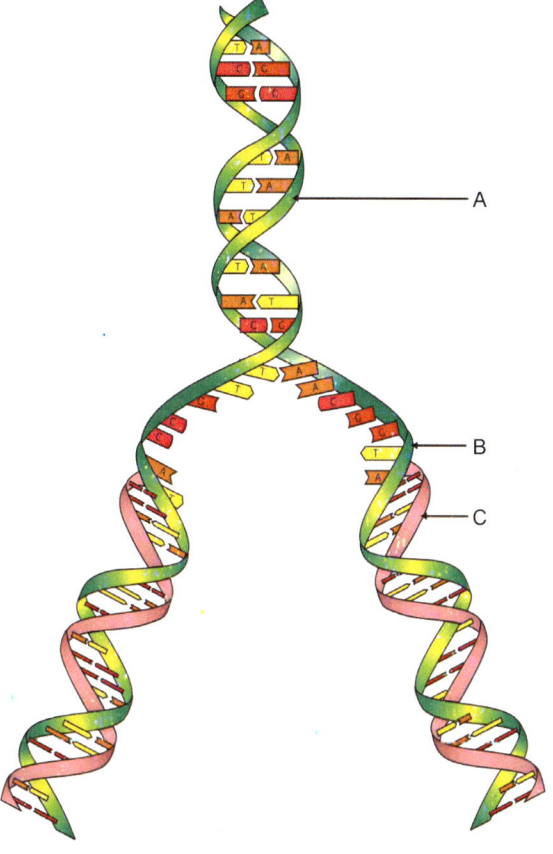

Figure 5-9. Semiconservative replication

After a helicase separates the DNA's double helix into two strands (DNA *templates*), several different enzymes must bind to the templates before replication of the templates can occur. One of these enzymes, called a **primase**, first brings in RNA nucleotides that are complimentary to the exposed DNA nucleotides on the template. Linking these RNA nucleotides together, the primase forms a short segment called the **RNA primer**. Once the RNA primer is in place, another enzyme, **DNA polymerase III**, moves in next to the primer. While moving along the DNA template, the DNA polymerase III pulls in free DNA nucleotides from the nucleoplasm and bonds them (via H-bonds) with complementary nucleotides on the DNA template. DNA polymerase III also forms covalent bonds between the new DNA nucleotides.

DNA polymerase can move along a DNA template only toward the template's 5' end; therefore, synthesis of a new DNA polymer occurs only in a 5' to 3' direction. As figure 5-10 shows, one template

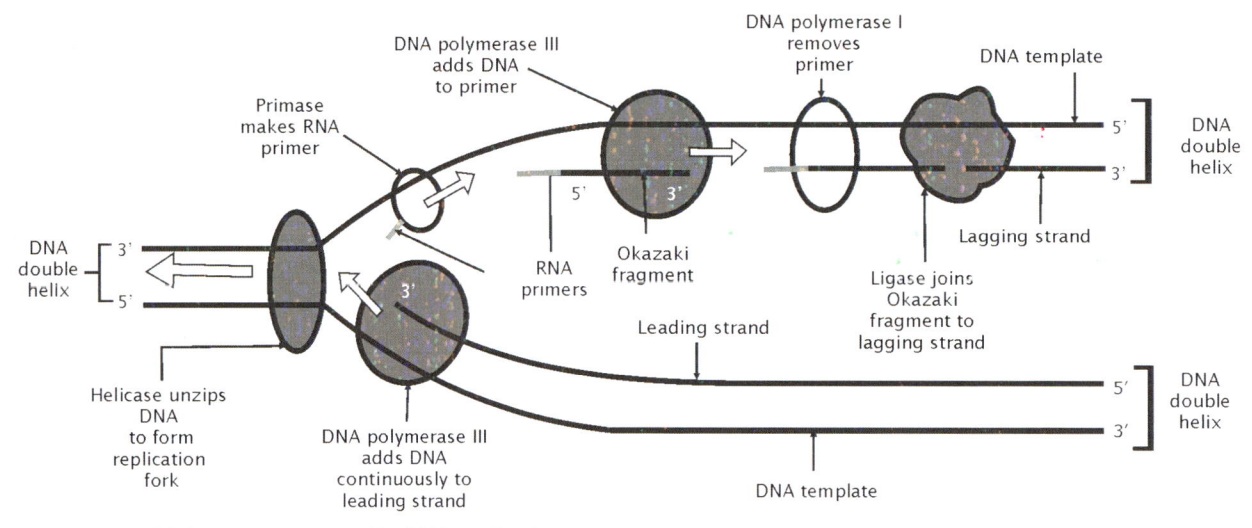

Figure 5-10. Major enzymes used in DNA replication

is replicated continuously in the direction of the replication fork; the new DNA polymer formed on this template is called the leading *strand*. The other template is replicated in short segments, called **Okazaki** (ō-ka-SOK-ē) **fragments**, away from the replication fork, but still in a 5' to 3' direction. The new DNA polymer formed on this template is the *lagging strand*. Before Okazaki fragments can join together to elongate the lagging strand, a different polymerase, **DNA polymerase I**, must first remove the RNA primers. After this happens, yet another enzyme, **DNA ligase** (LĪ-gās; *liga*, to join), must move in to join the Okazaki fragment to the lagging strand. Figure 5-10 shows the role of the major enzymes used in DNA replication.

DNA proofreading: To transfer genetic material accurately from parent cell to daughter cells, DNA replication must occur "letter for letter" without any mistakes. How can there be replication of a typical cell's several million genes, some of which contain several thousand nucleotide bases, with virtually no copying errors? The answer lies with yet another type of enzyme, **DNA polymerase II**, which moves along the leading and lagging strands to check the accuracy of the pairing between the new nucleotides and the DNA template. This process is called **DNA proofreading**. If DNA polymerase II detects a pairing mistake, such as A-G or T-C, it clips out the wrong nucleotide and brings in another one to pair with the complementary base on the template. Proofreading reduces the chance that daughter cells will inherit genetic mistakes (mutations) that could impair their ability to synthesize certain proteins.

Note: DNA proofreading fails to correct only about one error for every ten million base pairs replicated.

MUTATIONS

A **mutation** is a change in the base sequence of a gene. Since the order of the DNA triplets determines the order of amino acids in a protein, a change in the order of bases could have adverse effects on a protein's composition. Mutations include *substitutions*, *insertions*, and *deletions*.

A **substitution** mutation involves changing (substituting) one nitrogenous base in a triplet. As a result, a single amino acid in the resulting polypeptide may change, but the other amino acids are unaffected. However, since more than one codon can code for the same amino acid, a substitution mutation may have no effect on the amino acid sequence at all. Consider the sentence below that contains only 3-letter words. Substituting an "A" for the first "E" in the following sentence changes the sentence slightly, but the meaning is still understood.

TH**E**-CAT-ATE-THE-RAT
becomes
TH**A**-CAT-ATE-THE-RAT

THE NUCLEUS, DNA EXPRESSION, AND THE CELL CYCLE

Now let's consider how a single substitution mutation can alter a single gene triplet sequence. First, let's assume we have the following DNA sequence and its corresponding transcription and translation products:

DNA: CAT-CAT–CAT
mRNA: GUA-GUA-GUA
Polypeptide: Valine-Valine-Valine

Now, if a cytosine substitutes for the first adenine, notice how the amino acid sequence changes:

DNA: CAT-CAT–CAT
Mutation: **CCT**-CAT–CAT
mRNA: **GGA**-GUA–GUA
Polypeptide: **glycine**-valine-valine

This alteration of the protein's primary structure could also alter its secondary and tertiary structure, thereby, preventing it from functioning normally. An example of a substitution mutation is **sickle-cell anemia**. Hemoglobin (Hb) is a quaternary protein consisting of four of tertiary proteins. Each protein is 150 amino acids long. At a single location in two of these tertiary proteins, valine substitutes for glutamic acid, due to a single substitution in the gene coding for these proteins. This causes the hemoglobin to change the cell's shape when [oxygen] is low, resulting in clogged blood vessels.

An **insertion** mutation causes the reading sequence to shift, which can significantly affect the codon sequence and, ultimately the amino acid sequence in the protein. Notice how the insertion of an "A" after the first H in the following sentence greatly affects the meaning of the sentence:

TH**E**-CAT-ATE-THE-RAT
becomes
TH**A**-ECA-TAT-ETH-ERA

A **deletion** mutation occurs when a nucleotide is removed from the gene. Deletions also cause a shift in the reading sequence of the gene. In our example, a deletion of the first E greatly affects the meaning of the sentence:

TH**E**-CAT-ATE-THE-RAT
becomes
THC-ATA-TET-HER-AT

Insertions and deletions are **frameshift mutations** because they cause shifts in the reading sequence of the nucleotide bases. Substances that cause mutations are called *mutagens*. Mutagens that cause cancer are classified as *carcinogenic* (kar-sen-ō-JEN-ik).

CONTROL OF THE CELL CYCLE

A number of factors, both outside and inside a cell, are important in determining whether a cell will divide or not. Just as certain hormones and other chemicals released from surrounding cells can determine which genes a cell will transcribe, similar extracellular factors may either cause or prevent cell division. In addition, when normal dividing cells touch one another, they stop dividing. This external factor, called contact inhibition, is not a characteristic of cancer cells; therefore, cancer cells can divide uncontrollably producing large masses of abnormal cells (*tumors*) that can invade and destroy healthy tissues.

In recent years, cell biologists discovered that cells have a cell-cycle control system that operates through negative feedback and involves "molecular road blocks" at various stages or checkpoints in the cell's life. In other words, a cell will not proceed past a certain stage in its life cycle unless the cell-cycle control system gives the "Go ahead" signal. For example, if nutrient deficiency or other factor prevents a cell from doubling its size, the cell will not enter S phase. Furthermore, a cell will not enter G_2 and mitosis until the S phase is complete. The stop signal between G_1 and S phase allowing the cell to "check" its size prevents cells that are too small from dividing. This control mechanism prevents future daughter cells from becoming smaller than previous daughter cells. The stop signal between S phase and mitosis allowing the cell to check the status of DNA replication ensures that daughter cells have the same genetic material as the parent cell.

A major intracellular stimulus that causes a cell to proceed into different stages of the cell cycle involves the interaction of two groups of proteins: cyclins and certain enzymes called *cyclin-dependent kinases*. **Cyclins** (SĪ-klinz) are so-named because their concentrations fluctuate (cycle) in a regular pattern during the cell cycle. Cyclin concentration increases steadily during interphase and drops off dramatically at the end of cell division. **Cyclin-dependent kinases (Cdks)** have

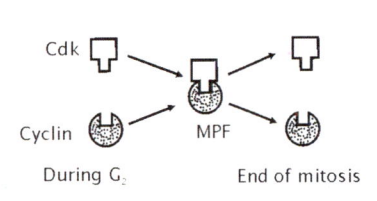

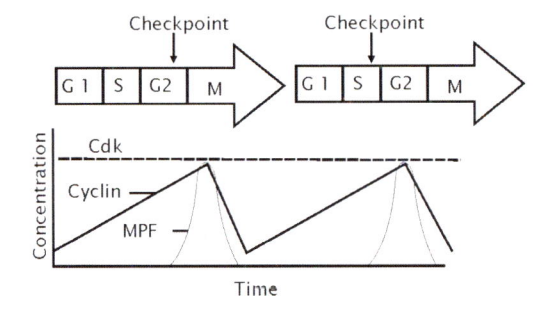

Figure 5-11. Regulation of the Cell Cycle

a relatively constant concentration throughout the cell cycle. Binding a certain cyclin with a certain Cdk produces a protein complex called **mitosis-promoting factor (MPF)** that can stimulate the cell to proceed into mitosis. After mitosis and cytokinesis, the MPF breaks apart and enzymes break down the cyclin. Then throughout interphase, cyclin concentrations increase until the cell can produce enough MPF to trigger the next mitotic division. Regulation of the cell cycle is illustrated in Figure 5-11.

PREDETERMINED LIMITS ON CELL DIVISION

Even under the best extracellular conditions, most human cells have a genetic limit on how many times they can divide. Current research has identified the length of *telomeres* on chromosomes as one explanation for this limit on cell division. A **telomere** (TĒ-lō-mēr) is a repeating sequence of DNA nucleotides located at each end of a chromosome. In human telomeres, the repeating base sequence is TTAGGG, and it may repeat as many as 2000 times. Telomeres do not code for proteins, but serve three important functions: (1) enable DNA polymerases to replicate genes near the ends of a DNA molecule; (2) protect the ends of the DNA molecule against degradation by certain enzymes located in the nucleus; and (3) prevent the ends of chromosomes from sticking together.

A decrease in telomere length over time will ultimately prevent a cell from dividing and can lead to cell death. During each S phase, the end of a telomere may lose about 15 TTAGGG segments because DNA polymerase is unable to replicate them. (The reason for this failure to replicate is that DNA polymerase cannot position itself properly near the end of the telomere.) If a telomere early in life began with 2000 repeating segments, there would be none left after 133 cell divisions. When a telomere becomes too short, certain proteins in the nucleus prevent the replication of the DNA molecules; consequently, the cell can no longer divide. Furthermore, without telomeres to protect them, functional genes near the end of a chromosome are more susceptible to damage.

As you have seen, the world of the cell is small but complex. However, like the crafted gears of a fine-tuned clock, the intricate components of the cell carry out their activities with amazing precision. Since every tissue and organ relies upon cells to function, the details you remember from this chapter will serve as a solid foundation for all chapters ahead. In the next chapter, you will learn about the body's tissues or groups of cells working together.

TOPICS TO KNOW FOR CHAPTER 5 (THE NUCLEUS, DNA EXPRESSION, AND THE CELL CYCLE)

3' end
5' end
A site
anaphase
anticodon
anucleate
autosomes
carcinogenic
cell cycle
cell division
cellular differentiation
central dogma of molecular biology
centromere
chromatid
chromatin
chromatin condensation
chromosome number
chromosomes
cleavage furrow
codons
contact inhibition
contraction ring
control of the cell cycle
cyclin-dependent kinases
cyclins
cytokinesis
daughter cells
deletion mutation
diploid number
direction of DNA replication
direction of RNA transcription
DNA expression
DNA ligase
DNA polymerase I
DNA polymerase II
DNA polymerase III
DNA proofreading
DNA replication
DNA template

exons
frameshift mutation
G0 phase
G1 phase
G2 phase
genes
genetic code
genetic material
genome
haploid number
helicase
histones
humans' 1N number
humans' 2N number
insertion mutation
interphase
introns
kinetochore
kinetochore fibers,
leader sequence
maternal chromosomes
messenger RNA
metaphase
metaphase plate
methionine
mitosis
mitosis-promoting factor
mitotic spindle
mRNA processing
multinucleate
mutagens
mutation
nuclear envelope
nuclear pores
nucleolus
nucleoplasm
nucleosome
nucleus
Okazaki fragments

one gene-one polypeptide theory
P site
paternal chromosomes
polar fibers
polyribosome
predetermined limits on cell division
primase
promoter
prophase
replicated chromosome
replication fork
ribosomal RNA
RNA polymerase
RNA primer
RNA transcript
S phase
semiconservative replication
sex chromosome
sickle-cell anemia
signal recognition particle
sister chromatids
sister chromosomes
start codon
steps in translation
stop codon
substitution
surface area to volume ratio
telomere
telophase
terminator
transcription
transcription factors
transfer RNA
translocation
triplets
tumors
uninucleate

CHAPTER 6

Membrane Structure and Function

The **plasma membrane**, or **cell membrane**, separates the cytoplasm from the surrounding extracellular fluid (ECF). The fluid part of the cytoplasm, called the **cytosol** (SĪ-to-sōl), has different chemical properties than the ECF, and maintaining these differences is essential to the life of a cell. The plasma membrane maintains the cytosol's chemical properties by regulating the types and amounts of molecules that enter or leave the cell. Moreover, features on the surface of the plasma membrane enable cells to interact with each other. Often, these surface features allow the cell to respond in a specific way when chemical triggers (such as hormones) appear in the ECF.

A cell's plasma membrane isn't a solid sheet like the transparent plastic wrap that you might use to cover a dish of leftovers. Like a mosaic, a picture made of tiny pieces, the plasma membrane is an assembly of macromolecules. In fact, it behaves more like a liquid because the plasma membrane's individual pieces can spin around and slide past each other. For this reason, biochemists call plasma membranes *fluid mosaics*. The structure and composition of a plasma membrane isn't static, either. Molecules constantly shuttle back and forth between the cytoplasm and plasma membrane. This steady flow of "molecular traffic" promotes survival, allowing a cell to change the make up of its plasma membrane in order to adapt to changing conditions. Look at Figure 6-1 to see the fluid mosaic plasma membrane.

MEMBRANE LIPIDS

Lipids account for less than half of the plasma membrane's *weight*, but they account for about 99 percent of the membrane's molecules. The two most abundant lipids in the plasma membrane of a human cell are phospholipids and cholesterol.

Phospholipids: A plasma membrane is a bilayer (two layers) of phospholipid molecules. Half of the bilayer faces the ECF while the other half faces the cytosol. Other macromolecules tunnel through the bilayer or cling to either face. Phospholipids are *amphipathic*, having parts that have opposite or dissimilar chemical properties. Each phospholipid molecule has a polar, hydrophilic ("water-loving") head made of glycerol and two nonpolar, hydrophobic ("water-fearing") tails made of long fatty-acid chains.

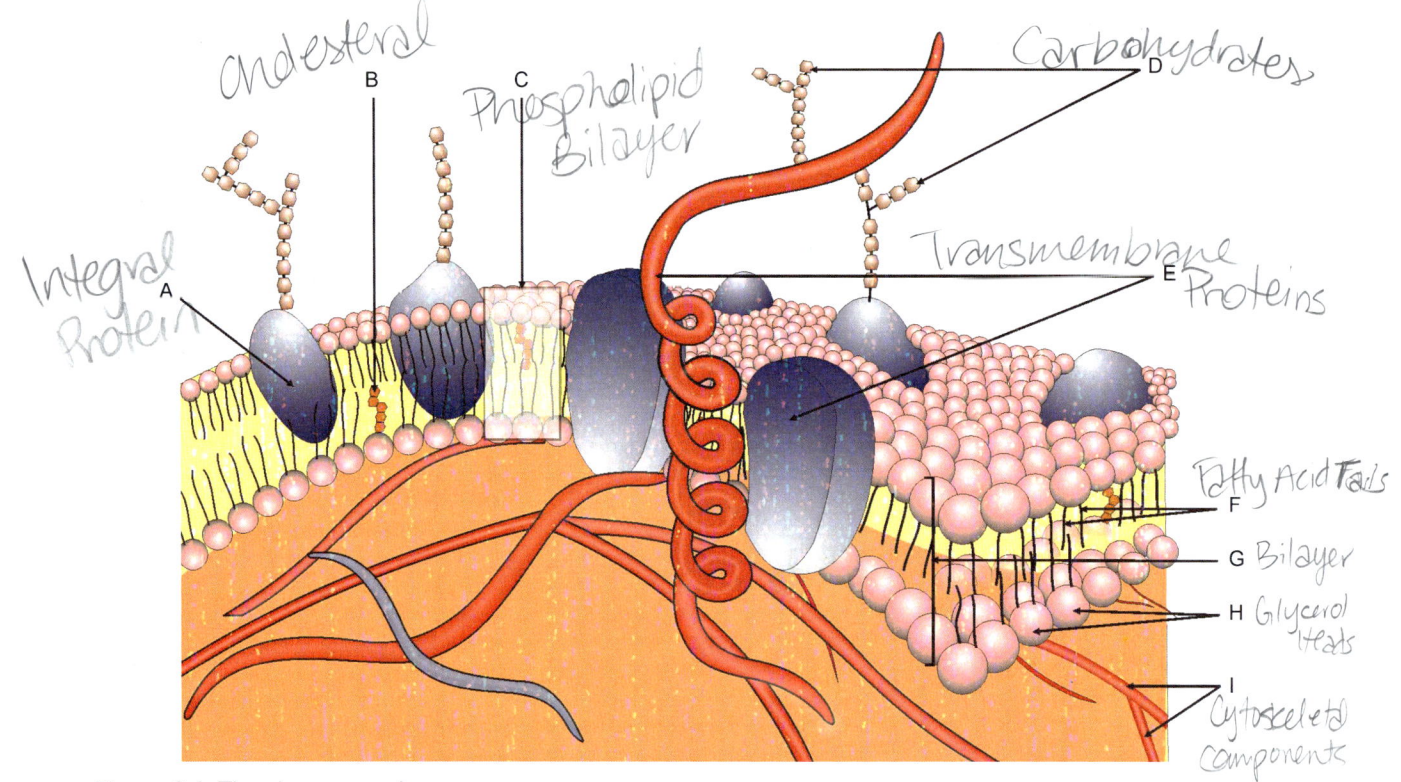

Figure 6-1. The plasma membrane

The amphipathic properties of phospholipid molecules enable them to self-organize into a bilayer. The slender fatty-acid tails cluster together in the center of the bilayer, forming a hydrophobic zone that squeezes out water and water-soluble substances. At the same time, the hydrophilic heads seek out the watery extracellular fluid or cytosol. The combined hydrophobic and hydrophilic attractions "pull" the bilayer into shape. But since the phospholipid molecules do not chemically bond to each other, they are free to spin on their axes and slide past one another, actions that give the plasma membrane its fluid properties. Membrane phospholipids rarely turn somersaults, however, so they do not flip-flop from one face of a bilayer to the other.

> **Note:** Model the lipid bilayer by drawing together the fingertips on each hand, and then move both hands together so the facing fingertips overlap near the distal finger joints. Since fatty-acid tails are always moving, wiggle your fingers a bit to set the model in motion.

Functionally, the amphipathic qualities of phospholipids are what make the plasma membrane an effective chemical barrier. The hydrophobic zone at the membrane's center largely prevents water molecules and water-soluble substances (including ions) from darting back and forth between the extracellular fluid and cytosol. At the same time, the polar hydrophilic heads on each face of the membrane tend to repel fat-soluble and non-ionized substances. The fluid-like nature of the plasma membrane is due primarily to the phospholipid molecules, and is important to the cell in three ways:

- A plasma membrane is self-repairing: Imagine the glycerol heads of the phospholipids as an unbroken sheet of ping-pong balls floating in a bucket of water. The balls move apart if you plunge your hand into the water then come together again as you pull back your hand. Like the ping-pong balls, if a few phospholipid molecules are bumped apart in the bilayer, they pull back together quickly, resealing the membrane.

- A plasma membrane is flexible: Membrane fluidity enables a cell to ingest large particles, to change shape, and to divide during cellular reproduction. A white blood cell, for example, traps invading microorganisms by encircling them with its plasma

MEMBRANE STRUCTURE AND FUNCTION

membrane. Oxygen-carrying red blood cells can squeeze through the narrowest blood vessels without rupturing. When it is time for a cell to reproduce, the plasma membrane's fluidity allows the cell to pinch itself in two without exposing the cytoplasm to the extracellular fluid.

- **A plasma membrane readily changes size**: Because "fat attracts fat," new phospholipids easily join the plasma membrane. You can witness a similar process by observing how the tiny fat droplets on the surface of a bowl of hot chicken soup eventually combine into a few large fat globules. The cytoplasm inserts or retrieves phospholipids from the plasma membrane in tiny hollow spheres called *vesicles*. In this way, the plasma membrane can enlarge as the cell grows, or it can supply molecules for use elsewhere inside the cell.

Cholesterol: Like tiny cars wedged between trucks in a parking lot, slender cholesterol molecules tuck themselves between the larger phospholipids along both faces of the plasma membrane. Given the frequent new reports about the dangers of excessive levels of cholesterol in the blood, is the cholesterol in a cell's plasma membrane a good thing? The answer is yes, because cholesterol stabilizes the fluidity of the membrane when the temperature changes. At low temperatures, fatty acids tend to pack together and stiffen. (This is why butter, which is high in fat, hardens in the refrigerator.) On a frigid day, a skin cell may be far colder than the body's core temperature. However, cholesterol in the skin cell's plasma membrane prevents membrane phospholipids from bunching up, keeping the membrane flexible. This is one reason why your skin doesn't quickly crack open when exposed to freezing temperatures.

Cholesterol also stabilizes the plasma membrane when the cell is warmer than the body's average temperature. At higher temperatures, fatty acids become even more fluid-like. (This is why butter melts in a pan on the stove.) So why doesn't the plasma membrane of skin cells "melt" if you have a fever or if you soak in a hot bath? In these situations, cholesterol molecules act like tiny anchors, snagging nearby fatty acid tails of the phospholipid molecules and slowing their side-to-side movement within the membranes. As you might have guessed, a cell controls the stiffness of its plasma membrane by adding or removing cholesterol molecules as conditions change.

MEMBRANE CARBOHYDRATES

A host of carbohydrates extends like tree branches from the extracellular face of the plasma membrane. Membrane carbohydrates are typically **oligosaccharides** (ol-i-gō-SAK-ar-īdz; *oligo*, few), short chains of simple sugars. Some oligosaccharides bond directly to membrane phospholipids forming **glycolipids**. More often, however, oligosaccharides bond to proteins that project from the membrane, forming **glycoproteins**.

All of the carbohydrate molecules that project from the extracellular face of the plasma membrane comprise the cell's **glycocalyx** (glī-kō-KĀ-lix; *glyco*, sugar; *calyx*, coat). The configuration of the glycocalyx differs according to cell type. Hence, the glycocalyx, along with proteins in the plasma membrane, give a cell a distinctive chemical nature by which other cells recognize it. The glycocalyx is the basis of *cellular recognition*, which guides how cells join to form distinct tissues and organs. The body's immune system cells also rely on cellular recognition to detect and kill "foreign" cells, such as bacteria, that may enter the body.

The importance of the plasma membrane's glycocalyx cannot be overstated. The body begins forming because a sperm cell recognizes the glycocalyx of an ovum (egg cell). Liver cells stay put in the liver because their glycocalyces (glī-kō-KĀ-li-sēz) hold them together. Too, the presence (or absence) of specific oligosaccharides in the glycocalyx of red blood cells determines a person's blood type. If someone receives an incompatible blood type during a transfusion, the recipient's immune system identifies the donated blood cells as having "foreign" glycocalyces and destroys them.

In addition to cellular recognition, the glycocalyx also protects cells from damage. For example, water readily sticks to the glycocalyx and makes the surface of some cells very slippery. The glycocalyx greatly reduces friction as red blood cells slide past one another inside tiny blood vessels. A slippery glycocalyx also allows certain white blood cells to squeeze out of blood vessels and prowl through the surrounding tissues in search of invading microorganisms and viruses.

MEMBRANE PROTEINS

Although not nearly as numerous as lipid molecules, proteins contribute more than 50 percent of the plasma membrane's weight. Each type of protein in the membrane has a unique size, shape, and chemical structure that is suited to its particular role.

Classification by Location

Cell biologists divide plasma membrane proteins into two categories based on their physical relationship to the membrane.

- **Integral proteins** anchor to the inner, hydrophobic layer of the membrane and tend to bob up and down between the phospholipid molecules like buoys in a harbor. Some integral proteins penetrate only part way through the bilayer, but most are *transmembrane proteins*, which span the membrane from the cytosol to the extracellular fluid.

- **Peripheral proteins** are completely outside the bilayer. They attach to the projecting ends of integral proteins or to lipid "anchors" sunk in between the phospholipids. Some peripheral proteins face the cytosol, while others face the extracellular fluid.

Classification by Function

In addition to location, cell biologists classify membrane proteins according to their functions as *channels, carriers, receptors, enzymes, adhesion proteins*, or *markers*. Read the following descriptions of these proteins and see them illustrated in Figure 6-2.

- **Channels** are tunnel-like transmembrane proteins through which molecules enter or leave the cell. Some channels are always open, like the entrance to a cave. Other channels have door-like "gates" that open and close in response to certain stimuli. Selected molecules move freely through open channels, without the need of energy from ATP. The movement of molecules through channels is like water flowing down an open drain.

- **Carriers** are transmembrane proteins that change shape and, by so doing, move a selected molecule across the membrane. Instead of opening a gate to let a substance pass through the membrane by itself, a carrier "escorts" the substance through the membrane. Most organic nutrients, such as glucose and amino acids, move into the cell with the help of carriers. Some carriers require energy from ATP to change shape, but others do not.

- **Receptors** are integral proteins that act like chemical switches that turn cellular processes on or off. To do this, a specific molecule in the extracellular fluid must attach to a receptor. After the right molecule attaches, the receptor changes shape, triggering chemical reactions within the membrane or cytosol.

- **Enzymes** are peripheral or integral proteins that catalyze (speed up) chemical reactions. The enzyme's substrate-binding site faces either the cytosol or the extracellular fluid (but not both). Most membrane enzymes perform hydrolysis reactions that break large molecules into smaller products.

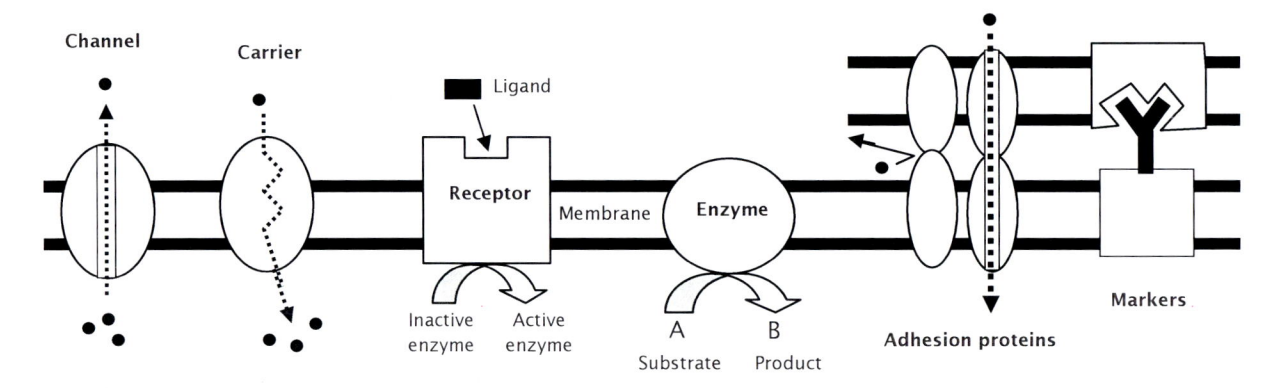

Figure 6-2. Membrane proteins classified by function

MEMBRANE STRUCTURE AND FUNCTION

- **Adhesion (linker) proteins** are integral proteins that bind cells to each other or to other structures in the extracellular fluid. Some adhesion proteins act like tiny "spot welds" that hold cells together. Other adhesion proteins look like thick belts around a cell's midsection and prevent molecules from slipping between the plasma membranes of adjacent cells. Still other adhesion proteins have channel-like properties that allow molecules to pass directly from one cell into another cell.

- **Markers (recognition proteins)** are integral proteins with attached oligosaccharides that act like cellular "I.D. tags." Except for identical twins, the protein markers on a person's cells are unique to each individual. Protein markers allow a person's immune system to recognize cells belonging to that person's body. Without these "self" markers, the immune system would attack the body's own cells.

> **Note:** While **TRICCS** can help you remember the functional classification of all proteins (see Chapter 2), use **CCREAM** to recall the functions of plasma membrane proteins: **C**hannels, **C**arriers, **R**eceptors, **E**nzymes, **A**dhesion proteins, **M**arkers.

MEMBRANE TRANSPORT

Now that you are familiar with the plasma membrane and the organization of the cytoplasm, it is appropriate to describe how the plasma membrane allows the cytoplasm to interact with the extracellular fluid. This section deals with **membrane transport**, the movement of materials across the plasma membrane. To maintain homeostasis, the plasma membrane must be highly selective in what it allows to pass into and out of the cell; in other words, the plasma membrane must have selective *permeability*.

MEMBRANE PERMEABILITY

The ability of a membrane to allow substances to pass through it is called **permeability**. A permeable membrane allows substances to pass through it, whereas an impermeable membrane does not. The plasma membrane is permeable to some things but impermeable to others; therefore, it is *semipermeable* or *selectively permeable*. Semipermeability allows the plasma membrane to regulate what gets into and out of the cell, much like a border crossing between two countries. Security guards and gates allow certain people and automobiles to cross the border but prohibit others from doing so. Similarly, phospholipids and integral proteins allow only certain types of particles to pass through the plasma membrane.

The plasma membrane's semipermeability is important to the cell in five ways. (1) It allows nutrients such as glucose, fatty acids, and amino acids to enter the cell, replacing those that the cell consumes during metabolic activities. (2) It prevents organelles and nutrients in the cytosol from leaking out of the cell. (3) It allows waste products to enter the extracellular fluid, thereby preventing them from accumulating in the cytosol and poisoning the cell. (4) It prevents many types of harmful substances from entering the cell. (5) It allows certain types of cells to release substances, such as hormones, into the extracellular fluid that can help the body maintain homeostasis. An example of such a secretion is insulin, which, when released from cells in the pancreas, enables other cells in the body to take in and use glucose as a source of energy.

Depending on the type of substance moving into or out of the cell, membrane transport may occur with or without cellular energy. If the membrane transport does not use up cellular energy, then the transport is a **passive process**. If the transport requires cellular energy (usually derived from ATP), it is an **active process**. Some substances move through the membrane by active and passive processes, but this always occurs in opposite directions. For instance, passive transport moves sodium ions (Na^+) into the cell, while active transport moves Na^+ out of the cell. One factor that determines whether a substance will move through a membrane passively or actively relates to the difference in concentration for that substance on opposite sides of the membrane.

GRADIENTS ACROSS A MEMBRANE

The plasma membrane's selective permeability is directly responsible for differences in the concentrations of various solutes in the cytosol and the extracellular fluid. Any difference in concentration of a substance at two locations is a **concentration gradient**. Think of this in terms of a highway's gradient (steepness), in which one section of the highway is higher than another section. Moreover, since ions are charged particles, a difference in their concentrations can cause some regions to become positively charged while other regions become negatively charged. An **electrochemical gradient** is a combination of an electrical gradient (difference in electrical charges) and a concentration gradient. Gradients across the plasma membrane can develop in several ways:

(1) A substance may pass into and out of the cell at different rates. For example, an active process moves Na^+ out of a cell faster than a passive process allows them to enter the cell. This unequal membrane transport creates a higher concentration of Na^+ in the extracellular fluid. Likewise, an active process moves potassium ions (K^+) into the cell faster than a passive process allows them to leave the cell; consequently, the concentration of K^+ is higher in the cytosol than in the ECF.

(2) The cell may accumulate or deplete a particular substance on one side of the membrane. For example, when oxygen molecules enter a typical cell, the mitochondria utilize them in oxidation reactions. This action causes the cytosol to have a lower concentration of oxygen than the extracellular fluid. In contrast, certain oxidation reactions in the cytoplasm generate carbon dioxide molecules (CO_2), causing the cytosol to have a higher CO_2 than the extracellular fluid.

As you might expect, the concentration gradient is a major factor in determining whether membrane transport of a particular substance will be passive or active. Passive transport moves substances from regions of higher concentration to regions of lower concentration without consuming cellular energy. Compare this to running out of gas at the top of a hill; you can still coast downhill. Oppositely, active transport can move substances from a region of lower concentration to a region of higher concentration. To move a car uphill, however, the engine must use gas.

Membrane transport can occur by three mechanisms: *simple diffusion*, *carrier-mediated transport*, and *vesicular transport*. A fourth mechanism, *filtration*, relates mostly to the movement of substances between cells.

DIFFUSION

To understand how some kinds of particles move through the plasma membrane, you must first understand why particles move in the first place. At temperatures above absolute zero (273° C), molecules and ions vibrate due to the kinetic energy of their subatomic particles. While this vibration causes individual particles to move about randomly, it causes groups of particles to distribute themselves evenly in an environment. The tendency of similar particles to distribute evenly is **diffusion** (di-FYOO-shun; to scatter).

When particles diffuse, they spread out from a region of higher concentration to a region of lower concentration like a car rolling downhill. For this reason, diffusing substances are said to move *down* or *along* their concentration gradient. You can see a dye such as food coloring diffuse through water in a graduated cylinder. The dye molecules spread out from the drop, where they are concentrated, to distribute themselves evenly throughout the water. Although the dye molecules continue to vibrate randomly, diffusion ceases when a concentration gradient no longer exists in the graduated cylinder (see Figure 6-3a).

What would happen if you added two or three different colors of dye to the water at the same time? Interestingly, each solute would diffuse independently of the other solutes; over time, the molecules of each color of dye would distribute themselves evenly throughout the glass of water. You can also see this happen when a semipermeable membrane separates different solutes (Figure 6-3b). If a solute can pass through the semipermeable membrane then it is called a *permeating* solute. Solutes that cannot pass through the membrane are *nonpermeating* solutes. In the next section we will examine how simple diffusion occurs through the plasma membrane.

MEMBRANE STRUCTURE AND FUNCTION

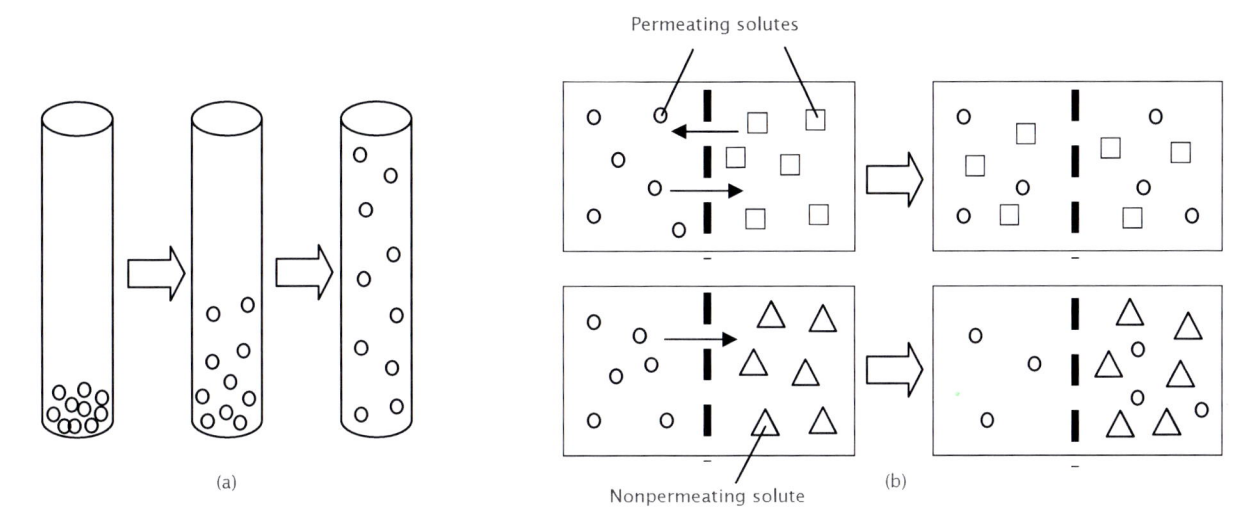

Figure 6-3. Diffusion along concentration gradients

Diffusion through a cell's membrane

Although many different kinds of particles move through the plasma membrane by simple diffusion, they do not all follow the same route. A substance moves into or out of a cell by simple diffusion in one of two ways: (1) between the membrane's phospholipid molecules and (2) through different types of membrane channels. The route taken by a diffusing substance through the plasma membrane depends on the lipid solubility of the substance.

Lipid-soluble molecules are nonpolar and hydrophobic, which allows them to diffuse through the phospholipid part of the plasma membrane. Examples of substances that diffuse in this manner include molecular oxygen (O_2), carbon dioxide (CO_2), nitrogen gas (N_2), fatty acids, steroids, fat-soluble vitamins (A, D, E, and K), and alcohol. In most tissues, oxygen is in a higher concentration in the extracellular fluid; therefore, it diffuses into the cells. Simultaneously, carbon dioxide is in a higher concentration in the cytosol, so it diffuses out of the cell.

Water-soluble substances are polar (hydrophilic) and cannot diffuse between the hydrophobic fatty acid "tails" of the phospholipid bilayer; therefore, these substances must diffuse through integral proteins. Examples of substances that diffuse through integral proteins include ions, glucose, amino acids, and nucleotides. Water molecules are unique in that although they are polar, a few of them can squirt between the phospholipid molecules of the bilayer. Because of their small size and high kinetic energy, water molecules bounce back and forth between the fatty acid tails in the bilayer and eventually reach the other side of the membrane.

Most membrane channels are *ion channels*, which have very small passageways and allow only ions and water molecules to diffuse through them. Furthermore, most ion channels are highly selective, allowing passage for only one kind of ion. Ion channels are classified either *leaky* or *gated*.

- **Leaky channels** (or **pores**) function like hollow pipes, allowing ions to diffuse through continuously. Examples include leaky sodium (Na^+) channels, which allow Na^+ ions to diffuse into the cell, and leaky potassium (K^+) channels, which allow K^+ ions to diffuse out of the cell.

- **Gated channels** have a portion of the integral protein that functions as a "gate." When the gate closes, no ions diffuse through the channel. When the gate opens, particular ions can diffuse through the channel. The stimuli that open particular gated channels vary. A chemical, generally called a *ligand*, opens a **ligand-gated channel**. A change in the electrical condition around a cell opens a **voltage-gated channel**. A mechanical stimulus, such as stretching the cell, opens a **stretch-activated channel** (also called *mechanically gated channel*). Examples of gated channels include ligand-gated

Na⁺ channels, voltage-gated K⁺ channels, and stretch-activated Ca²⁺ channels; however, not every type of cell in the body has every type of gated channel mentioned here. Gated channels stay open for only a short moment, closing quickly after the stimulus no longer exists.

While ion channels have names that denote their mode of action and the type of ion diffusing them, water is always the major substance diffusing through them. In addition, most, if not all, cells contain special channels called **aquaporins** (OK-wa-POR-inz), which are primary routes for the diffusion of water through the plasma membrane.

OSMOSIS: A SPECIAL CASE OF DIFFUSION

Now let's take a closer look at factors affecting the diffusion of water through a plasma membrane. When water *diffuses* through the plasma membrane or any other semipermeable membrane, the process is called **osmosis** (oz-MŌ-sis; *osmo-*, push through; *osis*, process). During osmosis, water molecules diffuse down their own concentration gradient; that is, from a region with a higher concentration of water molecules to a region with a lower concentration of water molecules. There is an inverse correlation between the concentration of water molecules in a solution and the concentration of solute particles dissolved in the water. In other words, as the concentration of solute particles increases, the concentration of water molecules decreases.

Cells are susceptible to swelling and rupturing if their cytosol has a higher concentration of solute particles than the extracellular fluid. If more water is moving into a cell than is moving out of it, the excess water in the cytosol exerts ever-increasing pressure on the inner face of the plasma membrane. The pressure exerted by water because of its volume or the effect of gravity is called **hydrostatic pressure**. In the case of a swelling cell, osmosis is "pulling" water into the cell, while hydrostatic pressure is attempting to push it out. If the hydrostatic pressure inside a cell becomes greater than the plasma membrane can resist, the cell will rupture and die.

To illustrate osmosis and hydrostatic pressure, consider an aquarium divided into two chambers (A and B) by a partition that has a semipermeable membrane at the bottom (see figure 6-4). If we add distilled water (contains no solutes) to both sides, then both sides have the same concentration of water per unit volume. If we add a solute, such as salt or sugar, to side B, then side B will have fewer water molecules per unit of volume compared to the distilled water because the solute particles take up space that was formerly occupied by water molecules. Due to osmosis, there will be a net movement of water from side A to side B; i.e., water will move from the side with more water molecules per unit of volume (side A) to the side with fewer water molecules per unit of volume (side B). This net movement of water causes the level of solution in side B to rise (see figure).

Osmolarity (OZ-mō-LAR-i-tē) is a measure of the concentration of solute particles in a solution, and it allows you to predict whether water will move into or out of a cell by osmosis. The standard units for osmolarity are **milliosmoles** of solute per liter of solution (written mOsm/L). Normal human tissue fluid usually contains a solute concentration of 280–300 mOsm/L. When comparing two solutions separated by a semipermeable membrane, the solution with the higher concentration of solute particles has a higher osmolarity. In our aquarium example, side B has a higher osmolarity than side A after we add solute to side B. Water always moves through a semipermeable membrane from a region of lower osmolarity (*higher* water concentration) toward a region of higher osmolarity (*lower* water concentration). The tendency of a solution to gain water because of its osmolarity is **osmotic pressure**. In the figure, side B shows a greater tendency to gain water than does side A; therefore, side B has a higher osmotic pressure than side A. More exactly, osmotic pressure is the force required to prevent osmosis. You could determine the osmotic pressure of solution B by measuring the amount of pressure exerted by a piston that prevents a net movement of water into side B (see figure 6-4).

When predicting how extracellular fluid will affect a cell's volume, or internal tension, it is common to use the term **tonicity** (tō-NI-si-tē; *tonic*, strength) instead of osmolarity. A solution's tonicity relates to its concentration of *nonpermeating* solutes. An **isotonic** (Ī-sō-TON-ik; *iso*, same) solution has the same concentration of nonpermeating solute particles

MEMBRANE STRUCTURE AND FUNCTION

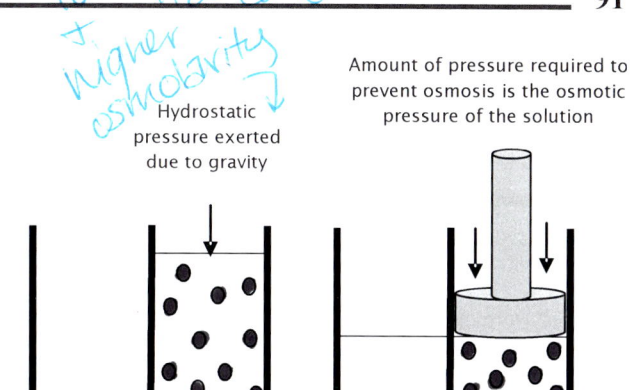

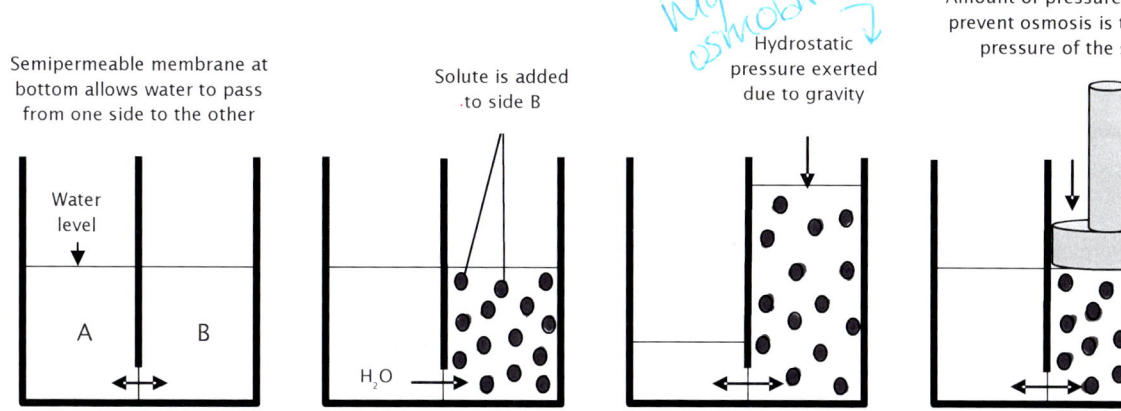

Figure 6-4. Osmotic and hydrostatic pressure

as the cell's cytosol. A 0.9% NaCl solution, which is approximately 280-300 mOsm/L, is isotonic to human cells because it does not cause the cells to lose or gain water. A **hypertonic** (*hyper*, high) solution has a higher concentration of nonpermeating solute than a cell and causes the cell to lose water. Cells that are losing water may often take on a "spiny" appearance: a condition called *crenation* (krē-NĀ-shun; notched). A **hypotonic** (*hypo-*, low) solution has a lower concentration of nonpermeating solute particles than the cell, and causes the cell to gain water and swell. In some cases, such as with red blood cells, a hypotonic solution can cause the cells to swell so much that they rupture: a phenomenon called *lysis* (LĪ-sis, loosening).

When considering how different solutes affect a solution's osmotic pressure, the *number* of particles is more important than the *type* of particles. In general, one small solute particle has the same effect on osmotic pressure as a larger solute particle. For example, although a single ion may be small, its strong electrical charge attracts numerous water molecules that form hydration shells around the ion. A polar molecule also attracts water molecules, but the attraction is only around the charged regions of the molecule. Therefore, a small ion with a "larger" hydration shell may tie up as many water molecules as a larger polar molecule with its "smaller" hydration shells (see Figure 6-5).

Although a 0.9% NaCl solution is isotonic to a human cell, it takes a 5% glucose (dextrose) solution to be isotonic to the same cell. Why does it take a little more than five times as much weight of glucose dissolved in water to make an isoosmotic solution compared to a 0.9% NaCl solution? The reason is that when one glucose molecule ($C_6H_{12}O_6$) dissolves in water (when surrounded by polar water molecules), it does not ionize. In contrast, when one NaCl dissolves, it ionizes to form one Na^+ ion and one Cl^- ion. Figure 6-6 illustrates this idea. The top left corner of the figure shows that 1 gram of substance *A* dissolves to yield eight "small" solute particles. Think of this as being like Na^+ and Cl^- dissolving out of a salt crystal. The top right corner shows that 1 gm of substance *B* dissolves to form two "large" solute particles. Think of this as being like glucose molecules dissolving out of a sugar crystal. Notice that compartments 1 and 2 both contain 8 solute particles per 100 mL of solution. However, compartment 2 contains 4 grams of substance B, while compartment 1 contains only 1 gram of substance A. Still, the number of solute particles in compartments 1 and 2 are the same; hence, they are isoosmotic (i.e., they have the same osmotic pressure). Compartment 3 shows a mixture of substances A and B, but the concentration is 10 particles per 100 mL, which makes it

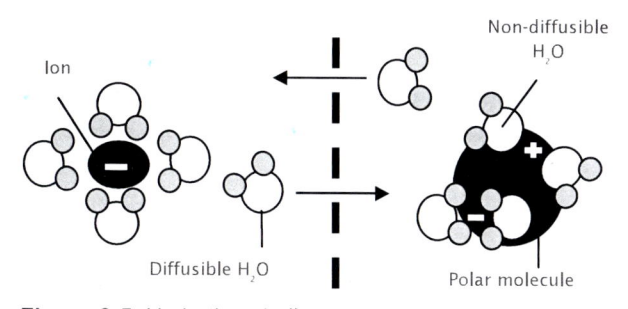

Figure 6-5. Hydration shells

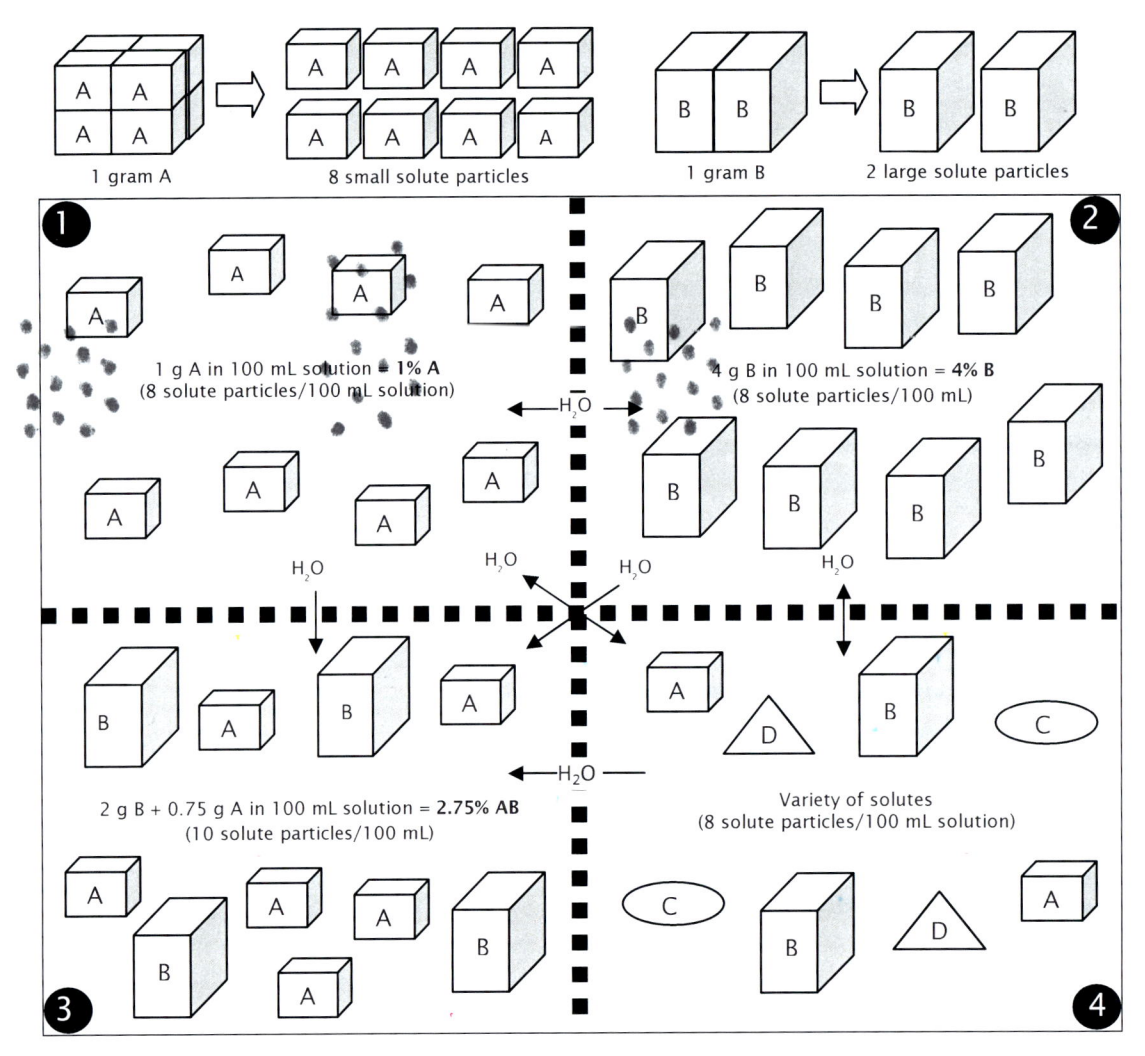

Figure 6-6. Effect of different solutes on osmolarity

hyperosmotic to compartments 1 and 2. Compartment 4 contains a variety of solutes, including A and B, but the total number of solutes per 100 mL is still 8; therefore, it is isoosmotic to compartments 1 and 2, and it is hypoosmotic to compartment 3.

Although a 5% glucose solution is initially isotonic to a human cell, it can become hypotonic because glucose is a **permeating solute**; that is, a cell may readily absorb it, thus, decreasing the solute concentration in the solution. Remember that NaCl is a nonpermeating solute because cells do not allow it to pass through the plasma membrane readily. Therefore, a 0.9% NaCl will remain isotonic to a living cell, whereas, a 5% glucose solution is initially isotonic but becomes hypotonic when glucose molecules enter the cell.

Figure 6-8 shows the effects that different salt and sugars solutions have on the osmotic pressure around a red blood cell. Remember that NaCl is a nonpermeating solute, whereas glucose is a permeating solute. What would the osmolarity of solution be if you mixed 100 mL of 5% glucose and 100 mL of 0.9% NaCl to yield a 200 mL solution? If you said it would be isotonic then you are correct. What would be the concentration of each solute in that isotonic solution? The answer is 0.45% NaCl and 2.5% glucose since each solute was diluted in half when it was mixed with the other solution.

Dialysis

Dialysis (dī-AL-i-sis; to separate) is a passive process involving the separation of different-size solute particles

MEMBRANE STRUCTURE AND FUNCTION

using a semipermeable membrane. Only smaller solute particles can pass through the membrane. Dialysis is used in artificial kidneys to cleanse the blood of patients whose kidneys no longer function efficiently. In Figure 6-7, some of the solutes are able to pass through the semipermeable membrane, while others are prevented; this is an example of dialysis. Notice in the figure how dialysis can also affect osmosis.

FACTORS AFFECTING DIFFUSION

Now consider factors that affect how fast diffusion occurs. This is important because if diffusion of nutrients into a cell or the diffusion of wastes out of a cell is too slow, the cell can suffer ill effects. The rate, or speed, of diffusion fluctuates in response to three major factors:

1. **Temperature**: When molecules and ions are warmer, their subatomic particles have more kinetic energy and vibrate faster. This, in turn, causes molecules and ions to diffuse faster through the plasma membrane. Moreover, warmer molecules within the plasma membrane vibrate faster and can "bump" diffusing substances through at a faster rate.

2. **Molecule size**: Large particles have more surface area than smaller particles and are more likely to bump into other particles while diffusing. Consequently, larger particles encounter more resistance and diffuse more slowly than smaller particles under the same conditions. Compare this to small scooters darting quickly between slow-moving cars in rush-hour traffic.

3. **Steepness of the gradient**: The greater the difference in concentration of a substance at two locations, the *steeper* the concentration gradient will be. In turn, the steeper the concentration gradient for a particular substance, the faster that substance will diffuse. As a comparison, a car will roll down a *steep* hill much faster than it will roll down a gentle (less steep) slope. Likewise, a greater difference in electrical charge at two locations (that is, the greater the electrochemical gradient), the faster ions will diffuse to regions of opposite charge.

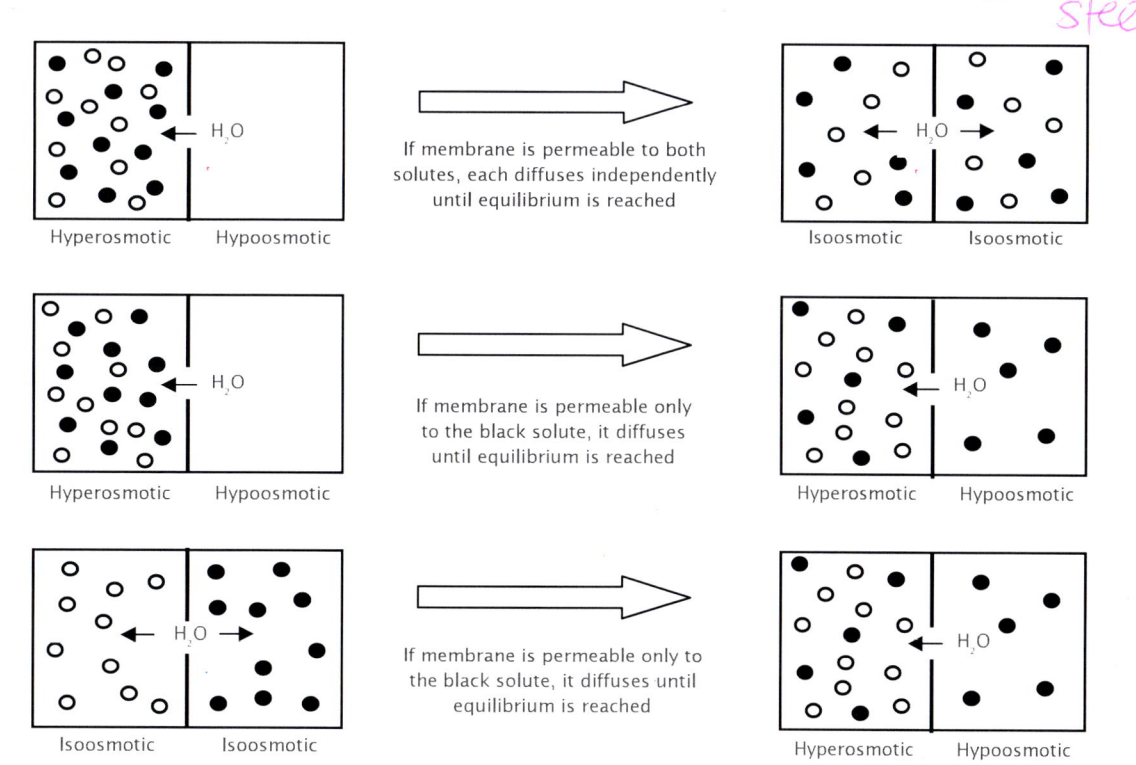

Figure 6-7. Dialysis

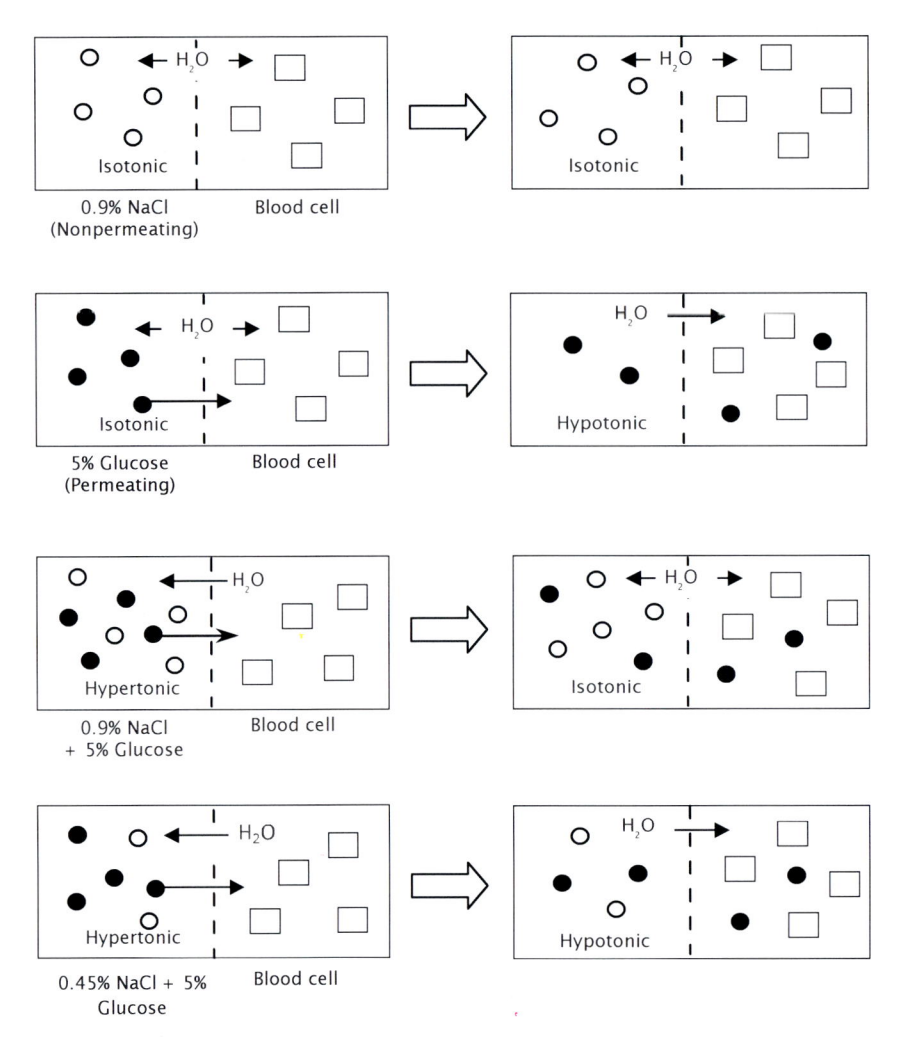

Figure 6-8. Effect of mixing permeating and nonpermeating solutes

CARRIER-MEDIATED TRANSPORT

Some substances enter or leave a cell without passing through the phospholipid bilayer or membrane channels. These substances are either (1) too large to pass through a channel, or (2) they must move *against* a concentration gradient. Most of these substances, called **substrates**, move through integral proteins called *carriers* in a process called **carrier-mediated transport**. There are two methods of carrier-mediated transport: *facilitated transport* and *active transport*.

Facilitated Transport

If a substrate can move through a carrier that does not require the cell to use ATP as a source of energy, the process is **facilitated transport**. The name implies that the carrier helps the movement of the substrate. When the substrate moves *down* a concentration gradient, facilitated transport is synonymous with *facilitated diffusion*. However, research has shown that facilitated transport can move a substrate through the membrane even when there is no concentration gradient. In either case, the cell does not use up energy to make this happen, so facilitated transport is a *passive* process.

To see how facilitated transport helps maintain homeostasis, consider the movement of glucose into and out of liver cells through the same carriers. When blood has a higher concentration of glucose than the liver cells, glucose *enters* the cells by facilitated transport. When the liver cells have a higher concentration of glucose than the blood, glucose leaves the cells by

MEMBRANE STRUCTURE AND FUNCTION

facilitated transport. In this way, facilitated transport helps maintain a relatively stable concentration of glucose in the blood. The steps in facilitated transport are as follows (see Figure 6-9a):

1. Substrate binds to receptor: The substrate binds to a site, called a **receptor**, located on the carrier. The binding is specific; only a certain kind of substrate can bind to the receptor, like a key fitting into a lock. Both sides of the carrier display receptors, thus, substrate molecules in the ECF or in the cytosol can attach to the carrier. However, the side with the higher concentration of substrate will bind more substrate molecules. As a result, there will be a net movement of the substrate *down* its concentration gradient.

2. Carrier changes shape: Binding of the substrate causes the carrier to change shape, and this action moves the substrate across the membrane. Notice the substrate is moving down its concentration gradient and no ATP energy is required to change the carrier's shape.

3. Substrate detaches from receptor: After moving down its concentration gradient through the carrier, the substrate detaches from the carrier and diffuses away from it. Since this side of the membrane has a relatively low concentration of substrate, it is unlikely that a substrate particle will be available to bind to the receptor on that side.

4. Carrier changes shape: After the substrate detaches, the carrier changes shape so the receptor returns to the side of the membrane with the higher concentration of substrate. Another substrate molecule attaches to the receptor and facilitated transport occurs.

The speed at which substrate particles move down their concentration gradient by facilitated transport is directly proportional to the steepness of the gradient. In other words, the greater the difference in concentration of substrate on either side of the membrane, the faster facilitated transport occurs. If the concentration of substrate is the same on either side of the membrane, facilitated transport still occurs, but in both directions at the same rate.

Although carriers can transport many substrate particles each second, they can only work so fast. The maximum number of substrate molecules that can pass through a carrier in a given amount of time is the carrier's **saturation point** (see Figure 6-9b). Compare this to the maximum number of people who can ride an escalator from the second floor to the first floor of a building each minute. Regardless of how many people are waiting on the second floor, no more than a maximum number can ride the escalator each minute. Why does our analogy need to have people riding *down* the escalator? The reason is that any *net* movement of substrate by facilitated transport will always be *down* a concentration gradient.

Active transport

While facilitated transport moves a substrate down a concentration gradient, **active transport** moves a substrate *against* a concentration gradient. In the same way that a car must burn fuel to move uphill, a cell must expend energy to move a substance

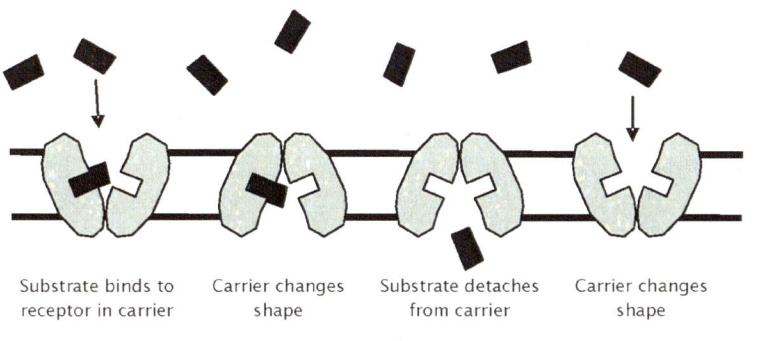

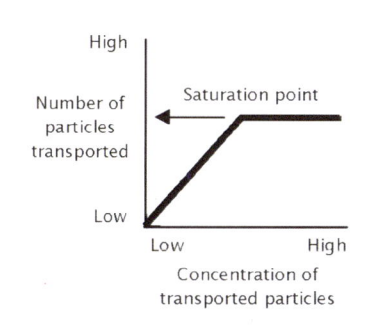

| Substrate binds to receptor in carrier | Carrier changes shape | Substrate detaches from carrier | Carrier changes shape |

(a)

(b)

Figure 6-9. Facilitated diffusion

from a region of low concentration into a region of higher concentration. Active transport helps maintain optimum concentrations of various solutes inside and outside of the cell, which is crucial to maintaining homeostasis. Like facilitated transport carriers, active transport carriers change shape to transport substrates across the membrane. Also, like the facilitated diffusion carrier, an active transport carrier can experience saturation. However, in our analogy, the people would be riding the escalator *up* to the second floor. Depending on whether the carrier expends cellular energy directly or indirectly, active transport is either *primary* or *secondary*, respectively.

Primary active transport uses energy derived from ATP molecules to change a carrier's shape in order to move a substrate across a membrane against a concentration gradient. Although there are variations, the general process occurs in three steps: First, a substrate attaches to a receptor site on the carrier. Second, an ATP molecule transfers one of its phosphate molecules to the carrier. In response, the carrier changes shape, allowing it to move the substrate across the membrane. Third, the carrier releases the substrate and the phosphate molecule. Losing the phosphate causes the carrier to change back to its original shape and the process repeats.

Active transport carriers function as membrane *pumps*, implying that they require energy to "push" a substrate against a concentration gradient. Compare this to a water pump that uses electrical energy to push water uphill because the water will not move "up" under its own power. The plasma membrane has a variety of pumps, but one of the most important is the **sodium-potassium (Na^+/K^+) pump** (Figure 6-10). Recall that Na^+ ions diffuse into the cell and potassium ions diffuse out of the cell through leaky channels. To counteract this diffusion, the Na^+/K^+ pumps move Na^+ ions out of the cell and move K^+ ions into the cell. Without Na^+/K^+ pumps, sodium would accumulate in the cell and make the cytosol hypertonic to the extracellular fluid; in turn, too much water would enter the cell causing the cell to swell and possibly rupture. Because Na^+/K^+ pumps are so important to all cells in the body, we will describe their activity. Identify the following steps in Figure 6-10:

1. **Sodium ions attach to pump:** Three Na^+ ions in the cytosol bind to receptors on the cytosolic side of the pump. At this time, the pump cannot bind K^+ ions.

2. **ATP phosphorylates the pump:** ATP transfers a phosphate group (PO_4^{3-}) to the pump. This step can occur only if the pump is holding three Na^+ ions.

3. **Pump changes shape:** Phosphorylation causes the pump to change shape, in essence, turning "inside out" so that the Na^+ ions now face the extracellular fluid.

4. **Pump releases Na^+ ions and bind K^+ ions:** The three Na^+ ions detach from the pump and enter the extracellular fluid. When this happens, the receptor sites for Na^+ change shape, preventing Na^+ ions from binding to the pump. At the same time, the receptor sites for K^+ ions become available, allowing two K^+ ions to enter the pump from the extracellular fluid.

5. **PO_4^{3-} detaches from the pump:** When the K^+ ions bind to the pump, the pump changes shape slightly, which, in turn, causes the PO_4^{3-} group to detach from the pump and enter the cytosol.

6. **Pump releases K^+:** Detaching the PO_4^{3-} group causes the pump to change shape again, virtually turning "outside in" so that the K^+ ions now face the cytosol. The K^+ ions quickly detach from the pump and enter the cytosol. The pump is now ready to accept three Na^+ ions, and repeat steps 1-6.

Two other examples of primary active transport carriers are calcium pumps and chloride pumps. **Calcium pumps** transport Ca^{2+} ions out of cells, maintaining a lower concentration of Ca^{2+} in the cytosol than in the ECF. **Chloride pumps** transport Cl^- ions out of the cell, maintaining a lower concentration of Cl^- ions in the cytosol than in the ECF. Although the cell must expend energy to maintain ion concentration gradients across membranes, these ions may diffuse back through the membranes and perform useful work for the cell. This energy tradeoff is like using an electric pump to push ("actively" transport) water into a tall tower so that later the water can flow passively

MEMBRANE STRUCTURE AND FUNCTION

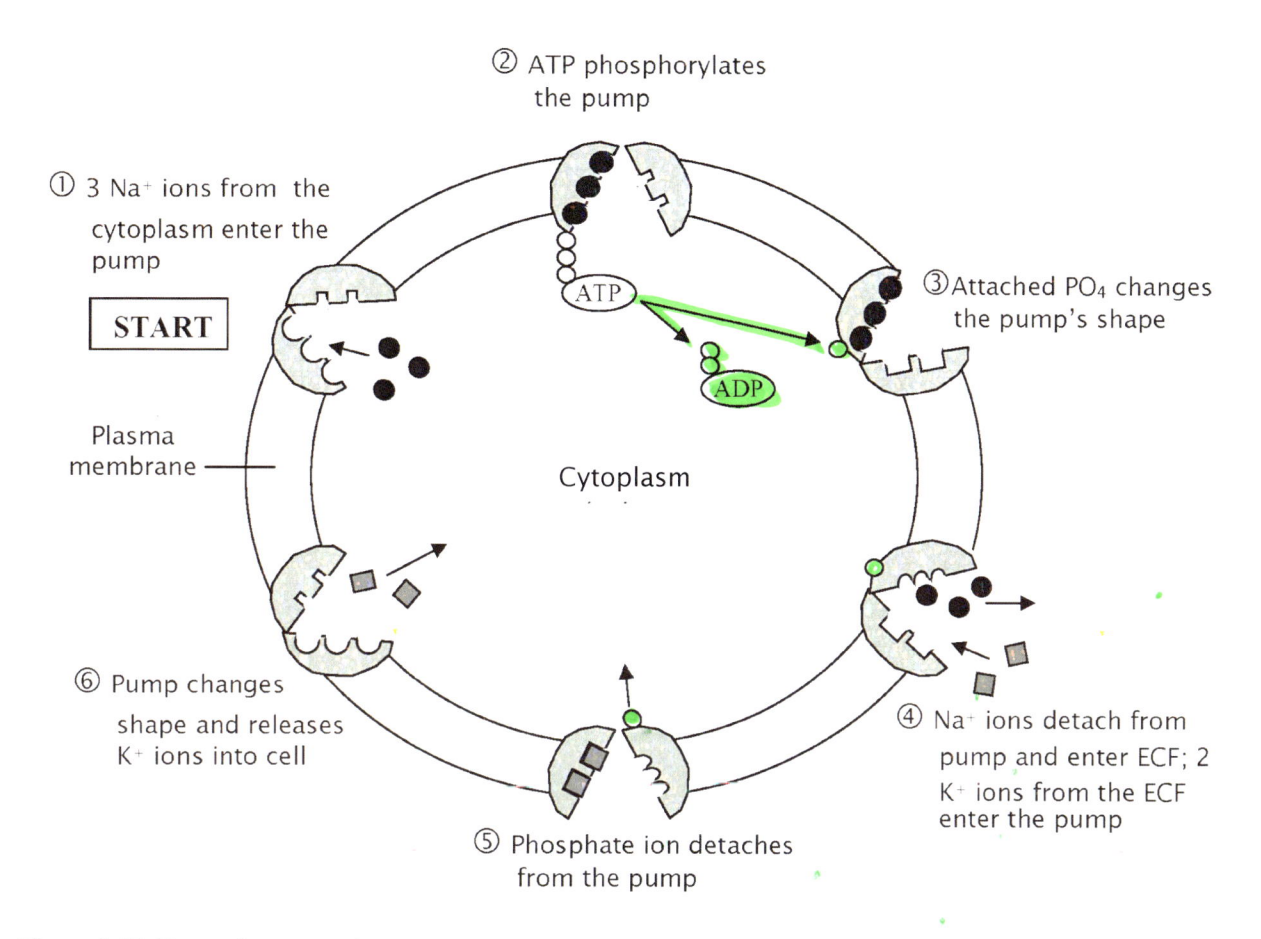

Figure 6-10. The sodium-potassium pump

down a pipe and through a showerhead, allowing you to take a shower. Like facilitated transport carriers, active transport pumps have a saturation point at which they cannot work any faster.

Secondary active transport uses the kinetic energy released during facilitated transport of one substance to move another substrate through the same carrier protein (see figure 6-11). During this process, a single carrier binds several substrates and transports them through the membrane simultaneously. One of these substrates always moves *down* its concentration gradient (passive transport), while the other substrate may move either *along* or *against* a concentration gradient. Most secondary active transport carriers have receptor sites for two different substrates, and both substrates must bind to the carrier before the carrier will change shape and transport them through the membrane.

A secondary active transport carrier does not derive energy from ATP directly; instead, it derives kinetic energy from the movement of one of its substrates down a steep concentration gradient. This kinetic energy is the "driving force" that moves the other substrate through the carrier against a concentration gradient. Most often, a Na^+ ion is the substrate that moves down its concentration gradient through a secondary active transport carrier. Since Na^+ ions are in a higher concentration in the ECF, they always move through a secondary carrier into the cytosol. Without a steep concentration gradient to promote the binding of Na^+ ions to its outside surface, a secondary carrier loses its source of kinetic energy. Consequently, these secondary carriers rely on Na^+/K^+ pumps, which *do* utilize energy from ATP directly, to maintain a steep concentration gradient for Na^+ across the membrane. In this way, secondary active transport derives energy indirectly from primary ("first") active transport.

Secondary active transport carriers are *coupled transporters* because they couple the transport of

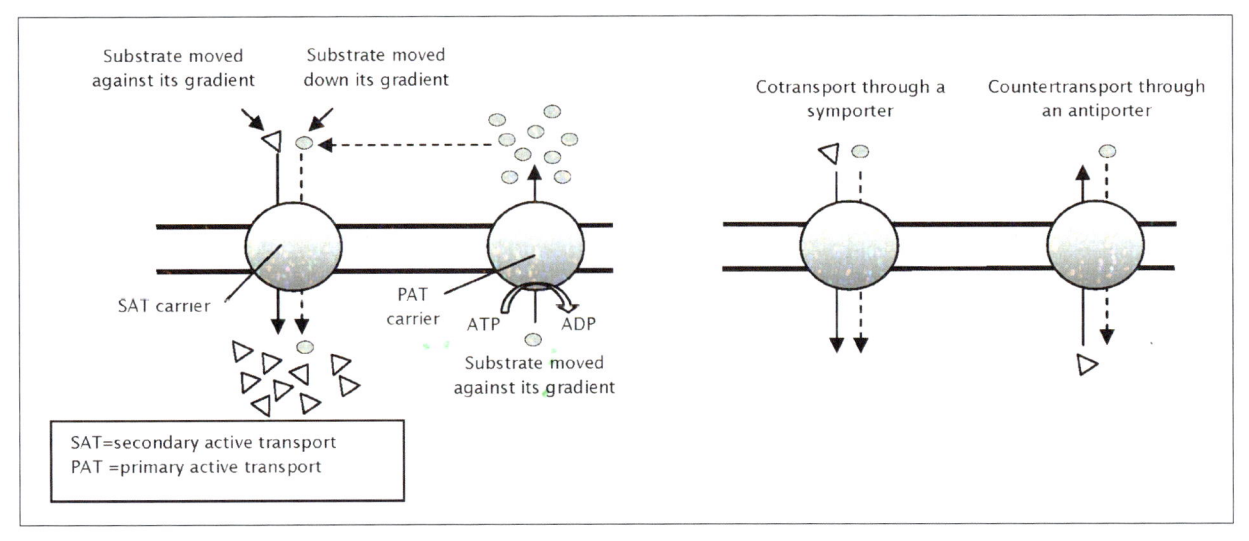

Figure 6-11. Secondary active transport

one substrate to the transport of another substrate. A coupled transporter is either a *symporter* or an *antiporter*. A **symporter** transports different substrates simultaneously in the same direction in a process called **cotransport**. Some symporters cotransport amino acids into a cell in conjunction with Na^+ ions. An **antiporter** transports different substrates simultaneously in opposite directions in a process called **countertransport**. One type of antiporter transports H^+ ions out of the cell while transporting Na^+ ions into the cell. Since H^+ ions are byproducts of normal metabolism, this antiporter prevents them from accumulating in the cytosol and lowering its pH below a normal level.

VESICULAR TRANSPORT

In certain situations, it is important for a cell to take in, or get rid of, substances that are too large to pass through the plasma membrane's lipid bilayer, its channels, or its carriers. These substances can enter or leave a cell by hitching rides inside of vesicles in a process called **vesicular transport** (also called **bulk transport**). Recall that a vesicle is a spherical, membranous sac that forms when a portion of an existing membrane pinches off. Some vesicles form at certain cytoplasmic organelles, while others form at the plasma membrane. Since vesicles arise from membranes, they can also fuse with them.

A cell uses its cytoskeleton to organize phospholipids molecules into a vesicle. To begin forming a vesicle, motor molecules pull on cytoskeleton microfilaments that are anchored to an existing membrane. Eventually, the microfilaments pull a small portion of the membrane off as a vesicle. While it is forming, a vesicle surrounds a substance that is waiting for transport. A motor molecule then binds to the vesicle and carries it along a microfilament. Since the motor molecules need ATP to form and transport the vesicles, vesicular transport is an *active* process. The two major types of vesicular transport are *endocytosis* and *exocytosis* (Figure 6-12).

Endocytosis

When a cell is ready to move a relatively large substance from the extracellular fluid to the cytosol, it performs a process called **endocytosis** (en-dō-sī-TŌ-sis; *endo*, inside). Endocytosis occurs in three ways: *phagocytosis*, *pinocytosis*, or *receptor-mediated endocytosis*.

Phagocytosis (fā-gō-sī-TŌ-sis; *phag*, to eat) is a type of endocytosis in which a cell ingests relatively large, solid particles. These particles may include dead or dying body cells, cellular debris, bacteria, viruses, or some other solid object. The cell first extends **pseudopodia** (projections of its plasma membrane) around the particle completely enveloping it. The pseudopodia come together to form an *endocytic vesicle* (EN-dō-SI-tik) called a **phagosome** (FĀ-go-sōm).

MEMBRANE STRUCTURE AND FUNCTION

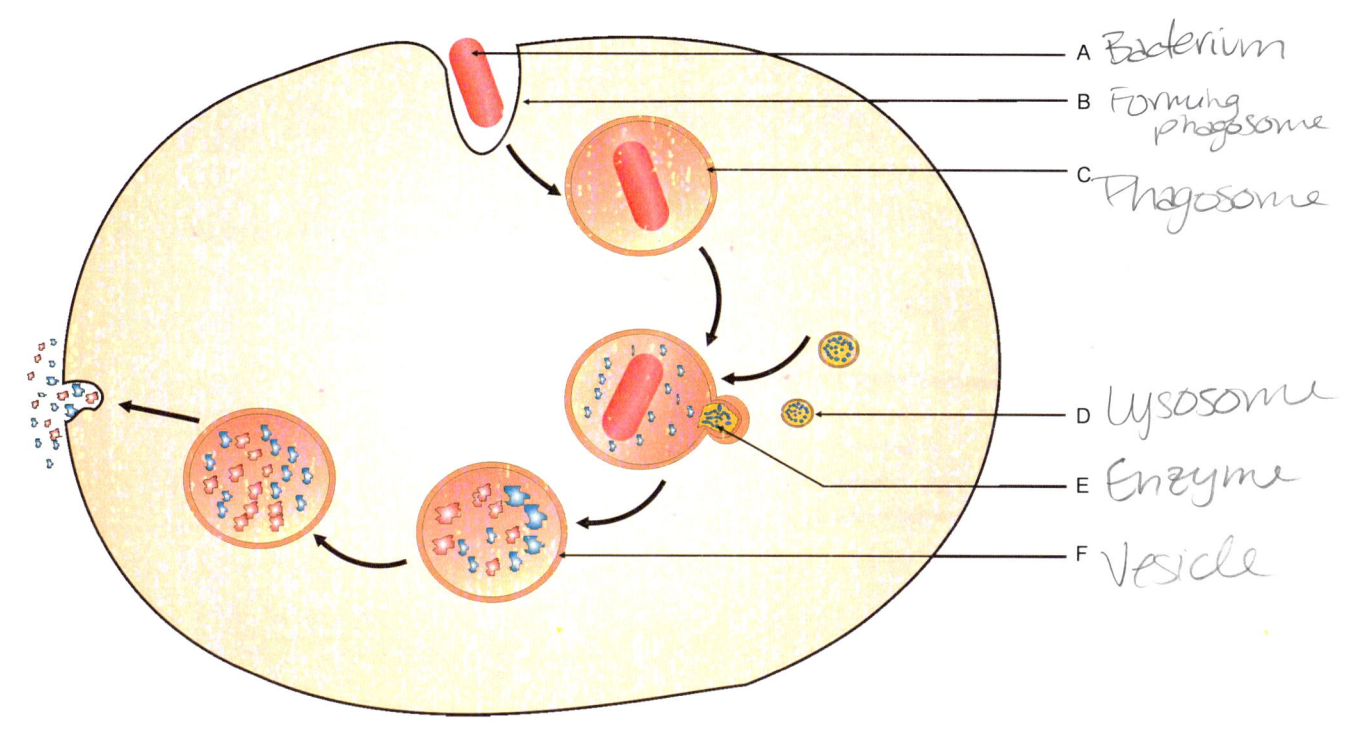

Figure 6-12. Endocytosis and exocytosis

Labels (handwritten):
- A — Bacterium
- B — Forming phagosome
- C — Phagosome
- D — Lysosome
- E — Enzyme
- F — Vesicle

The body uses cells called *phagocytic cells*, or *phagocytes*, as a defense against foreign particles. Phagocytes in the body are certain types of white blood cells. The type that has the most voracious appetite for bacteria and viruses is the **macrophage** (MAK-rō-fāj). A macrophage develops from a certain type of white blood cell that leaves the blood to move around in other tissues. In a sense, macrophages are like police officers who walk the streets looking for troublemakers; in most cases, the troublemakers are bacteria or viruses. Macrophages also use phagocytosis to clean up wounds by ingesting dead body cells.

Before a macrophage can ingest a particle by phagocytosis, there must be a receptor on the particle's surface for the macrophage to grab. Often the receptor is a chemical that attaches to the particle shortly after the particle enters the body. After phagocytosis, a motor molecule pulls the phagosome through the cytosol where it fuses with a lysosome. Digestive enzymes from the lysosome break down the contents of the phagosome into a variety of chemical products. The usable products enter the cytosol where the cell can use them for energy or for cellular components. The cell expels the unusable material through exocytosis (described shortly).

Pinocytosis (pin-ō-sī-TŌ-sis; *pino*, to drink) is a type of endocytosis in which a cell ingests a small amount of extracellular fluid. Unlike phagocytosis, pinocytosis does not use pseudopodia and it does not require recognition of receptors. Instead, the plasma membrane simply pulls inward and traps a small amount of extracellular fluid within an endocytic vesicle. Pinocytosis occurs continually and is the cell's way of "sampling" its surrounding environment. Various solutes leave the endocytic vesicle as it moves through the cytosol. A broader benefit of pinocytosis is that it allows cells in the intestines to absorb a variety of dissolved nutrients from food.

Receptor-mediated endocytosis forms a vesicle only after a substrate binds to a receptor (mostly glycoproteins) on the plasma membrane. Substrates ingested by this method include cholesterol, iron, and certain hormones and vitamins. Certain types of white blood cells use receptor-mediated endocytosis to ingest foreign particles that can cause illness. The receptors on the surface of these white blood cells are special protein called *antibodies*. An antibody is highly specific in that it will bind only to one type of foreign particle.

Receptor-mediated endocytosis (RME) is similar to pinocytosis in that there are no pseudopodia; the plasma membrane simply pulls inward to form a vesicle. However, there are three major differences between RME and pinocytosis. (1) Whereas pinocytosis occurs continually, RME occurs only when a certain substrate is present in the extracellular fluid. (2) Whereas pinocytosis is nonspecific and takes in whatever dissolves in the extracellular fluid, RME is highly specific, taking in only a certain type of particle. (3) Whereas pinocytosis makes vesicles that have the same concentration of particles as the extracellular fluid, RME makes vesicles that have a much higher concentration of particles than the extracellular fluid.

Now consider a specific example of receptor-mediated endocytosis, one in which a cell absorbs cholesterol for its plasma membrane. Hundreds of cholesterol molecules move together in the blood, surrounded by a shell of phospholipids and protein. This lipid-protein mass is a *lipoprotein*. Different lipoproteins have different molecular weights, but the type mainly responsible for transporting cholesterol is a *low-density lipoprotein*, or LDL. The method by which a cell absorbs and processes an LDL involves the following steps:

1. Binding of LDL to receptor: A protein on the LDL binds to a specific receptor (LDL receptor) on the outer surface of the plasma membrane.

2. Migration to a coated pit: The membrane receptor with its bound LDL moves along the plasma membrane until it reaches a small depression called a *coated pit*. **Clathrin** (KLĀ-thrin; lattice) is a protein that forms a net-like lining along the cytoplasmic side of this pit. Movement of more receptors with their bound LDLs into the pit concentrates the LDLs in one place.

3. Formation of a vesicle: Myosin motor molecules pull microfilaments that connect to the clathrin-coated pit, causing the pit to bow inward and form a vesicle. Shortly thereafter, the clathrin molecules disconnect from the vesicle and return to the plasma membrane. A motor molecule attaches to the vesicle and pulls it farther into the cytosol along microfilaments of the cytoskeleton.

4. Separation of LDL and receptor: The receptors and their bound LDLs separate from one another and the vesicle splits in two. The receptors end up in one vesicle and the LDLs in the other vesicle.

5. Migration of vesicles: The vesicle containing the LDL receptors migrates back to the plasma membrane and fuses with it. This causes the receptors to end up on the outer surface of the membrane. The vesicle containing the LDL fuses with a lysosome. Enzymes break up the LDLs and release the cholesterol molecules, which move to the plasma membrane and become part of it.

Exocytosis

The opposite of endocytosis is **exocytosis** (ex-ō-sī-TŌ-sis; *exo*, outside). During this process, a secretory vesicle releases its contents into the extracellular fluid after fusing with the plasma membrane. In addition, the phospholipids that make up the vesicle become part of the plasma membrane, which causes the membrane to grow. Since endocytosis removes part of the plasma membrane, if a cell is to maintain a constant size, the amount of exocytosis and endocytosis must be equal.

The cell uses exocytosis to secrete a variety of substances into the extracellular fluid. The secretory vesicles move along microfilaments and finally turn inside out when they fuse with the plasma membrane. This ensures that the vesicle releases its contents to the outside of the cell. The cell also uses exocytosis to rid itself of waste products that are too large to pass through channels or carriers. For example, after a lysosome breaks down solid particles inside other vesicles, it expels the indigestible pieces from the cell by exocytosis.

MEMBRANE STRUCTURE AND FUNCTION

TOPICS TO KNOW FOR CHAPTER 6 (MEMBRANE STRUCTURE AND FUNCTION)

1. Define each item in the following list.
2. On a sheet of paper, draw a "concept web" that includes each item in this list.

0.9 % NaCl solution
5% glucose (dextrose)
280-300 mOsm/L
active process
active transport
adhesion (linker) proteins
amphipathic
antiporter
aquaporins
bulk transport
calcium pumps
carrier receptor
carrier-mediated transport
carriers
CCREAM
cell membrane
cellular recognition
channels
chloride pumps
cholesterol
classification of membrane proteins
concentration gradient
cotransport
countertransport
coupled transporter
crenation
cytosol
dialysis
diffusion
electrochemical gradient
endocytic vesicle
endocytosis
enzymes
exocytosis
facilitated transport
factors affecting diffusion
fluid mosaics
gated channels

glycocalyx
glycolipids
glycoproteins
gradient steepness
gradients across a membrane
hydrostatic pressure
hypertonic
hypotonic
importance of fluid nature of membrane
importance of membrane semipermeability
integral proteins
ion channels
isotonic
leaky channels
ligand
ligand-gated channel
lipoprotein
lysis
macrophage
markers (recognition proteins)
mechanically-gated channel
membrane carbohydrates
membrane lipids
membrane permeability
membrane proteins
membrane pumps
membrane transport
method of absorbing LDLs
movement against a gradient
movement along a gradient
movement down a gradient
movement of lipid-soluble items
movement of water-soluble items
movement up a gradient
nonpermeating solute
oligosaccharides
osmolarity

osmosis
osmotic pressure
passive process
peripheral proteins
permeability
permeating solute
phagocytes
phagocytic cells
phagocytosis
phagosome
phospholipids
pinocytosis
plasma membrane
pores
primary active transport
pseudopodia
reasons why gradients develop
receptor-mediated endocytosis
receptors
saturation point
secondary active transport
selectively permeable
semipermeable
simple diffusion through a membrane
sodium-potassium (Na+/K+) pump
solute
solvent
steps for Na/K pump
steps in facilitated transport
stretch-activated channel
substrates
symporter
tonicity
transmembrane proteins
vesicle
vesicular transport
voltage-gated channel

CHAPTER 7

Tissues

Thus far, on our journey through the human body, we have made our way through the chemical and cellular levels of organization. The next stop along the way is tissues. A **tissue** (TISH-ū; woven) is a group of similar cells working together to perform a particular function. There are four major groups of tissues: *epithelial*, *connective*, *muscle*, and *nervous*. The study of tissues is **histology** (his-TOL-ō-jē; *histo*, tissue), and histologists are scientists who study tissues.

Although all tissues are groups of cells, some tissues have cells packed closely together, while others have cells more widely scattered. Before looking at specific types of tissue, let's look at some of the ways cells hold onto one another within a tissue.

CELL CONNECTIONS

Cells may be "stuck" together in a variety of ways, but the two most significant ways are: (1) via the "sticky" glycocalyx (sugar coats) on the surfaces of the cells; and (2) via specialized junctions, which include *desmosomes*, *tight junctions*, and *gap junctions* (Figure 7-1).

Desmosomes (DEZ-mo-sōmz; *desmo*, band; *somes*, bodies) are filamentous connections that not only hold adjacent cells together but also give internal structural support to the cells. Each desmosome contains a *plaque* (PLAK; plate) located on the cytoplasmic surface of the plasma membrane. The plaque consists of glycoproteins and resembles a tiny button. Externally, filamentous proteins called *cadherins* (kad-HAIR-enz) radiate out from the plaque and intertwine with cadherin filaments from the adjacent cell. Internally, intermediate filaments of the cytoskeleton attach to the plaques and anchor them to plaques on the opposite side of the cytoplasm. As a result, a pulling force on one side of the cell exerts tension throughout the cell's cytoskeleton and not just on the plasma membrane.

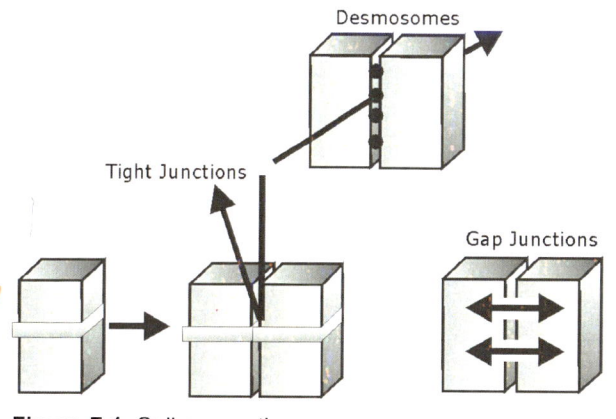

Figure 7-1. Cell connections

This internal support system reduces the likelihood that cells will tear apart.

Desmosomes are found in tissues that experience stretching, such as in the skin (in these cells, the intermediate filaments of the cytoskeleton are made of the protein *keratin*). Since desmosomes are filamentous (not densely packed globular structures) in the intercellular space, they do not prevent materials from passing in between the connected cells (see figure).

Tight junctions are continuous bands of protein that form an almost impenetrable barrier to prevent substances from passing through the intercellular space between connected cells. A tight junction consists of integral proteins called *occludins* (ō-KLŪ-denz) that extend out from the plasma membrane of adjoining cells and fuse together. In effect, these junctions function like thick belts around the cells. The fact that the "belt" of one cell fuses with a similar belt on an adjacent cell prevents materials from passing in between the cells. This is important in regions where it is important to keep fluids in one compartment from leaking freely into another compartment. In order for materials to get past the tight junction barrier, they must pass through the cytoplasm of the adjoining cells. In this way, the cells can modify the substances as they pass from one compartment to another. Tight junctions are found in cells that line the stomach and intestines, and in cells that line blood vessels in the brain.

Gap junctions are tiny channels that allow materials to pass from the cytoplasm of one cell into the cytoplasm of an adjacent cell. A gap junction forms when transmembrane proteins called *connexons* (ko-NEX-onz) in adjacent cells bind to one another. The result is a tiny tube between the joined cells. These connections are abundant in cardiac and smooth muscle cells.

EPITHELIAL TISSUE

Epithelial tissue (ep-i-THĒ-lē-al; *epithe*, added on), also called **epithelium**, forms thin membranous coverings around and inside various organs and it forms glands. For this reason, epithelial tissue is classified as either *membranous* or *glandular*.

Glandular Epithelium

Glandular epithelium forms specialized structures called **glands** that release substances beneficial to the body. The word **secretion** (sē-KRĒ-shun; *secret*, set apart) is a noun when it refers to the substance released from the gland, and it is a verb when referring to the process of releasing the substance. Histologists classify glands based on the destination of their secretions.

Endocrine glands (EN-dō-krin; *endo*, inside; *crine*, secretion) secrete chemicals called **hormones** into tissue fluid or the bloodstream. Hormones function as chemical messengers sent through the blood from endocrine glands to other organs in the body. The prefix *endo* implies that the secretions of these glands remain inside the body. You will learn about endocrine glands in a later chapter.

Exocrine glands (EX-ō-krin; *exo*, outside) expel secretions into a cavity or tube that has connections with the outside of the body. These glands are either *unicellular* or *multicellular*. The only example of a unicellular gland in the body is a *goblet cell*, which secretes mucus directly onto the surface of certain epithelial membranes. Multicellular glands expel their secretions into a tiny tube called a **duct** (literally, "to lead"). Histologists classify multicellular glands based on the structure of the gland and the method of secretion. Here we will consider only the method of secretion:

- **Apocrine glands** (AP-ō-krin; *apo*, off) make secretions consisting of portions of glandular cells that have broken off (notice the literal meaning of the name). Mammary glands that produce milk in the breasts are the only glands in humans that are apocrine type. You can remember apocrine glands by relating the first four letters of their name with their mode of secretion: A Piece of Cell is in the secretion.

- **Holocrine glands** (HŌ-lō-krin; "whole secretion") make secretions consisting of entire cell that have disintegrated. An example of a holocrine gland is a sebaceous (oil) gland in the skin. Remember holocrine glands have "whole" cells disintegrating to enter the secretion.

- **Merocrine glands** (MER-ō-krin; *mero*, part) make secretions by exocytosis. These are the most common type of exocrine gland and include sweat glands, salivary glands, and mammary glands.

TISSUES

Membranous Epithelium

Membranous epithelium (MEM-bruh-nus) exists on the free surfaces of various organs, including the skin where it forms the *epidermis* (the outer, visible part of the skin). It also covers the outside of visceral organs such as the stomach and intestines, and lines their internal cavities. Membranous epithelium functions in protection, absorption, filtration, and secretion. Unlike cell membranes, which are phospholipid bilayers, epithelial membranes are *multicellular*. Membranous epithelium has the following characteristics:

- Tightly packed cells: There is little extracellular space in membranous epithelium due to desmosomes and, sometimes, tight junctions that hold cells close together.

- Cells arranged in layers: Some epithelial tissues may consist of only one layer of cells, or it may have more than 30 layers, or *strata*; each layer is a *stratum*.

- Avascular (ā-VAS-ku-lar; *a*, without; *vascul*, vessel): There are no blood vessels in membranous epithelium. Nutrition for membranous epithelial cells arrives by diffusion from blood vessels in nearby connective tissues.

- Nerve supply: Epithelial tissues contain nerve fibers from the nervous system; therefore, we say the tissues are *innervated* (EN-er-vā-ted). As a result, damage or irritation of an epithelial tissue can cause pain.

- Polarity: All membranous epithelia exhibit anatomical and physiological differences between their cells located at the free surface (in contact with the outside of the body or a body cavity) and their cells in contact with underlying connective tissues. This characteristic is called *polarity*. An epithelium's **apical surface** is its outermost layer of cells in contact with the "free" surface; the epithelial cells in this region are the **apical cells**. An epithelium's **basal surface** is its deepest layer of cells; the epithelial cells in this region are **basal cells**.

- Basement membrane: A thin layer of glycoproteins and collagen fibers make up a basement membrane that separates membranous epithelium from underlying connective tissues. This membrane supports the overlying epithelial tissue and serves as a passageway for the diffusion of nutrients from the underlying connective tissue. The glycoprotein component of the basement membrane is secreted from the basal cells of the epithelium and is called the **basal lamina** (LAM-i-na; thin plate). The collagen protein component of the basement membrane is secreted from connective tissue cells lying beneath the epithelium. The collagen fibers in this region intertwine to form a net-like pattern; for this reason, this part of the basement membrane is called the **reticular lamina** (re-TIK-ū-lar; *reti*, net).

- Some house receptors: Special structures called *receptors* exist in some epithelia and allow the body to detect changes in the internal or external environment. In the nasal cavity, some receptors within epithelia are sensitive to odors, while others are sensitive to touch.

CLASSIFICATION OF MEMBRANOUS EPITHELIUM

Histologists classify membranous epithelium by *cell shape*, *cell arrangement*, and *location*.

Classification by Cell Shape (see Figure 7-2)

- **Squamous** (SKWĀ-mus; thin plate): cells are flat and resemble scales on a fish. The outer part of your skin consists of dead squamous cells.

- **Cuboidal** (kū-BOY-dal; *oid*, resembles): cells are cube shaped; example: lining of tiny tubes in the kidneys.

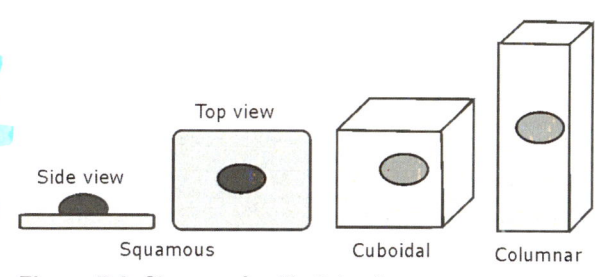

Figure 7-2. Shapes of epithelial cells

- **Columnar** cells are column-shaped; i.e., they are taller than they are wide. These cells are found in various glands of the body.
- **Transitional** cells can change shape from cuboidal to squamous and back to cuboidal, depending on the amount of compression exerted on the cells. These cells line the inside of the urinary bladder.

Classification by Cell Arrangement (see Figure 7-3)

- **Simple** epithelium has only one layer of cells; includes simple squamous, cuboidal, and columnar epithelium.
- **Stratified** epithelium has two or more layers of cells. The name for a particular stratified epithelium depends on the shape of the apical cells. Examples include stratified squamous, stratified cuboidal and stratified columnar epithelium.
- **Pseudostratified** epithelium (SU-dō-STRA-ti-fid) is actually a simple epithelium but it looks stratified (*pseudo*, false). The reason for this illusion is that although each cell in the epithelium rests on the basement membrane, not all of them reach the apical surface.

Classification by Location

- **Endothelium** (en-dō-THĒ-lē-um) is simple squamous epithelium that lines the inside of blood vessels and lymph vessels.
- **Serous membranes** (SĒR-us) are simple squamous epithelia that cover visceral organs and line major body cavities that do not have connections with the outside of the body. A serous membrane, also called **mesothelium** (mez-ō-THĒ-lē-um), secretes a watery liquid called **serous fluid** that reduces friction during movement. The word serous comes from the word *serum*, which means "whey," the liquid component of milk after the fat (curd) has been removed. Serous membranes include the peritoneal, pleural, and pericardial membranes.
- **Mucous membranes** (MU-kus) may be simple columnar, pseudostratified, or stratified squamous epithelia, but all line cavities that have a connection to the outside of the body. Examples include the linings of the nasal cavity, esophagus, trachea, stomach, intestines, and tubes associated with the urinary and reproductive systems. Mucous membranes contain **goblet cells** that secrete a viscous fluid called **mucus** (note the different spelling) onto the membrane's free surface. A protein called *mucin* gives mucus its thick viscous nature.

SPECIFIC MEMBRANOUS EPITHELIA

We will now describe various types of membranous epithelium and you can see them illustrated in Figure 7-4. Learn to recognize these tissues and know their locations.

Simple squamous epithelium consists of a single layer of flat cells and forms serous membranes, small sacs within the lungs, filtering devices within the kidneys, and endothelium. It protects underlying tissues by reducing friction (in the case of serous membranes) and allows diffusion of gases through the walls of capillaries and tiny sacs in the lungs.

Stratified squamous epithelium contains multiple layers of cuboidal or columnar cells, with flat apical cells covering the free surface. It exists on the surface of the skin and the inner linings of the mouth, esophagus, and vagina where it provides protection to underlying tissues.

Simple cuboidal epithelium is a single layer of cube-shaped cells and exists in tiny tubes of the kidney and certain glands, and on the surface of the ovary. It protects underlying tissues and allows passage of material between the blood and kidney fluid destined to become urine.

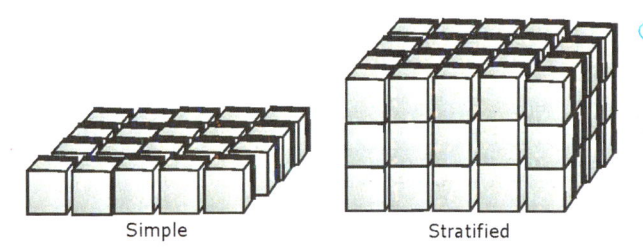

Figure 7-3. Arrangement of epithelial cells

TISSUES

(a) Simple squamous

(b) Stratified squamous

(c) Simple cuboidal

(d) Stratified cuboidal

(e) Simple columnar

(f) Stratified columnar

(g) Pseudo stratified columnar

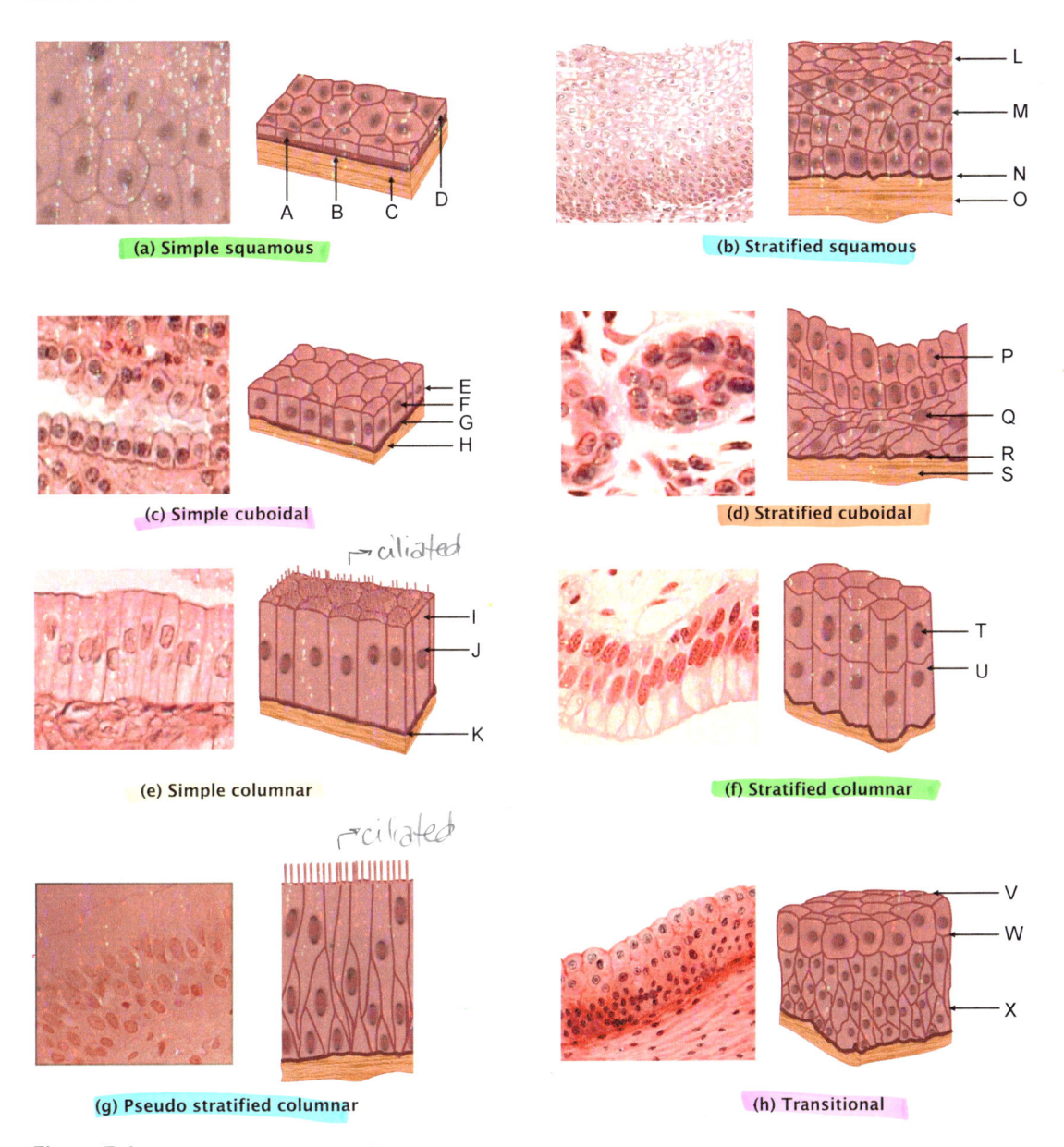

(h) Transitional

Figure 7-4.

Stratified cuboidal epithelium consists of multiple layers of cube-shaped cells and exists in the ducts of certain glands. Its primary function is protection of underlying tissues.

Simple columnar epithelium is a single layer of columnar cells interspersed with goblet cells. A *nonciliated* type makes up the inner lining of the digestive tract where it allows absorption of digested food molecules. A *ciliated* type lines the oviducts and the small tubes in the lungs, where it moves mucus that traps dust and other particles.

Stratified columnar epithelium has multiple layers of column-shaped cells and lines the male's urethra and ducts of some glands. It protects underlying tissues.

Pseudostratified ciliated columnar epithelium is a single layer of columnar cells in which some cells do not reach the free surface. It contains ciliated cells and goblet cells and lines the nasal cavity, trachea, and part of male's urethra. It protects underlying tissues by secreting and moving mucus.

Transitional epithelium is a stratified epithelium in which the apical cells change shape when compressed. It exists in the lining of the urinary bladder, ureters, and part of the urethra, where it allows these organs to expand.

CONNECTIVE TISSUE

Connective tissue is the most abundant tissue in the body and serves primarily to bind structures together. Other functions include support, protection, insulation, movement, shock absorption, transport of nutrients and metabolites, and storage. Histologists classify connective tissues according to the abundance of cells, amount of extracellular space, arrangement of extracellular fibers, and function. Major groups include connective tissue proper, cartilage, vascular tissue (blood), and osseous tissue (bone). All connective tissues arise from **mesenchyme** (MEZ-en-kīm), an undifferentiated, embryonic tissue. While most mesenchyme differentiates to form specific types of connective tissue, the mature body still possesses some mesenchyme that can replace damaged tissues when needed.

The major structural characteristics of connective tissue include *vascularization* and an extensive *matrix*. All connective tissues, except cartilage, are supplied with blood vessels, a condition known as **vascularization** (vas-kū-lar-ZĀ-shun). Loose connective tissues are the most vascularized, while vessels are sparsely scattered in dense connective tissues. Most connective tissues contain a significant amount of material in between the cells called **extracellular matrix**. The connective tissue matrix includes two components: *ground substance and extracellular fibers.*

Ground Substance of Connective Tissues

Ground substance is the fluid component of the matrix and contains water, ions, nutrients, metabolites, adhesion proteins, and proteoglycans. Adhesion proteins, the most common being *fibronectin* (fī-brō-NEK-tin), connect cells to extracellular fibers and the ground substance. Proteoglycans resemble bristle brushes used to clean bottles. The central "wire" of this proteoglycan "brush" consists of a filamentous protein, while the "bristles" include a variety of polysaccharides, collectively called **glycosaminoglycans** (GAGs; GLĪ-kōs-am-ē-nō-GLĪ-kanz); formerly called *mucopolysaccharides.*) Because they have the capacity to intertwine and trap water, GAGs contribute to the ground substance's viscosity (gel-like nature).

Two common polysaccharides (GAGs) associated with proteoglycans are *hyaluronic acid* and *chondroitin sulfate.* **Hyaluronic acid** makes ground substance very slippery and aids in lubrication, especially in joints. **Chondroitin sulfate** makes the ground substance more viscous and helps hold the matrix together, especially in cartilage and bone tissue.

Extracellular Fibers in Connective Tissues

Extracellular fibers are abundant in most connective tissues and exist throughout the ground substance of the matrix. These fibers provide structural support and strength for the connective tissue. The connective tissue cells synthesize the fiber's proteins at ribosomes then secrete them into the matrix where they intertwine to form coiled strands. There are three major types of protein fibers in various connective tissues:

- **Collagenous fibers** (ko-LAJ-e-nus) are made of the protein *collagen* and appear as *white fibers* in the matrix. They offer the connective tissue a great amount of resistance to tension (pulling force). Collagen is the body's most abundant protein, and it is the primary component of leather.

- **Reticular fibers** are very thin, highly branched collagenous fibers that give the matrix of certain connective tissues a net-like appearance (*ret*, net). Reticular fibers are abundant in the reticular lamina of the basement membrane that supports all epithelial tissues.

- **Elastic fibers** contain *elastin* protein and appear as *yellow fibers.* Their highly coiled structure allows certain connective tissues to recoil after stretching. Elastic fibers are abundant in stretchable organs, including the lungs, most blood vessels, and the skin.

TISSUES

CELLS IN CONNECTIVE TISSUES

Since all connective tissues arise from mesenchyme tissue, the mesenchyme cells must differentiate to give rise to the many unique connective tissues. The early developmental stage of any connective tissue involves highly active cells with names that end with *blast* ("to bud"). The blast cells of *most* connective tissues produce the matrix of the developing tissue (cells that give rise to blood cells are an exception). In many connective tissues, after the blasts surround themselves with matrix and become "mature" they become less active. The mature cells primarily associated with a particular connective tissue have names that end with *-cyte* (sīt; cell). Examples of blasts and cytes in various connective tissues include:

- **Fibroblasts** (FĪ-brō-blasts) produce the matrix of most connective tissues. In most cases, fibroblasts become **fibrocytes**, but in adipose (fat) tissue they become **adipocytes**.

- **Chondroblasts** (KON-drō-blasts) produce the matrix of cartilage and eventually become **chondrocytes**.

- **Osteoblasts** (OS-tē-ō-blasts) produce the matrix of bone and eventually become **osteocytes**.

- **Hemocytoblasts** (hēm-ō-SĪ-tō-blasts) are cells that give rise to different blood cells (described shortly) but do not produce the liquid matrix, or *plasma*, of blood.

In addition to the major cell types, there are a number of other cells associated with various connective tissues. These include *mast cells* and *macrophages*. **Mast cells** congregate around blood vessels and when stimulated by a variety of chemicals release the chemical *histamine* (HIS-ta-mēn). Histamine causes the blood vessels to dilate (open up) and become "leaky." As a result, fluid can leave the vessel and enter the surrounding tissues, causing them to swell. **Macrophages** (MAK-rō-fā-jez) are specialized white blood cells that once lived in the blood but squeezed out of the blood vessel into the surrounding tissues. Macrophages crawl around engulfing foreign particles and dead or damaged body cells.

Now we turn our attention to the major types of connective tissue in the body. These tissues can be grouped into four major classes: *connective tissue proper, cartilage, osseous tissue,* and *blood*.

CONNECTIVE TISSUE PROPER

Connective tissue proper includes all connective tissues except bone, cartilage, and blood, and it is subdivided into *loose connective tissues* and *dense connective tissues*.

Loose Connective Tissues

Loose connective tissues have loosely packed intercellular fibers and include *areolar*, *adipose*, and *reticular* tissue (see Figure 7-5).

Areolar tissue (a-RĒ-ō-lar; area) is the most widely distributed connective tissue. It has a gel-like matrix and contains collagenous, reticular, and elastic fibers produced by fibroblasts (Figure 7-5a). Large phagocytic cells called *macrophages* are abundant in this tissue and defend the body against foreign particles such as bacteria. Areolar tissue also contains mast cells that secrete histamine (mentioned earlier). Allergic reactions in skin and mucous membranes result when mast cells react to various "foreign" chemicals. **Lamina propria** (LAM-i-na PRŌ-prē-a) is areolar tissue beneath a mucous membrane.

Adipose tissue (AD-i-pōs; *adipo*, fat) is a loose tissue containing **adipocytes** (fat cells). The cytoplasm of adipocytes contains a large droplet consisting of triglyceride molecules (Figure 7-5b). Adipocytes form early in life and do not divide, but they can swell and shrink depending on the amount of lipid molecules stored in the cytoplasm. The functions of adipose tissue include energy storage, insulation, protection, and heat generation. Adipose (fat) tissue exists in two forms, *yellow* and *brown*.

- **Yellow fat** gets its characteristic yellow color from pigments such as *carotene* (common in many vegetables). Yellow fat is the most common fat in an adult, and is abundant just below the skin of the abdomen, buttocks, and thighs.

- **Brown fat** has a brown color due to pigments in its numerous mitochondria and an abundance of blood vessels coursing through the tissue. It is more abundant in infants than in adults. Brown fat

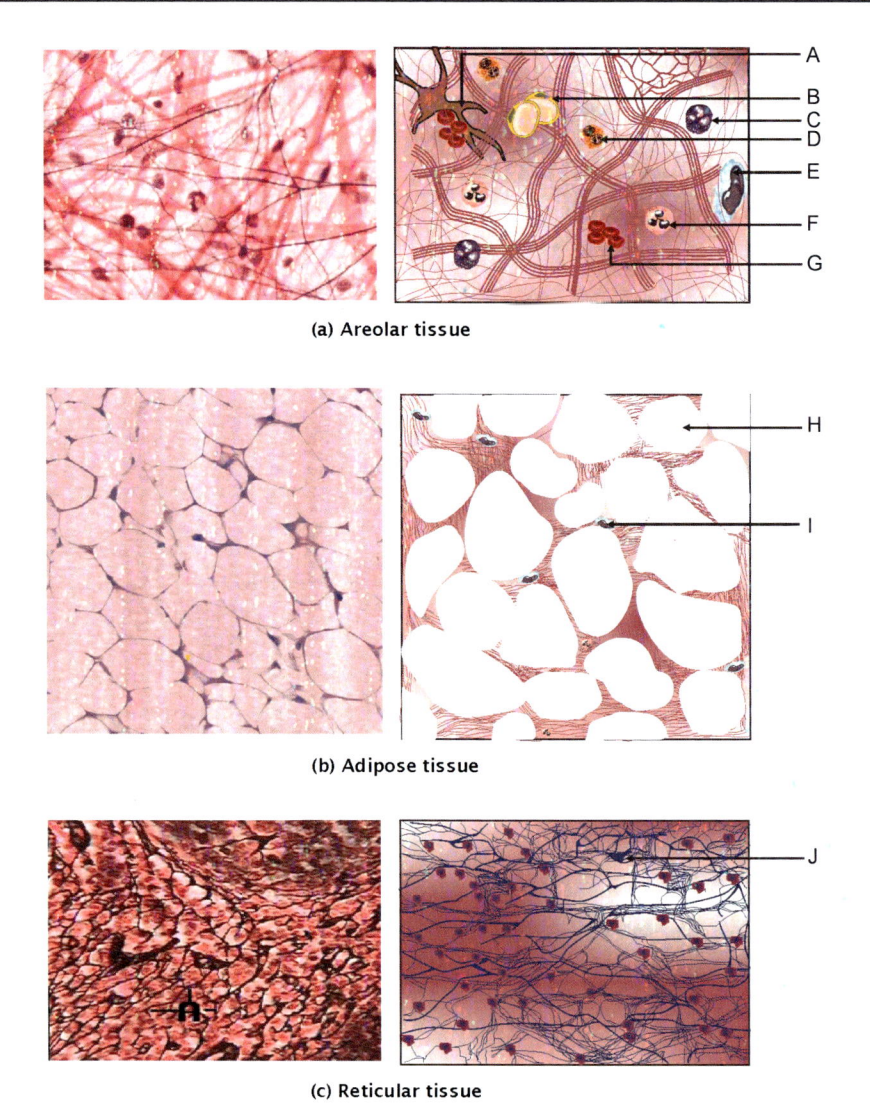

Figure 7-5. Loose connective tissues

is specialized to generate heat from fat catabolism. In the adult, brown fat is found primarily in the armpits, neck, and kidney regions.

Reticular tissue gets its name from the thin, highly branched collagen fibers that produce a net-like appearance (Figure 7-5c). The fibers intertwine in a loose fashion, but link together to form the internal framework, or *stroma*, of the liver, spleen, lymph nodes, and bone marrow.

Dense Connective Tissues

Dense connective tissues have protein fibers packed together tightly so that fibroblasts appear squeezed in between them. Dense connective tissues include *elastic*, *dense regular*, and *dense irregular* tissue (Figure 7-6).

Elastic tissue has many extracellular, elastin protein fibers. This tissue is strong and stretchable, providing elasticity to blood vessels, lungs, and vocal cords.

Dense regular tissue has collagen fibers arranged in a parallel fashion with fibroblasts squeezed in between them. It has a limited ability to stretch, but provides tremendous strength to tendons (tough fibrous bands that attach muscles to bones) and ligaments (similar bands that attach bones to other bones).

Dense irregular tissue gets its name because of its irregular arrangement of collagen fibers. This

TISSUES

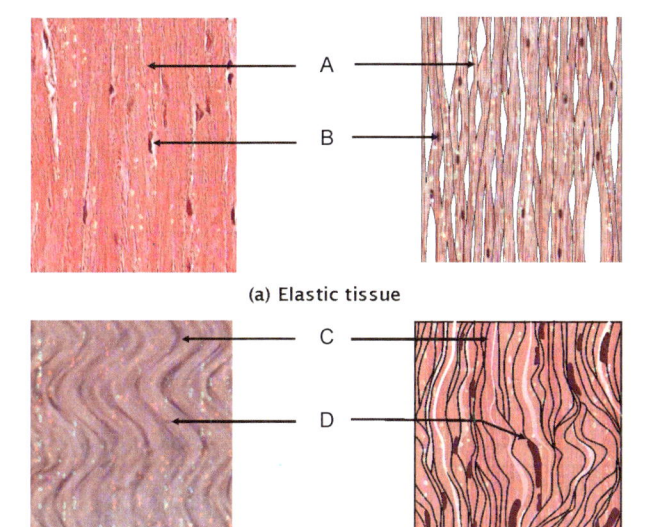

(a) Elastic tissue

(b) Dense regular tissue

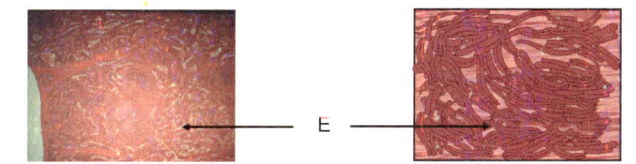

(c) Dense irregular tissue

Figure 7-6. Dense connective tissues

tissue offers structural strength and is more resilient (flexible) than dense regular tissue. Dense irregular tissue is abundant in the skin and coverings of the kidneys, bones, and testes.

CARTILAGE

Cartilage (KAR-ti-lij; gristle) is a strong, yet somewhat flexible, connective tissue that functions primarily in support. Cartilage is the only connective tissue that is *avascular* and it lacks nerve endings. During growth or repair of cartilage, cells called **chondroblasts** divide and secrete a matrix containing fine collagen fibers. The matrix traps the chondroblasts within tiny cavities called **lacunae** (la-KŪ-nā; bowl). After this happens, the trapped chondroblasts become **chondrocytes**. A fibrous membrane, the **perichondrium** (per-i-KON-drē-um) covers the surface of cartilage. Three types of cartilage include *hyaline, elastic*, and *fibrocartilage* (Figure 7-7).

- **Hyaline cartilage** (HĪ-a-lin; glassy) has very fine collagenous fibers that are virtually invisible with a light microscope. It has a "glassy" appearance and is the tissue that most people call *gristle*. Hyaline cartilage covers the ends of bones and reduces friction when the ends of bones rub against each other. This cartilage forms the "growth plates" of bones, allowing them to grow in length. It also forms parts of the nose, larynx (voice box), and trachea (windpipe).

- **Elastic cartilage** contains abundant elastic fibers, which make it very flexible. This cartilage maintains the shape of the ear and epiglottis (a flap that covers the opening to the trachea when you swallow).

- **Fibrocartilage** has a matrix packed with very thick collagen fibers. It provides tension (pulling) strength and compression strength for intervertebral discs (pads between the vertebrae), pubic symphysis (connection between the two

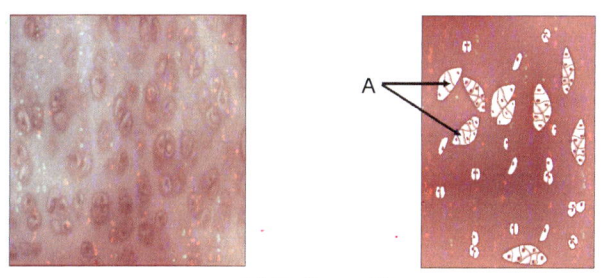

(a) Hyaline cartilage

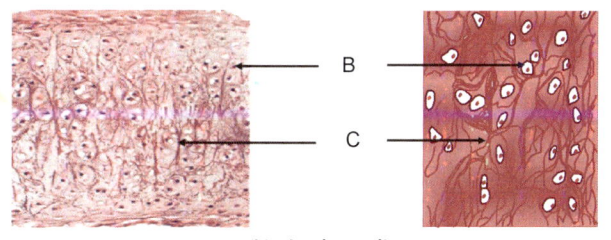

(b) Elastic cartilage

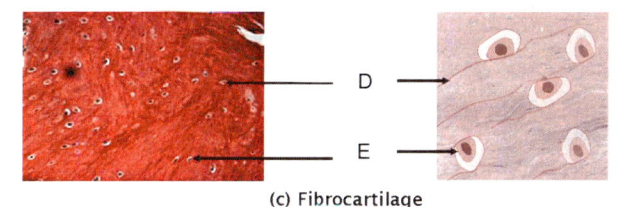

(c) Fibrocartilage

Figure 7-7. Types of cartilage

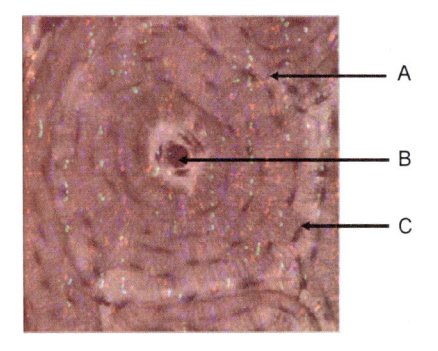

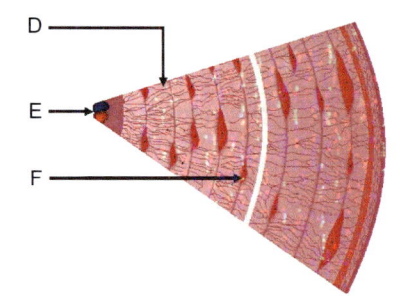

Figure 7-8. Osseous tissue

hipbones), and menisci (crescent-shaped pads in certain joints).

OSSEOUS TISSUE

Osseous tissue (bone) (OS-ē-us) is the connective tissue with the hardest matrix. **Osteoblasts** secrete an organic material, called *osteoid* (os-tē-OYD) that hardens when calcium salts precipitate within it. The hardened matrix eventually surrounds the osteoblasts, which then become **osteocytes** trapped within a *lacuna* (similar to a trapped chondroblast in cartilage) (Figure 7-8). Bones provide support for the body, attachment sites for muscles, storage sites for minerals and fat, and they contain marrow that manufactures blood cells.

BLOOD

Blood is a unique connective tissue in that it flows throughout the body; therefore, in a sense, it "connects" all parts of the body. Blood consists of two components: (1) *formed elements*, which are the cellular components, and (2) **plasma**, the liquid extracellular matrix that surrounds the formed elements (Figure 7-9). While it is flowing through the body, plasma does not contain extracellular fibers. However, when blood forms a clot, the extracellular fibers develop from soluble proteins already present in the plasma. The plasma transports gases, nutrients, and cellular metabolites (wastes, hormones, various proteins, and other chemicals). The kidneys help regulate the amount of plasma in the blood.

The blood's formed elements include *red blood cells*, *white blood cells* and *platelets*. **Red blood cells (RBCs** or **erythrocytes**: e-RITH-rō-sīts; *erythro*, red) are anucleate and transport oxygen from the lungs to the tissues throughout the body. The **white blood cells (WBCs** or **leukocytes**: LŪ-kō-sīts; *leuk*, white) are part of the body's defense system. Some of these leave the bloodstream, enter other tissues, and differentiate to become macrophages. **Platelets** (or **thrombocytes**: THROM-bō-sīts; thromb, clot) are small, anucleate cell fragments that release chemicals that promote blood clotting.

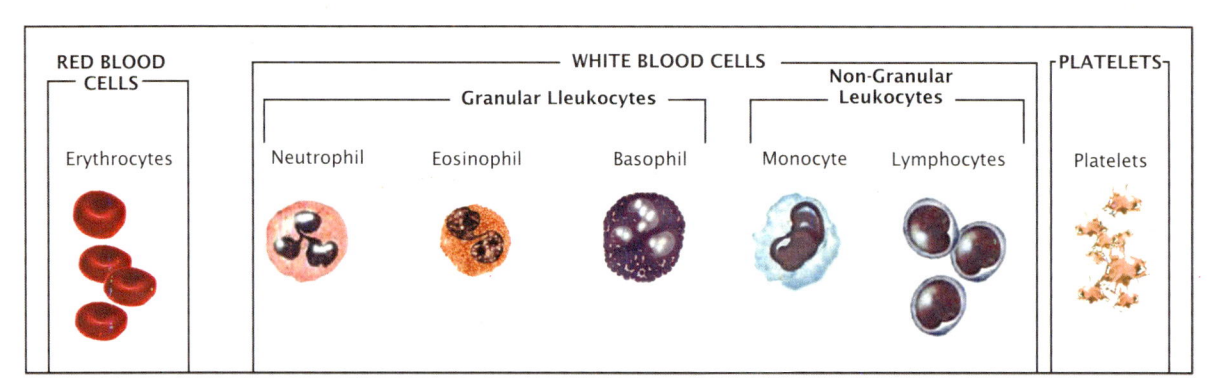

Figure 7-9. Blood

TISSUE HEALING

Shallow (superficial) wounds may damage only a membranous epithelium. In this case, healthy basal cells from nearby regions can proliferate and replace the lost or damaged cells. Shallow skin wounds, such as abrasions, non-bleeding cuts, and first-degree and second-degree burns, heal through division and migration of basal cells, which eventually fill in the lost tissue. When the two sides of the wound grow together, most cells stop migrating due to a phenomenon called **contact inhibition**.

When wounds are deeper and more extensive, the repair process is more complex. In the first step, blood clotting occurs. Platelets and damaged blood vessels in the wound release chemicals that cause the formation of fibers called **fibrin** (FĪ-brin). The fibrin fibers intertwine and form a netlike mesh in the broken vessel that traps blood cells. This collection of fibrin and the blood's formed elements is a **blood clot**, and it can help decrease the loss of blood from the vessel. Fibrin fibers also develop outside the vessel and help "wall off" the area, preventing bacteria from moving into other tissues. Mast cells release histamine that makes capillaries dilate and become "leaky." As plasma leaks out of the vessel, the surrounding tissues show **edema** (e-DĒ-ma; swelling).

Damaged tissues also release a variety of chemicals that attract WBCs to the damaged site. The movement of a cell toward a certain chemical is **chemotaxis**. When the WBCs in nearby blood vessels detect the chemicals released from damaged tissues, they begin to cling to the blood vessel's inner wall in a process called **margination** (mar-jen-Ā-shun). Then the WBCs exit the vessel in a process called **diapedesis** (dī-a-pe-DĒ-sis; *dia*, through; *pedesis*, leaping), whereby the cell squeezes between the vessel's endothelial cells. In the surrounding tissues, the WBCs engulf foreign particles and remove dead cells.

Various signs and symptoms, collectively known as **inflammation**, characterize a tissue soon after the tissue suffers damage. The signs of inflammation include heat, redness, and swelling, all of which result when chemicals released from damaged tissues cause local blood vessels to dilate. This vasodilation increases blood flow and provides more nutrients and oxygen to the damaged tissue. However, it also causes the tissues to swell as fluid leaks out of the dilated vessels. A symptom of inflammation is pain in and around the damaged tissue resulting, in part, from edema exerting pressure on local pain receptors.

The clotted blood and tissue fluid hardens to form a **scab** that protects the underlying tissue as it heals. Beneath the scab, fibroblasts produce fibers that help "bridge the gap" between the cut edges of the damaged tissue. At this time, capillaries, nerve endings, and other damaged structures begin to regenerate. Evidence of this tissue replacement process is a pink sensitive tissue called **granulation tissue**, located beneath the scab. As nerve tissue regenerates in the wounded area, they often send signals to the brain spontaneously, which causes the wound to itch.

Near the end of the healing process, a scar forms in a process called **fibrosis** (fī-BRŌ-sis), in which fibrous connective tissue replaces the damaged tissues. Closing a large wound with sutures (stitches) limits the amount of fibrosis. Allowing excessive fibrous tissue production results in raised scars known as *keloid scar*. During the healing process, blood platelets release **platelet-derived growth factors** (PDGFs) that stimulate fibroblasts to produce more fibers, thereby accelerating tissue repair.

TISSUE NECROSIS

Tissue death can occur in response to a number of factors, but one factor involves a lack of needed substances. Tissues deprived of oxygen or other nutrients for an extended time will die and decay. This process, called **tissue necrosis** (ne-KRŌ-sis; *necro*, corpse) is common during wound healing. However, when necrosis becomes extensive, a condition called **gangrene** (gan-GRĒN; "gnawing sore") develops and can lead to **septicemia** (sep-ti-SĒ-mē-a; *septi*, putrefying; *emia*, blood), also known as blood poisoning. As bacteria decompose tissues, various chemicals form, including **ptomaine** (tō-MĀN; "corpse"), which is a toxic alkaline material released when bacteria decompose certain amino acids. The foul smell of decaying tissue is most commonly due to a chemical called **cadaverine** (ka-da-ver-ĒN; *cadaver*, to perish), which forms when bacteria decompose the amino acid lysine.

TOPICS TO KNOW FOR CHAPTER 7 (TISSUES)

adipocytes
adipose tissue
apical cells
apical surface
areolar tissue
avascular
basal cells
basal lamina
basal surface
basement membrane
blood
blood clot
blood's formed elements
brown fat
cadaverine
cadherins
carotene
cartilage
cell connections
cells in connective tissues
characteristics of membranous epithelium
chemotaxis
chondroblasts
chondrocytes
chondroitin sulfate
ciliated epithelium
classification by location
classification of membranous epithelium
collagen
collagenous fibers
columnar cells
connective tissue
connective tissue matrix
connective tissue proper
connexons
contact inhibition
cuboidal cells
dense connective tissues
dense irregular tissue
dense regular tissue
desmosome plaque
desmosomes
diapedesis
edema
elastic cartilage
elastic fibers
elastic tissue
elastin
endocrine glands

endothelium
epithelial polarity
epithelial tissue
epithelium
exocrine glands
extracellular fibers
erythrocytes
fibrin
fibroblasts
fibrocartilage
fibrocytes
fibronectin
fibrosis
gangrene
gap junctions
gland duct
glands
glandular epithelium
glycosaminoglycans
goblet cells
granulation tissue
gristle
ground substance
hemocytoblasts
histamine
histology
holocrine glands
hormones
hyaline cartilage
hyaluronic acid
inflammation
keloid scar
lacunae
lamina propria
leukocytes
loose connective tissues
lysine
macrophages
margination
mast cells
membranous epithelium
merocrine glands
mesenchyme
mesothelium
mucin
mucous membranes
mucus
multicellular gland
nonciliated epithelium

occludins
osseous tissue
osteoblasts
osteocytes
osteoid
perichondrium
plasma
platelet-derived growth factors
platelets
proteoglycans
pseudostratified ciliated columnar epithelium
pseudostratified epithelium
ptomaine
red blood cells
reticular fibers
reticular lamina
reticular tissue
scab
secretion
septicemia
serous fluid
serous membranes
serum
simple columnar epithelium
simple cuboidal epithelium
simple epithelium
simple squamous
specific membranous epithelia
squamous cells
strata
stratified columnar epithelium
stratified cuboidal epithelium
stratified epithelium
stratified squamous epithelium
stroma
thrombocytes
tight junctions
tissue
tissue healing
tissue necrosis
transitional cells
transitional epithelium
unicellular gland
vascularization
white blood cells
white fibers
yellow fat
yellow fiber

CHAPTER 8

The Integumentary System

The skin is the most public, the most scrutinized of the body's organs. For better or for worse, no other organ system says so much to others about who you are as an individual. Your skin is, in fact, a cornerstone of your personal identity. The social importance of the skin typically surpasses its critical physiological importance in the day-to-day thinking of most people. Then again, when the skin is injured or diseased, its central importance to homeostasis becomes all-too-readily, and sometimes very painfully, apparent.

The skin is a stratified (layered) organ. Throughout this chapter, you will learn that the skin's stratified structure gives it many remarkable properties. Skin is *flexible*; it follows the body's contours and movements, and it can grow as thin or as thick as necessary to protect specific parts of the body. The skin's stratified structure enables it to be *self-renewing*; your skin replaces itself many times throughout your life, and it can usually repair itself if it is damaged. Finally, skin is *multifunctional*; its layers house many accessory organs, as well as organs that are parts of other body systems, all of which contribute to maintaining homeostasis.

First and foremost, the skin is a barrier, one that shields us physiologically from our ever-fluctuating external environment. Because it is a cornerstone of our personal identity, it's not too surprising that the skin also is an object of profound adoration, fascination, and disappointment. Given its undeniable importance to our pursuit of happiness, as well as to our very survival, it is fitting that we begin the study of human body systems by studying the skin.

INTEGUMENTARY SYSTEM OVERVIEW

If you were asked to name an organ, the skin likely would not be the first that comes to mind. But like all organs, the **skin**, or **cutaneous** (kū-TĀN-ē-us; *cutan*, skin) **membrane**, is composed of different tissues, is physically distinct from surrounding organs, and performs functions specific to its structure (Figure 8-1). The skin is the most prominent organ of the **integumentary** (in-teg-ū-MEN-ta-rē; "covering") **system**. The other organs that comprise the integumentary system are called *skin derivatives* (or *accessory organs*), which originate from modified skin cells early in fetal development. Skin derivatives include hairs, nails, and a variety of microscopically small glands, such as those that produce sweat.

The skin also houses structures that are part of other organ systems. These structures include blood vessels (the cardiovascular system), nerves and sensory receptors (the nervous system), and lymph vessels (the lymphatic system). Although they are distinct from the integumentary system, blood vessels and nerves in particular are integral components of the skin; in turn, they carry out some functions that are attributed to the integumentary system as a whole.

THE SKIN AS AN ORGAN

What is the actual extent of the skin? Skin covers the entire body and is continuous with every orifice that opens to the outside environment, such as the openings leading to the mucous membranes of the mouth and nose. The skin also envelops the ear canals, and is continuous with the mucous membrane that lines the inner surface of the eyelids. In fact, the skin is the body's largest organ in terms of its weight and surface area.

> **Note**: The skin of an average adult weighs about 2.7 kg (6 lbs.), or about 8 percent of the total body weight, and it covers a surface of 1.5 – 2.0 square meters

The exact surface area of the skin depends directly on a person's height and weight, but a woman could have more skin than a man does, even when both have identical heights and weights. How can this be so? Pound for pound, adipose tissue occupies more space than muscle tissue, and adipose tissue typically accounts for a higher percentage of a woman's body weight. (The opposite usually is true for a man.) Due to her higher percentage of adipose tissue, a woman's body occupies more space than a man's body of the same height and weight. Consequently, a woman's body requires more skin to cover it. A general estimate for a person's surface area can be calculated using the following equations*:

$$BSA\ (m^2) = SQRT([Height\ (in) \times Weight\ (lbs)] \div 3131)$$

$$BSA\ (m^2) = SQRT([Height\ (cm) \times Weight\ (kg)] \div 3600)$$

*From Mosteller RD: Simplified Calculation of Body Surface Area. N Engl J Med 1987 Oct 22: 317(17):1098 (letter)

LAYERS OF THE SKIN

Skin consists of two major layers: the epidermis and the dermis. The **epidermis** (ep-i-DER-mis; *epi*, on;

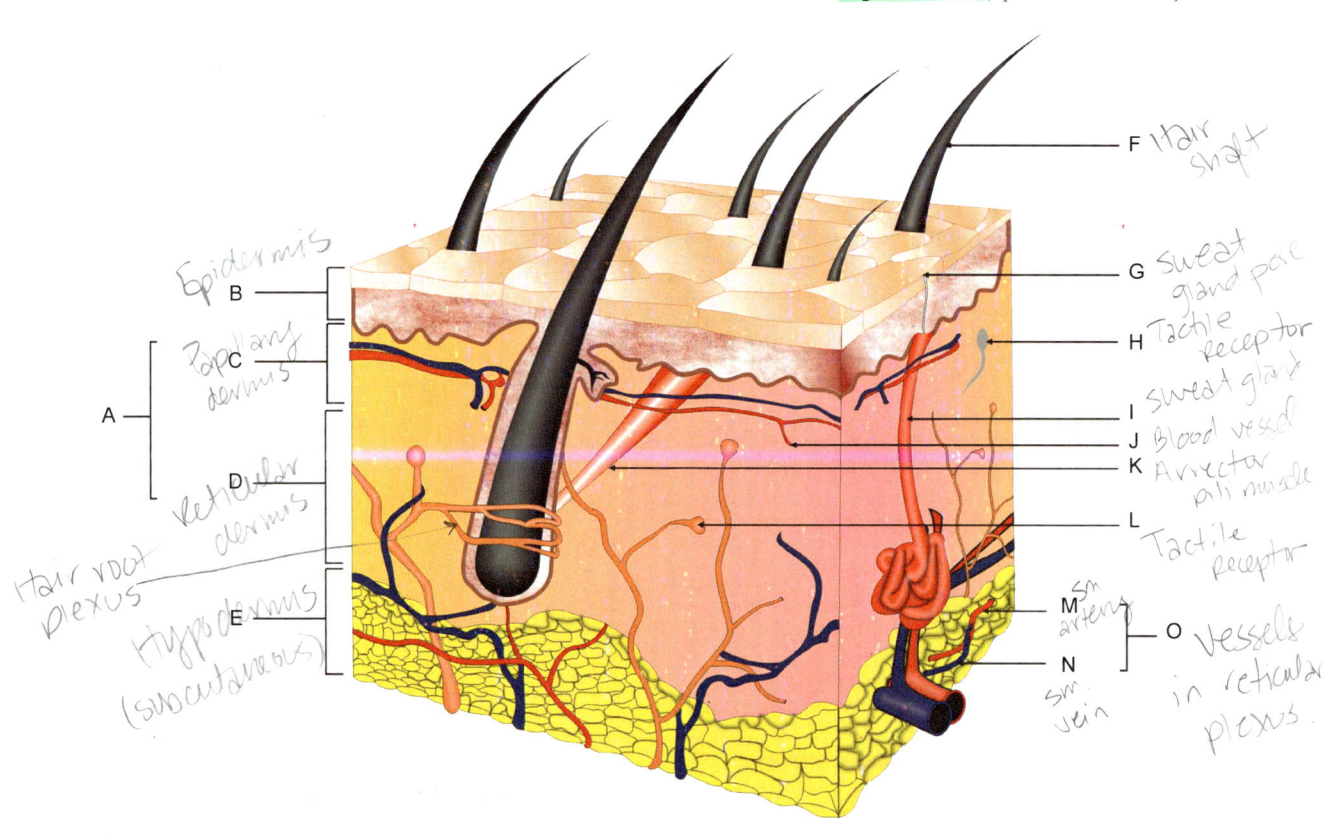

Figure 8-1. Structure of the skin

THE INTEGUMENTARY SYSTEM

dermis, skin) is the thinner, superficial layer of the skin, consisting of stratified squamous epithelium. It functions as a flexible, self-renewing barrier between the body and the external environment. The thicker layer, the **dermis**, lies deep to the epidermis and consists mostly of dense irregular and areolar connective tissues. The dermis is the strong-but-flexible, self-renewing scaffolding of the skin; the dermis gives skin its strength. In turn, the epidermis and dermis each consist of finer tissue layers called **strata** (STRA-ta; "layers"; singular is *stratum*—STRA-tum); hence, the skin is a *stratified* organ.

Underlying the skin is the **hypodermis** (hī-pō-DER-mis; *hypo*, below) or **subcutaneous tissue**. Although the hypodermis is not part of the skin, it supports and protects many parts of the integumentary system. This region is composed of areolar and adipose connective tissue, and its superficial margin fuses with the connective tissue of the dermis.

TYPES OF SKIN

Two types of skin cover the body. Anatomists draw a distinction between "thin skin" and "thick skin." Strictly speaking, this distinction is based solely on the relative depth of the epidermis (Figure 8-2). Over most of the body, the epidermis is about as thick as a sheet of paper in this book; on the palms and soles, the epidermis may be about five times thicker. In addition to thickness, thin skin and thick skin look different from one another in terms of their surface texture. The presence or absence of hair and the distribution of glands also distinguish thin and thick skin. For these reasons, thin skin and thick skin have noticeably different functional characteristics.

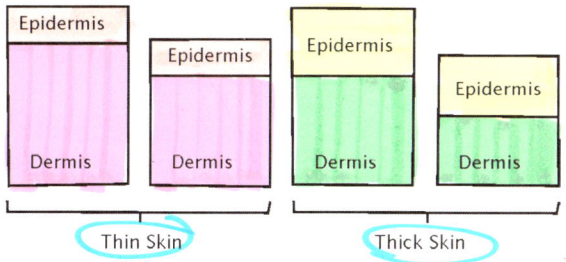

Figure 8-2. Thin and thick skin

Thin skin covers the entire body except the palms, the anterior surfaces of the fingers, the soles of the feet, and the plantar (inferior) surfaces of the toes. Thin skin has a relatively shallow, *four*-layer epidermis, numerous shallow creases on its surface, and the most variety of skin derivatives. Thin skin often contains hair, and for this reason it is sometimes called **hirsute** (HER-sūt; "hairy") **skin**. Sebaceous glands associated with each hair release oils that lubricate the hair and help waterproof the skin. In addition, thin skin may have two types of sweat glands. Finally, the dermis of thin skin has a light-but-even mix of the different sensory receptors (extensions of the nervous system that respond to stimuli such as touch and temperature change).

While you might describe somebody who is not easily offended as having "thick skin," anatomists reserve this term for skin that covers the anterior surface of the hands and fingers and the plantar surface of the feet and toes. **Thick skin** has a relatively deep, *five*-layer epidermis, a regular pattern of ridges and grooves on its surface, and fewer kinds of skin derivatives than thin skin. Most notably, thick skin lacks hair, which is why it is sometimes called **glabrous** (GLĀ-brus; "smooth") **skin**. Since thick skin lacks hair, it also lacks sebaceous (oil) glands. However, thick skin is well supplied with a type of sweat gland that can become overactive when you are nervous, causing your palms to sweat. Within its dermis, thick skin has numerous sensory receptors specialized to develop the sense of fine touch, which enables a person to detect subtle differences in texture. For example, fine touch is what allows someone to distinguish between an apple and an orange merely by comparing the feel of their surfaces.

> **Note**: The average depth of an adult's skin—epidermis and dermis together—is about 1.5 millimeters, or the thickness of 10 sheets of paper in this book.

Curiously, the skin with the greatest overall depth—epidermis and dermis together—is the skin on the back, which has a relatively thin epidermis; therefore, it's classified as thin skin. The skin on the palms and soles, however, is average in depth but has a relatively thick epidermis; consequently, it's classified as thick skin. If all this seems a bit confusing to you, just keep in mind that the dermis anywhere on the body is *always* thicker than the epidermis. Designations such as "thin skin" and "thick skin" only apply to the epidermis.

FUNCTIONS OF THE SKIN

The integumentary system is much more than a covering to wash and groom. On the contrary, it plays a variety of major and minor roles in maintaining homeostasis.

- **Protection**: Most importantly, the skin is a protective barrier, one that keeps harmful agents out of the body while holding in essential fluids and energy. The skin blocks infectious agents such as bacteria and viruses from penetrating to deeper tissues, and it even contains special cells that seek and destroy such agents. The skin also shields the body from many dangerous environmental chemicals and from the damaging ultraviolet (UV) rays of the sun. As a protective barrier, the skin prevents the body from dehydrating, and it helps conserve body heat.

- **Temperature regulation**: The skin is more than just a passive blanket that can trap body heat. Its dense network of blood vessels makes the skin an important site for regulating body temperature. In the same way that water and coolant deliver an engine's heat to the car's radiator, blood delivers the body's heat to the skin. In both cases, heat is brought to a surface where it can radiate (disperse) more efficiently into the environment. When your body's temperature rises above normal, blood vessels in your skin dilate (open wider), allowing more warm blood to flow through the skin. In addition, sweat evaporating from your skin's surface speeds up the rate at which heat is lost. Conversely, when your body temperature drops below normal, vessels in your skin constrict (become narrower) causing more warm blood to stay deep inside the body.

- **Emergency blood reserve**: The dense network of blood vessels that makes the skin an effective radiator also makes it an emergency blood reserve. During times of physiological stress, much of the skin's blood supply is diverted deep within the body to support the work of other organs. For example, if you suddenly lost a significant amount of blood, impulses from your nervous system would cause the blood vessels in your skin to constrict. The constricting vessels squeeze blood away from the skin and reduce the amount of blood flowing toward the skin. In this way, a normal volume of blood can continue to flow to vital organs such as the brain, heart, and lungs. In fact, the body may start diverting blood away from the skin at the first hint of trouble, as part of its "fight-or-flight" response. That is why watching a violent movie, or even thinking about that "make-or-break" A&P exam, may cause your skin to become cool and pale as your body prepares to deal with these "threats."

- **Excretion**: The skin is one of several organs in the body that expels wastes in a process called **excretion**. Secretory glands in the skin continuously remove excess water and salts, heavy metals (mercury, lead, and cadmium), and metabolic wastes (ammonia, carbon dioxide, urea, lactic acid, and uric acid) from the blood and excrete them from the skin in the sweat. You can see clear evidence of the skin's role in excretion in the chalky film of salts that may accumulate on your skin or clothing after you have been perspiring heavily.

- **Sensation**: The skin houses a variety of sensory receptors and nerve endings, most of which reside in the dermis. Each kind of sensory receptor is adapted to respond to a particular mechanical, chemical, or thermal stimulus originating from the external environment or from within the skin itself. Some sensory receptors give rise to the conscious sensations of touch that enable a person to determine the size, shape, and texture of objects. Other kinds of sensory receptors initiate sensations of pain or itching, while still other kinds of receptors give rise to sensations of heat or cold. Sensations may initiate a behavioral or physiological response that is necessary to maintain or reestablish homeostasis. For example, if you touch a hot stove, pain receptors initiate impulses that cause you to pull your hand away quickly, without even thinking about it, to prevent extensive tissue damage.

- **Vitamin D synthesis**: Ultraviolet light striking the skin converts a modified cholesterol molecule into an inactive form of vitamin D. The blood transports the vitamin through several other

THE INTEGUMENTARY SYSTEM

organs that convert it into its active form. Active vitamin D helps regulate how the body uses calcium and phosphorus, and so it is especially important for maintaining the health of bones, teeth, and muscles.

Other skin functions

The skin plays important roles in social identity and communication. Because skin is so conspicuous, it's not surprising that it plays important roles in human society and culture, roles that are quite different from the skin's contributions to homeostasis. We use the skin to identify one another, to communicate, to detect sexual differences, and as a means of diagnosing an illness.

- **Identification**: "I recognize your face, but I forget your name!" This isn't a surprising admission, because a portion of your brain is actually "wired" to remember the skin contours of other people's faces. Most people do this job so well that they can recognize someone's face after not having seen it for many decades. Of course, modern technology now allows us to record human fingerprints, which are unique to each person, as a means of authenticating personal identity.

- **Communication of emotions**: Long before people learn to talk, they learn to recognize the emotional states of others by studying facial expressions. The characteristic stretching and wrinkling of the skin that are associated with happiness (smiling) or sadness (frowning) represent a universal language that is recognized by individuals of all cultures. In addition, sudden changes in skin color, as might occur when a person blushes, can communicate to others the presence of intense negative emotions such as shame, fear, embarrassment, or rage.

- **Sexual differentiation**: The skin plays a role in helping individuals to detect and attract sexual partners. Characteristic differences in the skin texture and hair density on adult faces (part of what is called our "secondary sexual characteristics") help us to figure out who is male and who is female. Moreover, hair growth in the pubic and axillary regions is a signal of sexual maturity. In many cultures, the way in which men and women style their hair is an important factor in attracting and retaining a mate.

- **Diagnosing and treating health problems**: From earliest times, people looked to the skin for signs of illness elsewhere in the body. Even today, physicians are trained to examine the skin for color changes or telltale lesions (patches of altered tissue) in order to detect the presence of certain diseases. And while the skin is an effective barrier to most substances, in recent decades pharmacologists (scientists who study drugs) have developed technologies that can deliver medications slowly and steadily through the skin.

TOPICAL FEATURES OF THE SKIN

When you look closely at the surface of your skin, you will see an assortment of deep grooves, intersecting lines, and creases. The epidermal surface features found on average adult skin are classified into three groups: *surface pattern lines, flexure lines,* and *friction ridges.*

Surface pattern lines are extremely small, triangular or polygonal-shaped line patterns seen only on thin skin. These lines increase the skin's surface area, thereby allowing it to stretch more evenly during movement. **Flexure lines** are deeper than surface pattern lines and exist in regions where skin is flexed (bent) repeatedly. Examples include the "life lines" on the palms and the lines where fingers bend. Wrinkles and grooves on the face are flexure lines that develop because of frequent and prolonged muscle contraction during smiling and squinting. The pattern of flexure lines usually corresponds to the orientation of parallel bundles of collagen fibers in the underlying dermis. **Epidermal ridges**, or **friction ridges**, are slightly elevated, parallel lines separated by shallow grooves on the surface of thick skin. These ridges correspond to rows of tiny projections, called *dermal papillae,* located at the superficial margin of the dermis. The shallow grooves between epidermal ridges are **epidermal grooves**, which correspond to indentations of the epidermis, called *epidermal pegs,* into the dermis. Friction ridges are so named because they provide a rough surface that allows the fingers and palms to grip objects more effectively, and they help prevent the feet from slipping.

CHAPTER 8

The friction ridges on the anterior-distal ends of the fingers can leave **fingerprints**, telltale impressions of the ridges themselves. Fingerprints come in three basic patterns: whorl, loop, and arch. Glands beneath the skin secrete watery sweat and lipids that coat the peaks of the friction ridges. When you touch something, the secretions adhere to the object's surface in a pattern that matches the configuration of your friction ridges. Fingerprints are not genetically controlled and are, therefore, unique to every person, even identical twins. Consequently, fingerprints can be used to establish a person's identity. For example, forensic experts (specialists who collect physical evidence used in courts of law) employ a variety of techniques to detect and harvest fingerprints left at crime scenes. The discovered fingerprints can help investigators to identify individuals who may have witnessed or committed a criminal act.

> **Note**: Fingerprints develop when a fetus is about 3 months old; however, a small number of people (less than 1% of the population) are born without epidermal ridges and, therefore, can leave no fingerprints.

THE EPIDERMIS

The **epidermis** is the most superficial region of the skin, and as the name implies it lies superficial to the dermis. The junction between the epidermis and dermis is not flat, but consists of interlocking projections from both regions. The *downward* projections of the epidermis are called **epidermal pegs**, and the *upward* projections of the dermis are called **dermal papillae** (pa-PIL-lē; *papilla*, nipple) (see Figure 8-3). The epidermal pegs and dermal papillae greatly increase the amount of surface area contact between the epidermis and dermis. This structural arrangement has two advantages: (1) it firmly anchors the epidermis to the dermis, and (2) it increases the surface area over which nutrients can diffuse from dermal blood vessels to epidermal cells. The second advantage is crucial because the epidermis is epithelial in nature, and like all other epithelial tissues, it is *avascular* (lacks vessels). Thus, the epidermal cells rely solely on oxygen and nutrients diffusing from dermal blood vessels for survival.

If we cut off a piece of the epidermis, stain it, and examine it under a microscope, we would see four or five distinct regions of cells, collectively called **strata**. Each *stratum* (singular form) consists of one or more rows of similar-looking cells. Most cells within a stratum have the same size, shape, and they stain the same color. The epidermis of thin skin has four strata, and the epidermis of thick skin has five strata. The epidermal strata in their order from most superficial to deepest include the *stratum corneum, stratum lucidum* (seen only in thick skin), *stratum granulosum, stratum spinosum, and stratum basale* (Figure 8-3).

Most of the cells in the epidermis are **keratinocytes** (ker-a-TEN-ō-sīts), so named because they synthesize **keratin** (KER-a-tin; *kera*, horn-like). Keratin is a structural, filamentous protein, and as its root suggests, it is abundant in the horns of certain animals (particularly cows). Each stratum within the epidermis represents a different stage in the metabolic life of keratinocytes and keratin processing. Keratinocytes in the deeper strata are metabolically active, but activity slows and the cells take on a different role as they are pushed toward the apical surface. The more superficial strata consist of rows of dead or dying keratinocytes, varying from only a few rows of cells to more than 50 rows deep. The transformation of living keratinocytes, in the deeper strata, to dead flat cells full of keratin

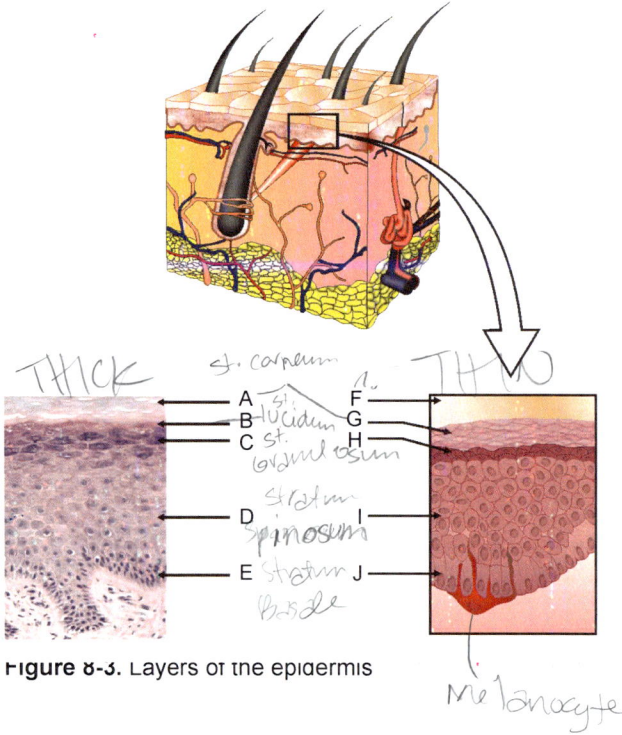

Figure 8-3. Layers of the epidermis

THE INTEGUMENTARY SYSTEM

protein, at the apical surface, is called **keratinization** (ker-a-ten-i-ZĀ-shun); this process requires about four weeks.

Stratum basale

The **stratum basale** (ba-SAL-ē; *basal*, bottom) is a single row of cells (most of these are keratinocytes) that form the base (*basal layer*) of the epidermis. Keratinocytes in the stratum basale have three important functions: (1) they synthesize part of the basement membrane; (2) they synthesize keratin polypeptides; and (3) they are the principal source of epidermal growth.

Keratinocytes comprising the stratum basale are called *basal cells*, and each is attached to neighboring basal cells by *desmosomes*. Basal cell keratinocytes synthesize proteoglycans and secrete them along their deepest edge, next to the dermis. The proteoglycans form the **basal lamina**, the superficial portion of a basement membrane that separates the epidermis from the dermis. Basal cell keratinocytes also synthesize keratin polypeptides, which combine to form the intermediate filaments of the cell's cytoskeleton. The intermediate filaments anchor the desmosomes found along the keratinocyte's plasma membrane.

After a basal cell keratinocyte divides (undergoes mitosis and cytokinesis), the deeper of the two daughter cells remains attached to the basement membrane by *hemidesmosomes*; the more superficial daughter cell is pushed outward to the stratum spinosum. Subsequent cell divisions in the stratum basale cause keratinocytes in the stratum spinosum to be pushed into the more superficial strata, and eventually onto the apical surface. In this way, basal cell keratinocytes are the ultimate source of all keratinocytes in the epidermis.

Between 5% and 25% of the cells in the stratum basale are **melanocytes** (MEL-a-nō-sīts) with the higher percentage occurring in parts of the body normally exposed to sunlight. These spider-shaped cells synthesize *melanin* (MEL-a-nin; *mela*, black), a chemical that darkens the skin and helps protect underlying tissues from the ultraviolet rays of the sun. The arm-like projections of a melanocyte, called *dendrites*, extend between adjacent basal cells and outward between keratinocytes in the stratum spinosum. The melanocytes package melanin into granules that are taken in by keratinocytes; this, in effect, causes the epidermis to darken. Melanocytes do not attach to other cells by desmosomes, but firmly attach to the basement membrane. Therefore, melanocytes remain in the stratum basale while adjacent keratinocytes are pushed into the stratum spinosum.

Merkel cells, thought to be modified keratinocytes, are also scattered throughout the stratum basale. These cells are in close contact with a nerve ending located in the upper region of the dermis. A single Merkel cell and the nerve ending beneath it are called a *Merkel disk*, and it functions as a receptor of light touch.

Stratum spinosum

The **stratum spinosum** (spī-NŌ-sum) contains eight to ten rows of keratinocytes, and is superficial to the stratum basale. When skin is prepared for microscopic examination, the cells in the stratum spinosum lose water and crenate (shrivel). Since desmosomes continue to hold adjacent cells together, the stretched plasma membranes appear to have spines; for this reason, keratinocytes in the stratum spinosum are sometimes called *spiny (prickle) cells*.

Nutrients reach keratinocytes in the stratum spinosum by diffusing between cells of the stratum basale. Keratinocytes in the deeper portion of this stratum are polygonal in shape and they are moderately active metabolically. Some of these cells are still capable of dividing, which means they can contribute to the outward growth of the epidermis. For this reason, the stratum basale and stratum spinosum together are sometimes referred to as the **stratum germinativum** (jer-men-ō-TĪ-vum; *germin*, give rise to). As the keratinocytes are pushed more superficially within the stratum spinosum, they begin to flatten and their metabolic activity decreases significantly.

> **Note**: The word *germinativum* is derived from "germinate," which refers to a seed sprouting forth (giving rise to) a new plant; likewise, cells of the stratum germinativum give rise to new epidermal cells.

In the stratum spinosum, more keratin polypeptides form within the keratinocytes and combine with existing intermediate filaments of the cytoskeleton. The resulting protein strands, called **keratin tonofilaments** (TŌ-nō-fil-a-mentz), are thicker and denser than the intermediate filaments found within the stratum basale.

The stratum spinosum contains **Langerhans cells** (LANG-er-hanz) that belong to a class of white blood cells called *macrophages*. Langerhans cells are motile and can perform phagocytosis to remove foreign particles from the epidermis. Consequently, they are important as a line of defense against bacteria and other microorganisms. Langerhans cells squeeze out of blood vessels in the dermis and migrate through the basement membrane and stratum basale. In the stratum spinosum, they continually squeeze between keratinocytes while searching for foreign particles. Langerhans cells manage to slip between all the interlocking desmosomes that bind the keratinocytes, a feat that is analogous to pushing a balloon through a rosebush without popping it!

Sensory receptors called **free nerve endings**, which are root-like branches of neurons, extend between the basal cells and into the stratum spinosum. These receptors are important in temperature detection and generation of pain signals when the epidermis is damaged.

Stratum granulosum

The **stratum granulosum** (gran-ū-LŌ-sum) is a thin region, containing only three to five rows of cells, and located immediately superficial to the stratum spinosum. The keratinocytes here are flatter than the spiny cells in the stratum spinosum, and most are dying and undergoing *autophagia*; that is, lysosomes in the cytoplasm are digesting other organelles. The reason why keratinocytes die in the stratum granulosum is not fully understood; some researchers attribute it to a lack of nutrients, while others say it is an example of programmed cell death (*apoptosis*).

As keratinocytes are pushed outward into the stratum granulosum, their keratin tonofilaments intertwine to form thick strands called **keratin fibrils** (FĪ-brilz; little fibers). In addition, granules of **keratohyalin** (ker-a-tō-HĪ-a-lin) attach to the keratin fibrils. During slide preparation, keratohyalin granules, which are part protein, absorb dye and cause the keratinocytes to appear dark and "grainy." Keratinocytes in the stratum granulosum also contain numerous, lipid-rich vesicles called **lamellar granules** (la-MEL-lar), so named because they stack like small saucers within the cell. Lamellar granules fuse with the plasma membrane and release their lipids into the extracellular spaces between the keratinocytes. The lipids, in turn, help waterproof the epidermis.

Stratum lucidum

The **stratum lucidum** (LŪ-si-dum; *lucid*, clear) is a thin, clear region seen only in the thick skin of the palm and sole. It is located immediately superficial to the stratum granulosum and contains three to five layers of keratinocytes. All of the keratinocytes in the stratum lucidum are dead, and their cytoplasmic components undergo changes that give these cells their distinctive, clear appearance when viewed under a microscope. Autophagia causes all of the organelles to disintegrate. Without nuclei, cells in this stratum allow light to pass through when they are viewed with a light microscope; this is how the stratum got the name "lucidum." In addition, enzymes transform the keratohyalin granules into a chemical called **eleidin** (e-LĒ-ō-den), causing the cell's cytoplasm to appear clear, not grainy. Keratinocytes in thin skin also experience a keratin-eleidin stage, but the layer in which keratohyalin transforms to eleidin is so thin that it cannot be seen with an ordinary light microscope.

Stratum corneum

The **stratum corneum** (KOR-nē-um; *corne*, horn-like) is the most superficial stratum of the epidermis, so it is what you see when you look at your skin. The relative thickness of the stratum corneum accounts for most of the difference between thick skin and thin skin. In thin skin, the stratum corneum consists of only a few layers of cells, while in the thick skin of the heel, it may consist of more than 50 layers of cells. The cells in the stratum corneum are dead, flattened keratinocytes, known as **squame cells** (skwām).

As keratinocytes move into the stratum corneum, their keratin fibrils join to form thick bundles. In fact, by the time a keratinocyte (squame cell) reaches the apical surface, it is little more than a plasma membrane enclosing these bundles of protein. The keratin fibril bundles cause the squame cells to take on a tough, "leathery" texture, and in this condition, the cells are *keratinized* (or *cornified*). A squame cell usually remains in the stratum corneum from two to four weeks.

THE INTEGUMENTARY SYSTEM

Eventually, the desmosomes holding adjacent squame cells together break, allowing the outermost cells to peel off, a process called **desquamation** (dē-skwa-MĀ-shun), or **exfoliation** (eks-fō-lē-Ā-shun; *ex*, off; *foli*, leaf). If the epidermis becomes too dry, large clumps of squame cells may detach together, causing the skin surface to look flaky. When this occurs on the scalp, it produces *dandruff*.

Note: A person may shed over 50 million squame cells per day, and 80 percent of airborne house dust you might see in a beam of light is desquamated (exfoliated) skin cells.

In review, **keratinization**, or **cornification** (kor-ni-fi-KĀ-shun), of epidermal cells involves five steps:

(1) Synthesis of keratin and formation of intermediate filaments in the stratum basale

(2) Formation of keratin tonofilaments in the stratum spinosum

(3) Binding of tonofilaments with keratohyalin to form keratin fibrils in the stratum granulosum

(4) Conversion of keratohyalin to eleidin (in the upper stratum granulosum or stratum lucidum)

(5) Aggregation of keratin fibrils into bundles in the stratum corneum

Protective Function of the Epidermis

The epidermis is the body's first line of defense against invasion by disease-causing agents from the external environment. The fact that a tiny cut or abrasion on the skin can become infected with bacteria rather quickly reveals the protective role of a healthy epidermis. For example, you have millions of bacteria living on your epidermis at this very moment, and merely washing with soap will not remove all of them. Most of these bacterial "residents" are harmless as long as the epidermis is unbroken. There is even evidence that some bacteria residing on the skin may actually help restrict the growth of more dangerous bacteria by competing with them for nutrients on the skin's surface. If any bacteria manage to penetrate deeper into the epidermis, they will likely encounter the phagocytic Langerhans cells of the stratum spinosum.

Note: While stratum corneum cells are dead and beyond hope of rejuvenation, they effectively prevent most substances from reaching the living cells of the stratum germinativum; this is why topical skin lotions, no matter how expensive or exotically crafted, cannot successfully reinvigorate and renew chronically damaged skin.

In addition to keeping out microorganisms, the epidermis is a barrier that slows the movement of water between the dermis and the outside environment. The outer epidermis is somewhat water resistant due to lipids in the extracellular spaces. Some of these lipids are secreted from the keratinocytes in the stratum granulosum, and others are secreted from sebaceous glands in the dermis. The epidermis is not waterproof, however, so in a dry environment, water constantly diffuses out of the skin. Because you are unaware of this water loss, it is called *insensible perspiration*, as distinguished from *sensible perspiration* (sweating). In other words, insensible perspiration is water lost by diffusion through the epidermis.

Under normal conditions, you lose about 500 ml of water each day through insensible perspiration. However, this rate would be much higher without keratin and lipids to make the epidermis water-resistant. The crucial role of the epidermis as a water barrier is exemplified in severely burned patients who have lost large amounts of skin. If the burned regions of the body are not covered, these patients can quickly die from dehydration. To counteract the loss of water, burned patients usually receive large amounts of fluid introduced intravenously (directly into the blood). The epidermis also acts as a barrier to restrict the passage of ultraviolet (UV) radiation from the sun. The extent to which the epidermis absorbs UV radiation, thereby preventing its passage to deeper tissues, is positively correlated with the amount of melanin present. Melanin makes the epidermis darker, and in effect, acts like an umbrella to shade deeper tissues. Without melanin, UV radiation can penetrate deep into the skin where it can cause ionization damage to DNA.

Vitamin D Synthesis

Although overexposing your epidermis to the sun's ultraviolet rays may increase your chances of developing skin cancer, a small amount of UV exposure can have healthy benefits. Ultraviolet B (UVB) radiation converts a compound called **dehydrocholesterol** (dē-hī-drō-kol-ES-ter-ol), found inside keratinocytes of the stratum germinativum, into **cholecalciferol** (kōl-e-kal-SIF-er-ol). Cholecalciferol is also known as **vitamin D₃** and is added to milk to promote good health. The keratinocytes synthesize dehydrocholesterol from cholesterol. The vitamin D₃, which is an inactive (unusable) form of vitamin D, diffuses into the blood and travels to the liver. The liver converts the vitamin D₃ into **calcidiol** (kal-si-DĪ-ol), which travels through the blood to reach the kidneys. Finally, the kidneys convert the calcidiol into the active (usable) form of vitamin D, called **calcitriol** (kal-si-TRĪ-ol). Calcitriol's name suggests the importance of this vitamin to calcium homeostasis.

THE DERMIS

The **dermis** or **stratum corium** (KOR-ē-um; hide) is deep to the epidermis and forms the bulk of the skin (by weight and volume). Most of the dermis consists of dense, irregular connective tissue, with collagen fibers accounting for about 70% of the total weight of the dermis. Collagen fibers provide significant pulling strength to the dermis, making it difficult to tear. The dermis is divided into a thin *papillary region* and a thicker *reticular region*. The papillary region is adapted for passing nutrients to the epidermis, and its cells secrete proteins that help bond the dermis to the epidermis. The reticular region is mainly the structural scaffolding of the skin, the part that gives it strength.

> **Note**: The stratum "corium" should not be confused with the stratum "corneum" of the epidermis; as its name implies, the stratum corium of certain animals is used to make leather goods (*corium*, leather).

The papillary region

The papillary region anchors and nourishes the epidermis. The **papillary region** of the dermis is located deep to the basement membrane of the epidermis, and is named for its tiny projections, the **dermal papillae**, which interlock with the epidermal pegs. In thin skin, the dermal papillae are relatively small and are evenly distributed. In thick skin, the dermal papillae are relatively large and may gather into clumps that are responsible for epidermal ridges. The papillary region is important to the epidermis for two reasons: (1) it secures the epidermis to the dermis, and (2) it provides nutrients to the cells of the epidermis.

Dermal papillae consist of areolar connective tissue that contains fibroblasts, mast cells, very thin collagenous and elastin fibers, tiny loops of capillaries, and one or more sensory receptors. Dermal papillae increase the surface area between the dermis and epidermis and, indirectly, help bond together both divisions of the skin. However, the basement membrane contains the actual "glue" that welds the epidermis to the dermis. The basement membrane consists of a dense web of collagen proteins, glycoproteins, and proteoglycans. Fibroblasts within the dermal papillae secrete compounds that form the bottom half, or *reticular lamina* portion, of the basement membrane (basal keratinocytes in the stratum basale secrete the superficial half, or *basal lamina* portion of the basement membrane).

Because the areolar tissue within dermal papillae has a "loose" arrangement of protein fibers, substances can easily diffuse between them. For this reason, oxygen and nutrients can easily diffuse from the capillary loops and across the basement membrane where they can be absorbed by cells of the stratum germinativum. In addition, the dermal papillae increase the surface area through which nutrients can reach these epidermal cells. If the epidermis is torn away from the papillary region, such as in the case of blisters, the cells in the detached stratum germinativum will starve.

The reticular region

The reticular region is the scaffolding of the skin. The fibrous **reticular region** of the dermis is located between the papillary region and the hypodermis, and it is the thickest part of the dermis. Consistent with its structural role, the reticular region consists of dense irregular connective tissue, composed mostly of thick collagenous and elastin fibers. Fibroblasts synthesize collagen strands and then expel them into the extracellular matrix. In the extracellular matrix, the strands intertwine to form thick, collagenous fibers resembling a twisted rope.

THE INTEGUMENTARY SYSTEM

Most of the collagen fibers in the reticular region are irregularly arranged, but others are organized into bundles that align in parallel rows. These bundles usually align in the same direction that the skin stretches, which is why they are known as dermal **tension lines**, or **lines of cleavage**. So-called "frown lines" that develop on different parts of the face, and the "life lines" on the palm of the hand are examples of tension lines. These lines develop due to years of muscle contractions that cause the skin to crease in those locations. This is like creasing a piece of paper; the crease can be seen even after the paper is unfolded. Bend your palm and you will see the skin crease along several major tension lines.

Knowledge of how dermal tension lines are oriented is important during surgery. Incisions made across the long axis of tension lines tend to pull apart readily and result in more noticeable scarring. An incision made parallel to tension lines results in less side-to-side stretching of the wound, and the incision is less likely to tear open. As a result, there is less tissue damage and less scarring.

Even the skin of infants and children exhibit tension lines; however, **wrinkles** are skin creases that become more prevalent as we get older, when the epidermis and the dermis become thinner. In older adults, the fibroblasts within the reticular region of the dermis synthesize less collagen and elastin protein, resulting in looser, sagging skin. Thinner skin also allows more water to diffuse to the outside environment, resulting in drier skin. Skin wrinkling due to loss of moisture can be compared to a drying grape developing "wrinkles" on its way to becoming a raisin.

Dermal blood vessels

Blood vessels are organs of the cardiovascular system, but their functions in the skin are critical to homeostasis. The largest vessels in the skin are sandwiched between the reticular dermis and the hypodermis. Here, they appear as a "braided" network called the **reticular plexus** (PLEK-sus; braid). Blood enters the reticular plexus through arteries in the hypodermis and underlying muscles. Numerous arterioles (small arteries) branch off of the reticular plexus. Some of these arterioles extend deep and nourish cells in the hypodermis, including cells of sweat glands and hair follicles present in that region. Other arterioles extend superficially into the reticular region, where they nourish fibroblasts, sweat glands, sebaceous glands, hairs and hair follicles, arrector pili muscles, and nerve endings. The reticular plexus branches into ever-smaller divisions through the reticular region until it reaches the papillary region.

Arterioles at the junction between the reticular and papillary regions of the dermis form an even finer network, called the **papillary plexus**. Small loops of capillaries extend superficially from the papillary plexus into the dermal papillae, where nutrients diffuse across the basement membrane into the epidermis. A parallel network of small veins accompanies the arterioles throughout the skin and returns blood to larger veins in the hypodermis and underlying muscles.

At rest, about 5% of the blood flowing out of your heart goes to your skin's blood vessels, and this amount is about ten times more than your skin needs to survive. Why is it important to have "extra" blood flowing through the skin? The reason is that the skin's vessels play a key role in regulating body temperature, and they serve as a blood reservoir. Both functions are possible because the nervous system controls the diameter of dermal vessels. In a process called **vasodilation** (VĀ-so-dī-LĀ-shun; *vaso*, vessel; *dilat*, open up), rings of smooth muscle that surround the dermal arterioles relax, causing the vessels to widen. Dermal blood flow increases, so more heat radiates to the external environment from blood in the capillary loops beneath the epidermis. During vasodilation, as much as 30% of the blood flowing out of your heart may go to your skin.

In an opposite process called **vasoconstriction**, ring-like muscles surrounding the dermal arterioles contract, causing the vessels to narrow. Dermal blood flow decreases, and less heat radiates from the blood to the external environment. Vasoconstriction squeezes blood out of the dermis, making it available for circulation to other regions of the body. A significant amount of vasoconstriction in your skin while you are at rest could increase the amount of blood flowing to other parts of your body by as much as 5%. This amount may not seem like much, but in a physiological crisis, it could be the difference between life and death.

THE HYPODERMIS

The **hypodermis**, or **subcutaneous tissue**, is not part of the skin. However, it is closely associated with some of the structures and functions of the skin, and it helps attach the skin to the body. The hypodermis consists primarily of areolar and adipose connective tissue. Some skin appendages such as hair roots and the bases of glands project deep into this region. Functionally, the hypodermis cushions the skin against pressure from hard, deep structures such as bones, and it physically shields underlying organs. Because the hypodermis is superficial to underlying muscles, it sometimes is called the **superficial fascia** (FA-sha; band). Its adipose tissue insulates the body and typically stores half of the body's fats in the form of triglycerides. The normal distribution of adipose tissue within the hypodermis varies among men and women.

CUTANEOUS SENSATION

Your ability to experience different *cutaneous sensations* (awareness of stimuli in the skin) is made possible by a variety of **cutaneous receptors**, or nerve endings, in your epidermis, dermis, and hypodermis. When stimulated, a cutaneous receptor initiates an impulse that passes along a nerve to the brain, where the impulse is interpreted. Depending on which type of receptor is stimulated, the brain will interpret the impulse as touch, pain, temperature change, or some other sensation such as a tickle or itch.

Cutaneous Receptors

We can classify cutaneous receptors on the basis of their structure and the type of stimulus to which they respond. Structurally, there are three types of cutaneous receptors:

(1) **Encapsulated nerve endings** are surrounded by a well-defined "shell" of connective tissue.

(2) **Free nerve endings** consist of a nerve endings not surrounded by a capsule of connective tissue.

(3) **Epidermal nerve endings** attach to a specific type of cell in the epidermis, or a structure that is derived from epidermal cells.

Categorized by the type of stimulus to which they respond cutaneous receptors fall into one of three groups:

(1) A **mechanoreceptor** (me-KAN-ō-rē-sep-tor) responds to mechanical forces, such as compression and stretch. A *tactile (touch) receptor* is a mechanoreceptor that generates an impulse when something makes light contact with the skin. A *deep pressure receptor* is a mechanoreceptor that generates an impulse when something presses hard enough against the skin to compress the hypodermis. Most mechanoreceptors are encapsulated nerve endings.

(2) A **nociceptor** (NŌS-ē-sep-tor; *noci*, pain) is a free nerve ending that generates an impulse interpreted as pain. Nociceptors are stimulated most often by tissue damage, resulting from a wound, extreme hot or cold temperature, or stretching. In addition, certain chemicals, whether foreign or those released from surrounding tissues, can stimulate nociceptors.

(3) A **thermoreceptor** generates an impulse in response to changes in temperature. Most thermoreceptors are free nerve endings.

Types of cutaneous receptors

The degree to which thin skin and thick skin is sensitive to particular stimuli depends on the type and abundance of specific cutaneous receptors present. For example, thick skin on the fingertips has a greater density of tactile receptors than does the thin skin on the back. Therefore, fingertips are more sensitive to light touch than is the skin on the back. Some types of receptors are common to both thin and thick skin, while other receptors are found in only one type of skin.

Free nerve endings (FNEs) are the only cutaneous receptor found in both the epidermis and the dermis, and they are found in both thin skin and thick skin. FNEs resemble the roots of a tree as they branch throughout the dermis and extend through the basement membrane into the stratum basale and stratum spinosum. Most FNEs are nociceptors, but some function as mechanoreceptors or thermoreceptors. FNE nociceptors in the epidermis are responsible for the burning pain of a superficial

THE INTEGUMENTARY SYSTEM

scrape on your knee and the sharp pain of a shallow "paper" cut on your finger.

Merkel discs, or **tactile discs**, are epidermal nerve endings that attach to Merkel cells in the stratum basale of both thin and thick skin. When something makes light contact with the skin, the Merkel cell causes its corresponding Merkel disc to initiate an impulse, which you feel as a light touch. A number of Merkel discs branch from a single nerve fiber in the dermis and extend to the base of an epidermal peg. Here, each Merkel disc attaches to the base of a separate Merkel cell. To demonstrate this arrangement, if you balance this book on your fingertips, the book is like the epidermis, your fingertips are like the Merkel discs, and your arm is like the nerve fiber.

Meissner corpuscles (KOR-pus-ulz; "little bodies"), or **tactile** (TAK-tĭl; "touch") **corpuscles**, are mechanoreceptors sensitive to light touch, and are found mainly in the dermal papillae of thick skin. These receptors are most abundant in your fingertips where they are probably responsible for your ability to distinguish the fine texture of an object. A Meissner corpuscle is a fluid-filled, encapsulated receptor, consisting of several layers of flat epithelial cells intertwined with a single nerve ending. The corpuscle has an outer covering made of fine elastic fibers and fibroblasts. The corpuscle at the end of its nerve fiber looks sort of like a balloon at the end of a string.

Hair receptors, or **hair root plexuses**, are found only in thin skin containing hair follicles, the tubes from which individual hairs grow. The hair follicle is derived from epidermal cells; hence, hair receptors are epidermal nerve endings. A hair receptor consists of numerous nerve endings, some of which run parallel to the hair follicle while others wrap around the follicle. The hair receptor does not reach the hair, but when something touches the hair hard enough to bend its follicle, the hair receptor initiates an impulse allowing you to feel the hair move.

Pacinian corpuscles (pa-SEN-ē-un), or **lamellated corpuscles**, are the largest cutaneous receptors (up to 2 mm in length), and respond to deep pressure and vibration. A few Pacinian corpuscles are found deep in the dermis of both thin and thick skin, but most are found in the hypodermis, where they are examples of *subcutaneous* receptors. Pacinian corpuscles are encapsulated mechanoreceptors. The capsule surrounding the nerve ending consists of flat fibroblasts arranged in concentric layers, called *lamellae*, which look like the layers of an onion. The fibroblasts produce collagen fibers that extend between the lamellae. As we get older, the amount of collagen increases, which may decrease the corpuscle's sensitivity to deep pressure.

Ruffini's endings (rū-FĒ-nēz) are located mainly in the lower dermis of both thin and thick skin, and in the hypodermis, where they respond mostly to skin stretch and vibration. Ruffini endings resemble a cylinder, consisting of a connective tissue shell (fibroblasts and collagen fibers) surrounding one or two nerve endings. When you wrap your fingers around an object, the skin stretches at your finger joints and stimulates Ruffini endings. The combination of impulses from different Ruffini endings allows your brain to interpret the shape of the object.

SKIN COLOR

No feature of human skin is more noticed — for better or worse — than its color. It is not surprising then that some of the earliest scientific studies of the human body sought explanations for the basis and purpose of skin color. Recent physiological investigations have given rise to hypotheses about the adaptive advantages of skin color that seem plausible, but they are not conclusive.

Human skin varies in color from purplish-black to pinkish-white. In most people, skin color is a mixture of brown, red, and yellow hues. Pigments deposited in epidermal cells or nearby tissues influence skin color. In the body, a **pigment** is an organic molecule that gives color to a cell, tissue, or organ. The story of skin color is largely one about the pigment melanin.

Melanin

Melanin is the only endogenous skin pigment; that is, it is the only pigment made by the skin itself. Melanocytes in the stratum basale synthesize melanin, which is a complex polymer derived from the amino acid tyrosine. Melanocytes can make two kinds of melanin. **Eumelanin** (Ū-mel-a-nen; *eu*; true), the darkest and most common form, is brown-to-black in color. The other form of melanin, **pheomelanin**

(FĀ-ō-mel-a-nen; *pheo*, dusky) is red-to-amber in color. The ratio between the two types of melanin produced is genetically determined and accounts for all the variations in skin color that characterizes different human populations. Darker-skinned people typically produce more eumelanin, while light-skinned people produce more pheomelanin.

> **Note: Freckles** and **moles** have larger, more active melanocytes than pale skin, but pale skin usually has more melanocytes in each square centimeter of skin area.

Inside melanocytes, melanin molecules (granules) are packaged into vesicles called **melanosomes** (MEL-a-nō-sōmz). The melanosomes are drawn to the ends of a melanocyte's branch-like extensions, which snake between keratinocytes in the stratum basale and stratum spinosum. The keratinocytes use phagocytosis to engulf the dendritic tips containing the melanosomes (Figure 8-4). The melanosomes may remain intact once they are inside the keratinocytes, or they may release their granules into the cytoplasm. In any event, a keratinocyte tends to arrange the melanin it gathers on the "sunny" (superficial) side of its nucleus. In this way, the melanin shades the nuclear DNA against the damaging effects of ultraviolet (UV) radiation in sunlight. As keratinocytes push closer to the apical surface of the epidermis, the melanin granules disintegrate. Consequently, melanin production must take place continuously to maintain your skin color.

Although the number of melanin granules that each keratinocyte collects determines the depth and hue of a person's skin color, exposure to UV light can cause the skin to darken (tan) further. Tanning happens in two ways. Like photographic film, melanin molecules within keratinocytes and melanocytes oxidize and darken after only a few minutes' exposure to UV light. Over the longer term, UV light causes keratinocytes to release a growth factor (a kind of hormone) that stimulates neighboring melanocytes to grow and form larger granules. Even dark-skinned people tan following sunlight exposure, although the effects may not be readily evident. The skin of most people noticeably lightens during the winter months when sunlight is less intense and melanocytes are less active.

Some researchers hypothesize that the predominant skin color in a human population may represent an outcome of a selection process that balanced the need to shield skin from UV damage against the body's need to synthesize and preserve essential nutrients. On the one hand, too much melanin shielding can block the UV light needed to kick off the chemical chain reaction that forms vitamin D. On the other hand, too little melanin shielding can admit enough UV light to destroy folic acid (a B-vitamin) in the blood. Folic acid is essential for the formation of normal red blood cells, and it is crucial for the formation of the nervous system during fetal life. Over time, light-skinned populations may have been selected in higher latitudes where sunlight is weak, while darker-skinned populations may have been selected in lower latitudes where sunlight is intense. In

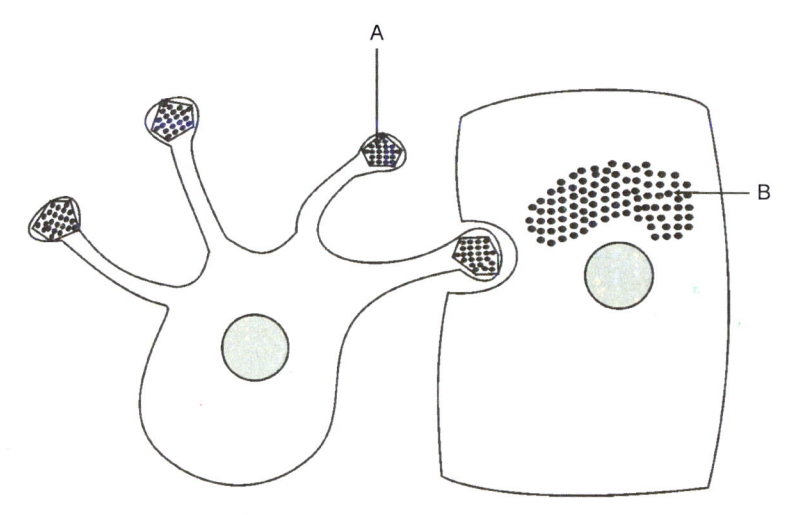

Figure 8-4. Melanin transfer to a keratinocyte

both cases, the population's predominant skin color may have represented a "happy balance" between adequate vitamin D synthesis and the need to protect bodily stores of folic acid.

Other skin pigments

Two pigments not produced in the skin, *heme* and *carotene*, may faintly tint a person's skin. **Heme** is a constituent of **hemoglobin** (HĒ-mō-glō-ben), the oxygen-carrying molecule in red blood cells. Oxygenated hemoglobin has a vivid red color, while deoxygenated hemoglobin has a purplish hue. Especially in lighter-skinned people, the color of the red blood cells flowing within the dermal capillaries projects outward through the epidermis, giving their skin a noticeably pinkish cast. Dramatic evidence of heme's ability to tint the skin occurs during *blushing*, the rapid reddening of the face that sometimes happens when a person feels embarrassed. Blushing is caused by a sudden rush of blood through temporarily dilated dermal capillaries.

The other pigment, **carotene** (KER-ō-tēn) is a yellow-orange, lipid–soluble precursor to vitamin A. Carotene can diffuse from the blood into keratinocytes of the epidermis and adipocytes of the hypodermis. The amount of carotene deposited in these cells is proportional to the amount consumed in the diet. The effect of carotene on skin color is extremely subtle and only noticeable in the most light-skinned of people.

SKIN DERIVATIVES

The skin protects underlying tissues but also produces glands, hairs, and nails that contribute to its own protection and help maintain homeostasis. At the beginning of the chapter, we referred to these organs as *skin derivatives* or *accessory organs* of the skin. More specifically, they are also called *epidermal derivatives*, because they develop from epidermal cells. In fact, if the epidermis is damaged, cells from hair follicles and the ducts of skin glands can supply cells to regenerate the epidermis. We will first look at the skin derivatives most responsible for maintaining homeostasis: skin glands.

If you're a typical North American consumer, by the time you reach your thirties you will likely have spent a small fortune for deodorants to mask your normal human scent; acne preparations to cleanse clogged pores; and shampoos to remove scalp oils and waxes. If you're physically active, you may have spent even more on sports drinks that claim to protect you when you sweat. The sources of this drain on your income are all tiny glands within your skin–epidermal derivatives. Although you may sometimes regard them as cosmetic nuisances, all of your skin glands are essential to the health and homeostasis of your body. We will consider three different skin glands: *eccrine glands, apocrine glands*, and *sebaceous glands*. Each type of gland releases a unique secretion.

Eccrine sweat glands

Due to their role in regulating body temperature and in excretion, **eccrine sweat glands** (EK-rin; to secrete) are the most important skin derivatives. They also are the most numerous; you have over two million of them in your skin. Although eccrine sweat glands are found in thin and thick skin, they are more prevalent in the palms and soles of the feet and within the skin of the axillary regions. The sweat-forming portion of the gland is a tightly coiled tube housed in the reticular region of the dermis. The gland's secretions are released into a single tubular duct that opens directly onto the skin's surface through a tiny **sweat pore**. The duct has two parts: a *straight* part in the dermis, and a *spiraled* part in the epidermis. Because it produces sweat, an eccrine sweat gland is a type of **sudoriferous gland** (sū-dōr-IF-er-us; *sudori*, sweat).

Eccrine sweat is derived from tissue fluid, specifically from the plasma (watery portion) of the blood. Hence, eccrine sweat is about 99% water. The remaining 1% includes ions (mostly Na^+ and Cl^-), an assortment of metabolic wastes, and even heavy metals, such as mercury, lead, and aluminum. The presence of all these substances testifies to the role of eccrine glands as excretory organs. The watery portion of eccrine sweat is an important source of *evaporative cooling*, the release of heat that takes place when water evaporates off the skin surface. However, prolonged periods of heavy sweating can remove so much water from the blood plasma that blood pressure can drop to life-threatening levels. Moreover, heavy sweating can pull enough ions out of the plasma that the normal operation of muscles and nerves is disturbed. For both reasons, it is essential to remain well hydrated during hot weather or prolonged physical activity and to replenish the salts the body loses due to sweating.

> **Note**: Eccrine sweat glands are **simple, coiled tubular** (one duct and one coiled tube-like gland). They are also **sudoriferous** (produce sweat), **exocrine** (have a duct and release secretions to the outside of the body), and **merocrine** (release secretions by exocytosis) glands.

The autonomic (involuntary) nervous system controls the release of sweat from eccrine sweat glands. Consequently, sweating is an involuntary bodily response. As body temperature rises, nerve impulses stimulate the production of sweat in the base of the glands. Sweating usually begins on skin of the face and then spreads outward to the extremities. Strong emotions or stress can jangle the autonomic nervous system, too, which in turn will stimulate the eccrine sweat glands. This nervous system response explains why you may break out in a "cold sweat" when you are anxious or startled by something. Moreover, the nervous system stimulates specialized contractile cells, called **myoepithelial cells** (mī-ō-ep-ē-THĒ-lē-al; *myo*, muscle), which surround the secretory cells at the base of the gland. When the myoepithelial cells contract, they squeeze the sweat into the duct leading to the hair follicle. These muscles work sort of like your fingers when they squeeze toothpaste from a tube.

Apocrine sweat glands

Apocrine sweat glands (AP-ō-krin; to separate) are unique sweat glands that function in ways that are not completely understood. Most of these glands are attached to hair follicles, and are found only in thin skin of the axillary, anal, areola (nipple), and pubic regions. Like an eccrine sweat gland, the sweat-forming portion of an apocrine sweat gland is a highly coiled tube, but it is usually found much deeper in the dermis or in the hypodermis. The sweat-forming portion of apocrine glands may be up to 2 mm in diameter, which is significantly larger than eccrine glands. In addition, most apocrine sweat glands do not secrete sweat directly onto the skin's surface; instead, they secrete sweat into the hair follicle to which they are attached.

Apocrine sweat contains lipids and proteins, which make it more viscous (thicker) than eccrine sweat. Fresh apocrine sweat is odorless, but it acquires a foul odor when resident skin bacteria decompose its lipids and proteins. For this reason, adults with active apocrine glands have a more distinct odor than young children do. Apocrine sweat glands were originally thought to produce secretions by releasing small pieces of glandular cells; hence, the name "apocrine" gland seemed applicable. However, recent evidence suggests that apocrine sweat glands are actually merocrine glands, but use of the former term persists as a way to differentiate them from eccrine sweat glands.

Apocrine glands are inactive before puberty, but they enlarge and become active under the influence of increasing levels of sex hormones in early adulthood. These glands secrete sweat in response to various hormones, particularly sex hormones, and in response to stimulation from the nervous system. During sexual activity and under emotional stress, such as fear and anger, the nervous system stimulates the apocrine glands to secrete sweat. Like eccrine glands, apocrine sweat glands have myoepithelial cells surrounding their secretory cells that squeeze sweat into the secretory ducts.

Two kinds of modified apocrine glands are located within specific body structures. **Ceruminous glands** (se-RŪ-mi-nus; *cerumen*, wax) are located within the skin of the external ear canals. Their waxy secretion, called **cerumen** (se-RŪ-men) or *earwax* waterproofs the ear canal and may help repel tiny insects. **Mammary glands** located within the breasts produce milk, but this occurs only during a *lactation period* following childbirth. Various hormones in the female affect the development and activity of mammary glands.

Sebaceous glands

Sebaceous glands (se-BĀ-shus), also called **oil glands**, secrete an oily fluid called **sebum** (SĒ-bum; oil), which lubricates hair within hair follicles and helps make the hair and epidermis water resistant. Like apocrine sweat glands, most sebaceous glands are attached to the "leaning" side of hair follicles. Together the hair follicle and sebaceous gland is called a **pilosebaceous unit** (PĪ-lō-se-BĀ-shus; *pilo*, hair). In contrast, **free sebaceous glands** do not attach to hair follicles, but secrete sebum directly onto the skin's surface. Free sebaceous glands are found in the skin of the eyelids, certain regions on the external genitalia, and in the areola of the nipples. Both types of sebaceous glands are globular masses of large cells that look sort of like clusters of grapes. Some of these cells disintegrate and enter the sebum, making a sebaceous gland an example of a holocrine gland.

Sebum is a viscous secretion, consisting mostly of triglycerides and free fatty acids that serve three main purposes: First, the fatty acids decrease the sebum's pH, which can inhibit the growth of certain types of bacteria and fungi on the skin's surface. Second, after entering a hair follicle, sebum coats the hair inside making it more flexible and able to repel water. Third, when sebum reaches the skin's surface, it coats the epidermal cells and helps keep them flexible and water-resistant as well. So why do your fingers and toes wrinkle like prunes if you keep them in water for a long time. You do not have sebaceous glands on your palms or soles, so these regions lack that water-resistant, oily covering present on other parts of your body. Consequently, water can infiltrate into your epidermis in these regions, causing it to swell both vertically and horizontally; the result is wrinkling.

Sebaceous glands are similar to apocrine sweat glands in the way they are stimulated to develop and become more active. During childhood, when sex hormone levels are low, sebaceous glands are relatively small; therefore, children do not produce much sebum. During puberty, increasing levels of sex hormones causes sebaceous glands to enlarge and become more active. Male hormones are the most potent stimulators of these glands, causing a man's skin to be oilier than a woman's skin. Temperature can also affect sebaceous gland activity. Low outside temperature cools the skin and causes sebaceous glands to become less active. With less sebum to keep your stratum corneum cells soft and pliable during cold weather, your skin may become dry and flaky.

Hair

Hairs, also called **pili** (PIL-ī) grow from tube-like structures called hair follicles and consist of densely packed keratinized cells. Most thin skin contains about 60 hairs per cm², but the face has about ten times as many. The integumentary system has two types of hairs. **Vellus hairs** (VEL-us; fleece), often called "peach fuzz," cover most of the body and are about one-eighth as thick as this sheet of paper. Most vellus hairs lack pigment, and those on the eyelids do not extend beyond their follicles. **Terminal hairs** are about eight times thicker than vellus hairs (or about as thick as this sheet of paper), and usually contain pigment. At puberty, terminal hairs develop from vellus hairs in the axillary and pubic regions of both sexes, and in the face of males. Examples of terminal hairs include scalp hairs, eyebrows, eyelashes, axillary and pubic hairs, and hairs on the arms and legs. Hairs perform a variety of functions:

- Scalp hairs shield the scalp, the skin that covers the skull, from the damaging effects of UV radiation. Scalp hairs also help to insulate the scalp from heat and cold.

- Eyebrows reduce glare around the eyes, and eyelashes prevent foreign particles from reaching the surface of the eyes.

- Hairs help keep dust and other foreign objects from entering the eyes, nasal cavities and ear canals.

- Hairs in the axillary regions reduce friction while the arms are swinging, and hair in the pubic region reduces skin friction during sexual intercourse.

Hair Follicles

A **hair follicle** (FOL-i-kul; bag) is a tube-like organ that produces a hair (Figure 8-5). As its Greek root suggests, a hair follicle is a pouch-like extension of the epidermis that plunges deep into the superficial region of the hypodermis in some cases. The deepest part of most hair follicles usually is located within the reticular region of the dermis. At birth, a person has all the hair follicles he or she will ever have, about five million of them, including about 100,000 on the scalp. Over time, the skin that covers the scalp spreads out, causing the follicle density (number of follicles per square centimeter of surface) on the scalp to decrease. In reality, though, a person probably has about the same number of scalp follicles that he or she had at birth.

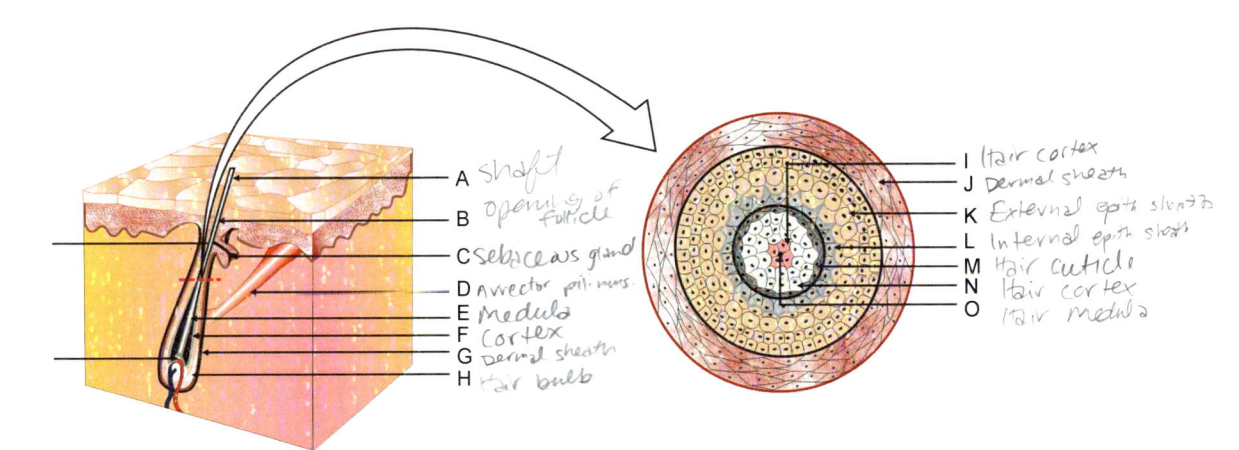

Figure 8-5. Hair follicle and hair

> **Note**: On average, each square centimeter of skin on the arm contains 10 hair follicles, 15 sebaceous glands, 100 sweat glands, 1 meter of blood vessels, 2 meters of nerves, and over 3,000 sensory receptors.

A hair follicle looks sort of like an onion plant, with a narrow cylindrical portion extending to the skin's surface from a swollen base embedded in the dermis or hypodermis. The base, or **hair bulb**, fits like a cup over the **hair papilla**, which consists of areolar connective tissue and blood vessels. During fetal development, a fingerlike projection of epidermal tissue grows into the dermis or hypodermis and surrounds a papilla. This explains why the hair bulb is wider than the more superficial part of the follicle. Blood vessels in the hair papilla provide nutrients to the hair bulb in the same way that blood vessels in dermal papillae provide nutrients to the epidermis. The hair bulb contains mostly keratinocytes, but it also contains a few melanocytes and Langerhans cells.

A closer look at the wall of a hair follicle reveals its kinship with the overlying epidermis. From outside in, we see four major layers: the *dermal root sheath*, the *glassy membrane*, the *outer root sheath*, and the *inner root sheath*. The **dermal (fibrous) root sheath** consists of collagen fibers and fibroblasts, and serves to anchor the hair follicle to the surrounding dermal tissue. The basement membrane separating the epidermis from the dermis extends into the hair follicle as the **glassy membrane**, named for its clear appearance. Like the basement membrane above, the glassy membrane separates epidermal tissue (in this case, the outer root sheath) from dermal tissue (in this case, the dermal root sheath). The **outer root sheath** lies between the glassy membrane and the inner root sheath. It contains mostly keratinocytes, and is continuous with the stratum basale. The **inner root sheath** contains mostly keratinocytes and is continuous with the stratum spinosum. The inner root sheath makes contact with the hair from the hair bulb to about the level of the sebaceous gland, but at the sebaceous gland, the inner root sheath disintegrates.

In addition to hair receptors, sebaceous glands, and in some cases, apocrine sweat glands, a slender **arrector pili** (a-rek-tor PIL-ī) muscle attaches to the dermal root sheath of most hair follicles. It extends from just below the sebaceous gland to the papillary region of the dermis. This tiny smooth muscle always is located on the "leaning" side of the hair follicle. When the arrector pili contracts in response to cold temperature or intense emotions, it yanks the follicle and its hair into a vertical position. This process, called *piloerection*, pushes the skin around the hair into a little peak called a *goose bump*, so named because it resembles the little dimples that cover the skin of a plucked goose. Hairs "standing on end" in this way trap warm air and help insulate the skin from cold, rather like putting on an insulated jacket.

> **Note**: The physiological name for "goose bumps," resulting from cold, fear, or tactile stimuli is **cutis anserina**.

Piloerection probably benefited our distant human ancestors, who likely were much hairier than the average person is today. Still, these muscles generate a small amount of heat when they contract, and their contractions may help squeeze sebum into your hair follicles. Follicles of facial hair, eyebrows, eyelashes, axillary and pubic hairs do not have arrector pili muscles.

Parts of a Hair

Along its length, a hair has two regions: the *shaft* and the *root* (Figure 8-5). The **hair shaft** is the part you see above the skin's surface, but it also extends into the skin to about the level of the sebaceous gland. The **hair root** is the deeper part that is firmly attached to the inner root sheath of the hair follicle. The root extends from the hair shaft into the hair bulb. If you pull a scalp hair out "by the root," you may see part of the bulb at its base, and the white cylindrical mass above the bulb is part of the internal root sheath.

Along its width, a hair's shaft has two major regions: the *cuticle* and the *cortex*. The **cuticle** (KŪ-ti-kul; "skin") is a hair's outer covering and consists of five to ten layers of dead, flattened keratinocytes (squamous cells). These cells overlap one another like shingles on a roof, with their free edges facing toward the distal end of the hair. If you comb hairs toward the scalp (that is, "tease" the hair), the comb lifts the free edges of the cuticle cells. In turn, the cuticle cells of adjacent cells interlock and stick to one another, giving hair that "frizzy" look. Cuticle cells contain *hard keratin*, which has more sulfide bonds and twists more tightly than "soft" keratin found in the epidermis. Hard keratin strengthens the desmosomes so that the cuticle cells do not peel off (desquamate). The **cortex** ("bark") forms the bulk of a hair, and it is responsible for the hair's strength and color. The cortex consists of cylindrical keratinocytes that contain hard keratin. A third region, the **medulla** (me-DŪ-la; "marrow") forms a narrow central core that is seen only in the root of thick terminal hairs. The medulla consists of loosely packed keratinocytes filled with soft keratin and interspersed with air spaces.

The cells that form the different layers in a hair arise from the portion of the hair bulb called the **hair matrix** (*matrix*, womb). As its name suggests, the matrix is where the hair is "born," but it also gives rise to parts of the hair follicle. The hair matrix consists of several layers of modified epidermal cells (mainly keratinocytes) that cover the apical and lateral surfaces of the hair papilla. Cells covering most of the papilla give rise to the hair root, while cells at the deepest portion of the matrix give rise to the inner and outer root sheaths of the hair follicle. When matrix cells nearest the papilla divide, the growing daughter cells push older cells away from the papilla. As the hair cells and inner sheath cells move together toward the skin's surface they remain attached by desmosomes. However, when both groups of cells reach the sebaceous gland, the inner root sheath disintegrates. Without connections to the hair follicle, the hair root is now called the hair shaft.

As soon as hair cells and sheath cells move out of the matrix, they begin the slow process of keratinization. Differences in gene expression likely cause the cellular differentiation responsible for the different layers of the hair and its follicle. When hair cells reach the sebaceous gland, they are dead and highly keratinized. (Recall this series of events is similar to what happens to keratinocytes moving through the epidermal strata).

Cycles of Hair Growth

Try as you might, it's unlikely that you'll ever be able to grow your scalp hair long enough so that it reaches the floor when you're standing. The reason you're denied this singular accomplishment is because hair follicles don't grow hairs continuously. Instead, they roll through repeated cycles of growth, shrinkage, and rest. The **hair growth** cycle consists of three phases — anagen, catagen, and telogen — during which a hair follicle grows a hair, sheds it, and then begins forming a new hair.

Anagen (AN-a-jen; *ana*, up; *gen*, generate) is the first and longest phase of the hair growth cycle. During this stage, the hair is growing from dividing cells in the hair matrix, and the hair is pushing through a fully developed hair follicle. Anagen for scalp hairs typically lasts 2 – 6 years, whereas it lasts only 1-2 months for eyelash and eyebrow hairs. The actual length of this phase for your own hair is determined by your genetic inheritance and by situational factors such as your diet and general state of health. Even the changing seasons can affect the rate of hair growth. Hair grows fastest at the start of anagen and slowly tapers off as the second phase nears. On average, a scalp hair grows about 1 centimeter in a month.

Catagen (KA-ta-gen; *cata*, cast down) is the second and shortest phase of the hair growth cycle, lasting only 2 – 4 weeks for scalp hairs. During this period, the base of the hair follicle shrinks toward the epidermis, eventually diminishing to about one-sixth its original length. The matrix cells die, and the hair bulb detaches from the hair papilla resulting in a *club hair*, so named because it looks like a club-shaped mass under a microscope. As the hair follicle shrinks, it slowly pushes the club hair toward the surface of the skin, creating the illusion of growth in a hair that's now totally dead.

Telogen (TĒL-ō-jen; *telo*, end) is a hair follicle's resting phase. During this final period of the hair growth cycle, the base of the follicle has shrunk to the point that it is very near the surface of the epidermis. At this time, the club hair may be shed from the follicle. Your scalp loses 80–100 hairs each day as follicles enter telogen. This resting phase lasts about 5–6 weeks for scalp hairs, but may last for several months for eyelashes and eyebrows.

> **Note**: The record for the longest scalp hair is 5.15 meters; even if you never again cut your scalp hair, it is unlikely that you could grow it this long, because in most people, the anagen phase of hair growth simply doesn't last long enough.

At the start of the next anagen phase, cells in the mid-portion of the hair follicle divide and drill deep into the dermis to form a new bulb around the hair papilla. New matrix cells develop and start producing a new hair. If the club hair is still lingering in the follicle at this time, the new hair will dislodge it. In an average adult, about 85% of all hairs are in anagen, while 10-15% are in telogen. The hair growth cycle slows progressively as you get older, and by age 50 about one-third of the scalp hair follicles are permanently in telogen.

Hair Texture and Color

Hair texture depends on its cross-sectional shape, which in turn depends on the cross-sectional shape of the follicles. Round hairs are straight and emerge from straight hair follicles. Oval hairs are wavy, whereas flatter hairs are more curly or kinky; these types emerge from curved follicles. Straight hairs, because of their greater diameter, are usually stronger and less likely to break than curly hairs.

Natural hair color is due primarily to the amount and particular shade of melanin present. Melanocytes in the hair matrix contribute to hair color in the same way that epidermal melanocytes contribute to skin color. When melanocytes make large amounts of eumelanin, hair is dark. When more pheomelanin is present, hair is varying shades of brown or blonde. An iron-rich form of pheomelanin called **trichosiderin** (trik-ō-SID-er-in; *tricho*, hair; *sideri*, iron) makes hair red, while white hair lacks pigment altogether. "Gray" hairs may have a small amount of pigment, but most often, they are white hairs; however, because they are interspersed among dark hairs, there is an illusion that some hairs are gray. Graying is more noticeable in people who have dark hair to start with because there is greater contrast between the white hairs and the dark hairs.

Nails

If you dropped a dime on a smooth tabletop, you'd have a hard time retrieving it – or even feeling it distinctly – if the digits of your hands lacked fingernails. Nails allow your fingers to develop leverage around small objects so you can lift them, and they act as pressure plates that magnify your sense of fine touch at the fingertips. So apart from their obvious role of protecting the ends of the digits, fingernails may be used to accomplish a host of manual skills—from typing to manipulating a pencil—activities you may not associate with thin, translucent plates of keratin. Figure 8-6 shows the parts of a nail.

Like the cuticle of hairs, your nails (whether fingernails or toenails) are formed from stacked plates of hard keratin. But, instead of growing in a follicle, nails form in a pocket of the epidermis called the **proximal nail fold**, located at the end of a digit. At the nail fold's margin, the epidermis tucks beneath itself, becoming the **dorsal matrix**, which then wraps distally forming the **ventral matrix**. The nail starts forming at the **nail root**, and the dorsal matrix and ventral matrix add more keratinocytes to complete the **nail plate**, the shovel-shaped body of a nail. The longer the nail matrix, the thicker the resulting nail will be. Adding keratinocytes to the proximal end of the nail plate nudges the nail distally along its **nail bed**. Dense collagenous fibers firmly anchor the nail bed to the underlying bony structure of the digit. At its lateral margins, the nail plate curves inferiorly to form

THE INTEGUMENTARY SYSTEM

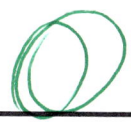

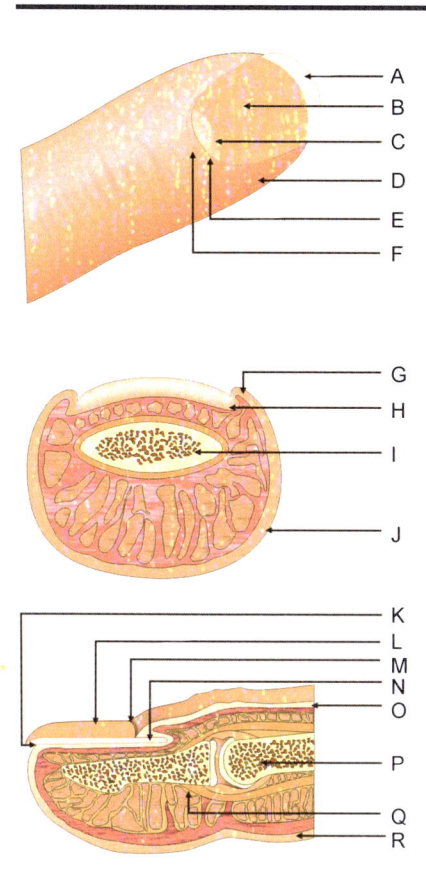

Figure 8-6. Parts of a nail

the **lateral nail groove**. The **free edge** of the nail is the part used to grasp or pinch objects.

Unlike hairs, your nails grow continuously, although their growth rate is affected by factors such as your diet, general state of health, and age. As the nail plate creeps along the nail bed, bands of the stratum corneum from the surrounding epidermis stick to the nail's superior margins, forming the **eponychium** (ep-ō-NIK-ē-um; *epo*; above; *onyx*, nail). The eponychium helps to seal the nail matrix and nail bed from the external environment. An actively growing part of the nail is visible as the **lunula** (LŪN-ū-la; moon), a pale, crescent-shaped disc that extends beyond the proximal nail fold. The lunula is the distal portion of the ventral nail matrix; it is lighter in color than the rest of the nail bed because the thick matrix tissue hides underlying blood vessels. The nail's free end may extend beyond the tip of the digit. Clumps of stratum corneum form the **hyponychium** (hī-pō-NIK-ē-um; *hypo*, below), which helps to seal the inferior margin of the free end. Nails grow about 0.1 mm a day, and the progression from nail root to free end takes about six months.

> **Note**: Curiously, the nails on your longer digits grow faster than the nails on your shorter digits.

SKIN REPAIR

Your skin is exposed on a daily basis to many hazards from the external environment and must be capable of repairing itself when damaged. Depending on the depth to which damage occurs, skin wounds are classified as either *epidermal* or *deep*.

Epidermal wounds do not penetrate deeper than the basement membrane of the epidermis. Since the epidermis is avascular, these wounds do not bleed; however, free nerve endings in this region can cause you to feel pain. Repairing epidermal wounds involves repeated cell divisions of nearby, undamaged epidermal. If the stratum germinativum (stratum basale and stratum spinosum) is still intact at the wound site, the superficial strata simply re-grow from these cells. If the stratum germinativum is damaged, however, undamaged epidermal cells from the stratum germinativum surrounding the wound divide and the daughter cells spread to fill in the wound. This process is called **epidermal migration**. In addition, the cells that form hair follicles and ducts of sweat glands can migrate above the basement membrane to replace the damaged stratum germinativum. In this ironic twist, the new epidermis is actually "derived" from epidermal derivatives.

Deep wounds are those that penetrate into the reticular region of the dermis, but they may extend well into the hypodermis. Deep wounds damage much more integumentary tissue than epidermal wounds, and so require more extensive repair. Repair of deep wounds involves three main stages: *inflammation, proliferation, and remodeling* (Figure 8-7).

(1) The **inflammation stage** of deep wound repair can be likened to disaster crews who seal off a storm-ravaged town and start clearing away debris. Inflammation is a specific physiological response to an injury or tissue damage, and serves two major functions: (1) to restrict the movement of

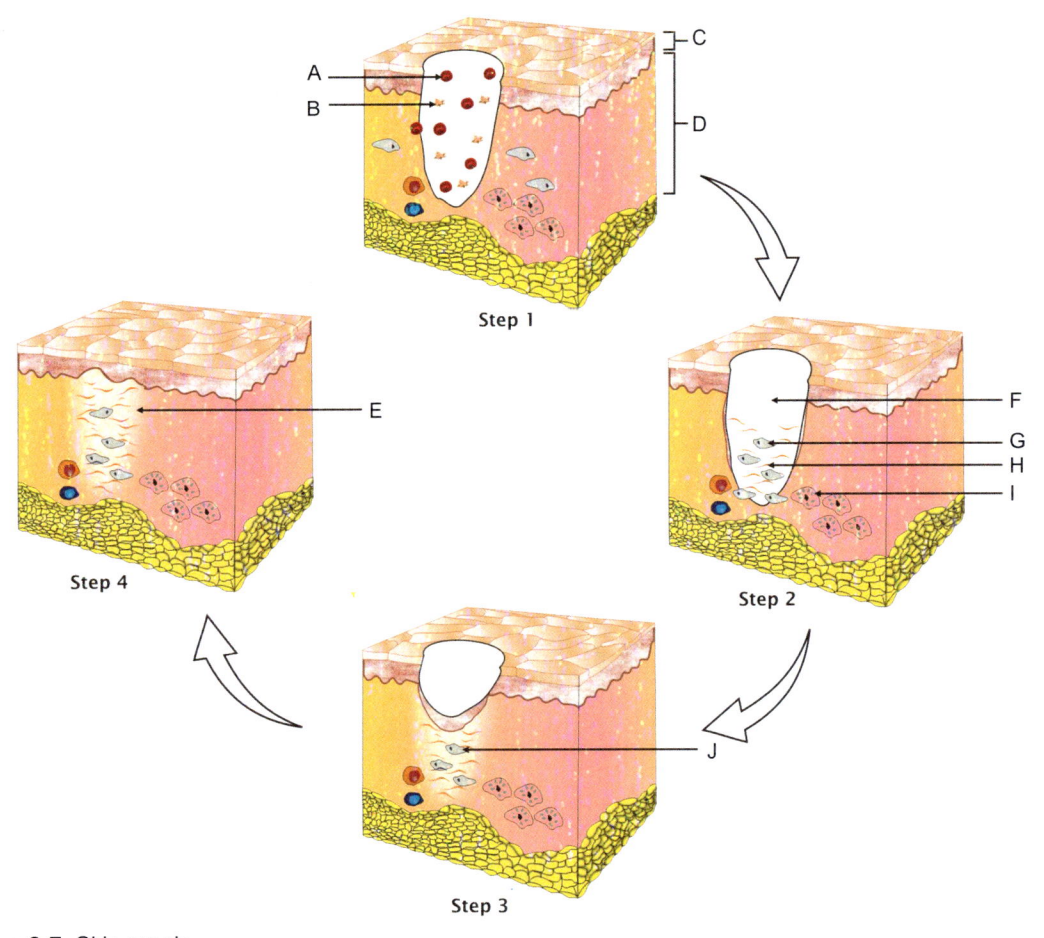

Figure 8-7. Skin repair

harmful agents, such as bacteria, from the wound site; and (2) to seal off damaged tissues so they can be cleaned up. Within minutes after a deep wound occurs, chemical reactions in the blood convert a soluble blood protein into an insoluble form called **fibrin**. Strands of fibrin interlock, forming a "net" that traps blood cells in the broken vessels and helps reduce blood loss. The fibrin strands and trapped blood cells form a **clot**. The part of the clot at the wound's surface soon hardens, forming a **scab**, which protects the wound against bacteria and prevents the underlying tissue from dehydrating.

In response to tissue damage, mast cells in the region of the wound release *histamine*, a substance that dilates blood vessels. As a result, more blood flows through the skin's vessels, and the skin turns red (**erythema**; ar-e-THĒ-ma; *eryth*, red) and feels warm to the touch. Histamine also causes the vessels to leak blood plasma into surrounding tissues causing them to swell; this is called **edema** (e-DĒ-ma; "swelling"). The swollen tissue may press on sensory receptors resulting in pain around the wound. White blood cells squeeze out of nearby blood vessels and infiltrate the wound, engulfing dead tissue and foreign particles by phagocytosis.

(2) During the **proliferation stage**, damaged integumentary system structures begin to regrow. This stage can be compared to the arrival of construction workers who start rebuilding the storm-ravaged town after the disaster crews depart. Cells from the stratum germinativum migrate across the wound along the inferior

margin of the scab and begin replacing the epidermis. Fibroblasts in the dermis secrete collagen that twists into thick fibers and ties the edges of the wound together. The collagen fibers can be compared to scaffolding that surrounds and supports the walls of a building under construction. The pink, sensitive tissue around and beneath the scab during this stage is called **granulation tissue**, because it does not have a well-defined structure. During this stage, severed blood vessels are reconnected, and damaged nerves are regenerated. If the scab is removed before the proliferation stage is finished, the newly formed vessels and nerves may tear. In this case, the wound re-enters the inflammation stage, and the healing process must start over.

(3) The final part of deep wound repair, the **remodeling stage**, can be compared to the rebuilt town undergoing final cleanup and remodeling. This stage may last for several months or several years, depending on the extent of the wound. Fibroblasts in the dermal zone of the wound continue to produce collagen fibers that arrange themselves in large irregular bundles. The proliferation of collagen fibers during this stage is called **fibrosis**, which is the source of **scar tissue**, and the more fibrosis, the more scar tissue. Scar tissue helps strengthen the site of the wound, but it may be problematic because it is usually much less flexible than an undamaged dermis. Over time, collagen fibers in the scar tissue arrange themselves in a more regular pattern, similar to the pattern in dermal tension lines.

TOPICS TO KNOW FOR CHAPTER 8 (THE INTEGUMENTARY SYSTEM)

accessory skin organs
anagen
apocrine sweat glands
apoptosis
arrector pili
autophagia
basal lamina
blushing
calcidiol
calcitriol
carotene
catagen
cerumen
ceruminous glands
cholecalciferol
clot
club hair
cornification
cornified cells
corpuscle lamellae
cutaneous membrane
cutaneous receptors
cutaneous sensations
cutis anserina
dandruff
deep pressure receptor
deep wound repair
dehydrocholesterol
dermal (fibrous) root sheath
dermal blood vessels
dermal papillae
dermis
desquamation

dorsal nail matrix
eccrine sweat glands
edema
eleidin
encapsulated nerve endings
epidermal grooves
epidermal migration
epidermal nerve endings
epidermal pegs
epidermal ridges
epidermal strata
epidermal wound repair
epidermis
eponychium
erythema
eumelanin
evaporative cooling
exfoliation
factors affecting skin gland secretion
fibrin
fibrosis
fingerprints
flexure lines
freckles
free nerve endings
free sebaceous glands
friction ridges
functions of hair
functions of papillary dermis
functions of reticular dermis
functions of the epidermis
functions of the skin
glabrous skin

glassy membrane
granulation tissue
gray hair
hair
hair bulb
hair cortex
hair cuticle
hair follicles
hair growth cycle
hair matrix
hair medulla
hair papilla
hair receptors
hair root
hair root plexuses
hair shaft
hair texture and color
hard keratin
heme
hemidesmosomes
hemoglobin
hirsute skin
histamine
hypodermis
hyponychium
inflammation stage
inner root sheath
insensible perspiration
integumentary system
keratin
keratin fibrils
keratin tonofilaments
keratinization

keratinized cells
keratinocytes
keratohyalin
lamellar granules
lamellated corpuscles
Langerhans cells
lateral nail groove
layers of the skin
lines of cleavage
lunula
mammary glands
mechanoreceptor
Meissner corpuscles
melanin
melanin granules
melanocyte dendrites
melanocytes
melanosomes
Merkel cells
Merkel discs
moles
myoepithelial cells
nail bed
nail free edge
nail plate
nail root
nails
nociceptor
oil glands
outer root sheath
Pacinian corpuscles
papillary plexus

papillary region
pheomelanin
pili
piloerection
pilosebaceous unit
prickle cells
proliferation stage
properties of skin
proximal nail fold
remodeling stage
reticular lamina
reticular plexus
reticular region
Ruffini endings
scab
scar tissue
sebaceous glands
sebum
sensible perspiration
skin
skin color
skin derivatives
skin glands
skin pigments
skin repair
spiny cells
squame cells
steps of keratinization
stratum basale
stratum corium
stratum corneum
stratum germinativum

stratum granulosum
stratum lucidum
stratum spinosum
subcutaneous receptors
subcutaneous tissue
sudoriferous gland
superficial fascia
surface pattern lines
sweat pore
sweating
tactile corpuscles
tactile discs
tactile receptor
telogen
tension lines
terminal hairs
thermoreceptor
thick skin
thin skin
topical features of the skin
trichosiderin
types of skin
ultraviolet B
vasoconstriction in skin
vasodilation in skin
vellus hairs
ventral nail matrix
vitamin D synthesis
vitamin D3
wrinkles

CHAPTER 9

Osseous Tissue

Imagine a house occupied at the same time by competing construction and demolition crews. Day after day, the construction workers assemble the building's features with meticulous craftsmanship and care. But at the same time, the hard-hatted workers chip away at the walls and floors, pulverizing pieces into dust and carting away the debris. The house grows or comes apart, depending on which crew has the upper hand. But most times the competing crews work at the same steady and reliable pace, so the house stands solid and useful, but it's never really finished.

This construction-versus-demolition story can apply to the physiology of your bones. Every year, between 10 and 30 percent of the substance of adult skeletal bones "turns over." In other words, one group of bone cells (osteoclasts) methodically destroys bone matter while a different group of bone cells (osteoblasts) deposits fresh bone matter to replace what was lost. It really shouldn't surprise you to discover that your seemingly solid bones are in a constant state of flux. A recurring theme of this book is that the body is built to adapt to ever-changing conditions, and bones are no exception. Bone turnover makes it possible for the body to grow, and it enables bones to repair themselves from daily wear-and-tear.

Just as important, bone turnover releases minerals that other organs, especially muscles and nerves, need to function normally.

After an introduction to the skeletal system, this chapter looks at the structure and function of bones as individual, living organs. We will start by noting how anatomists classify bones by shape. Next, we will discuss what bones are made of and introduce the cells that build up bone and tear it down again. Bone cells don't work without a plan, so it's equally important to recognize the patterns of bone growth that can occur in the body. As with our discussion of the skin, we finish this chapter by looking at how damaged bones repair themselves.

OVERVIEW OF THE SKELETAL SYSTEM

Together bones, ligaments, and cartilages comprise the **skeletal system**. Every bone in this system is a living organ composed of a variety of tissues, all of which contribute to the bone's function. A bone is made mostly of **osseous tissue**, otherwise known as "bone." Osseous tissue consists of cells that live on or within a matrix of collagen fibers, ground substance, and calcium salts. The calcium salts give bones their remarkable qualities of hardness, durability, and strength. The living cells in bones include ones that build osseous tissue and ones that break it down. Bones also contain dense connective tissue, adipose tissue and blood-forming tissue, and some bones contain cartilage. In addition, numerous blood vessels and nerves surround and penetrate deep into living bones.

Collectively, bones form the **skeleton**, the body's rigid internal framework. A typical adult skeleton consists of 206 bones that anatomists divide into two sets: the axial skeleton and the appendicular skeleton. The **axial skeleton** includes the bones that form the head, neck, spine, and rib cage. The term "axial" signifies that these bones form a vertical axis or column through the body. In the same way that a trunk forms the structural core of a tree, the axial skeleton forms the body's structural core.

The **appendicular skeleton** includes the shoulder bones and hipbones, and the bones of the upper and lower limbs. The shoulder bones attach the upper limbs to the axial skeleton, while the hipbones attach the lower limbs to the axial skeleton. Hence, this division of the skeleton is so named because its bones are appended to (hang from) the axial skeleton. In this respect, the appendicular skeleton is like the branches that successively divide from a tree trunk. Appendicular skeletal bones make it possible for a person to move about and manipulate objects in the surrounding environment.

ACCESSORY PARTS OF THE SKELETAL SYSTEM

Individual bones meet and interact at **joints** or **articulations**. Many joints are freely moveable; that is, the bones that form the joint can easily change position with respect to one another. Perhaps the most familiar freely moveable joints are those that form the elbows and knees. Other joints are only slightly moveable, such as those between the vertebrae, the bones that make up the spine. Still other joints, such as those that connect the skull bones, are completely immovable. Bones at joints would either pull apart from each other or damage one another when rubbing together if it weren't for the presence of the skeleton's ligaments and cartilages.

Ligaments

A **ligament** (LIG-a-ment; band) is a strip of dense, regular connective tissue that holds bones together at a joint. Some ligaments may cross between bones deep within a joint, while other ligaments extend around a joint, forming a capsule-like enclosure. Relatively long ligaments hold bones together at freely moveable joints. In contrast, microscopically short ligaments are present between bones at immovable joints. These tiny ligaments act like glue, bonding the bones together so tightly that virtually no movement is possible at the joint.

Skeletal Cartilages

A skeletal **cartilage** is an avascular connective tissue consisting of chondrocytes living in a matrix of collagen fibers and ground substance. A thin, dense connective tissue membrane called the *perichondrium* covers the cartilage. The skeletal system has hyaline cartilage at most of its joints, fibrocartilage at some joints, both hyaline and fibrocartilage at a few joints, and elastic cartilage at several locations. Skeletal cartilage attaches and protects bones at joints, and serves as a substitute for bones in certain parts of the skeleton where flexibility is needed as much as mechanical strength. Functions of cartilage include:

- Attaching bones: Like ligaments, some cartilages connect bones at joints by acting like braces. For example, the *costal cartilages,* made of hyaline cartilage, connect the anterior ends of the ribs to the sternum (breastbone). Fibrocartilage pads called *intervertebral discs* act like flexible glue to hold the vertebrae together yet allows them to bend and twist. The *pubic symphysis* is a fibrocartilage pad that holds together the anterior portion of the pelvis.

- Protecting bones: Skeletal cartilages prevent bones at movable joints from damaging each other by reducing friction and absorbing impacts. For example, thin *articular cartilages* cover the ends of bones at freely moveable joints. These hyaline cartilages are smooth and slippery, which allows the ends of moving bones to slide back and forth over one another. Some joints have fibrocartilage pads that further reduce joint friction by keeping bones properly aligned as they move. Finally, skeletal cartilages keep adjacent bones from pulverizing one another by acting like rubber shock absorbers inside the joint. In particular, the springy fibrocartilage that makes up the intervertebral discs helps absorb and dissipate the physical pounding the spine receives when a person walks or runs.

- **Acting like bones:** Some cartilages act like bones at places where mechanical flexibility is important, and they help to protect underlying organs. For example, the costal cartilages at the ends of ribs enable the rib cage to expand and contract to produce breathing. These cartilages also shield organs in the lower thoracic and upper abdominal cavities. The *nasal cartilages* that form the nose are flexible, interlocking hyaline cartilages. The external ears consist mainly of elastic cartilages that surround the entrance to the external ear canals; short ligaments anchor these cartilages to the skull.

FUNCTIONS OF THE SKELETAL SYSTEM

Like the internal framing of a house, the skeleton determines a person's size and shape. Moreover, the arrangement of the facial bones largely determines a person's characteristic facial features. Apart from how it influences one's appearance, the skeletal system plays critical structural and physiological roles in the body. Structurally, the skeleton offers physical support and protection, and it allows for body movement. Physiologically, the skeleton is the site of blood formation in adults, and it serves as a storage site for minerals and fats.

- **Support:** Healthy bones can withstand tremendous pushing, pulling, and bending forces. Their strength makes bones well suited for supporting the body's soft tissues, which account for about 80 percent of an average adult's weight. Even the smallest skeletal bones, such as those that form the ankles and wrists are strong enough to support the body's full weight without breaking. In most cases, organs and soft tissues hang from the bones much like clothing suspended on hangers. But at some places, the body's soft tissues rest on a bony platform. The brain, for example, rests in a cradle of bones that form the base and sides of the skull.

- **Protection:** The bones of the axial skeleton surround the body's most delicate organs. For example, the bones that form the skull enclose the brain, making it possible for a boxer to survive a punch to the head. The rib cage surrounds and shelters the heart and lungs. The sturdy vertebrae along the spine not only support the trunk, but also enclose the spinal cord, the nervous system's communications pathway between the brain and most of the body.

- **Facilitating movement:** Bones that meet at movable joints act like *levers*, simple machines that can transmit mechanical force. Contracting muscles pull on bones, which then move in relationship to joints and facilitate body movement. For example, to curl your lower arm toward your chest, muscles and their tendons pull on bones of the arm and forearm that meet at the elbow joint. And when you chew food, sets of powerful facial muscles pull against the lower jawbone, which moves at hinge-like joints at the back of the jaw.

- **Blood formation:** Blood, the body's softest tissue, forms inside bones, the body's hardest organs. Blood cells form and differentiate in a process called **hemopoiesis** (HĒ-mō-poy-Ē-sis; *hemo*, blood; *poiesis*, making). In adults, blood cells form in *red marrow*, a specialized connective tissue that is concentrated inside certain bones. Red marrow produces all of the body's oxygen-carrying red blood cells, its clot-forming platelets, and practically all of its disease-fighting white blood cells.

- **Lipid storage:** Cavities deep within many bones are filled with *yellow marrow*. This connective tissue is yellow because it consists almost entirely of lipid-filled adipocytes (fat-storing cells). Yellow marrow comprises part of the body's chemical energy reserves.

- **Mineral storage:** Bones are the body's "mineral bank." Just as banks store and distribute money, bones store and release minerals depending on the body's needs. The "currency" that is deposited

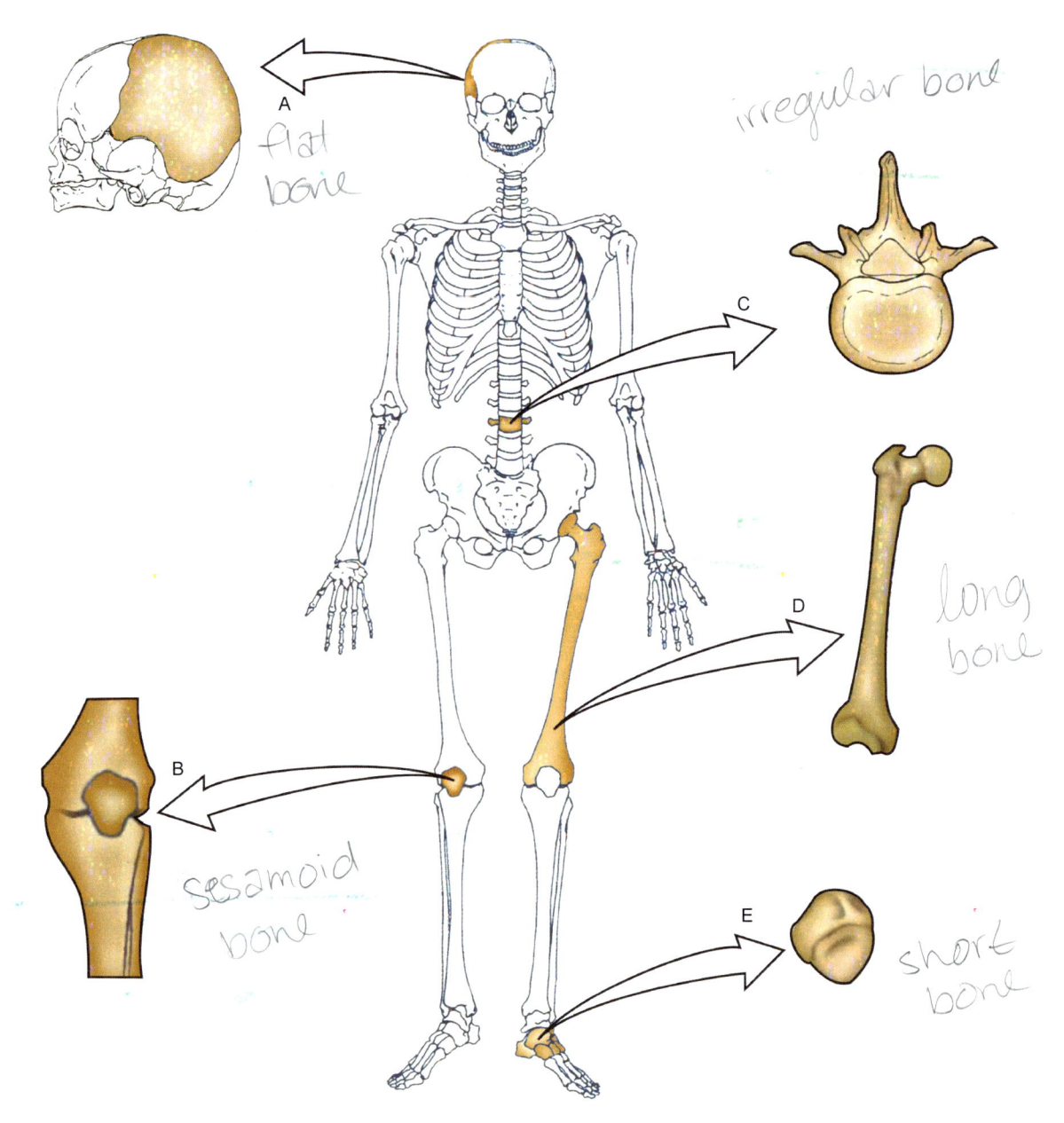

Figure 9-1. Bone shapes

in bones and can later be withdrawn consists of calcium and phosphorus ions. You probably have read that dietary calcium is required to build strong bones; it's true – the skeleton contains 99 percent of all the body's calcium. But organs such as muscles and nerves need steady levels of calcium in the blood and tissue fluids in order to work properly. Bones release calcium ions when blood calcium levels drop, and they tend to take in calcium ions when the blood calcium levels rise.

CLASSIFICATION OF BONES

Bones come in many shapes and sizes. But a closer look at their surface and interior reveals that all bones are derived from a basic blueprint. No two bones in the body are quite alike. But many bones share common physical traits, a fact that enabled anatomists to develop a simple bone classification method based on shape. The four shape-related categories of bones include *long bones, short bones, flat bones,* and *irregular bones* (Figure 9-1).

OSSEOUS TISSUE

Long Bones are rod shaped and are always longer than they are wide. All long bones are part of the appendicular skeleton, and comprise most of the bones that form the upper and lower limbs. The longest long bone is the *femur* in the thigh, and the shortest is the bean-like *distal phalanx* at the end of the little toe. Long bones function as levers that facilitate body movements.

Short Bones are wedge-shaped bones and form the wrists and ankles. These little bones can slide over one another, giving the hands and feet a wide range of motion. The *cuneiform bones* of the ankle typify the structure of a short bone. Special short bones develop solely in *tendons*, the connective tissue bands that attach muscles to bones. These are **sesamoid bones** (SES-a-moyd), so named because they look like sesame seeds. The patella, or kneecap, is the largest sesamoid bone, but rice-sized sesamoid bones may form inside tendons of the hands and feet. It is thought that sesamoid bones stabilize tendons by preventing them from slipping from side to side, as they cross a joint.

Flat Bones have a broad, smooth surface, and it's always thinner than it is long or wide. Despite their classification, many flat bones are curved. The bowl-like *parietal bone*, for example, forms part of the curved dome of the skull. Most flat bones are part of the axial skeleton and shield underlying organs and soft tissues. Some people have extra flat bones between their sutures, the zigzagging joints that hold together the major flat bones of the skull. These tiny bony islands are called **sutural bones** (Wormian bones).

Irregular Bones. Like the "none-of-the-above" selection from a multiple-choice question, irregular bones have unique and bizarre shapes. These bones may exhibit a variety of projections, indentations, notches, and holes. Ultimately, the odd shapes of irregular bones relate to their functions. For example, a typical vertebra has a hole through its vertical axis that allows for passage of the spinal cord. In addition, the vertebra's antler-like projections are sturdy attachment points for powerful back muscles that control posture and trunk movements.

While considerable variation in design exists among short bones, flat bones, and irregular bones, the long bones show the least variation in design. For this reason, we will use a long bone as a model for describing the gross anatomical features of a bone (Figure 9-2).

ANATOMY OF A LONG BONE

While long bones come in a wide range of lengths, they all have three external features in common:

- **Diaphysis** (dī-AF-i-sis; growing between): the relatively long shaft that forms the middle section of the long bone

- **Epiphysis** (e-PIF-i-sis; upon growth): the enlarged region at the end of the diaphysis. An epiphysis is specified as either *proximal* or *distal*, depending on its relative distance from the body's torso. In most long bones, both epiphyses are covered with articular cartilages (described earlier).

- **Metaphysis** (me-TAF-i-sis; between growth): the cone-shaped, transition region between the diaphysis and the epiphysis. The proximal or distal metaphysis of both regions in an adult may contain one or two *epiphyseal lines*, which are remnants of growth zones that existed when the bone was developing.

In addition, all long bones have a *periosteum, compact bone, spongy bone, endosteum, medullary cavity*, and a rich supply of *blood vessels* and *nerves*, and *marrow*. We will take a closer look at each of these features, beginning on the outer surface of the bone and working inward.

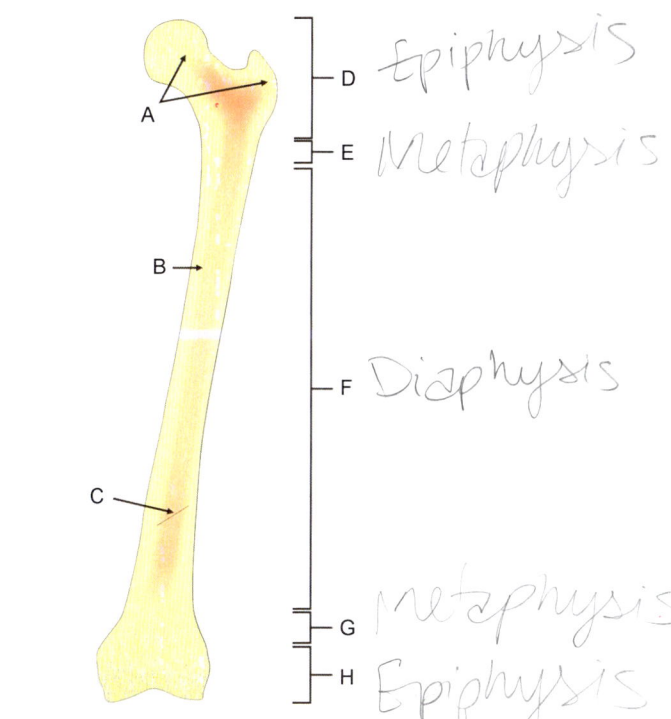

Figure 9-2. Parts of a long bone

The periosteum

When bones are cleaned, dried, and sterilized for display in a lab, all that remains is hard osseous tissue. However, living bones appear white because a tough membrane called the **periosteum** (per-ē-OS-tē-um; *peri*, around; *oste*, bone) covers them. This membrane consists of two layers that are structurally and functionally different from one another. The periosteum has an outer *fibrous layer* that consists of dense regular connective tissue. The inner *osteogenic layer* contains several types of bone cells. The periosteum is important to the bone in three ways:

- Protection: Densely packed collagen fibers make the fibrous periosteum an effective barrier that separates osseous tissue from surrounding tissues. If bacteria infect a nearby tissue, the periosteum can help prevent their spread into the osseous tissue. However, the periosteum cannot prevent bacteria from entering the bone through blood vessels. The fibrous periosteum also acts like a stretch-resistant jacket that helps prevent bones from bending excessively.

- Attachment site: The fibrous layer of the periosteum is the attachment site for tendons, ligaments, and blood vessels. In fact, the collagen fibers of the fibrous periosteum are continuous with those of tendons and ligaments. Short collagenous fibers, called **perforating fibers** (Sharpey's fibers) attach the periosteum firmly to the underlying hard osseous tissue. When tendons or ligaments pull on the bone, the perforating fibers prevent the periosteum from tearing away. Blood vessels and nerves also attach to the fibrous periosteum, and they are distributed throughout this layer.

- Bone growth: The osteogenic layer of the periosteum contains several types of bone cells, including *osteoblasts* and *osteoclasts*. Osteoblasts add hard osseous material to the bone's surface, while osteoclasts remove this material.

Compact Bone

Compact bone (dense bone) is osseous tissue that is solid and heavy, much like concrete (Figure 9-3). It forms the hard exterior, or cortex, of the bone; for this reason, compact bone is also called *cortical bone* (KOR-tik-al; *cortex*, bark). Due in part to its high density, compact bone is very strong and able to withstand enormous physical pressure and stress. As you might imagine, strength is an essential property of weight-bearing bones, such as those in your lower limbs. When running or jumping, the forces exerted on these weight-bearing bones in the average adult male may approach 550 kg (~ 1200 lbs.)! However,

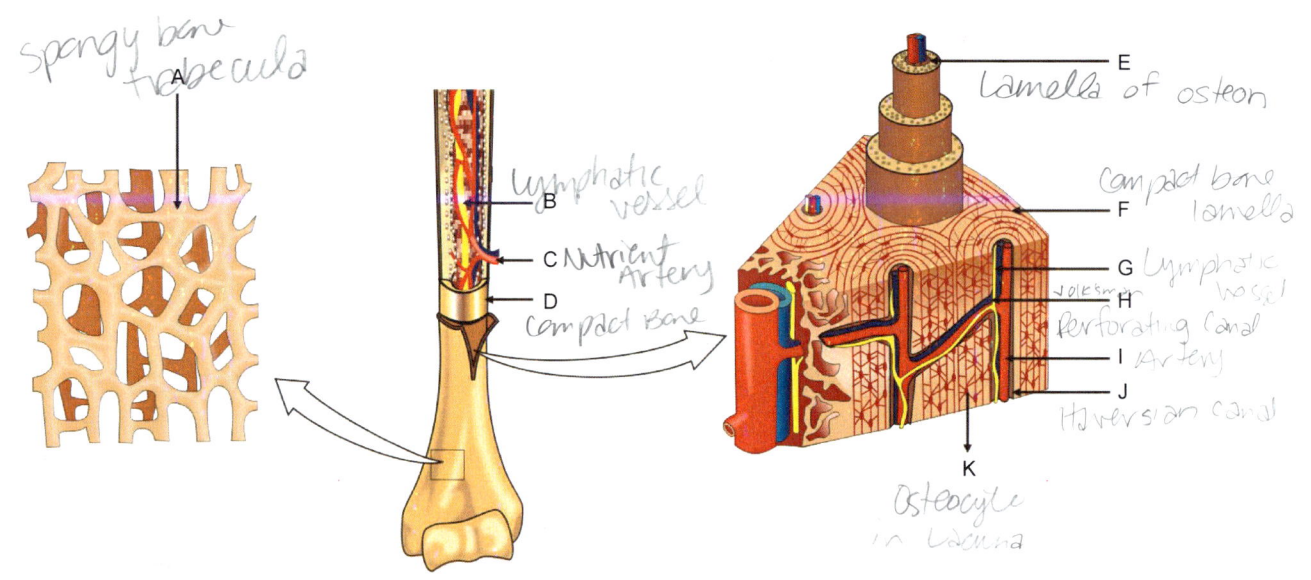

Figure 9-3. Compact and spongy bone

OSSEOUS TISSUE

even bones that seldom support much weight can experience intense compression and bending forces as your muscles contract and relax. For example, simply unscrewing a tight jar lid can apply tremendous pressure to the two long bones within your forearm.

Spongy bone

Spongy, or **cancellous bone** (KAN-se-lus; lattice), is osseous tissue that makes up all or part of the interior of bones. In long bones, it makes up most of the epiphyses and lines a tube-like **medullary cavity** within the diaphysis (shaft). Spongy bone consists of short interlocking struts of osseous tissue called **trabeculae** that separate numerous tiny cavities. A thin membrane, the **endosteum**, covers all trabeculae, but unlike the periosteum, the endosteum lacks a fibrous layer. In adult bones, either red or yellow bone marrow may fill the cavities between the trabeculae. Spongy bone reduces a bone's total weight without overly reducing its strength; in fact, spongy bone actually helps to distribute the stress and strain that bones undergo as muscles pull on them.

Blood vessels, lymphatics, and nerves

Bones, like other organs, contain a rich supply of blood vessels (arteries and veins), lymphatic vessels, and nerves that play important roles in bone homeostasis. Arteries deliver nutrients to the bone, while veins remove substances that the bone releases into the tissue fluid. In most long bones, one **nutrient artery** enters the diaphysis through an opening called a **nutrient foramen** (for-Ā-men; opening). The nutrient artery enters the medullary cavity before it branches into smaller arteries that transport blood toward the epiphyses; however, these vessels do not extend past the epiphyseal line. Smaller arteries branch off of the medullary arteries and pass into the inner layers of compact bone in the diaphysis. These small arteries branch into still smaller arteries that transport blood toward the epiphyses. The periosteum has numerous arteries that penetrate and nourish the outer layers of compact bone in the diaphysis. On the other hand, the epiphyses have a blood vessel supply that is separate from that nourishing the metaphyses and diaphysis.

Running essentially parallel to the arteries are veins that transport blood out of the bone.

Lymphatic vessels accompany blood vessels along the periosteum and pick up excess tissue fluid that seeps out of the bones. Thus far, however, lymphatic vessels have not been shown to penetrate into bones. Tiny nerves run alongside the bone's periosteal blood vessels and lymphatic vessels. In addition, tiny nerve branches extend into the medullary cavity and the tiny passageways inside compact bone. When a bone tissue is damaged, nerves alert the person to the damage by sending pain signals to the brain.

Bone marrow

Bone marrow is a soft, gelatinous material that fills the medullary cavity of long bones and the spaces between trabeculae in spongy bone. There are two types of bone marrow: *red marrow* and *yellow marrow*.

- **Red marrow** consists of blood vessels and *hemopoietic tissue* (HĒ-mō-poy-e-tik), the latter being responsible for making blood cells. Hemopoietic tissue contains highly branched fibroblasts that produce very delicate collagen filaments. These filaments intertwine in the extracellular fluid to form a network of collagen fibers. The network of fibers support specialized cells called *hemopoietic stem cells* that divide repeatedly to form blood cells. During fetal development, red marrow occupies the marrow cavities of all bones, but by age 25, most of the skeleton's red marrow has changed to yellow marrow. In the adult, red marrow exists mainly in the axial skeleton and in the proximal end of the upper arm bones and the thighbones.

- **Yellow marrow** consists mostly of adipose tissue that arises from red marrow. Beginning at about age 5, some of the hemopoietic cells in red marrow change into adipocytes. The adipocytes fill with lipid droplets, causing the cells to appear yellow. In the adult, most of the skeleton's yellow marrow is found in the medullary cavities of long bones. The conversion of red marrow to yellow marrow begins first in the distal bones of the upper and lower limbs. Lipids stored in yellow marrow provide energy for the bone and for other body tissues.

ANATOMY OF SHORT BONES, FLAT BONES, AND IRREGULAR BONES

While these bones come in an assortment of shapes and sizes, they all differ from long bones by not having a diaphysis, epiphyses, or medullary cavity. However, like long bones, they all have an outer layer of compact bone covered with periosteum. Since there is no medullary cavity, the interior of these bones is filled with spongy bone. Endosteum covers the trabeculae, and marrow fills the spaces between the trabeculae. In most flat bones and certain irregular bones (vertebrae), red marrow persists throughout adulthood.

Flat bones consist of equally thick layers of compact bone and spongy bone. In the parietal bone of the skull, for example, two layers of compact bone sandwich an equally thick layer of spongy bone called **diploë** (DIP-lō-ē; double). Short bones and irregular bones are made mostly of spongy bone surrounded by a thin shell of compact bone. In terms of their composition, short bones and irregular bones look much like the epiphyses of long bones.

OSSEOUS TISSUE

As fascinating as an individual bone may look, its gross anatomy barely hints at the constant chemical tug-of-war that takes place in its osseous tissue. A bone can grow, and it can rearrange its tissue to help it withstand mechanical stress. These qualities are due to the actions of different kinds of bone cells, and the extracellular environment in which they act. Moreover, the microscopic structure of both compact bone and spongy bone reveals that bone cells act in a coordinated manner. In this section, we will describe the stuff that makes up bones and how bone cells assemble osseous tissue into characteristic patterns.

Bone matrix

The strength of osseous tissue is an attribute of its extracellular material, called **bone matrix**. Like the matrix of other connective tissues, bone matrix has two parts: (1) a homogeneous ground substance, and (2) a fibrous portion. The ground substance, which makes up about 65% of the bone matrix, consists of inorganic and organic materials. The most abundant inorganic material in the ground substance of bone matrix is *hydroxyapatite*, a mineral salt containing calcium phosphate, $Ca_3(PO_4)_2$. The major organic components of the ground substance are proteoglycans, which contain chondroitin sulfate and hyaluronic acid. Collagen fibers make up the fibrous portion of bone matrix. The entire organic component of bone matrix, including the collagen fibers and proteoglycans, is called **osteoid** (OS-tē-oyd; *ost*, bone; *oid*, resembles).

A bone receives two benefits of having its bone matrix as a mixture of mineral salts and collagen fibers:

(1) Since mineral crystals bind tightly to collagen fibers, they cannot easily shift or slide past one another under stress.

(2) Collagen is less dense than mineral salts, so a mixture of collagen and minerals is lighter than an equal amount of minerals alone. Altogether, the arrangement of mineral salts and collagen fibers in bone matrix helps bones to resist compression, *tension* (pulling-forces), and *torsion* (twisting forces).

The balance of mineral salts and collagen in the matrix is crucial to maintaining a bone's physical integrity. If the concentration of either component in the matrix falls below normal, the bone may become either too brittle or too soft. On the one hand, a bone deficient in bone salts would be too flexible; it would twist or warp when stressed, just as a rubber dog bone would. On the other hand, a bone that is deficient in collagen would still be very hard, but it might shatter like glass when bent.

Classification of Bone Matrix

Based on the arrangement of the ground substance and collagen fibers in its bone matrix, osseous tissue is classified as either *woven bone* or *lamellar bone*.

- **Woven bone** is so named because it contains delicate, interlacing strands that look like threads in woven cloth. The tiny strands that make up woven bone contain irregularly arranged collagen fibers surrounded by tiny crystals of hydroxyapatite. Woven bone is found in the embryonic skeleton or in broken bones that are healing, and it represents the earliest stage of bone development.

OSSEOUS TISSUE

- **Lamellar bone** (la-MEL-lar; *lamella*, plate) has parallel collagen fibers surrounded by ground substance that is assembled in layers called **lamellae**. Lamellar bone is "mature" bone tissue, and it comprises almost all of the osseous tissue in the adult skeleton. Depending on how the lamellae are arranged, lamellar bone is classified as either *compact bone* or *spongy bone*. These two types of osseous tissue have strikingly different patterns of lamellae, and these patterns determine how nutrients travel through the osseous tissue. Most compact bone is nourished from the "inside out," while spongy bone is nourished from the "outside in."

Compact bone and osteons

The lamellae of compact bone form groups of tiny cylinders called **osteons**, or Haversian systems. Researchers estimate that the adult skeleton contains around 20 million osteons. The average osteon has about 30 **concentric lamellae**, giving it the appearance of a sliced onion when viewed in cross section. The innermost lamella surrounds a narrow tunnel called the **central canal**, or Haversian canal, through which blood vessels and nerves run. Smaller branches extend from these vessels and nerves and pass into small **perforating canals** (Volkmann's canals) that lead to the bone's surface or into the medullary cavity. Nutrients from blood vessels in the central canal diffuse outward through tiny canals, called **canaliculi** (kan-a-LIK-ū-lī; little canals) to reach tiny cavities called **lacunae**, which house bone cells called *osteocytes*. Cellular wastes diffuse in the opposite direction; osteocytes in the outer lamella of an osteon are seldom more than 1/2 mm from the central canal.

The lamellae of compact bone form other patterns besides the concentric circles that identify osteons. **Circumferential lamellae** make up a few layers of a bone's outer surface, and they are formed by osteoblasts in the osteogenic layer of the periosteum. After they are surrounded by calcified bone matrix, the osteocytes in circumferential lamellae are nourished through canaliculi that communicate with blood vessels in the periosteum. In addition, wedge-shaped features called **interstitial lamellae** exist within compact bone. These structures are the remains of older osteons that were destroyed as the result of *bone resorption* (discussed shortly).

Osteons are one reason why bones, especially long bones, are strong. Imagine that you could pull out the lamellae of an osteon like the tubes of a telescope. The osteon would look like a series of tubes-within-tubes. The outer lamellae reinforce the inner ones, an arrangement that helps an osteon to withstand tremendous compression. A spiraling pattern of collagen fibers within each lamella also resists tension. Also, the orientation of the collagen fibers alternates from one lamella to the next helping an osteon resist torsion. When a force twists an osteon clockwise, all the collagen fibers that spiral clockwise tighten and oppose the force. This is similar to the way a wet towel becomes progressively harder to twist as you add more twists to it. Half of an osteon's lamellae have collagen fibers spiraling in one direction, while the remaining lamellae have fibers spiraling in the opposite direction. This allows an osteon to be resistant to torsion applied from any direction.

Spongy bone and trabeculae

Whereas lamellae form osteons in compact bone, they form **trabeculae** in spongy bone. The lamellae in a trabecula look like irregular or flattened ovals when viewed in cross section, and they seldom stack more than a few layers deep from center to edge. Unlike that of an osteon, the innermost lamella of a trabecula does not surround a central canal with a nourishing blood vessel. Instead, osteocytes within trabeculae receive nutrients through canaliculi that open through the endosteum to the bone marrow. This means that the osteocytes inside trabeculae are nourished from "outside in," compared to the osteocytes in the osteons of compact bone, which are nourished from "inside out." The outer lamella of a trabecula is covered by the endosteum, which consists of different kinds of bone cells, including *osteoblasts* and *osteoclasts*. We will discuss these cells, along with osteocytes, in the context of how osseous tissue is built up and broken down. Table 9-1 summarizes the characteristics in spongy and compact bone tissue.

Table 9-1. Comparison of trabeculae and osteons

Characteristic	Trabeculae in spongy bone	Osteons in compact bone
Lamellae	Present; irregular	Present; concentric
Lacunae	Present	Present
Osteocytes	Present	Present
Canaliculi	Present	Present
Central canals	Absent	Present
Surrounding material	Endosteum	Other lamellae
Source of nutrients	Blood in marrow	Blood in central canal
Flow of nutrients	Outer lamella to inner lamella	Inner lamella to outer lamella

BONE DEPOSITION BY OSTEOBLASTS

Bone deposition refers to the formation of osseous tissue, and this process requires the (1) the formation of osteoid secreting bone cells, (2) the secretion of osteoid, and (3) the precipitation of calcium salts in the osteoid to form a hard matrix. These steps are described below:

1. Development of osteoblasts. **Osteoblasts** are cells that secrete osteoid, the organic component of the bone matrix (Figure 9-4). Osteoblasts develop from **osteogenic cells**, unspecialized stem cells in the osteogenic layer of the periosteum and in the endosteum. Osteogenic cells are the only cells that divide in osseous tissue. Prior to secreting osteoid, the osteoblasts develop long cytoplasmic projections that extend in all directions to connect with adjacent osteoblasts. The tips of these projections contain gap junctions through which materials pass from one osteoblast into another.

2. Secretion of osteoid. Spider-shaped osteoblasts begin bone deposition by secreting (depositing) osteoid, the bone's organic matrix, into the extracellular space. The osteoid spreads around the cell's "body" (containing the nucleus) and around the cell's cytoplasmic extensions. At the same time, osteoblasts secrete enzymes that cause the bone matrix to harden. One such enzyme is **alkaline phosphatase**, which increases the concentration of phosphate ions (PO_4^{3-}) in the osteoid.

3. Calcification of the osteoid. The abundance of PO_4^{3-} ions in the osteoid causes mineral salts, particularly calcium phosphate, to crystallize and precipitate like snow in the osteoid; this process

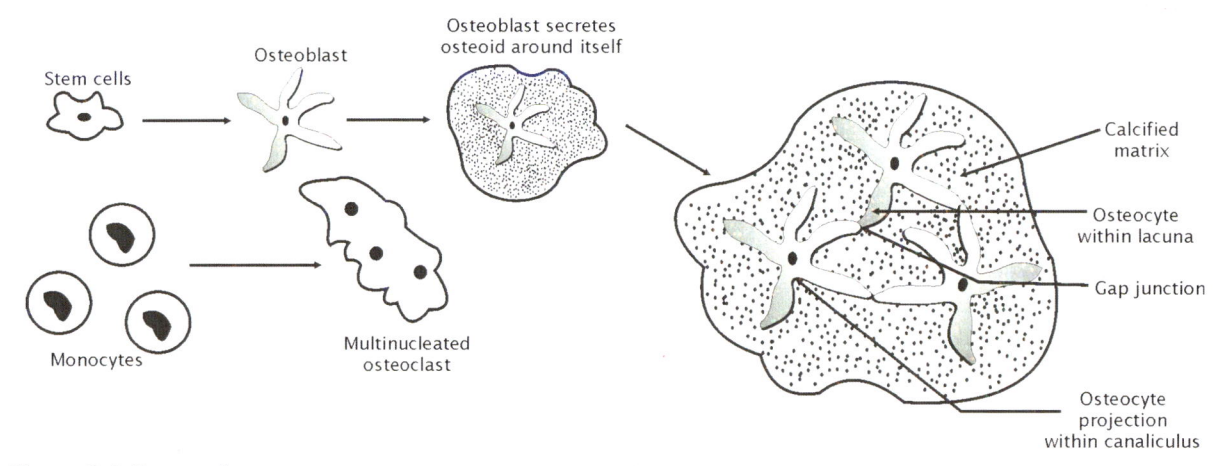

Figure 9-4. Bone cells

OSSEOUS TISSUE

149

is called **calcification**. As osteoid calcifies, the osteoblast's body becomes trapped within a lacuna, and its cytoplasmic extensions become enclosed within canaliculi. After being "buried alive" in bone matrix, the osteoblasts are called **osteocytes**. Osteocytes are the most abundant cells in osseous tissue, and represent the "building superintendents" of bones, patiently maintaining and recycling the bone matrix. They do this by secreting enzymes that can dissolve mineral salts from the matrix or ones that cause mineral salts to precipitate in it. Osteocytes receive nutrients through the canaliculi and through gap junctions with adjacent osteocytes.

BONE RESORPTION BY OSTEOCLASTS

Just as it is necessary to withdraw money from a bank account periodically, under certain conditions, it is necessary to "withdraw" minerals from the calcified matrix of bones. The destruction of bone matrix and subsequent diffusion of its minerals into the blood is called **bone resorption**. The term "resorption" implies that the bone's minerals are being absorbed into the blood a second time. This is true since they entered the body in food and were first absorbed into the blood through the intestines. Osteocytes can cause a small amount of bone resorption, but most resorption involves cells called *osteoclasts*.

1. Development of osteoclasts: **Osteoclasts** are the most important matrix-destroying cells. These multinucleated cells are found mostly in the endosteum, but small numbers live in the periosteum's osteogenic layer (Figure 9-4). In the marrow, specialized blood cells, called *monocytes*, fuse to form a single osteoclast. Like a tiny scrubbing brush, the part of an osteoclast's plasma membrane that is in contact with the bone surface has hundreds of tiny finger-like processes, collectively known as a *ruffled membrane*. The ruffled membrane greatly increases the amount of osteoclast surface in contact with the bone surface, thereby increasing its ability to destroy bone matrix.

2. Secretion of acids and enzymes: Osteoclasts begin bone resorption by secreting acids and enzymes onto a bone surface. The acids dissolve mineral salts within the ground substance of the matrix, while the enzymes break down the collagen fibers distributed throughout the ground substance. The ruffled membrane also engulfs pieces of digested bone matrix by phagocytosis.

3. Formation of resorption pit: As an osteoclast does its work, it leaves behind a little dimple in the bone surface called a resorption pit, or *Howship's lacuna*. Much of the calcium freed during bone resorption enters the blood; therefore, when osteoclasts become more active, the amount of calcium ions in the blood rises.

DEVELOPMENT AND GROWTH OF BONES

Our discussions to this point have focused on the osseous tissue in an adult human body. Now consider an X-ray that reveals what your body probably looked like when you were a fetus only 12 weeks old. There are no bones to be found! What you can see instead are cloudy patches of membranes and little bone-shaped pieces of cartilage that together look like a human skeleton. Two processes take place that transform this tiny skeleton-to-be into a network of sturdy bones. First, the soft fetal "models" of bones seen in the X-ray must ossify. Second, the ossified bones must keep growing in a coordinated fashion until adulthood.

To trace out the processes of bone development and growth, we will start by describing **ossification** (os-i-fi-KĀ-shun), or **osteogenesis** (os-tē-ō-JEN-e-sis; *osteo*, bone; *genesis*, creating), the process in which hard bones arise from soft tissues during fetal life. Then we will examine two ways in which bones grow and look at the activities of osteoblasts and osteoclasts that make bone growth happen. Bones can neither ossify nor grow, however, without precise hormonal controls and the right balance of nutrients, so we will discuss these topics to finish this section.

Ossification starts early during fetal life when connective tissues arrange themselves into *bone models*. These models consist of soft tissues but look something like future bones. The models for bones have two different origins: some bones arise from mesenchymal membranes, but most arise from hyaline cartilage. Keep in mind that regardless of their origin, bones ossify in two main steps: (1) osteoblasts secrete osteoid into the bone model; and (2) the osteoid calcifies. But since bones arise from two kinds of bone models, physiologists distinguish between two kinds of ossification: *intramembranous ossification* and *endochondral ossification*.

Intramembranous ossification

A few bones in the skeleton develop through **intramembranous ossification** (en-tra-MEM-bra-nus). As the name implies, this form of ossification occurs "within a membrane;" in this case, the membrane consists of dense irregular connective tissue. Intramembranous ossification begins around the eighth week of fetal development and forms the flat bones of the skull, parts of the lower jaw, and the diaphyses of the collarbones. In the skull, the process begins after fibroblasts weave a dense fibrous membrane, consisting mostly of collagen fibers, between the scalp and brain. Intramembranous ossification unfolds in four steps.

1. Formation of ossification center: Some osteogenic cells in the membrane differentiate to become osteoblasts. The site where this occurs is called an ossification center. The osteoblasts secrete osteoid, which calcifies to form threadlike trabeculae around the collagen fibers of the membrane.

2. Development of woven bone: The first trabeculae in the ossification center consist of only one layer of bone matrix. As more of these "nonlamellar" trabeculae emerge, they interconnect to form a delicate net-like tissue called **woven bone** (described earlier). At the same time, blood vessels within the fibrous membrane become trapped in between the trabeculae.

3. Development of lamellar bone and periosteum: The osteoblasts on the surface of woven bone secrete osteoid, which calcifies to form another layer of bone matrix. Now, the woven bone is becoming lamellar bone. Meanwhile, a periosteum develops as fibroblasts and collagen fibers cluster together along the perimeter of the fibrous membrane model. Osteoblasts in the periosteum deposit layers of bone matrix that form a shell of compact bone around the membrane.

4. Formation of marrow: As the trabeculae grow thicker, the spaces between them (and around the intertwining blood vessels) get smaller and the tissue is called spongy bone. In flat bones of the skull, this spongy bone is also called **diploë**. Eventually, blood vessels between the trabeculae give rise to red marrow (hemopoietic tissue) and begin making blood cells.

At birth, not all of the flat bones in the skull are completely ossified. Where certain flat bones will eventually connect to one another, sections of the fibrous membrane remain and are called **fontanels** (fon-ta-NELZ; little fountains), or "soft spots." Fontanels allow the skull to deform slightly as it passes through the birth canal, and they allow the skull to expand as the brain grows. Fontanels completely ossify within 1-2 years after birth.

Endochondral ossification

Most bones in the skeleton develop through a process called **endochondral ossification** (en-dō-KON-dral). As the name implies, this process occurs "inside cartilage" tissue. We will discuss the steps of endochondral ossification using a "generic" long bone as an example (Figure 9-5).

1. Formation of cartilage model: Prior to the sixth week of fetal development, chondroblasts (cartilage cells) gather at the site of the bone-to-be and secrete a cartilage matrix. The matrix forms a hyaline cartilage model, a soft, miniature version of a bone, and the chondroblasts within the matrix become chondrocytes. At the same time, dense fibrous connective tissue condenses around the cartilage model, forming a tough covering, the *perichondrium*. As the cartilage model grows, nutrients cannot reach the chondrocytes deep inside the model fast enough to sustain them. Malnutrition and a lack of oxygen cause the chondrocytes to swell and release alkaline compounds into the cartilage matrix. As the matrix pH rises in those areas, calcium salts precipitate, causing the cartilage to calcify.

OSSEOUS TISSUE

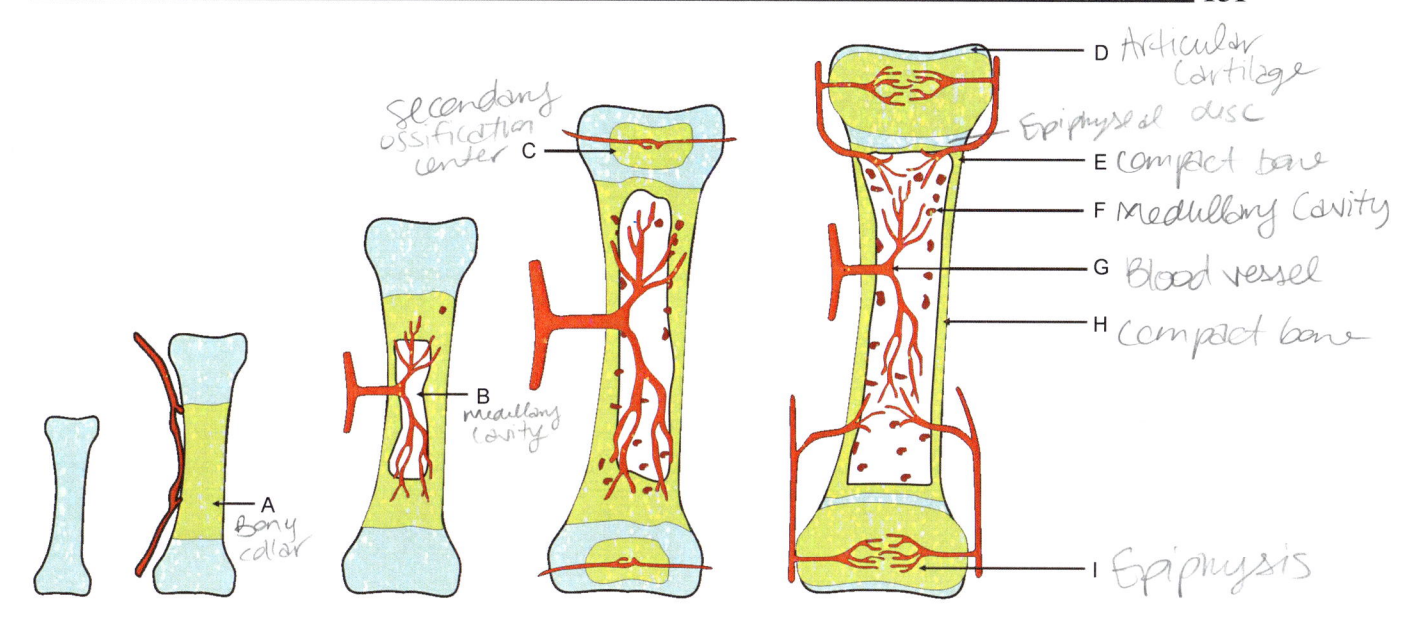

Figure 9-5. Endochondral ossification

Labels (handwritten):
- A — Bony collar
- B — medullary cavity
- C — secondary ossification center
- D — Articular cartilage
- E — Epiphyseal disc / Compact bone
- F — Medullary cavity
- G — Blood vessel
- H — Compact bone
- I — Epiphysis

2. <u>Formation of primary ossification center</u>: At 6-8 weeks of fetal development, blood vessels penetrate and grow throughout the **perichondrium** in the diaphysis of the cartilage model. Shortly thereafter, osteogenic cells in the perichondrium differentiate and become osteoblasts. After this happens, the **perichondrium is now called the periosteum**. The osteoblasts secrete osteoid onto the cartilage surface, which calcifies to form a hard **bone collar** around the diaphysis. The bone collar (1) prevents the cartilage from growing wider, and (2) effectively stops the diffusion of nutrients to the deepest cartilage. Consequently, the chondrocytes deep within the diaphysis swell, expand their lacunae, and die. This deep portion of the diaphysis is the first place where bone will replace cartilage, so it is called the **primary ossification center**.

3. <u>Formation of spongy bone in the inner diaphysis</u>: Blood vessels, along with osteoblasts and osteoclasts, penetrate the primary ossification center. Osteoclasts begin destroying some of the **calcified cartilage**, causing large cavities to develop. At the same time, osteoblasts secrete osteoid that calcifies to form woven bone (simple trabeculae without lamellae) around any remaining calcified cartilage.

4. <u>Formation of medullary cavity</u>: Osteoblasts in the periosteum create osteons by depositing concentric layers of bone matrix around periosteal blood vessels. The compact bone along the diaphysis continues to thicken as the bone collar spreads toward the epiphyses. Deep in the diaphysis, osteoclasts begin removing some of the woven bone that was deposited by the osteoblasts. Eventually, a large hollow channel, the **medullary cavity** (MED´-ū-lar-ē; *medulla*, marrow) emerges, but spongy bone remains along the inside wall of this cavity. In addition, hemopoietic cells brought into the bone by blood vessels divide rapidly and fill the medullary cavity with red marrow.

5. <u>Formation of secondary ossification centers and epiphyseal plate</u>: Near the time of birth, chondrocytes deep in the epiphyses swell and die; this event marks the beginning of **secondary ossification centers**. Blood vessels and osteoblasts enter the cavities left by the departed chondrocytes. The osteoblasts produce spongy bone, which spreads outward to the edges of the epiphyses. Eventually, only two structures in the maturing bone consist of cartilage from the original model: (1) an **epiphyseal plate** (ep-i-FIZ-ē-al), or growth plate, a thin layer of

cartilage in one or both metaphyses, and (2) **articular cartilage** covering the end of one or both epiphyses.

PATTERNS OF BONE GROWTH

Although ossification starts early in fetal life, most bones in the body keep growing long after they initially ossify from either a fibrous membrane or cartilage model. Interestingly, long bones have two independent growth processes: one that makes the bone longer, and one that makes the bone wider.

Longitudinal growth

Most long bones face the daunting challenge of having to grow longer (experience **longitudinal growth**) even as they bear weight or endure other types of physical stress. Amazingly enough, the way a long bone grows longer can be compared to making a skyscraper grow taller by simultaneously stuffing in additional floors part way from the top and bottom of the building. In a long bone, these "action sites" of growth are the epiphyseal plates. An *epiphyseal plate* in a long bone has four zones, each of which contributes to longitudinal growth.

1. Growth zone: the cartilage expands: The layer of the epiphyseal plate that faces the epiphysis is where cartilage grows most quickly, and it is where a long bone lengthens. Until early adulthood, the chondrocytes closest to the nourishing blood vessels in the epiphysis undergo mitosis and cytokinesis. Like one acrobat climbing atop the shoulders of another, the daughter cells push apart to form long stacks or rows of chondrocytes that stretch from the epiphysis toward the diaphysis. The recently divided chondrocytes secrete fresh cartilage matrix into the growth zone, which pushes the epiphysis away from the diaphysis. This action is sort of like squeezing a toothpaste tube with a loose cap. The rising mass of toothpaste (cartilage matrix) pushes the cap (the epiphysis) up and away from the neck of the tube (the diaphysis).

2. Transformation zone: the cartilage calcifies: As the cartilage matrix grows, the epiphysis and its nourishing blood vessels move away from the rows of chondrocytes. Consequently, the chondrocytes that are farthest from the epiphysis begin to starve, and in response, they swell up. (Recall that this is the fate suffered by the chondrocytes in the diaphysis of a long bone during endochondral ossification.) During this transformation, the swollen chondrocytes release alkaline substances into the surrounding matrix, which causes the pH of the matrix to rise. Mineral salts precipitate into the cartilage, causing it to calcify.

3. Osteogenic zone: the calcified cartilage ossifies: Eventually, the chondrocytes farthest from the epiphysis die within their lacunae. Osteoclasts digest some of the calcified cartilage, leaving behind long finger-like projections of calcified cartilage that point toward the medullary cavity of the diaphysis. New blood vessels grow between these projections, bringing with them osteoblasts that deposit layers of spongy bone; hence, the projections of calcified cartilage ossify.

4. Remodeling zone: the medullary cavity expands: The spongy bone that is deposited in the osteogenic zone doesn't last very long. Osteoclasts resorb the spongy bone and digest the remaining calcified cartilage at the tips of the projecting calcified cartilage. This action causes the medullary cavity to grow longer as the bone grows longer. Notice, too, that the thickness of the epiphyseal plate remains fairly constant as the bone grows longer; cartilage is piled up on the epiphysis side of the plate while bone disappears from the diaphysis side. In essence, the medullary cavity "chases after" the epiphysis that is being pushed away from the diaphysis.

As a person nears adulthood, cartilage formation at the growth zone slows while activity within the other zones continues at a steady pace. When this occurs, ossification on the diaphysis side of the epiphyseal plate eventually "overtakes" the growth zone. When the growth zone ossifies, the epiphyseal plate is "fused" and longitudinal growth ceases. Most epiphyseal plates fuse by age 20, and after fusion, they are called **epiphyseal lines**. Table 9-2 shows the approximate ages that epiphyseal plates become epiphyseal lines in different bones.

OSSEOUS TISSUE

Table 9-2. Age at time of growth plate fusion

Bone	Age
Thigh, leg, foot, ankle, toes	18-22
Arm, forearm, wrist, hand, fingers	17-20
Clavicle	20-30
Pelvic bones	18-23
Scapula (shoulder blade)	18-20
Sternum (breastbone)	23-30+
Vertebrae (bone in neck and back)	25

Appositional growth

Although fusion of an epiphyseal plate means a bone cannot get longer, the bone can still grow wider, a process called **appositional growth** (ap-ō-ZISH-un-al; to place at). This type of growth occurs whenever osteoblasts add matrix to the bone's outer surface faster than osteoclasts can remove it. Appositional growth occurs fastest during childhood and adolescence but continues at a very slow pace through most of adulthood. For a growing child, appositional growth is especially important in developing the weight-bearing bones of the lower limbs. Without appositional growth to accompany longitudinal growth, these long bones would likely bend and break.

Of course, thicker bones can better support the body's weight. But wouldn't appositional growth cause bones to be significantly more dense and heavier? Interestingly, the answer is no. As osteoblasts add bone matrix to the periosteal side of the bone, osteoclasts remove bone matrix from the endosteal side; therefore, as a long bone's outside diameter widens, its medullary cavity also widens. However, the rate of bone deposition along the periosteum slightly exceeds the rate of bone resorption along the endosteum. The result is a thickening of the compact bone in the diaphysis region as the overall diameter of this region increases. But the medullary cavity's diameter also increases, which allows the bone to remain lightweight while providing additional room for bone marrow (see Figure 9-6).

During appositional growth, new osteons develop as infoldings of the periosteum and circumferential lamellae. The growth process takes place in four steps:

1. Formation of bone ridges. Osteoblasts in the periosteum deposit bone matrix that forms a bony ridge on either side of a periosteal artery, vein, and nerve.

2. Fusion of bone ridges. Osteoblasts continue to deposit bone matrix, causing the ridges to rise above and over the vessel. Eventually, the ridges fuse, enclosing the vessel within a tunnel. The enclosed vessels and nerve maintain connections with surface vessels and nerves by way of branches within perforating (Volkmann's) canals.

3. Formation of concentric lamellae. Osteoblasts lining the inside of the tube deposit bone matrix in a series of circular layers (concentric lamellae). As each new lamella is added, the tunnel around the vessel gets smaller. The lining of this tunnel was derived from the periosteum but is now called endosteum.

4. Completion of osteon. In time, a final, innermost lamella forms around the vessel and the central

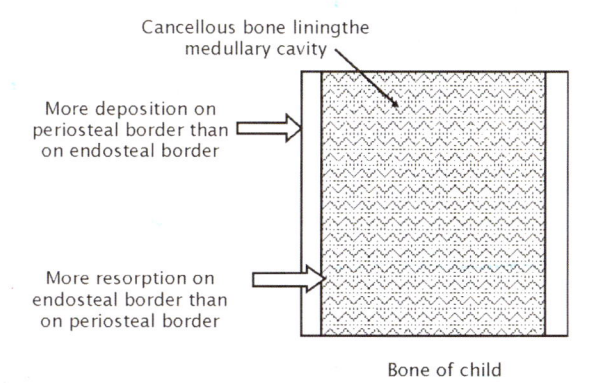

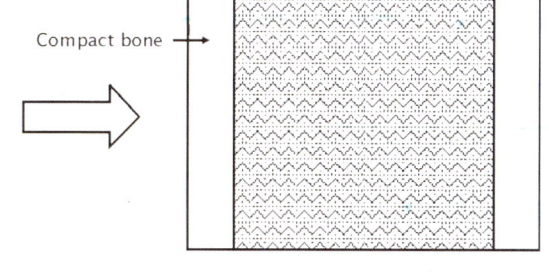

Figure 9-6. Appositional bone growth

(Haversian) canal is complete. Several layers of circumferential lamellae are laid down on the bone's surface, while new osteons begin forming. The entire process repeats at another vessel nearby, forming another osteon.

From beginning to end, construction of an osteon takes about 100 days. Periodically, osteoclasts erode grooves in the surfaces of a bone and in the process cut into old osteons. When new osteons form in these regions, the remnants of the old osteons remain as interstitial lamellae. The average life expectancy of an osteon in a middle-aged man is about 15 years.

Now that you know how a long bone grows in length and width, you may be wondering how short bones, flat bones, and irregular bones grow. While a bone must have an epiphyseal plate in order to have longitudinal growth as described earlier, bones of all shapes can experience appositional growth in the manner just described.

FACTORS AFFECTING BONE DEVELOPMENT

Although all tissues need an assortment of nutrients to stay healthy, a few nutrients are especially important to bone health.

- **Proteins**: Strong, resilient bones and cartilages contain a significant amount of collagen protein. Proteins in the diet are broken down in the intestines to their basic building blocks, amino acids. In turn, osteoblasts and chondroblasts use amino acids to make collagen.

- **Minerals**: In particular, **calcium** and **phosphorus** are needed to form the inorganic mineral salts that harden the bone matrix. Chondrocytes use **sulfur** to make chondroitin sulfate, which stiffens the hyaline cartilage located on the ends of bones and in epiphyseal plates. Sulfur also forms sulfide bonds in collagen, increasing its durability and providing flexibility to the collagen fibers.

- **Vitamins:** Two vitamins that play noteworthy roles in bone growth and maintenance are vitamins C and D. **Vitamin C** promotes the formation of cross-links between adjacent collagen fibers. The cross-links hold the fibers together and contribute to a bone's tensile (pulling) strength. **Calcitriol** (kal-si-TRĪ-ol), or active **vitamin D**, promotes bone deposition by stimulating osteoblasts to secrete more osteoid. It also stimulates cells in the intestine to make a protein called *calbindin*, which binds to calcium in food, thereby allowing the calcium to enter the blood. Without calbindin, most of the calcium a person might eat would pass right through the intestines and never reach the bones.

Although calcitriol functions as a hormone, other hormones that play significant roles in bone development include growth hormone, thyroxine, and the sex hormones.

- **Growth hormone (GH)**: The pea-sized pituitary gland at the base of the brain releases this hormone that stimulates cells to absorb amino acids and other chemicals from the blood, and it promotes protein synthesis. As the name suggests, growth hormone promotes growth; however, it does this in a roundabout way. Growth hormone causes the liver and muscles to secrete a group of proteins called **insulin-like growth factors – IGFs**, or **somatomedins**. The IGFs promote bone growth by stimulating chondrocytes to make cartilage at epiphyseal disks.

- **Thyroxine** (thī-ROK-sēn): The thyroid gland in the neck releases this hormone, also called **thyroid hormone (TH)**, which increases the metabolic activity of cells. Thyroxine also enhances growth hormone's effect on chondrocytes and osteoblasts.

- **Sex hormones**: The gonads (ovaries and testes) and the adrenal glands near the kidneys release sex hormones, including **estrogen** and **testosterone**. Sex hormones stimulate longitudinal bone growth, as evidenced by the dramatic growth spurt that occurs at the time of puberty. However, sex hormones also promote the calcification of epiphyseal disks. Females usually stop growing sooner than males due to the effect of high estrogen levels at puberty. Estrogen has a greater effect than testosterone in causing the fusion of epiphyseal plates.

OSSEOUS TISSUE

BONE REMODELING

Having learned about how bones develop, it might seem logical to compare bones to concrete. Concrete begins as a soft mixture that becomes extremely hard over time. Likewise, bones begin as either a soft membrane or a cartilage model that hardens over time, but there the analogy ends. Unlike concrete, which may not change for decades, bones are always changing. New bone matrix is constantly added to bones, and at the same time, old matrix is constantly removed from them. This simultaneous bone deposition and bone resorption is called **bone remodeling**. First, we will discuss the importance of remodeling as part of a bone's response to physical stress. Next we will discuss how remodeling is important to calcium homeostasis, and then we conclude with a look at how bones repair themselves after injury.

BONE REMODELING AND BONE DENSITY

Bone density is a measure of a bone's mineral (mainly calcium salt) content, and it has a positive effect on the bone's structural strength. In other words, as a bone's mineral content increases, so does the bone's density and strength. Bone remodeling can significantly alter bone density, but in most young and middle-aged adults, the rates of bone deposition and bone resorption are roughly equal. The result is that most bones in these individuals maintain a nearly constant shape and size. However, if a bone experiences higher-than-normal physical stress, such as compression or bending, the rate of bone deposition can exceed that of bone resorption. This explains why leg bones of a long-distance runner may be significantly more dense and stronger than leg bones of a sedentary person.

While physical stress increases the rate of bone deposition, a lack of physical stress increases the rate of bone resorption. You can see this effect in a person who has had a broken leg immobilized by a cast. During the healing process, a broken leg bone may become significantly less dense than the similar bone in the healthy leg. In addition, bone density in the healthy leg may increase if those bones have to support more body weight while the broken bone heals. Applying stress to the healed bone increases bone deposition and can return the bone's density to normal.

So how does a bone "know" when it is being stressed? There are various hypotheses that attempt to answer this question. Osteocytes within lacunae may react to minute *electrical currents* generated when the bone's mineral salts are compressed. Geologists have noted that mineral salts, such as quartz, generate minute electrical currents when compressed, a response called the *piezoelectric effect*. The minerals in bone matrix also exhibit a piezoelectric effect when compressed. Simply standing up could stress a leg bone enough to "shock" its osteocytes. In response, the osteocytes can stimulate osteoblasts on the bone's surface (by way of gap junctions), which respond by secreting more osteoid. The response of immobilized bones to artificially produced electric fields supports the piezoelectric hypothesis. Exposing an immobilized bone to electrical fields, which are the same intensity as those generated naturally under stress, can cause bone deposition to increase.

A second hypothesis for how bones detect mechanical stress relates to changes in *hydrostatic pressure*. When osseous tissue is squeezed, the pressure of liquids inside lacunae and canaliculi increases. Osteocytes may respond to this change in hydrostatic pressure by stimulating the osteoblasts as described previously. Osteoblasts may also be responding to increasing temperature that bones experience when under physical stress. It is likely that bones may respond to all of these factors.

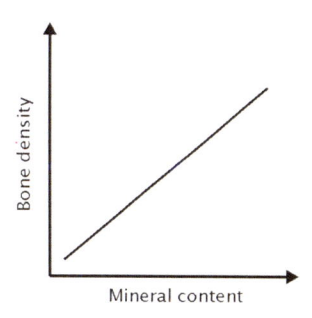

So why don't all bones respond the same way to stress? Some bones, such as those on top of the skull are rarely stressed. According to hypotheses, these bones should disappear because of resorption. Since this does not happen, it is apparent that not all bones respond to stress in the same way. While bones generally respond to periodic changes in stress by increasing deposition, some bones respond to *constant* stress by increasing resorption. Orthodontists take advantage of this fact when using braces to straighten protruding teeth. Applying constant pressure to the anterior side of a tooth causes resorption on the posterior side of the tooth's socket. This allows room for the tooth to move posteriorly.

BONE REMODELING AND Ca²⁺ HOMEOSTASIS

Not only does bone remodeling reshape bones to adapt them to the demands of physical stress, it is also important in maintaining optimum calcium concentration in the blood. Calcium is required for muscle contraction, transmission of nerve signals, blood clotting, and many other processes. Therefore, the role of the skeletal system in supplying calcium to the blood cannot be understated. Bones store 99% of the body's calcium, and remodeling causes about 25% of the calcium in the blood to exchange with calcium in bones every minute. All in all, remodeling accounts for about 10% of the skeleton being recycled each year. Two hormones, *parathyroid hormone* and *calcitonin*, regulate blood calcium levels, and they do this, in part, by affecting bone remodeling (Figure 9-7).

Parathyroid hormone (PTH) is made in four small parathyroid glands on the posterior surface of the thyroid gland. PTH increases blood calcium concentration (Ca^{2+}) in several ways, but one way is by increasing bone resorption. The parathyroid glands secrete PTH into the blood when the blood calcium concentration (Ca^{2+}) is lower than optimum. When PTH reaches the bones, it stimulates osteoclasts. The osteoclasts respond by releasing more acids that dissolve the mineral salts in bone matrix. Some of the liberated calcium ions diffuse into nearby blood vessels, thereby increasing blood Ca^{2+}.

Calcitonin (CT) is made in the thyroid gland, and it lowers blood Ca^{2+}. The thyroid gland secretes CT into the blood when blood Ca^{2+} is higher than optimum. When CT reaches the bone, it affects bone remodeling in two ways: (1) it stimulates osteoblasts to secrete more osteoid. Calcification of the osteoid removes calcium from surrounding tissue fluids including the blood. (2) It inhibits osteoclasts, thereby slowing the rate of bone resorption. The effect of calcitonin on the bone and blood Ca^{2+} opposes that of parathyroid hormone; therefore, CT and PTH are said to be **antagonists**.

REPAIR OF FRACTURES

In order for bones to function in the ways described at the beginning of the chapter, it is essential that

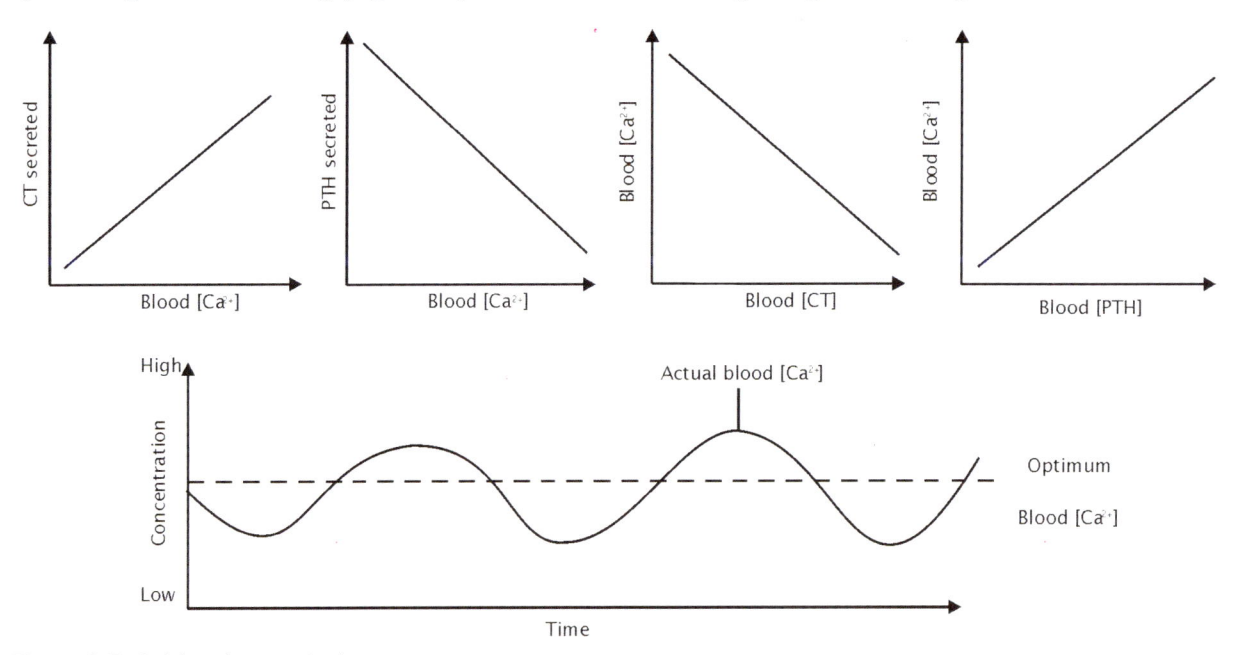

Figure 9-7. Calcium homeostasis

OSSEOUS TISSUE

they be repaired when damaged. Therefore, it is appropriate to conclude this chapter with a discussion of how broken bones heal. A break in a bone is called a **fracture**, and the healing of a fracture involves four stages: hematoma, fibrocartilage callus, bony callus, and remodeling.

1. **Hematoma stage**: When a bone breaks (fractures), blood vessels rupture and blood spills out into the surrounding tissues. Blood loss from the vessel is called *hemorrhage*. Chemical reactions in the blood cause numerous protein fibers to form at the injury site. The fibers traps blood cells to form a mass called a **hematoma** (hē-ma-TŌ-ma; *hema*, blood; *oma*, tumor), or **blood clot**. This process is called **coagulation** (kō-ag-ū-LĀ-shun; curdle). The hematoma helps prevent further loss of blood from the broken blood vessels. At this time, the damaged tissues release a variety of chemicals that promote **inflammation**. Signs of inflammation include swelling, redness, and heat. Specialized white blood cells called *macrophages* move through the wound removing dead tissue, any bacteria that might be present, and generally "cleaning up" the wound.

2. **Fibrocartilage callus stage**: A few days after the fracture, blood vessels grow into the area and mesenchyme cells differentiate to become fibroblasts. Fibroblasts secrete collagen proteins that form a network of collagen fibers in the interstitial spaces. At the same time, other mesenchyme cells become chondroblasts that secrete cartilage matrix. The cartilage matrix hardens around the collagen fibers creating a mass called a **fibrocartilage callus**. The fibrocartilage callus acts like a "bridge" to hold the broken ends of the bone together. In time the fibrocartilage callus calcifies, which sets the stage for the deposition of bone matrix. The wound now looks similar to the early stages of endochondral ossification (described earlier).

3. **Bony callus stage**: Eventually, the calcified fibrocartilage callus is replaced by osseous tissue to form a **bony callus**. This happens after osteogenic cells and osteoclasts migrate into the fibrocartilage callus. Osteoclasts begin digesting the calcified cartilage, while osteogenic cells differentiate to become osteoblasts. Within a month after the fracture, osteoblasts begin secreting osteoid within the fibrocartilage callus. The initial osseous tissue that forms in the wound is woven bone, which is similar to that formed in the medullary cavity during endochondral ossification. In time, more layers of bone matrix are added to the trabeculae, converting the woven bone to lamellar bone.

4. **Remodeling stage**: Normally, more bone matrix is deposited during the healing process than is needed, so resorption by osteoclasts removes excess osseous material. Ultimately, the final shape of the bone will be influenced by patterns of stress.

TOPICS TO KNOW FOR CHAPTER 9 (OSSEOUS TISSUE)

- accessory parts of the skeletal system
- alkaline phosphatase
- anatomy of a long bone
- anatomy of non-long bones
- antagonists
- appendicular skeleton
- appositional growth
- articular cartilage
- articulations
- axial skeleton
- blood clot
- bone collar
- bone density
- bone deposition
- bone deposition by osteoblasts
- bone marrow
- bone matrix
- bone models
- bone remodeling
- Ca2+ homeostasis
- bone repair
- bone resorption
- bony callus stage
- calbindin
- calcification
- calcitonin (CT)
- calcitriol
- canaliculi
- cancellous bone
- cartilage
- central canal
- chondroitin sulfate
- circumferential lamellae
- classification of bone matrix
- classification of bones
- coagulation
- collagen fibers
- compact bone
- comparison of trabeculae and osteons
- compression strength
- concentric lamellae
- cortical bone
- development and growth of bones
- diaphysis
- endochondral ossification
- endosteum
- epiphyseal lines
- epiphyseal plate
- epiphysis
- estrogen
- factors affecting bone development
- fibrocartilage callus stage
- fibrous periosteum
- flat bones
- fontanels
- function of periosteum
- functions of skeletal cartilages
- functions of the skeletal system
- growth hormone
- growth zone
- Haversian canal
- Haversian systems
- hematoma
- hematoma stage
- hemopoiesis
- hemopoietic stem cells
- hemopoietic tissue
- Howship's lacuna
- hyaluronic acid
- hydroxyapatite
- inflammation
- inorganic matrix
- insulin-like growth factors
- interstitial lamellae
- intramembranous ossification
- irregular bones
- joints
- lacunae
- lamellae
- lamellar bone
- ligament
- long bones
- longitudinal growth
- lymphatics of bone
- macrophages
- medullary cavity
- mesenchyme membranes
- metaphysic
- mineral salts
- monocytes
- nutrient artery
- nutrient foramen
- organic matrix
- osseous tissue
- ossification
- ossification center
- osteoblasts
- osteoclasts
- osteocytes
- osteogenesis
- osteogenic cells
- osteogenic layer
- osteogenic zone
- osteoid
- osteons
- parathyroid hormone (PTH)
- patterns of bone growth
- perforating canals
- perforating fibers
- primary ossification center
- proteoglycans
- red marrow
- remodeling stage
- remodeling zone
- repair of fractures
- resorption pit
- ruffled membrane
- secondary ossification centers
- sesamoid bones
- sex hormones
- Sharpey's fibers
- short bones
- skeletal system
- skeleton
- somatomedins
- spongy bone
- suture bones
- tension strength
- testosterone
- the periosteum
- thyroxine
- torsion strength
- trabeculae
- transformation zone
- vessels in bone
- vitamin C
- vitamin D
- Volkmann's canals
- Wormian bones
- woven bone
- yellow marrow

ion
CHAPTER 10

The Axial Skeleton

Have you ever studied the names of towns or cities printed on a road map or travel atlas? You might have noticed that the names of some municipalities offer interesting clues to important geographic features in the surrounding area. A town named Big Bend turns out to be situated along a sweeping curve in a river. If you're driving to Chapel Hill, you might expect to find a church on a bluff overlooking the town. And in Desert Hot Springs, well…you shouldn't expect to find a landscape covered with lush forests.

Just as names on a map can tell you something worth knowing about the geography of a place that you might like to visit, learning the names of the bones of the skeleton will make it easier for you to locate and remember many other structures in the human body. For instance, the *frontal* lobe of your brain, where you think about anatomy and physiology, is deep to the *frontal* bone of your skull. Your *radial* artery, where you can feel your pulse, runs alongside the *radius* bone in your forearm. Nerves are also named for nearby bones; for example, your *tibial* nerve runs alongside your *tibia*, one of the bones in your leg. In fact, a particular nerve in your body is sometimes called a "bone" in everyday speech. This nerve, the *ulnar* nerve, runs alongside your *ulna*, a bone that parallels the radius bone in your forearm. If you get a tingling sensation throughout your forearm and hand after hitting your elbow, it's because you've hit the ulnar nerve, your "funny bone."

OVERVIEW OF THE SKELETON

The typical adult skeleton contains 206 bones, along with an assortment of ligaments and cartilages. The qualifying phrase "typical adult" is important for two reasons: (1) The number of bones in the skeleton rises and falls from birth to adulthood. (2) The final number of bones in an adult skeleton may vary from person to person. Why is this so? Recall that a child's skeleton has more bones than an adult skeleton since some of the child's bones exist as segments separated by epiphyseal discs. In addition, sesamoid bones may develop in various tendons and the skull of an adult may have a varying number of sutural bones. The skeleton is divided into two parts: the *axial skeleton* and the *appendicular* skeleton.

In this chapter, you will learn the names and identify the unique features of individual bones. Apart from having a characteristic shape, each bone displays a unique assortment of surface markings that provides clues about how the bone interacts with other bones and organs. A bone may have projections (such as knobs, ridges, bumps, or spines) where it articulates (joins) with another bone or to which ligaments and tendons attach. In addition, a bone's surface may be marked by holes or carved by depressions and grooves through which blood vessels and nerves travel. Table 10.1 lists the variety of bone features that you will learn to recognize in this chapter.

The **axial skeleton** is related to the entire skeleton like a trunk is related to a tree. It forms the vertical "axis" of the skeleton upon which the "limbs" attach. The axial skeleton of a typical adult contains about 80 bones (40% of the total number in the body). Of these, 28 bones are part of the *skull*, 1 hyoid bone is in the neck region, 26 bones are in the *vertebral column* (spine), and 25 bones are in the *thoracic cage* (Figure 10-1).

Table 10 - 1: Bone features

PROJECTIONS WHERE BONES ARTICULATE WITH OTHER BONES	
Condyle (KON-dil; knuckle)	Smooth, rounded knob
Facet (FAS-et; face)	Smooth, flat surface
Head	Large, rounded epiphysis at end of narrow neck
Neck	Constricted region between the epiphysis and diaphysis of certain long bones
PROJECTIONS WHERE MUSCLES, LIGAMENTS, OR TENDONS ATTACH	
Crest	Prominent narrow ridge
Epicondyle	Projection above a condyle
Line	Slightly raised, narrow ridge
Process	Any bony projection
Protuberance (pro-TU-ber-ans)	A bony prominence
Ramus (RA-mus; branch)	Part of irregular bone forming an angle
Spine (spinous process)	Sharp, slender projection
Tubercle (TU-ber-kl; swelling)	Small, rounded projection
Tuberosity (tu'-ber-OS-i-ti; lump)	Small, roughened projection
OPENINGS, CANALS, AND CAVITIES	
Fissure (FISH-ur; deep furrow)	A slit-like opening
Foramen (fo-RA-men; opening)	Round or oval-shaped hole
Meatus (me-A-tus; passage)	Tube-like canal within a bone
Sinus	Air-filled cavity within a skull bone
DEPRESSIONS AND GROOVES	
Fossa (FOS-ah; ditch)	Shallow depression
Fovea (FO-ve-ah; pit)	Shallow pit
Notch	U-shaped indentation
Sulcus (SUL-kus; ditch)	Narrow, slit-like groove on a bone's surface

THE AXIAL SKELETON

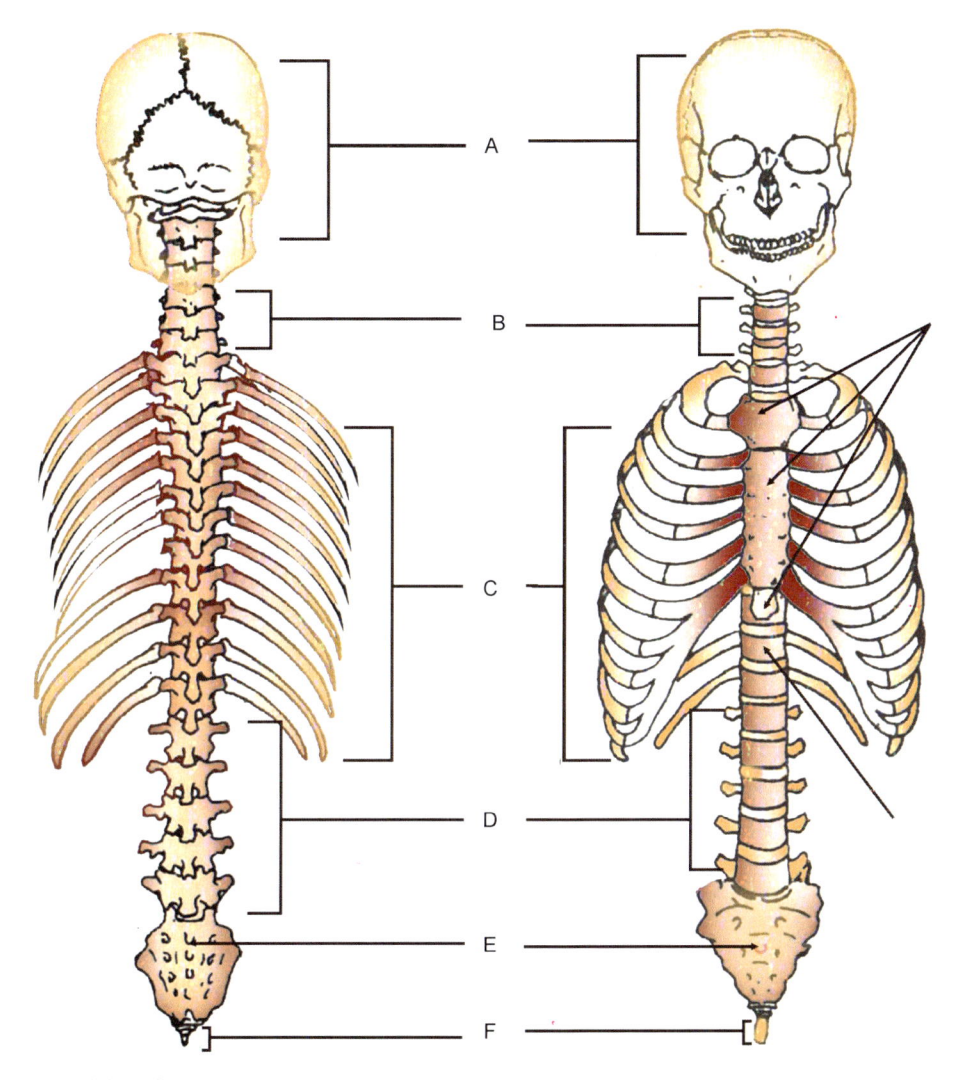

Figure 10-1. The axial skeleton

In addition to its role in maintaining homeostasis, the axial skeleton is important in several ways: (1) it surrounds and protects the brain, spinal cord, and soft visceral organs of the thorax. (2) It houses the sensory receptors for vision, smell, hearing, and taste that allow monitoring of the external environment. (3) It supports entrances and structures that function in the respiratory and digestive systems. (4) It provides attachment sites for skeletal muscles that allow you to speak, breathe, swallow, turn your head, and make facial expressions. (5) It provides attachment sites for your appendicular skeleton and the skeletal muscles that allow you to bend your back and move your shoulders and hips. Let's begin with the bones that form the axial skeleton's superior end, the skull.

THE SKULL

The **skull** is the most complex part of the skeleton, containing a wide assortment of flat and irregular bones that lock together like pieces of a 3-dimensional jigsaw puzzle (Figure 10-2). The skull of a typical adult consists of 22 bones plus 6 tiny *auditory ossicles* (3 in each ear) involved in hearing. For the most part, the skull is very rigid; the *mandible* (lower jaw) and the auditory ossicles are its only moving parts. You move your mandible up and down to grind food between your teeth. So when you can chew gum and listen to music at the same time, then all of your skull's movable bones are in motion.

The most distinctive features of the skull are its large domed region made up of *cranial bones* and its flattened, elongated anterior portion made up of *facial bones*. Together the skull bones form six cavities: the large cranial cavity that holds the brain, the right and left orbital cavities (eye sockets) that shield the eyes, the right and left nasal cavities that facilitate breathing, and the oral cavity that houses the tongue and teeth. Visualizing these cavities while you study can help you to remember the specific structural roll of each bone in the skull as well as the relationship of each skull bone to its neighbors.

Bones of the skull

Cranial bones are part of the *cranium* (KRĀ-ne-um; "helmet"), a term that can refer to different things. In this text, the **cranium** means only the skull bones that touch the brain's protective coverings, and excludes the auditory ossicles. The cranial bones include:

- 1 frontal bone
- 2 parietal bones
- 2 temporal bones
- 1 occipital bone
- 1 sphenoid bone
- 1 ethmoid bone

Just as the cranial bones form the cranium, the 14 facial bones form the *face*, the anterior part of the skull. Equally important, the facial bones connect with one another and with the cranium to form five smaller cavities beneath the face: the inferior portions of both orbital cavities, the left and right nasal cavities, and the oral cavity. Like some cranial bones, some of your facial bones occur in pairs (mirroring one another on each side of the skull). The facial bones that you can see from the skull's surface include:

- 2 maxillae
- 2 nasal bones
- 2 zygomatic bones
- 1 mandible

The remaining facial bones are deep to the face, and thus can't be seen from the surface of the skull. These bones include:

- 2 lacrimal bones (orbits)
- 2 palatine bones (oral cavity)
- 2 inferior nasal conchae (nasal cavity)
- 1 vomer (nasal cavity)

Recognizing and recalling the names of the different skull bones and their features, and remembering why all of these structures are important will take some time, so be patient. To make your task a little easier, skull bones are color-coded to help you learn the bones and their special features. All parts of a particular skull bone will have its own unique color throughout this chapter.

Sutures

All skull bones, except the mandible, connect tightly to adjacent skull bones at immovable joints. Most of these joints are called **sutures** (SŪ-cherz; *sutur-*, seam). The sutures' zigzag pattern makes skull bones look like they have been stitched together with a sewing machine. Sutures contain dense regular connective tissue consisting of very short collagenous fibers that "glue" the skull bones together and prevent them from shifting. Without strong sutures, your skull could flatten out on one side if you laid your head on a pillow. The four longest sutures are also the easiest ones to locate on the cranium exterior:

- The **coronal suture** is named for its orientation in the coronal (frontal) plane on the superior surface of the cranium. It occurs where the frontal bone meets the parietal bones.
- The **sagittal suture** is also named for its orientation, which is in the sagittal plane on the superior surface of the cranium. It occurs where the right parietal bone meets the left parietal bone.
- The **squamous sutures** (*squam-*, plate or scale) may have been given their name because the temporal bones around them look like plates or scales on a fish. The squamous suture runs along the lateral sides of the cranium where the temporal bone meets the parietal bone.
- The **lambdoid suture** (LAM-doyd) resembles the Greek letter, *lambda* (Λ). This suture is found on the posterior surface of the cranium where

THE AXIAL SKELETON

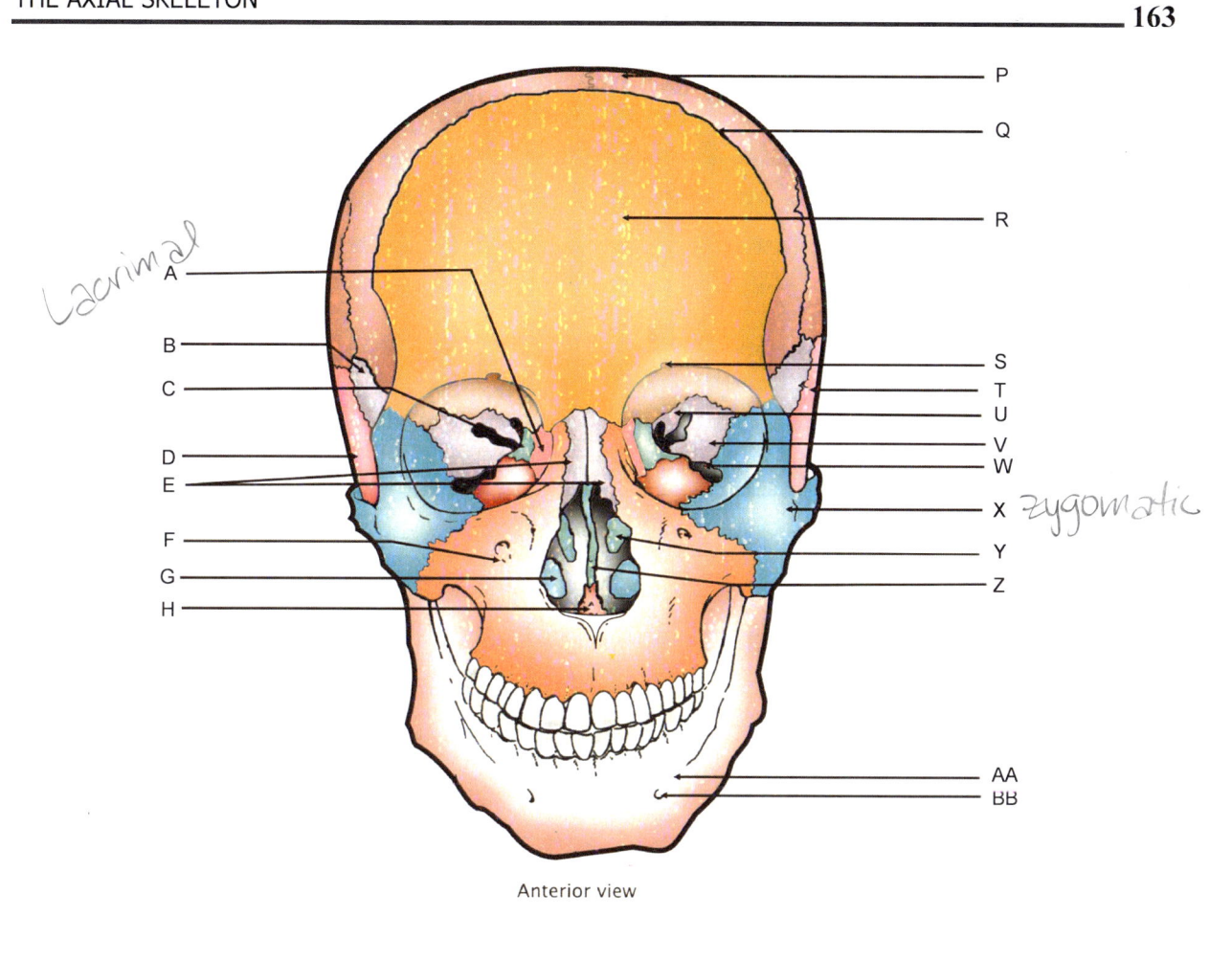

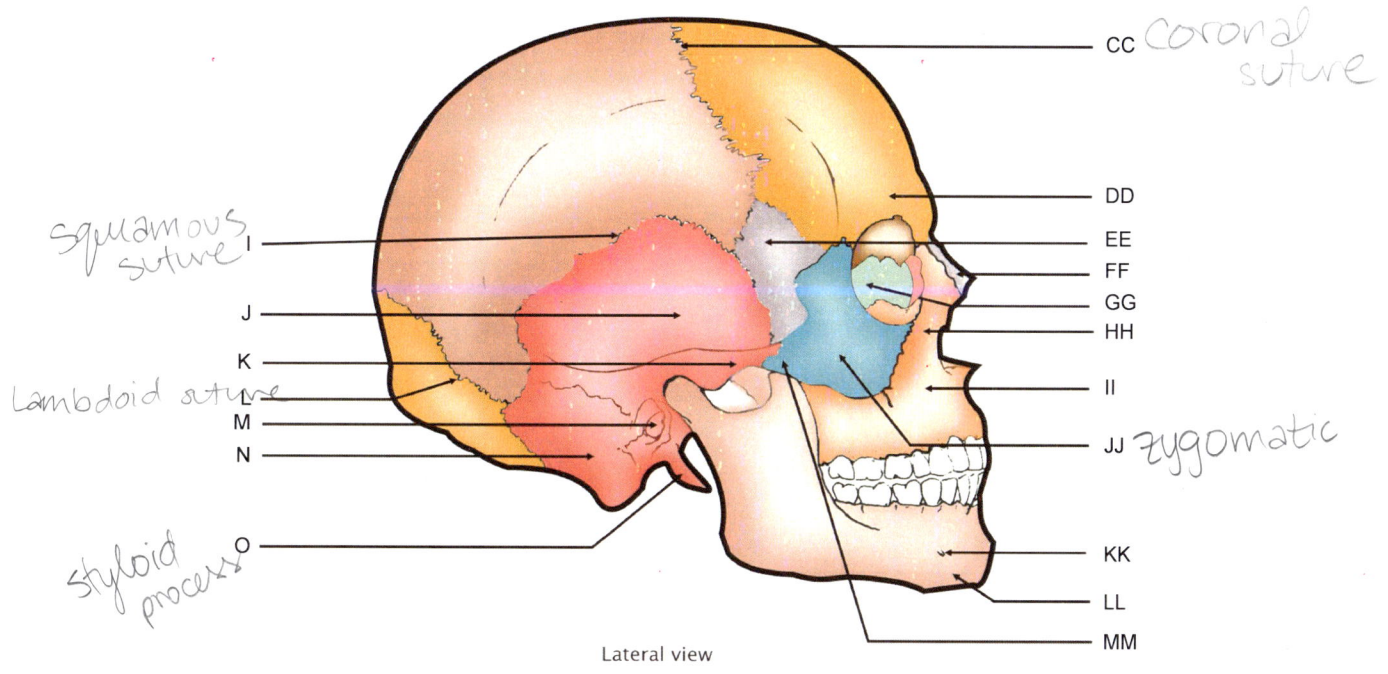

163

Figure 10-2. The skull

Anterior view

Lateral view

Handwritten annotations:
- A — Lacrimal
- X — zygomatic
- CC — coronal suture
- I — squamous suture
- Lambdoid suture (near L)
- O — styloid process
- JJ — zygomatic

164

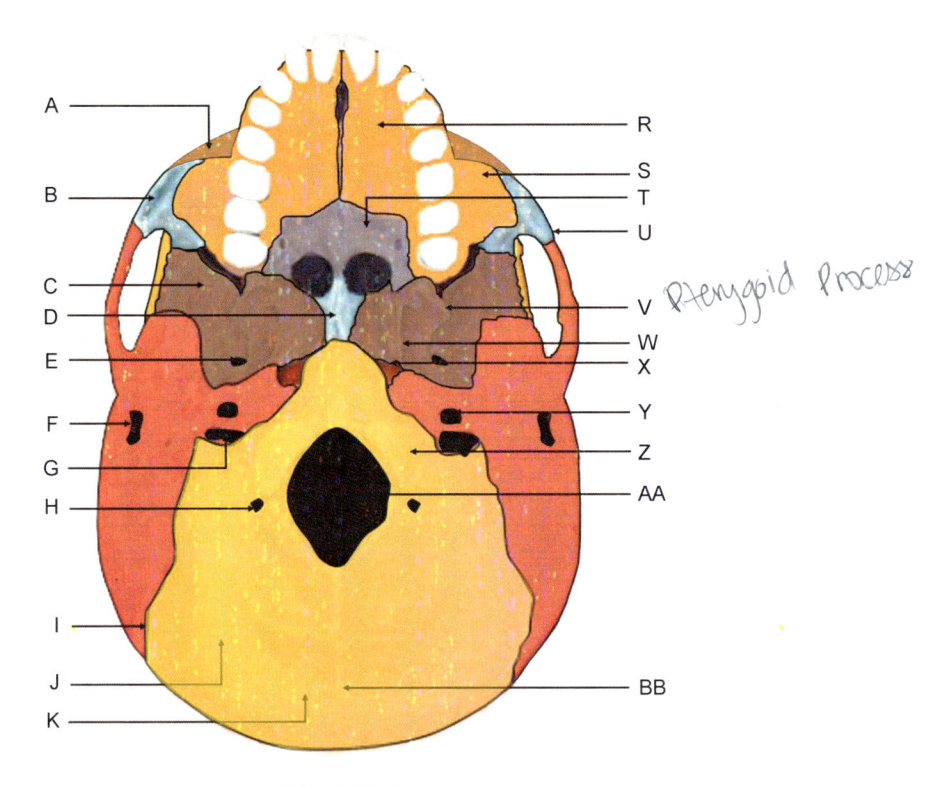

Inferior View

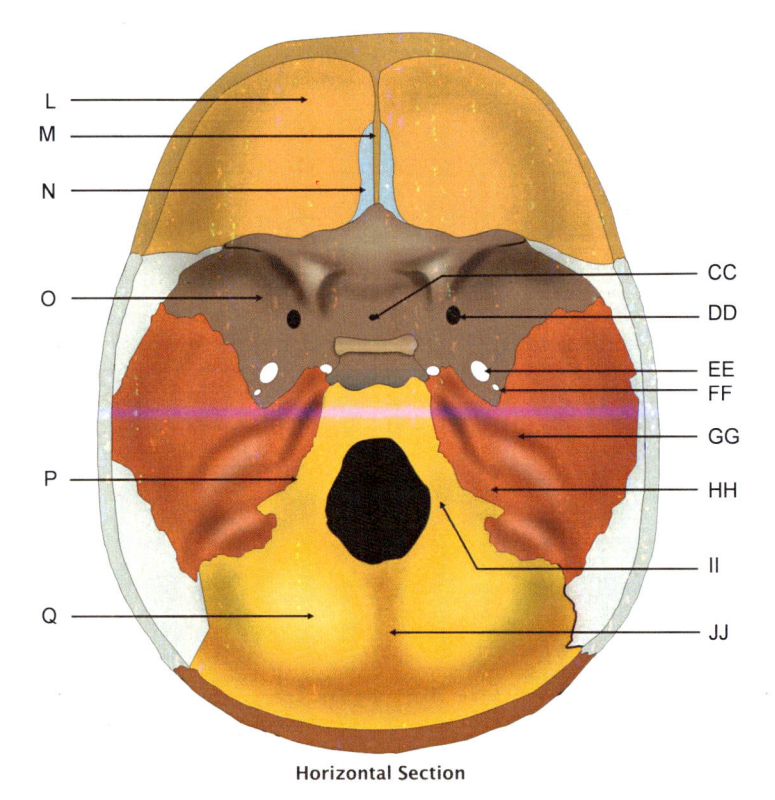

Horizontal Section

Figure 10.2 (continued)

(handwritten annotation near V: "Pterygoid Process")

the occipital bone meets the parietal bones. The superior point of the lambdoid suture intersects the sagittal suture. The lambdoid suture is the most common location for the occurrence of small flat bones known as *sutural* (or *Wormian*) bones.

The calvaria and skull base

Each of the four major sutures helps hold together a portion of the skull's superior half, also known as the **calvaria** (kal-VAR-ē-a; *calvar-*, skull) or *skullcap*. The calvaria consists of the frontal and parietal bones, and the superior halves of the occipital and temporal bones. In certain types of brain surgery, a neurosurgeon removes the calvaria to operate on the brain.

Whereas the calvaria forms the superior half of the skull, the **base** forms the inferior half. The external surface of the base consists of cranial bones and facial bones (except for the mandible), and you can see these when the skull is turned upside-down. However, removing the calvaria from a dry skull (one without a brain) reveals the skull's internal base, which consists only of cranial bones.

The skull's largest cavity is the **cranial cavity**, and it houses the brain. The calvaria encloses the cranial cavity superiorly and laterally, while the internal base encloses the cavity inferiorly and laterally. The relatively smooth, internal surfaces of the cranial bones help prevent the brain from being scratched if the head suddenly moves.

The skull's internal base consists of three large depressions, called *cranial fossae*. Each fossa is at a different level, like three steps of a staircase, and supports a different region of the brain. The **anterior cranial fossa** lies at the base of the frontal bone and a small portion of the ethmoid bone; this fossa supports the frontal lobe of the brain. The anterior cranial fossa is the most superior of the three cranial fossae, so it is like the "top step" in the staircase. Portions of the sphenoid and the right and left temporal bones form the **middle cranial fossa**, so it is like the "middle step" in the staircase. This fossa primarily supports the temporal lobes of the brain. The occipital bone forms the **posterior cranial fossa**, which is the most inferior of the three fossae; therefore, it is like the "bottom" step in our staircase analogy. This fossa primarily supports the cerebellum.

Cranial bones

Although the bones of the skull work together as a single, tightly knit unit, it's useful studying them individually, too. For example, forensic specialists (professionals who gather evidence for law courts) and archeologists (scientists who study past human cultures) often need to identify bones or bone fragments in isolation from the rest of a skull. But in general, studying individual skull bones is useful because they have markings, openings, and sinuses that will prepare you to learn about the muscles, blood vessels, nerves, and respiratory structures you will study later in this book. Indeed, the skull is like a 3D jigsaw puzzle.

FRONTAL BONE

The **frontal bone** (FRUN-tal; *front-*, forehead or brow) forms the anterior portion of the cranium, the superior wall of the orbital cavities, and most of the anterior cranial fossa. The posterior margin of the frontal bone articulates with the parietal bones at the *coronal suture*, while the inferior margins articulate with the sphenoid, zygomatic, ethmoid, lacrimal, maxilla, and nasal bones. Notice the part of the frontal bone that articulates with the zygomatic bone of the face. This process is the **zygomatic process**, so named not because it is part of the zygomatic bone, but because it articulates with the zygomatic bone. The *squamous part* of the frontal bone forms the forehead. Muscles that wrinkle the forehead's skin and move the eyebrows attach to the squamous part of the frontal bone.

> **Note**: It is common in anatomy to name a bony feature after the bone with which the feature interacts, not after the bone of which it is a part. This fact can help you to learn and remember the relationship of one bone in the skeleton with another.

The frontal bone forms a ridge, the **supraorbital margin**, at the superior edge of each orbit; an eyebrow lies over each supraorbital margin. The region between the supraorbital margins, where the forehead meets the nose, is the **glabella** (gla-BEL-a). The glabella (*glab-*, smooth or hairless) gets its name because eyebrows do not usually grow over that region of the skin. A pointed *nasal spine* projects inferiorly from the glabella, but in an intact skull, it is hidden behind the nasal bones. **A supraorbital foramen** in each supraorbital margin marks the passageway for an artery that delivers blood to the eyebrows and upper eyelids. Often the supraorbital foramen is merely a small notch in the supraorbital margin. On the superior wall of each orbit, posterior to the supraorbital margin, is a slight depression called a **lacrimal fossa**. A tear gland resides within the lacrimal fossa, and secretes tears to lubricate and protect the surface of the eyeball.

> **Note**: The frontal bone develops from a right and left half, but these segments normally fuse to form single bone. Sometimes fusion does not occur, and a *metopic (frontal) suture* (mē-TOP-ik; *metop-*, forehead) joins the two halves of the frontal bones.

Cavities lined with mucous membranes often develop within the frontal bone and these cavities are called **frontal sinuses**. Mucus from the frontal sinuses drains into the nasal cavity and helps trap dust and other airborne particles, preventing them from passing farther into the respiratory system.

PARIETAL BONES

The right and left **parietal bones** (pa-RĪ-e-tal; *parie-*, wall) form most of the cranium's superior and lateral walls. Each parietal bone articulates with the other parietal bone at the sagittal suture; with the frontal bone at the coronal suture; with the temporal bone at the squamous suture; and with the occipital bone at the lambdoid suture. Structurally, the parietal bones are the simplest cranial bones, resembling a square bedspread with its corners turned inward. The external surface is relatively smooth, with only two slightly raised *temporal lines* that serve as attachment sites for muscles that move the lower jaw. The internal surface of a parietal bone resembles a roadmap drawn in the sand, because it contains numerous shallow grooves in which blood vessels lie that supply the coverings of the brain.

TEMPORAL BONES

Each of the oddly shaped right and left **temporal bones** (TEM-pô-ral; "temple") look somewhat like an elephant's ears, which is an apt comparison because these bones house the organs of hearing. The temporal bones form parts of the cranium's lateral walls and base. Each temporal bone articulates with 3 cranial bones (sphenoid, parietal, and occipital) and 2 facial bones (zygomatic and mandible). The temporal bones are the only skull bones that articulate with the mandible.

Externally, the inferior half of the temporal bone has a coarse texture, but the superior half, the **squamous part**, is very smooth and is relatively thin-walled. In fact, if you hold a skull next to a light and look through the squamous part of the temporal bone, you will likely see the shadows of your fingers on the opposite side. Because a temporal bone's squamous part is so thin, it is relatively easy to fracture. This fact should suggest why it's important to wear a helmet when engaging in activities that could expose the skull to trauma.

The **external acoustic meatus** (a-KOOS-tik; "hear"; mē-Ā-tus; "passage") is a prominent opening just inferior to the squamous part of the temporal bone. This tube-like structure directs sound to the *tympanum* (eardrum), located deeper inside the temporal bone. For this reason, the region around the meatus is called the **tympanic part** of the temporal bone, and is considered part of the *external ear*. Looking at the internal surface, the **petrous part** (PET-rus; *petr-*, rock) of the temporal bone is a thick, bony ridge inside the cranial cavity that separates the middle cranial fossa from the posterior cranial fossa. The petrous part contains a *middle ear* and an *inner ear* cavity. The middle ear cavity contains the auditory ossicles that pass sound vibrations deeper into the temporal bone to the inner ear. The inner ear, in turn, contains the sensory organs for hearing and equilibrium (balance). Several nerves that conduct impulses from the inner ear to the brain pass through a tube, the **internal acoustic meatus**, on the posterior surface of the petrous part.

Each temporal bone contains three distinctive processes that anchor skeletal muscles. The **zygomatic process** (zī-gō-MAT-ik) is the most conspicuous of the three. This process is so named (*zygoma-*, yoke) because it looks like the crossbar used to attach a horse to a plow or wagon. The zygomatic process extends anteriorly from the squamous portion to connect with the *temporal process* on the zygomatic bone. Together, the zygomatic process on the temporal bone and the temporal process on the zygomatic bone form the *zygomatic arch*. A muscle that closes the mouth extends from the zygomatic arch to the mandible. You can feel your own zygomatic arches as ridges running between your ears and cheeks. The **mandibular fossa** lies at the posterior, inferior end of the zygomatic process, just anterior to the external acoustic meatus. This fossa articulates with the mandible's condyle and this is the only movable joint between skull bones.

The **mastoid process** (MAS-toyd) is the most posterior of the three processes, and is so-named because it resembles a breast (*mast-*, "breast"). You can feel the mastoid process as a bony knob immediately posterior to your ear. A large neck muscle pulls on the mastoid process to turn your head to the side. Although externally the mastoid process may appear to be a solid knob, it contains numerous air-filled spaces called *mastoid air cells* that help lighten the skull.

The **styloid process** (STĪ-loyd) looks like a sharp spike (*styl-*, "pillar") and extends anteriorly from the base of the mastoid process. The styloid process anchors skeletal muscles that move the tongue, pharynx (throat), and hyoid bone. Because of its slender shape and exposed position, the styloid process is often broken off and missing from dry skulls in the lab.

Externally, several openings are visible on the temporal bone's inferior surface. As its name implies, the **stylomastoid foramen** lies between the styloid process and the mastoid process. A nerve passing through this foramen stimulates certain facial muscles to contract. Lying posterior and medial to the styloid process is the **jugular foramen** (JUG-ū-lar; *jugul-*, throat). Three nerves and the large *jugular vein* pass through this opening; the jugular vein transports blood from the brain toward the heart. Slightly anterior and medial to the jugular foramen is the **carotid canal** (ka-ROT-id). The carotid artery, which delivers most of the brain's blood supply, passes through this canal.

OCCIPITAL BONE

The **occipital bone** (ok-SIP-i-tal; *occiput-*, "back of head") forms most of the cranium's posterior wall and much of its posterior base; internally this bone forms most of the posterior cranial fossa. The occipital bone articulates with the parietal bones at the *lambdoid suture*, and with the right and left temporal bones at the *occipitomastoid sutures*, which appear to be a continuation of the lambdoid suture. The occipital bone's most anterior part, the **basilar part** (BĀ-si-lar; also called the **basioccipital process**; bā-ē-ok-SIPP-i-tal), slopes superiorly and articulates with the sphenoid bone and vomer. The smooth sloping surface of the occipital bone's basilar part and sphenoid bone in the posterior cranial fossa is called the **clivus** (KLĪ-vus; "slope"). The anterior portion of the brain stem that connects to the spinal cord rests on the clivus.

The occipital bone is the only skull bone that articulates with the spine. Two large, rounded knobs on the occipital bone's inferior surface, the **occipital condyles**, articulate with the first cervical vertebra (the *atlas*). Occipital condyles enable you to nod your head to make the "yes" sign (but do not allow you to shake your head from side-to-side to make the "no" sign).

There are several distinguishing projections on the occipital bone's external surface. The **external occipital protuberance** is the site where the long *nuchal ligament* (NOO-kul; *nuch-*, back of neck), also called the *ligamentum nuchae* (lig-a-MEN-tum), attaches the skull to all cervical vertebrae (neck bones). You can feel this protuberance as a rounded bump on the posterior part of your head, where the skull begins to curve inward. Two horizontal ridges, the *nuchal lines*, are near the occipital protuberance and serve as attachment sites for skeletal muscles extending from the neck and back; these muscles keep your head in a raised position.

The occipital bone contains several foramina and forms a portion of two others. Between the occipital condyles is the **foramen magnum** (MAG-num; "large"), the skull's largest foramen, where the brain and spinal cord connect. Flanking the foramen magnum on the right and left side is a **hypoglossal canal**, through which a nerve passes that controls tongue movement. Some skulls have a *condylar canal* at the posterior end of each occipital condyle; this hole serves as a passageway for a small vein that drains blood from the brain. The occipital bone forms the posterior rim of the right and left **jugular foramen**, while the temporal bones form the anterior rims.

SPHENOID BONE

The **sphenoid bone** (SFĒ-noyd) has the most elaborate shape of all skull bones. From an anterior view it looks like a swooping bird of prey with its legs extended. The sphenoid bone lives up to its name (*sphen-*, wedge), because it is wedged in among most of the other skull bones. It articulates with all of the other cranial bones and 7 facial bones (maxillae, zygomatic, and palatine bones on both sides, and the single vomer). The sphenoid contains two air-filled **sphenoid sinuses**. Mucous membranes that line the sphenoid sinuses contribute mucus to the nasal cavity. The sphenoid sinuses also lighten the skull, and affect the sound of the voice. The **sella turcica** (SEL-a, "saddle"; TER-si-ka, "Turkish") is a saddle-shaped structure on the superior surface of the sphenoid that supports the hypophysis (pituitary gland) of the brain.

The sphenoid bone contains three prominent processes: the *greater wings*, the *lesser wings*, and the *pterygoid processes*. The **greater wings** extend laterally from the inferior portion of the sphenoid's body, and then curve slightly superiorly. Externally, the greater wings are visible as a rectangular-shaped bone in the temple region, between the frontal bone and temporal bone. The greater wings also form a portion of each orbit's posterior wall. Anterior to the sella turcica, the **lesser wings** extend laterally from the sphenoid's body and taper sharply to meet the frontal bone. The lesser wings form a ridge that marks the anterior, superior border of the middle cranial fossa. They also form part of each orbit's superior wall.

Despite the fact that their name means "wing," two **pterygoid processes** (TER-i-goyd; *ptery*-, wing) look more like extended legs. These processes extend inferiorly from the sphenoid's body and from the medial portion of each greater wing. The pterygoid processes are attachment sites for the pterygoid muscles that move the mandible in a horizontal plane (side-to-side).

Intricate bone that it is, the sphenoid contains a host of openings, including canals, fissures, and foramina. The **optic canals** (OP-tik; "eye") pass through the superior portion of the sphenoid body, and each canal supports an optic nerve and blood vessel from the eyeball. Within the cranial cavity, the optic canal opens just anterior to the sella turcica. The optic canal is also visible on the sphenoid's *orbital surface*, inside the superior, medial wall of each orbit. Also within the orbit, and lateral to the optic canal, is the **superior orbital fissure**. This slit-like groove is the space between the sphenoid's greater and lesser wings, and it serves as a passageway for several nerves and blood vessels leading to the face.

On the sphenoid's superior surface, three foramina are aligned in a diagonal row on each greater wing. The most anterior of these, the **foramen rotundum** (ro-TUN-dum; "round"), is a round opening inferior and slightly lateral to the sella turcica. It serves as a passageway for a nerve leading to the maxilla. Looking posteriorly and laterally, you can see the **foramen ovale** (ō-VĀ lē; "egg"), an egg-shaped (oval) opening near the posterior edge of the greater wing. It serves as a passageway for a nerve leading to the mandible. Slightly posterior and lateral from the foramen ovale is the **foramen spinosum** (spi-NO-sum; "thorn"), so-named because it is next to a short spine on the external surface of the cranial base. The foramen spinosum supports small blood vessels that lead to the membranous coverings that surround the brain.

The temporal bone and sphenoid bone each form part of the **foramen lacerum** (LA-ser-um; *lacer*-, to tear). This foramen's irregular edges look as if they were torn like paper; hence, the name "lacerum" is appropriate. The carotid artery emerges from the carotid canal and passes through this foramen before entering the cranial cavity.

ETHMOID BONE

The **ethmoid bone** (ĒTH-moyd; *ethm*-, sieve) has a strange, irregular shape that is difficult to compare with anything else, and much of the bone is hidden behind other bones. Its name relates to a sieve, a device with small holes used to strain or sift materials. Numerous **ethmoid air cells** inside the ethmoid bone resemble the holes of a sieve.

The ethmoid bone forms the superior portion and much of the lateral portion of the nasal cavity, most of the nasal septum, most of an orbit's medial wall, and a small portion of the anterior cranial fossa. Although the ethmoid is a cranial bone, it articulates with only two other cranial bones (the frontal and sphenoid), while articulating with more facial bones than any other cranial bone. The ethmoid articulates with the right and left nasal bones, lacrimal bones, maxillae, palatine bones, inferior nasal conchae, and the vomer.

The midline portion of the ethmoid bone consists of the *crista galli* and the *perpendicular plate*. The **crista** galli (KRIS-ta, "crest;" GAL-ē; "rooster") is a pyramid-like ridge resembling a rooster's comb on the ethmoid's superior surface. It serves as an attachment site for one of the membranous coverings of the brain. Extending inferiorly from the crista galli is the broad, flat **perpendicular plate**. The plate forms the superior half of the bony *nasal septum*, a vertical partition that divides the nasal cavity into right and left halves. The posterior portion of the perpendicular plate articulates with the vomer, which forms the inferior half of the nasal septum. In the living body (not a dried skull), a vertical plate of hyaline cartilage connects the perpendicular plate to the vomer to complete the nasal septum.

The lateral portions of the ethmoid bone consist of the *cribriform plate*, *lateral masses*, and *nasal conchae*. The **cribriform plate** (KRIB-ri-form; *cribri-*, sieve) is a narrow, horizontal shelf on either side of the crista galli. Numerous **olfactory foramina** perforate the cribriform plate and mark the passageways for the olfactory nerves leading from the nasal cavity; these nerves function in smelling. The lateral masses contain the ethmoid air cells.

Parts of the ethmoid bone extend inferiorly as two plate-like projections called *nasal conchae* (KON-kē, shells; singular is concha, KON-ka). The smaller, more superior conchae are the **superior nasal conchae**; the larger more inferior conchae are the **middle nasal conchae**. In the living body, the nasal conchae are enveloped in a cartilaginous structure and covered with a mucous membrane, which warms and moistens the air flowing through the nasal cavity on its way to the lungs. The mucus also helps trap airborne particles, thereby acting like an air filter.

Table 10-2 summarizes the cranial bones and their major features.

Facial bones

Compared to the cranial bones, some of the skull's facial bones are small and less easy to locate. A helpful way to keep track of the facial bones is to group them according to the three sets of facial cavities with which they are associated. For example, the maxillae, palatine bones, and mandible form the entire oral cavity. The maxillae, vomer, nasal bones, inferior nasal conchae, and lacrimal bones contribute to the nasal cavity. Finally, the maxillae, zygomatic bones, and lacrimal bones contribute to the orbits. (Notice the maxillae and lacrimal bones contribute to several facial cavities.)

MAXILLAE

The **maxillae** (mak-SIL-ē, "jaws;" singular is maxilla) form the anterior and superior portions of the oral cavity, but they touch almost every other facial bone and contribute to the orbits and nasal cavities, too. In fact, just as the sphenoid bone is said to "anchor" the cranial bones, the maxillae anchor the skull's facial bones. The maxillae form the upper jaw, and their inferior surfaces articulating at the *intermaxillary suture* form the anterior two-thirds of the *hard palate* (PAL-et, "roof of the mouth"). Near the posterior end of the hard palate, the maxillae articulate with the palatine bones, which form the remainder of the hard palate. The right and left maxillae articulate with all other facial bones on the same side of the face except the mandible. Each maxilla also articulates with the frontal bone and the ethmoid bone of the cranium.

Each maxilla forms several parts of an orbit. The superior portion of the maxilla, its *orbital surface*, forms most of the orbit's inferior surface, and the medial, inferior part of the orbit's inferior edge, the **infraorbital margin**. On the floor of the orbit, the maxilla forms the anterior edge of a slit-like groove, the **inferior orbital fissure**; the sphenoid bone's greater wing forms the posterior edge. Inferior to the infraorbital margin on the maxilla's anterior surface is a small opening, the **infraorbital foramen**. A nerve and a blood vessel leading to the face pass through this foramen. The maxilla also forms the lateral wall of the nasal cavity.

The most superior portions of the maxillae extend as wing-like **frontal processes** that articulate with the frontal bone. The medial edges of the frontal processes articulate with the nasal bones. The medial, anterior edge of each maxilla encloses the inferior half of the **nasal aperture**, the large opening into the nasal cavity. At the base of the nasal aperture, the maxillae join to form the **anterior nasal spine**.

Lateral to the nasal cavity and inferior to the orbit, each maxilla contains a large air-filled space, the **maxillary sinus**. Mucus secretions from the maxillary sinuses drain into the nasal cavity. Extending laterally to articulate with the zygomatic bone is the **zygomatic**

Table 10-2: Summary of CRANIAL BONES and their major features

Ethmoid bone	
Cribriform plate	Site of olfactory foramina
Crista galli	Projection for attachment of dura mater (covering of brain)
Ethmoid air cells	Small sinuses within ethmoid bone's lateral masses
Middle nasal conchae	Increases surface area of nasal cavity wall
Olfactory foramina	In cribriform plate; passage for olfactory nerves
Perpendicular plate	Forms upper two-thirds of nasal septum
Superior nasal conchae	Increases surface area of nasal cavity wall
Frontal bone	
Frontal sinus	May or may not be present inside frontal bone
Glabella	Smooth region between the orbital ridges
Supraorbital foramen	Sometimes this is just a notch; passage for vessels
Supraorbital margin	Upper rim of orbit; also called the *brow ridge*
Zygomatic process	Articulates with zygomatic bone
Parietal bones (2): forms most of lateral walls of skull	
Occipital bone	
Basilar part	(Basioccipital process) Most anterior part of occipital bone
Clivus	Smooth, sloping portion of basilar part on which brain stem rests
External occipital protuberance	Site of attachment for *nuchal ligament*
Foramen magnum	Passage for medulla oblongata, spinal cord, accessory nerves (XI), vertebral arteries
Hypoglossal canal	Passage for hypoglossal nerve (XII)
Jugular foramen (part)	Passage for internal jugular vein, glossopharyngeal nerve (IX), vagus nerve (X), accessory nerves
Occipital condyles	Articulate with the first cervical vertebra (the atlas)
Sphenoid bone	
Foramen lacerum (part)	Passage for internal carotid artery
Foramen ovale	Passage for mandibular branch of trigeminal nerve
Foramen rotundum	Passage for maxillary branch of trigeminal nerve
Foramen spinosum	Passage for blood vessels to meninges
Greater wing	Form part of the orbit
Inferior orbital fissure (part)	Passage for maxillary branch of trigeminal nerve and vessels to orbit
Lesser wing	Form part of the border for the middle cranial fossa
Optic canal	Passage for optic nerve
Pterygoid process	Attachment site for muscles that move mandible side-to-side
Sella turcica	Holds pituitary gland
Superior orbital fissure	Passage for oculomotor nerve (III), trochlear nerve (IV), ophthalmic branch of trigeminal nerve (V), abducens nerve, and ophthalmic vein

THE AXIAL SKELETON

Temporal bones (2)	
Carotid canal	Passage for internal carotid artery
External acoustic meatus	Passage for sound waves to middle ear
Foramen lacerum (part)	Passage for internal carotid artery
Internal acoustic meatus	Passage for vestibulocochlear nerve (VIII) and facial nerve (VII)
Mandibular fossa	Articulates with the condylar process of the mandible
Mastoid process	Attachment site for neck muscle
Petrous portion	Bony ridge that contains the inner ear components
Squamous part	Smooth, superior half of temporal bone
Styloid process	Attachment site for neck muscle
Stylomastoid foramen	Passage for facial nerve
Tympanic part	Rough, inferior half of temporal bone
Zygomatic process	Articulates with temporal process of zygomatic bone

process. (Recall that the temporal bone also has a zygomatic process.)

Making a V-shape around the anterior and lateral edges of the hard palate are **alveolar processes** (al-VĒ-ō-lar; *alveoli-*, socket), which form the rim around the **alveolar sockets** holding the teeth. Along the midline immediately posterior to the front teeth is the **incisive fossa** (in-SĪ-siv, "to cut"), named for the incisors (front teeth). This fossa leads to a foramen through which a blood vessel and nerve pass through to the soft tissues covering the hard palate.

PALATINE BONES

Two additional facial bones complete the roof of the oral cavity. The **palatine bones** (PAL-a-tīn; *palat-*, roof of mouth), one on each side of a midline plane, form the posterior one-third of the hard palate, as well as a tiny portion of each orbit. Each palatine bone articulates with four other facial bones: a maxilla, inferior nasal concha, vomer, and the other palatine bone. Each one also articulates with two cranial bones: the sphenoid and the ethmoid. Viewed anteriorly, each palatine bone is L-shaped, but the two bones together resemble a "crooked U."

MANDIBLE

The **mandible** (MAN-di-bul, "jaw") is the lower jaw forming the floor of the oral cavity. The mandible is the only movable skull bone (excluding the middle ear bones). It can move inferiorly, superiorly, and laterally to allow you to chew food, speak, and even make different facial expressions. A mandible of a typical adult contains 16 teeth. The mandible has three distinct landmarks on both of its superior, posterior ends: the *condylar process*, the *coronoid process*, and the *mandibular notch*.

The **condylar process** is a rounded knob that articulates with the mandibular fossa of the temporal bone. Anterior to the condylar process is the pointed **coronoid process** (KOR-ō-noyd; *coron-*, crow's beak). As the term suggests, this process looks like a bird's beak. The large temporalis muscle extends from the lateral side of the skull through the zygomatic arch to attach to the coronoid process. When the muscle pulls on the process, the anterior end of the mandible moves superiorly and the mouth closes. The U-shaped gap between the condylar process and coronoid process is the **mandibular notch**.

Extending inferiorly from the mandibular notch is a vertical portion of the mandible, the **ramus** (RĀ-mus, "branch"). The mandible's **angle** at the inferior, posterior end of each ramus is where the ramus meets the more horizontal part of the mandible, the **body**. The superior portion of the mandible's body contains *alveolar sockets*, which normally contain teeth. The rim around each socket is the *alveolar margin*. Superior projections along the alveolar margin are called *alveolar processes*. The inferior half of the mandible body's anterior tip curves outward, forming the **mental protuberance** (MEN-tul), or "chin." The midline region of the mandible's body is the **mandibular symphysis**.

The mandible displays four major foramina (two on each side). The **mandibular foramen** is found on the medial surface of the ramus. Blood vessels and nerves supplying the mandible's teeth pass through this foramen. The **mental foramen** is on the mandible body's external surface, slightly lateral and posterior to the mandibular symphysis. Nerves and blood vessels serving the chin and lower lip pass through this foramen.

NASAL BONES

Turning next to the facial bones that solely border the nasal cavity, the **nasal bones** form the bridge (superior portion) of the nose. The right and left nasal bones articulate with one another medially at the **internasal suture**, along the midline of the face. In addition, each nasal bone articulates with the frontal bone, superiorly; with a maxilla, laterally; and with the perpendicular plate of the ethmoid bone, posteriorly. The inferior edges of the nasal bones form the superior rim of the large nasal aperture leading to the nasal cavity.

VOMER

The **vomer** (VŌ-mer, "plow") is a long, thin bone that resembles the blade of a plow or knife. The vomer's vertical plate forms the inferior one-third of the bony nasal septum. The superior portion of the vomer articulates with the perpendicular plate of the ethmoid bone. Beginning anteriorly and moving posteriorly along the midline, the inferior edge of the vomer articulates with the maxillae and palatine bones. The superior, posterior end of the vomer displays two **alae** (Ā-lē; "wings"), each of which articulates with the sphenoid bone.

INFERIOR NASAL CONCHAE

Unlike the superior and middle nasal conchae, which are processes of the ethmoid bone, the **inferior nasal conchae** are independent bones that protrude from the lateral walls of the nasal cavity. Most of an inferior nasal concha's lateral surface articulates with a maxilla, while a small portion near its posterior end articulates with a palatine bone. A very tiny portion articulates with a lacrimal bone, superiorly.

Each inferior nasal concha tapers on its anterior and posterior ends. The medial surface is slightly convex and the lateral surface is slightly concave, like the blade of an airplane propeller. This shape causes inhaled air to "spiral," which enables it to be more evenly warmed by the nasal mucosae.

ZYGOMATIC BONES

Of the facial bones that contribute solely to the orbits, the **zygomatic bones** (zī'-gō-MAT-ik, "bar") are the largest. On each side of the face, a zygomatic bone forms the superior, protruding part of the cheeks and lateral walls of the orbits. The superior portion of each zygomatic bone articulates with the frontal bone at the *frontozygomatic suture*, while the inferior portion articulates with the maxilla at the *zygomaticomaxillary suture*. The medial, posterior portion of the zygomatic bone articulates with the sphenoid bone, and the lateral, posterior portion, called the **temporal process**, articulates with the zygomatic process of the temporal bone to complete the zygomatic arch. Viewing the skull inferiorly, the zygomatic arches look like handles of a kitchen pot.

LACRIMAL BONES

The **lacrimal bones** (LAK-ri-mal, tear) are the smallest facial bones and form a portion of the anterior, medial wall of the orbits. Each of these small, rectangular-shaped bones articulates with the frontal bone, superiorly; with a maxilla anteriorly and inferiorly; and with the ethmoid bone, posteriorly. At the medial edge of the infraorbital margin, the maxilla and lacrimal bone together form a narrow tube, the **nasolacrimal canal.** This canal surrounds a membranous *nasolacrimal duct* that drains tears from the lower eyelid into the nasal cavity. The anterior portion of a lacrimal bone forms half of the **lacrimal groove** (the maxilla forms the other half), which feeds into the nasolacrimal canal.

THE AXIAL SKELETON

THE ORBITS AND NASAL CAVITY

As you studied the cranial and facial bones, you probably noticed that the orbits and nasal cavity are amazingly intricate complexes of bones. Why such complexity? As with the cranial cavity, the many bony plates and splinters that make up the facial cavities allow these oddly shaped chambers to maintain their proportions as the skull grows. Because the orbits and nasal cavities will figure prominently in your study of the eyes and the respiratory tract, it's worth taking a second look at these structures individually and summarizing the bones that form them.

Orbits. Staring into the depths of an orbit is perhaps the closest you might get to experiencing what a hatching chick "sees" as it breaks free from its shell – a fractured assembly of curved plates. The orbits house the eyeballs. Between the orbital walls and the eyeball are skeletal muscles that move the eye, a cushioning layer of adipose tissue, as well as blood and lymphatic vessels, nerves, and a lacrimal (tear) gland.

Parts of three cranial bones (frontal, sphenoid, and ethmoid) and four facial bones (maxilla, zygomatic, lacrimal, and palatine) form the orbital walls. The protruding rim of each orbit (formed by the frontal bone, maxilla, and zygomatic bone) is quite sturdy, but the orbital floor is relatively fragile (Figure 10-3).

Table 10-3 summarizes the facial bones and their major features.

The nasal cavity. A vertical partition, the **nasal septum**, divides the nasal cavity into right and left sides. From a medial view, the nasal septum looks like three relatively flat plates. Anteriorly, the nasal septum consists of a hyaline cartilage plate, the **septal cartilage**. The septal cartilage tapers to a point near the posterior end of the nasal septum. The anterior end of the septal cartilage forms the medial portion of the nose that is covered by skin. The perpendicular plate of the ethmoid bone forms most the nasal septum's superior half, while the vomer forms the septum's inferior half (Figure 10-4).

The walls of each nasal cavity are formed, in part, by five facial bones (maxilla, palatine, inferior nasal concha, nasal, and lacrimal bones) and three cranial bones (ethmoid, frontal, and sphenoid). Three ridge-like *nasal conchae* protrude from the lateral walls of the nasal cavity. The two smaller ridges, the *superior nasal conchae* and *middle nasal conchae*, are part of the ethmoid bone. The *inferior nasal conchae* are separate bones and the largest nasal conchae. They are located inferior to the middle nasal conchae and extend anteriorly to meet the nasal spine of the maxilla.

The *cribriform plate* of the ethmoid bone forms most of the nasal cavity's superior border (roof), while the frontal bone and the nasal bones form a small portion of the roof near the anterior end. Nerves that function in the sense of smell pass from the superior portion of the nasal cavity through numerous tiny olfactory foramina of the cribriform plate and enter the brain in the anterior cranial fossa. The maxillae and palatine bones form the inferior border (the floor) of the nasal cavity, while the sphenoid bone forms most of the posterior wall.

PARANASAL SINUSES

As described earlier, five skull bones contain internal cavities called sinuses, and since these sinuses border the nasal cavity, they are collectively called **paranasal sinuses** (*para-*, alongside). The paranasal sinuses include the *frontal sinus*, the *sphenoid sinus*, the *ethmoid air cells*, and the *maxillary sinuses* (one in each maxilla). The paranasal sinuses lighten the skull and affect the sound of the voice. Each sinus is lined with a mucous membrane that secretes mucus, which drains into the nasal cavity. Normally a paranasal sinus is filled with air, but excessive mucus or watery tissue fluid in the sinus can change the resonance of the voice. This is similar to the difference in sounds that is apparent if you tap a spoon on an empty water glass, and then tap the glass again after filling it with water.

FONTANELS

So far, we have been describing the anatomy of the adult skull. A human infant, however, is born without fully developed cranial bones, a situation which is actually helpful. First, a partially formed skull is flexible, which helps an infant's head squeeze through its mother's birth canal. Second, a partially formed skull accommodates the explosive growth of the brain that occurs during the first few years after birth. An infant's cranial bones are relatively thin, and they aren't ossified

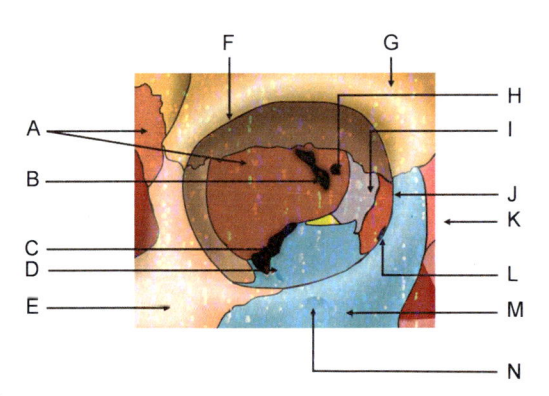

Figure 10-3. Bones of the orbit

Table 10-3: Summary of FACIAL BONES and their major features

Inferior nasal conchae (2): increases surface of nasal mucosa	
Lacrimal bones (2)	
Nasolacrimal canal (part)	Formed with maxilla; passage for tears into the nasal cavity
Mandible	
Angle	Site where ramus meets body of mandible
Body	Straight portion of mandible that contains alveolar sockets
Condylar process	Also called the mandibular condyle; articulates with temporal bone
Coronoid process	Site of muscle attachment
Mandibular foramen	Passage for nerve and vessels
Mandibular notch	U-shaped gap between the condylar process and coronoid process
Mandibular symphysis	Anterior, midline portion of mandible
Mental foramen	Passage for mental nerve and branch of the mandibular nerve
Mental protuberance	The "chin" portion
Maxillae (2)	
Alveolar processes	V-shaped projections around alveolar sockets
Alveolar sockets	Cavities that hold teeth
Frontal processes	Articulate with frontal bone
Incisive fossa	Passage for nerve and vessel
Inferior orbital fissure	Passage for maxillary branch of trigeminal nerve and vessels to orbit
Infraorbital foramen	Passage for infraorbital nerve and artery
Infraorbital margin	Lower rim of orbit
Maxillary sinus	Cavity within each maxilla
Nasal aperture (inferior half)	Opening of nasal cavity
Nasal spine	Formed where maxillae join; projection at inferior rim of nasal aperture
Nasolacrimal canal (part)	Formed with lacrimal bone; passage for tears into the nasal cavity
Zygomatic process	Articulates with zygomatic bone
Nasal bones (2)	
Internasal suture	Articulation site between the two nasal bones
Palatine bones (2): forms posterior portion of hard palate	
Vomer: forms inferior portion of nasal septum	
Zygomatic bones (2): form the "cheeks"	
Temporal process	Articulates with zygomatic process of temporal bone

THE AXIAL SKELETON

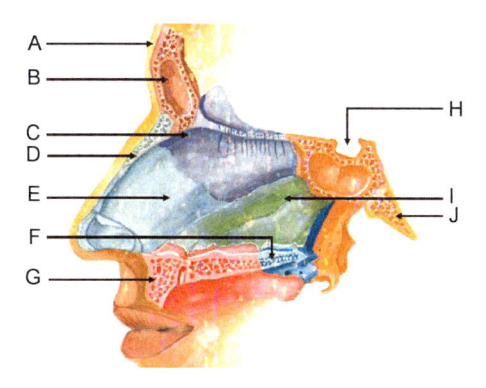

Figure 10-4. Bones of the nasal cavity

to the edges of the cranial sutures. In place of sutures, an infant's cranium has patches of fibrous membranes called **fontanels** (fon-ta-NELZ) or "soft spots" (Figure 10-5). The fontanels are what remain of the membrane model from which the cranial bones begin to form by intramembranous ossification. Eventually the cranial bones grow together to form sutures; the last fontanel usually ossifies by about age 2.

> **Note**: The French word, *fontanel*, literally means "fountains," but the sense of the word for English-speakers has a meaning closer to "wellspring," a source or origin of something.

There are six major fontanels present in an infant's skull at the time of birth. The **anterior fontanel** is the largest fontanel, and is found where the coronal suture and the sagittal suture meet. A smaller **posterior fontanel** is found at the intersection of the sagittal suture and the lambdoid suture. A **sphenoidal fontanel** is found in each temple region, where the squamous suture and coronal suture intersect. The **mastoid fontanel** is located superior to the mastoid process of the temporal bone, where the lambdoid suture meets the squamous suture.

THE HYOID BONE

Before turning to the rest of the axial skeleton, we will describe the only bone in the skeleton that does not articulate with another bone; this is the hyoid bone (HĪ-oyd, *hy-*, U-shaped). The U-shaped **hyoid bone** is found in the anterior cervical (neck) region, inferior to the mandible. Several muscles extend superiorly from the hyoid bone; two support the hyoid from the styloid process of each temporal bone, and the other moves the tongue. Muscles also extend inferiorly to support the larynx (voice box). In essence, the hyoid bone is a suspension device, much like a coat hanger or a curtain rod. What "hangs" from the hyoid are muscles that attach to and "lift" the larynx when a person swallows.

GENERAL STRUCTURE OF THE SPINE

Like a plant's stem, which supports its flower and branches, the vertebral column supports the skull and appendicular skeleton. In addition, the vertebral column surrounds and protects the spinal cord, and it provides attachment sites for muscles that move the skull, back, shoulders, arms, hips, and thighs.

Regions of the vertebral column

The **vertebral column** (VER-te-bral), or **spine**, of a typical adult consists of 33 bones stacked vertically along the body's midline, from the base of the skull

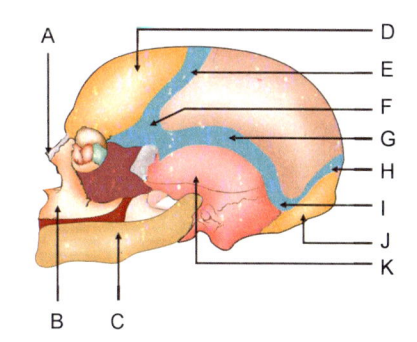

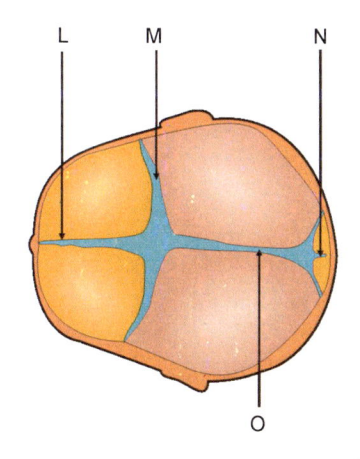

Figure 10-5. Fontanels

through the pelvis (Figure 10-6). The bones of the vertebral column are irregular in shape and are called **vertebrae** (VER-te-brā; *vertebr-*, a joint; singular is vertebra).

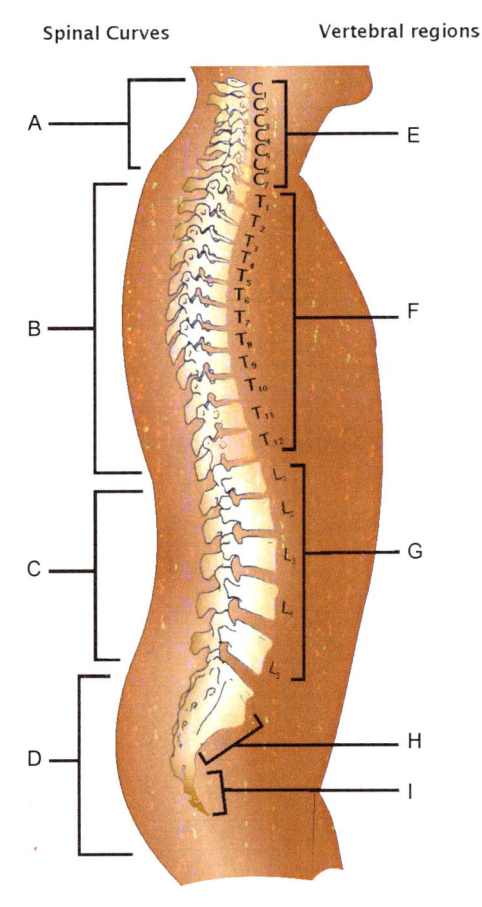

Figure 10-6. The vertebral column

Anatomists divide the vertebral column into five groups of vertebrae beginning at the skull and moving inferiorly. The groups include the *cervical, thoracic, lumbar, sacral,* and *coccygeal* vertebrae. There are 7 **cervical vertebrae** (SER-vi-kal) in the neck, and they are numbered C_1 (for the most superior cervical vertebra) through C7 (for the most inferior cervical vertebra). Twelve **thoracic vertebrae** (thō-RAS-ik; *thora-*, chest), numbered T_1 through T_{12}, run the length of the upper and middle back. The lower back has 5 **lumbar vertebrae** (LUM-bar), numbered L_1 through L_5. The next five vertebrae, the **sacral vertebrae** (SĀ-krul), fuse during childhood to form a single bone, the **sacrum** (SA-krum). Inferior to the sacrum are three to five **coccygeal vertebrae** (kok-SIJ-ē-al) that fuse to form a single bone, the **coccyx** (KOK-siks).

Just as a flower stem may bend as it supports its load, the vertebral column bends in a characteristic shape to help it support the body's weight. There are four major bends in the vertebral column of an adult, and these bends are called *spinal curvatures*. The **thoracic curvature** in the back and the **sacral curvature** in the pelvis are the two *primary curvatures* of the vertebral column. These are so named because they are the two curvatures a person is born with. The primary curvatures are convex; that is, they bow posteriorly, away from the body's ventral cavity. In the fetus, however, the other parts of the vertebral column are also convex, making the entire vertebral column appear as a single curve.

The **cervical curvature** in the neck and the **lumbar curvature** in the lower back are two *secondary curvatures*, because they develop within the first year after birth. The secondary curvatures are *concave*; that is, they bow anteriorly, toward the body's ventral cavity. Without secondary curvatures, the weight of the upper body would shift forward, causing more bending stress on the convex portions of the vertebral column. The secondary curvatures allow the upper body's weight to balance on the vertebral column and over the lower limbs. Think about how a weight lifter balances a heavy weight directly overhead. This technique distributes the weight throughout the vertebral column and to the lower limbs. Holding the weight too far forward would place excessive stress on the back, especially the lumbar curvature, possibly causing intense pain. Developing the cervical curvature allows a baby to hold its head upright, and developing the lumbar curvature allows it to learn to walk.

Characteristics of a "typical" vertebra

The vertebrae in the cervical, thoracic and lumbar regions of the vertebral column are unique in several ways, but they all have certain features in common. They all have a *body, vertebral arch,* and several *processes* (Figure 10-7).

The **vertebral body** is the thick, anterior part of a vertebra that bears the weight of structures superior to it. In a superior view, the vertebral body appears somewhat oval-shaped, whereas in a lateral view it appears more rectangular. In the living body, a thin

THE AXIAL SKELETON

(a) Lateral and inferior view

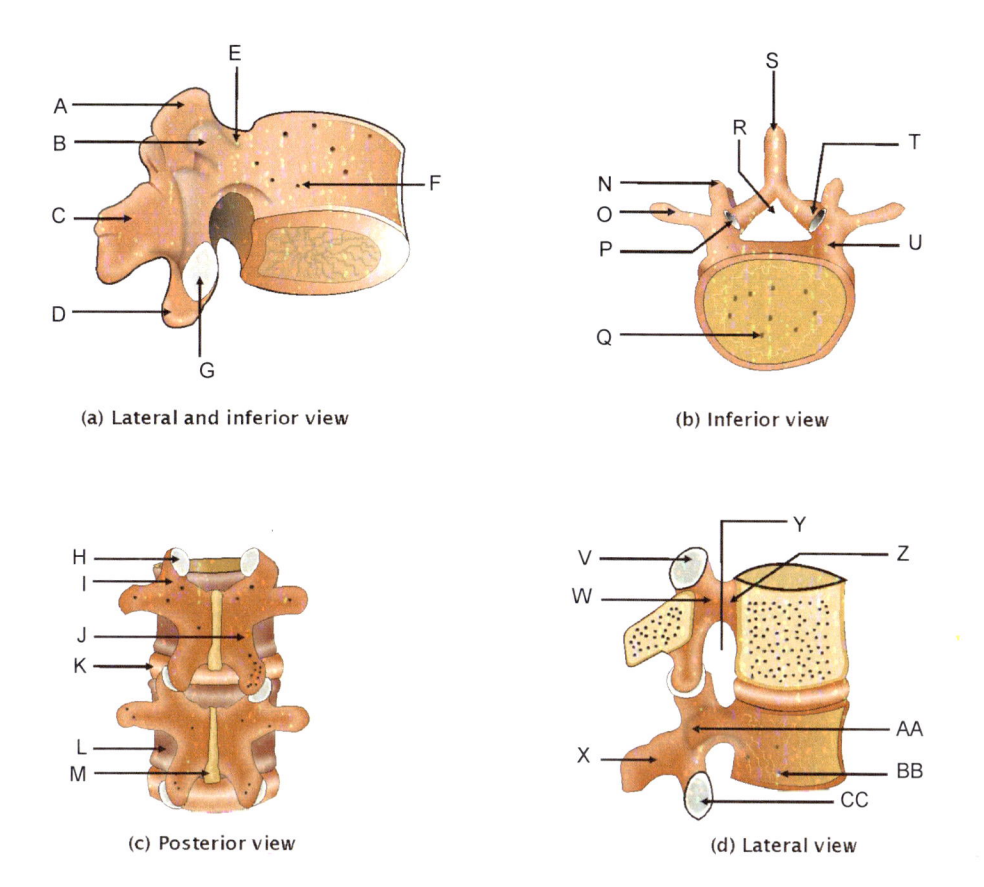

(b) Inferior view

(c) Posterior view

(d) Lateral view

Figure 10-7. Features of vertebrae

layer of compact bone tissue covers the sides of the vertebral body, while pads of fibrocartilage, called *intervertebral discs*, cover its superior and inferior surfaces. Spongy bone tissue comprises the internal portion of the vertebral body; this spongy tissue is easily visible on a dried vertebra that no longer has intervertebral discs attached to it. Cervical vertebrae have the smallest bodies; thoracic vertebra have medium-sized bodies; and lumbar vertebrae have the largest bodies. You can easily discern an increase in vertebral body size as you scan down the vertebral column from the skull to the sacrum. This progressive increase in size is logical since vertebrae that are more inferior in position must support more weight than vertebrae that are more superior in position.

The **vertebral arch** is posterior to the vertebral body and, along with the vertebral body, forms a large opening, the **vertebral foramen**. Within the vertebral column, vertebral foramina of the cervical, thoracic, and lumbar vertebrae align to form the *vertebral canal*, through which the spinal cord passes. The right and left vertebral **pedicles** (PED-i-kulz, *pedic-*, little feet) form the lateral walls of the vertebral arch and extend from the posterior, lateral sides of the vertebral body. Two prominent notches are visible on each pedicle's superior and inferior surface, respectively. The superior notch of one vertebra lines up with the inferior notch of the next highest vertebra to form an **intervertebral foramen**, which serves as a passageway for a spinal nerve. Remember that a *single* vertebra has a vertebral foramen, but it takes two vertebrae to make an intervertebral foramen. The right and left vertebral **laminae** (LAM-i-nē; "thin plates," singular is **lamina**) form the posterior walls of the vertebral arch.

Individual vertebrae display a number of processes, which may include a *spinous process, transverse processes*, and *articular processes*. A **spinous process** (SPĪ-nus; "thorny"), a tapered projection extending posteriorly from the vertebral arch, arises from the junction of the right and left laminae. The knobby projections that are visible beneath the skin covering your backbone are spinous processes of your vertebrae. Two **transverse processes** (one on each lateral side of the vertebra), arise at the junction of a pedicle and a lamina. The transverse processes are so-named because they orient along the vertebra's transverse (horizontal) plane. The spinous process and the transverse processes are important as attachment sites for muscles that bend the vertebral column.

Cervical, thoracic, and lumbar vertebrae each have four *articular processes*, which allow them to interact with adjacent vertebra. Each articular process has a smooth surface, an **articular facet** (FAS-et; "little face"), which articulates with an adjacent bone. Facets on superior articular processes of one vertebra articulate with facets on inferior articular processes of the vertebra immediately superior to it. (An exception is the first cervical vertebra (C_1), which articulates with the occipital condyles of the skull.) Vertebral facets act like little doorstops; that is, they work together to *restrict* movement of the spine. The facets are one (but not the only) reason why your spinal column doesn't topple over like a stack of dominoes. When you hyperextend your spine (i.e., bend backwards), for example, the superior and inferior vertebral facets of adjacent vertebrae "lock" together, resisting further movement.

Intervertebral discs and longitudinal ligaments

In an adult, pads of fibrocartilage called **intervertebral discs** separate most vertebrae from one another; exceptions are the first and second cervical vertebrae, and the sacral and coccygeal vertebrae. Altogether, intervertebral discs comprise about a fifth of the vertebral column's length. An intervertebral disc does not adhere directly to a vertebra, but rests on a thin layer of hyaline cartilage that attaches to the body of the vertebra. The superior and inferior surfaces of the vertebral body are also concave, with a slightly elevated ridge around the rim. This shape allows an intervertebral disc to penetrate slightly into the body of the vertebrae. Consequently, the vertebrae can "grip" the intervertebral disc and are less likely to experience excessive side-to-side or front-to-back sliding.

Intervertebral discs are thinnest in the thoracic region and thickest in the lumbar region, but they all have two major regions: an outer *annulus fibrosus* and an inner *nucleus pulposus*. The **annulus fibrosus** (AN-ū-lus, "ring;" fī-BRŌ-sus) consists of a thin outer layer of dense, fibrous connective tissue surrounding a thicker layer of fibrocartilage. The **nucleus pulposus** (pul-PŌ-sus; *pulp-*, flesh) at birth consists of a soft, gelatinous material, but this is gradually replaced by fibrocartilage after about age 10. Intervertebral discs cushion the vertebral bodies and allow the vertebral column to bend. Two extremely strong bands of dense regular connective tissue, the *longitudinal ligaments*, hold adjacent vertebral bodies together.

CERVICAL VERTEBRAE

The seven cervical vertebrae, numbered C_1 (most superior in position) through C_7 (most inferior), are the smallest and lightest of the nonfused vertebrae. Their relatively compact size reflects that the cervical vertebrae only need to support a small percentage of the body's weight that is comprised by the head. Although cervical vertebrae are relatively small, they have the largest vertebral foramina. This structural feature accommodates the spinal cord, which is widest near the head. The first two cervical vertebrae (C_1 and C_2), are "atypical" cervical vertebrae, because each has unique features.

The Atlas. The **atlas (C_1)** is the most superior cervical vertebra. Just as Atlas, a giant in Greek mythology, supported the world on his shoulders, the cervical atlas supports the base of the skull on its facets. The atlas lacks a vertebral body and a spinous process; therefore, it also lacks pedicles and laminae. Instead, the atlas has an **anterior arch** and a **posterior arch** that connect to two **lateral masses**. The arches and lateral masses join to form a large, circular vertebral foramen. The atlas has the largest vertebral foramen of all vertebrae; which is necessary because the spinal cord passing through it is thickest near the foramen magnum of the skull.

There are no articular processes on the atlas. In their place, each lateral mass has a large **superior articular facet** that articulates with an occipital condyle on the occipital bone. This articulation allows you to nod your head up and down (but not side-to-side). A

THE AXIAL SKELETON

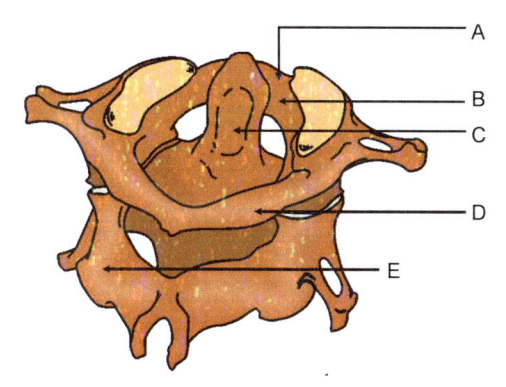

Figure 10-8. Atlas and axis

transverse process containing a transverse foramen extends laterally from each lateral mass. Each lateral mass also possesses an inferior articular surface that articulates with a superior articular surface of the axis.

The Axis. The **axis (C_2)**, the second cervical vertebra, is more similar to other cervical vertebrae (C_3-C_7), because it has a vertebral body, spinous process, pedicles, and laminae. The axis is slightly heavier or more "massive" than the atlas, which it supports on two superior articular surfaces. A prominent projection, the **dens** (denz; "toothlike") or **odontoid process** (ō-DON-toyd), extends superiorly from the body of the axis into the vertebral foramen of the atlas. A small facet on the anterior arch of the atlas articulates with the dens. This articulation between the atlas and the dens of the axis acts as a pivot, allowing you to rotate (twist) your head from side-to-side. A transverse ligament holds the dens against the anterior arch of the atlas, allowing the head to turn side to side. Like most of the other cervical vertebrae, the axis has a *bifid* (BĪ-fid; "split") spinous process. Extending inferiorly from the vertebral body where each pedicle and lamina unites is an inferior articular process, which contains an inferior articular facet. These two facets articulate with the superior articular facets of C_3.

C_3 to C_7. Vertebrae C_3-C_7 are considered "typical" cervical vertebra, because they share similar features. In superior view, the body of a typical vertebra looks oval shaped. The anterior surface is slightly convex, while the posterior surface is either flat or slightly concave.

As with the axis, the spinous processes of C_3-C_6 are bifid. In some cases, the spinous process of C6 tapers to a single blunt end. The spinous process of C_7 is noticeably longer than those of the other cervical vertebrae and can be seen or felt as a distinct knob on the inferior, posterior neck. For this reason, C_7 is called the **vertebra prominens** (PROM-i-nenz; "projecting"). It serves as a landmark that indicates the boundary between the cervical and thoracic portions of the spine. The *nuchal ligament* connects the posterior arch of the atlas and the spinous processes of the axis and other typical cervical vertebrae to the occipital bone, and it assists skeletal muscles in holding the head upright. Various skeletal muscles also attach to the spinous processes of the cervical vertebrae.

The right and left transverse processes of all seven cervical vertebrae have an opening, the **transverse foramen**, through which vertebral arteries and veins pass into and out of the brain. No other vertebrae have foramina in their transverse processes. Immediately posterior to each transverse process are the superior and inferior articular processes, each of which has a smooth articular facet.

THORACIC VERTEBRAE

The 12 thoracic vertebrae numbered T_1 (most superior) through T_{12} (most inferior) form the middle and longest portion of the vertebral column. T_1 articulates superiorly with C_7; and T_{12} articulates inferiorly with the first lumbar vertebra (L_1). Thoracic vertebrae are larger than cervical vertebrae and have nearly circular vertebral foramina. The two transverse processes project slightly posteriorly, and each bears a facet that serves as part of the posterior articulation for a rib. Thoracic vertebrae have relatively long spinous processes, some of which (T_2 – T_8) project at steeply inferior angles. You may be able to feel (or view in a mirror) the thoracic spinous processes as a vertical row of bumps along your spine.

Each thoracic vertebra has left and right inferior articular processes at the points where the pedicles join the laminae. The *inferior* articular processes have facets that articulate with the *superior* articular facets on an adjacent, inferior thoracic vertebra. The pairs of articular facets meet in a nearly vertical (frontal) plane, a configuration that enables the thoracic vertebrae to rotate around the spine's vertical axis. In other words, the thoracic vertebra's inferior and superior articular facets make it possible for you to twist your torso from side to side. In addition to their articular facets, thoracic vertebrae have **costal facets** (KOS-tal; "rib"), which articulate with the ribs. Vertebrae $T_1 – T_9$ each have six costal facets.

LUMBAR VERTEBRAE

The five lumbar vertebrae, numbered L$_1$ (most superior) through L$_5$ (most inferior), form the "lower back" portion of the vertebral column, between the thoracic region and the sacrum. The body of a typical lumbar vertebra is much more massive than the body of any other type of vertebra. This is advantageous because the lumbar vertebrae must support most of the body's weight above the hips. The lumbar vertebral body is oval shaped with a relatively flat superior and inferior surface. The lumbar vertebral foramina are triangle shaped and larger than those of thoracic vertebrae (but smaller than in cervical vertebrae).

Although the spinous and transverse processes of a lumbar vertebra are shorter than the same processes on the thoracic vertebrae, they are much wider in the vertical plane. In other words, if you were sculpting these processes in clay, you could create this flattened look by pinching the clay between your thumb and index finger. This structural feature creates more bone surface to which large skeletal muscles can attach. These muscles exert tremendous tension on the spinous and transverse processes to maintain the lumbar curvature and to maintain an erect posture.

Like thoracic vertebrae, lumbar vertebrae have articular processes containing vertically pitched facets that articulate with adjacent vertebrae. However, the articular facets of lumbar vertebrae face each other in different planes than those of the thoracic vertebrae. Between adjacent thoracic vertebrae, an anterior-facing superior articular facet meets a posterior-facing inferior articular facet. But between adjacent lumbar vertebrae, a medial-facing superior articular facet meets a lateral-facing inferior articular facet. Consequently, very little rotational movement is possible. On the other hand, the orientation of the lumbar articular facets does not impede anterior or posterior bending of the lumbar spine. You can demonstrate this with a simple experiment: Press your medially facing palms ("superior articular facets") firmly against the sides of an immovable object, such as a refrigerator ("inferior articular facets"). While keeping your shoulders perpendicular to your palms, try twisting your torso back and forth; it can't be done. However, you can bend forward or back if you let your hands slide up and down along the sides of the refrigerator.

The vertebral foramen of a lumbar vertebra is diamond shaped, and it is smaller than that of a cervical or thoracic vertebra. The smaller size of the lumbar foramen reflects the fact that the spinal cord at the lumbar level of the vertebral column is relatively narrow. In an adult, the spinal cord ends at the level of L$_1$ or L$_2$; however, numerous nerves extend inferiorly through the vertebral foramina of L$_3$-L$_5$, through the sacrum and to the coccyx.

THE SACRUM

Moving inferiorly from the lumbar region, we find a large, heart-shaped bone, the **sacrum** (SĀ-krum) (Figure 10-9).

In ancient cultures, the sacrum was considered a sacred bone (*sacr-*, sacred), one that could not be destroyed but would be part of the body after a person rises from the dead. During childhood, five

(a) Posterior Surface (b) Lateral Surface (c) Anterior Surface

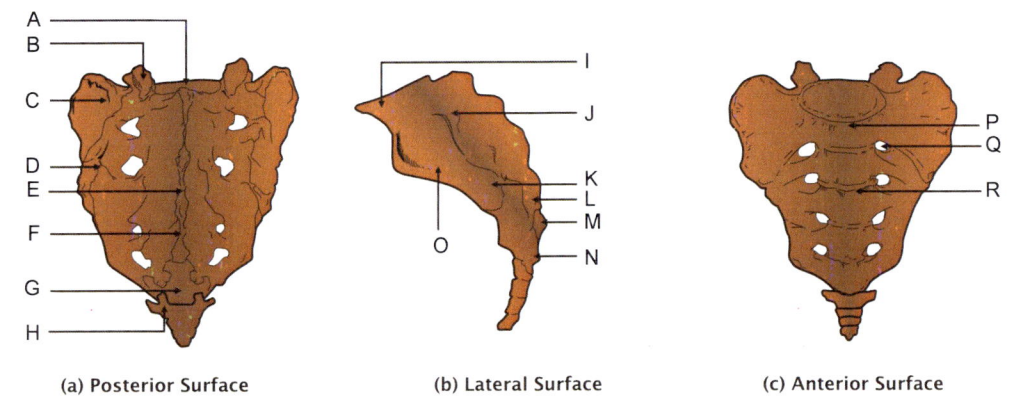

Figure 10-9. The sacrum

THE AXIAL SKELETON

sacral vertebrae, numbered S_1 (most superior) through S_5 (most inferior), grow as separate bones. However, during the mid-to-late teenage years, the sacral vertebrae fuse into a single bone, the sacrum. Its odd-looking wedge shape makes the sacrum a sturdy attachment point that divides the weight of the body supported by the vertebral column between the lower limbs (via the pelvic bones).

The sacrum is widest at its superior end, the **base**, and it is narrowest at the inferior end, the **apex**. You may recognize these terms as applying to a triangle. In this case, the sacrum would be like an upside-down triangle. The transverse processes of adjacent sacral vertebrae fuse together to form a sacral wing or **ala** (Ā-la; "wing") on each side of the sacrum. When viewed anteriorly, the alae (Ā-lē) resemble the spread wings of a bat.

The superior, anterior edge of the vertebral body of S_1 forms a circular lip, the **sacral promontory** (PROM-on-tor-ē). The extent to which the sacral promontory projects anteriorly is useful in distinguishing a female's pelvis from a male's pelvis. The sacral promontory projects shallowly in a female pelvis, which is advantageous because it allows more room within the pelvic cavity for a developing fetus.

A tube called the **sacral canal** passes internally through the sacrum, from the base to the apex. The superior opening of the sacral canal is between the two superior articular processes and is posterior to the sacral promontory. The canal's inferior opening is the **sacral hiatus** (hī-Ā-tus; *hiat-*, gap), visible near the apex on the posterior surface. Small horn-like projections, the **sacral cornua** (KOR-noo-a; singular is *cornu*; "horn"), guard the lateral edges of the sacral hiatus. The cornua are vertebral lamina of S_5 that did not fuse. Numerous nerves extending inferiorly from the spinal cord, which ends near L_2, pass through the sacral canal. Some nerves exit through the sacral hiatus, but most pass through *intervertebral foramina* in the lateral walls of the sacral canal and then exit through the **sacral foramina**. Four sacral foramina align vertically on each side of the midline between the medial and lateral sacral crests.

COCCYX

The **coccyx** (KOK-siks) is a triangular-shaped bone inferior to the sacrum and consists of 3-5 fused *caudal vertebrae* (KAW-dal; *caud-*, tail). The coccyx is so named (*coccy-*, cuckoo) because it looks like the bill of a cuckoo bird, but most people simply call it the *tailbone*. The small caudal vertebrae, numbered Co_1 (most superior in position) through Co_4 (most inferior), usually fuse when a person is in the mid-to-late twenties. The coccyx is one attachment site for the gluteus maximus muscles on which you sit, and for several muscles that support the visceral organs in the pelvic cavity. Table 10-4 summarizes the vertebrae and their features.

Table 10-4. Comparison of Cervical, Thoracic, and Lumbar Vertebrae

Feature	Cervical Vertebrae	Thoracic Vertebrae	Lumbar Vertebrae
Location	Neck	Posterior chest	Inferior back
Articulations	Occipital bone, C-vertebrae, T1	Ribs, C1, T-vertebrae, L1	T12, L-vertebrae, sacrum
Vertebral body	Smallest (absent in C_1), oval	Medium, heart shaped, Facets for ribs	Largest, oval shaped
Vertebral foramen	Largest, triangular	Medium size, circular	Smallest, diamond-shaped
Transverse foramen	Present	Absent	Absent
Spinous process	Short (absent in C1), some are split, project down	Long, pointed, project down	Short, blunt, project out
Transverse processes	Have transverse foramina Articular facets	No foramina Additional facets for ribs	No foramina Articular facets

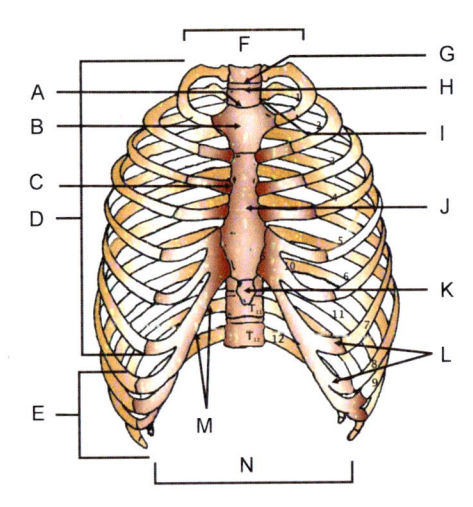

Figure 10-10. The ribs and sternum

THE THORACIC CAGE

Whereas a treasure chest surrounds and protects valuable jewels, your body's chest, called the **thorax** (THŌ-raks, "chest"), surrounds and protects vital organs such as your heart and lungs. The part of the axial skeleton that forms the thorax is the **thoracic cage** (thō-RAS-ik), so named because most of its bones, the *ribs*, appear like the bars of an animal cage. In addition to protecting internal organs, the thoracic cage supports parts of the appendicular skeleton and provides attachment sites for muscles of the neck, torso, and arm.

The thoracic cage forms four major parts: the *thoracic vertebrae*, the *ribs*, their *costal cartilages*, and the *sternum*. As we discussed earlier, thoracic vertebrae (T_1-T_{12}) form the posterior, midline portion of the thoracic cage, and they anchor the ribs posteriorly.

The ribs

A **rib** is a flexible, curved, flat bone that forms the bony wall of the thoracic cavity and serves as an attachment site for skeletal muscles (Figure 10-10). Certain skeletal muscles pull the ribs farther apart, which causes the thoracic cage to "expand" (move outward), drawing air into the lungs. Other skeletal muscles pull the ribs closer together, which causes the thoracic cage to "collapse" (move inward), forcefully expelling air out of the lungs. You can easily see the out-and-in movements of your own thoracic cage when you take deep breaths.

No two ribs look exactly alike. They are all flat bones, however, consisting of a layer of spongy bone (diploë) sandwiched between two layers of compact bone. The most superior ribs on each side curve gently. The superior pair of ribs, their *costal cartilages*, the first thoracic vertebra, and the superior part of the sternum form the boundary of the **superior thoracic aperture**; this is the opening where the neck and thoracic cavity meet. The most inferior pair of ribs, along with the cartilages extending from the inferior six pairs of ribs, form the rim of the **inferior thoracic aperture**. The muscular *diaphragm* attaches to this rim and separates the thoracic cavity from the abdominal cavity.

There are twelve pairs of ribs, numbered 1 (most superior pair) through 12 (most inferior pair). The anterior end of a rib consists of varying lengths of hyaline cartilage, the **costal cartilage**, which may or may not articulate with the sternum. Ribs 1-7 are called the **true ribs**, or *vertebrosternal ribs* (VER-te-brō-STER-nal), because their costal cartilages articulate directly with the sternum, forming a complete or "true" cage-like structure. Ribs 8-12 are called the **false ribs**, because their costal cartilages do not articulate directly with the sternum. Each of the costal cartilages of ribs 8-10 attaches to the costal cartilages of the immediately superior rib; therefore, false ribs 8-10 are also called *vertebrochondral ribs* (VER-te-brō-KON-dral). Because the costal cartilages of false ribs 11 and 12 do not attach to other costal cartilages, these ribs are often called *floating ribs* or *vertebral ribs*.

STERNUM

The **sternum** (STER-num; "breastbone") is the sword-shaped, flat bone on the anterior side of the thoracic cage (see Figure 10-10). The sternum anchors the costal cartilages of ribs 1-7, and serves as attachment sites for several skeletal muscles from the head and neck. In children and young adults, the sternum consists of three individual bones: the *manubrium*, *body*, and *xiphoid process*; in older adults, these bones fuse to form a single bone.

The **manubrium** (ma-NOO-brē-um; "handle") is the diamond-shaped, superior portion of the sternum. If the two inferior bones of the sternum look like a sword, then the manubrium looks like its handle. Each superior, lateral edge of the manubrium contains a

THE AXIAL SKELETON

broad depression, called a **clavicular notch** (kla-VIK-ū-lar), which articulates with the medial end of a clavicle (collarbone). At the superior end of the manubrium, between the clavicular notches, is a depression called the **jugular notch** (JUG-ū-lur; "throat"). You can feel this notch where your throat meets the top of your chest.

Each lateral edge of the manubrium contains two shallow depressions, called **costal notches** that articulate with *costal cartilages* on the ends of ribs. The costal cartilage of rib 1 articulates with a costal notch near the middle edge of the manubrium. A portion of the second rib's costal cartilage articulates with a costal notch at the inferior, lateral end of the manubrium. Two large muscles that turn the head right or left attach to the manubrium's superior, anterior portion. In addition, several smaller muscles that aid in swallowing extend from the throat and attach to the manubrium.

The sternum's long, middle portion is its **body**. The **sternal angle** is the site where the inferior end of the manubrium meets the superior end of the sternal body. You can feel the sternal angle as a slight projection. The costal cartilages of rib pairs 2-7 attach to costal notches along the lateral margins of the sternal body. The **xiphoid process** (ZĪ-foyd; *xiph*, sword) is the pointed, inferior end of the sternum. A portion of the muscular respiratory diaphragm attaches to the xiphoid's deep surface. A large abdominal muscle attaches to the xiphoid's superficial surface.

TOPICS TO KNOW FOR CHAPTER 10 (THE AXIAL SKELETON)

alae
alveolar processes
alveolar sockets
annulus fibrosus
anterior arch
anterior cranial fossa
anterior fontanel
anterior nasal spine
articular facet
articular processes
atlas
axial skeleton
axis
basilar part of occipital
basioccipital process
bones of the skull
calvaria
carotid canal
caudal vertebrae
cervical curvature
clavicular notch
clivus
coccygeal vertebrae
coccyx
condylar process
condyle
coronal suture
coronoid process
costal cartilage
costal facets
costal notches
cranial bones
cranial cavity
cranium
crest

cribriform plate
crista galli
dens
epicondyle
ervical vertebrae
ethmoid air cells
ethmoid bone
external acoustic meatus
external occipital protuberance
facet
facial bones
false ribs
fissure
floating ribs
fontanels
foramen
foramen lacerum
foramen magnum
foramen ovale
foramen rotundum
foramen spinosum
fossa
fovea
frontal bone
frontal processes
frontal sinus
frontozygomatic suture
glabella
greater wings
hard palate
head of rib
hyoid bone
hypoglossal canal
importance of axial skeleton
incisive fossa

inferior nasal conchae
inferior orbital fissure
inferior thoracic aperture
infraorbital foramen
infraorbital margin
intermaxillary suture
internal acoustic meatus
internasal suture
intervertebral discs
intervertebral foramen
jugular foramen
jugular notch
lacrimal bones
lacrimal fossa
lacrimal groove
lambdoid suture
lamina
lateral masses
lesser wings
ligamentum nuchae
line
longitudinal ligaments
lumbar vertebrae
mandible
mandible angle
mandible body
mandibular foramen
mandibular fossa
mandibular notch
mandibular symphysis
manubrium
mastoid air cells
mastoid fontanel
mastoid process
maxillae

maxillary sinus
meatus
mental foramen
mental protuberance
metopic (frontal) suture
middle cranial fossa
middle nasal conchae
middle nasal conchae
nasal aperture
nasal bones
nasal cavity
nasal septum
nasal spine
nasolacrimal canal
neck
notch
nuchal ligament
nuchal lines
nucleus pulposus
occipital bone
occipital condyles
occipitomastoid sutures
odontoid process
olfactory foramina
optic canals
orbits
palatine bones
paranasal sinuses
parietal bones
pedicles
perpendicular plate
petrous part of temporal bone
posterior arch
posterior cranial fossa
posterior fontanel
process
protuberance

pterygoid processes
ramus
regions of the vertebral column
rib
true ribs
sacral canal
sacral cornua
sacral curvature
sacral foramina
sacral hiatus
sacral promontory
sacral vertebrae
sacrum
sacrum apex
sacrum base
sagittal suture
sella turcica
septal cartilage
sinus
skull
sphenoid bone
sphenoid sinuses
sphenoidal fontanel
spine
spine
spinous process
squamous part of frontal bone
squamous sutures
sternal angle
sternal body
sternum
structure of the spine
styloid process
stylomastoid foramen
sulcus
superior articular facet
superior nasal conchae

superior orbital fissure
superior thoracic aperture
supraorbital foramen
supraorbital margin
sutural bone
suture
temporal bones
temporal lines
temporal process
thoracic cage
thoracic curvature
thoracic vertebrae
thorax
transverse foramen
transverse processes
tubercle
tuberosity
tympanic part of temporal bone
typical vertebra
vertebra prominens
vertebrae
vertebral arch
vertebral body
vertebral canal
vertebral column
vertebral foramen
vertebral laminae
vertebral ribs
vertebrochondral ribs
vertebrosternal ribs
vomer
wormian bone
zygomatic arch
zygomatic bones
zygomatic process
zygomaticomaxillary suture

CHAPTER 11

The Appendicular Skeleton

You could visualize the axial skeleton as two containers on a stick; i.e., the skull and thoracic cage attached to the vertebral column. But the skeleton's other division, the **appendicular skeleton** (ap-en-DIK-û-lar; *append-*, hang upon), could be thought of as a set of powerful tools. Your upper limbs (arms, forearms, and hands) and lower limbs (thighs, legs, and feet) help you to interact with your surroundings. The chief use of the upper limbs is to manipulate objects. But humans are *bipeds* (two-legged walkers) who chiefly use their lower limbs for locomotion and bodily support. As a set of tools, the limbs are so functionally sophisticated that at birth an infant doesn't know how to work them. From the earliest twitches of a newborn's fingers, to a toddler's comical waddle, to a teenager's nerve-wracking attempts learning to drive, people spend nearly the first two decades of life perfecting the use of their limbs.

The functional capabilities of the limbs are the result of the interaction of bones, muscles, and nervous tissue. In this chapter, we will discuss the bones of the limbs and the girdles that attach the limbs to the axial skeleton. The appendicular skeleton consists of 126 bones (about 60% of the body's bones). Anatomists classify appendicular skeletal bones into four groups: the *pectoral girdle*, *upper limbs*, *pelvic girdle*, and *lower limbs* (Figure 11-1).

THE PECTORAL GIRDLE

The **pectoral girdle** (PEK-to-ral; *pector-*, breast) or **shoulder girdle**, connects the upper limbs to the thoracic cage of the axial skeleton. A "girdle" is a belt-like structure; indeed, the pectoral girdle forms a semi-circular ring around the superior part of the thoracic cage. The right and left halves of the pectoral girdle each consist of a **clavicle** (KLAV-i-kl), or collarbone, and a **scapula** (SKAP-ū-la), or shoulder blade. Each scapula articulates with the bone in the proximal end of the arm. In addition, the pectoral girdle serves as an attachment site for skeletal muscles that move the upper limbs and the head.

Think about the flexibility and wide range of motion that your shoulders display when you shrug, throw a ball, or lift something over your head. These actions would be impossible (or at least difficult) if the pectoral girdle's bones were rigidly attached to the thoracic cage. (To appreciate this, lock one shoulder firmly in place, and using the arm on the same side try to touch the end of a pencil to your nose!) The

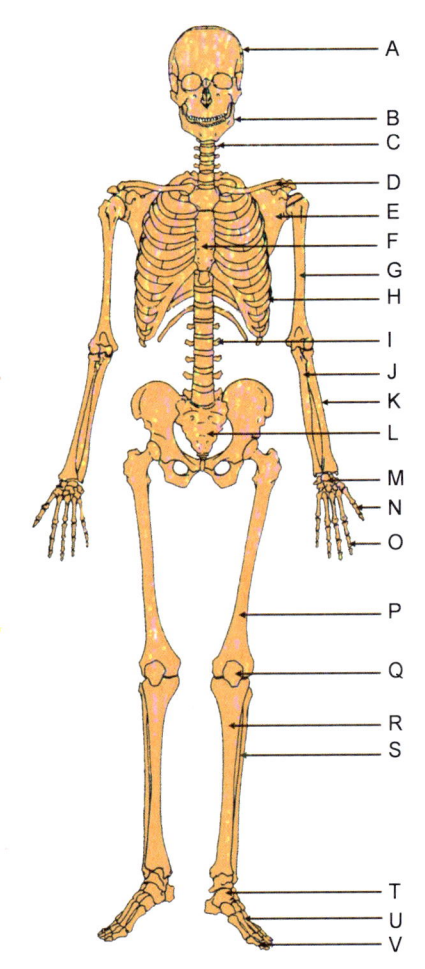

Figure 11-1. Appendicular skeleton

pectoral girdle articulates with the thoracic cage only at the manubrium. Ligaments and skeletal muscles in the shoulders, back, and anterior part of the chest hold the rest of this girdle in place. In a sense, much of the pectoral girdle "floats" above the thoracic cage, and these relatively loose attachments are what give your shoulders their exceptional mobility.

CLAVICLES

The two **clavicles** are slender, curved bones that anchor the pectoral girdle to the sternum (Figure 11-2).

Each clavicle lies horizontally along the anterior, superior surface of the thoracic cage. A clavicle's lateral, **acromial end** (a-KRŌ-mē-al; *acro-*, tip; *-omos*, shoulder) is flattened and articulates with the acromial process of the scapula. The acromial end of the clavicle looks like the flat handle of a key, which can help you remember the root meaning of clavicle (*clavic-*, key). Just as a key inserts into a lock, the medial, **sternal end** of the clavicle inserts into the clavicular notch of the manubrium. In a sense, the manubrium is the "lock" in the axial skeleton that holds the pectoral girdle in place.

Clavicles act as lateral supports. As the shoulder attempts to move anteriorly or medially, the clavicle presses against the sternum, restricting excessive movement. Pushing objects with the arms exerts compression stress on the clavicles, and it will cause the body of the clavicle to thicken over time. However, excessive compression force, as could occur when breaking a fall with an outstretched arm, can break the clavicle. In the same way that a broken rafter (brace) can cause a roof to collapse, a broken clavicle can cause the shoulder to collapse.

> **Note:** The clavicles of a bird articulate with each other, but not the sternum, thus forming the bird's "wishbone." This arrangement allows a greater range of motion in the pectoral girdle that a bird needs to beat its wings.

SCAPULAE

The two **scapulae** are large, triangular-shaped, flat bones lying on the posterior surfaces of ribs 2-7. Scapulae anchor the upper limbs to the pectoral girdle and serve as attachment sites for skeletal muscles of the back and shoulder. A scapula looks like the blade of an axe or shovel, which is how it gets its common name, the shoulder blade (Figure 11-3).

The anterior surface of the scapula rests over the posterior ribs and forms a slightly concave depression, the **subscapular fossa**. A major skeletal muscle that helps rotate the arm attaches to this fossa. The sharp edges of the body are called *borders*. The **lateral border** is closest to the axillary (armpit) region, the **medial border** is closest to the vertebral column, and the **superior border** forms the more horizontal edge superiorly.

Laterally, the superior border ends in an abrupt indentation, the **suprascapular notch**, through which a nerve passes. Lateral to the scapular notch, a **coracoid process** (KOR-a-koyd; *corac-*, beak) extends anteriorly and laterally; this process is an attachment site for

THE APPENDICULAR SKELETON

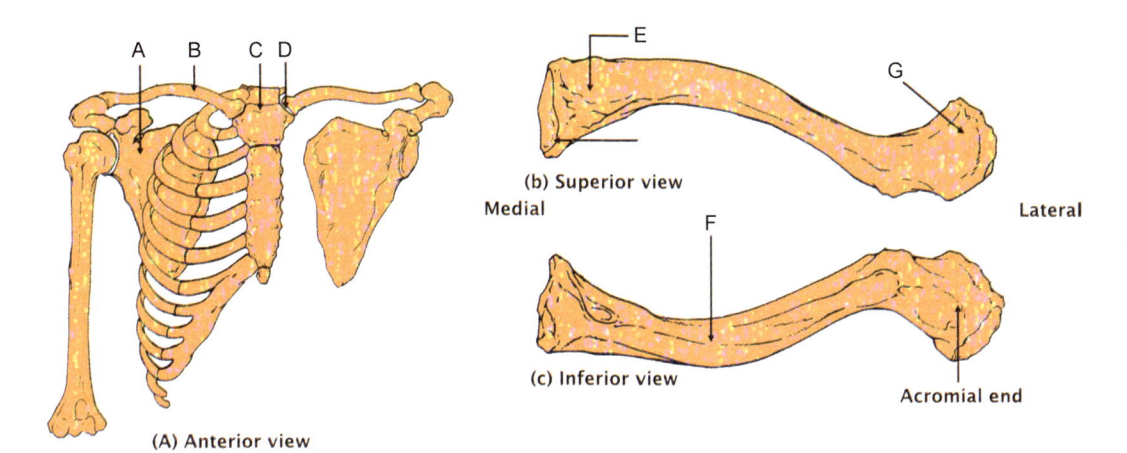

Figure 11-2. The pectoral girdle

several arm muscles. A circular depression, called the **glenoid cavity** (GLEN-oyd; *glen-*, socket), at the lateral angle receives the head of the humerus (arm bone).

Posteriorly, the scapula has a prominent ridge, the **spine** that ends laterally as the **acromion** (a-KRŌ-mē-on). The acromion forms the bony tip of the shoulder and articulates with the acromial end of the clavicle. The ditch-like depression superior to the spine is the **supraspinous fossa** (soo-pra-SPĪ-nus; *supra-*, above); whereas, the surface inferior to the spine forms the **infraspinous fossa** (in-fra-SPĪ-nus; *infra-*, below). Each of these fossae is an attachment site for a major skeletal muscle that rotates the arm.

THE UPPER LIMB

In the same way that the branches of a tree become progressively smaller farther away from the trunk, the bones in the upper limb become progressively smaller farther away from the pectoral girdle. Each upper limb consists of 30 bones, including 1 large bone in the arm, 2 slightly smaller bones in the forearm and 26 small bones in the hand (including the wrist). All of the bones in the upper limb, except for the wrist bones, are *long bones*; whereas the wrist bones are *short bones*.

HUMERUS

The **humerus** (HŪ-mer-us; "shoulder") is the longest and thickest bone in the upper limb, and it is the only bone in the arm, extending from the shoulder to the elbow (Figure 11-4).

The humerus articulates with the scapula proximally (superiorly), and with the forearm bones distally (inferiorly). The proximal epiphysis of the humerus has a smooth, rounded **humeral head** that articulates with the glenoid cavity of the scapula.

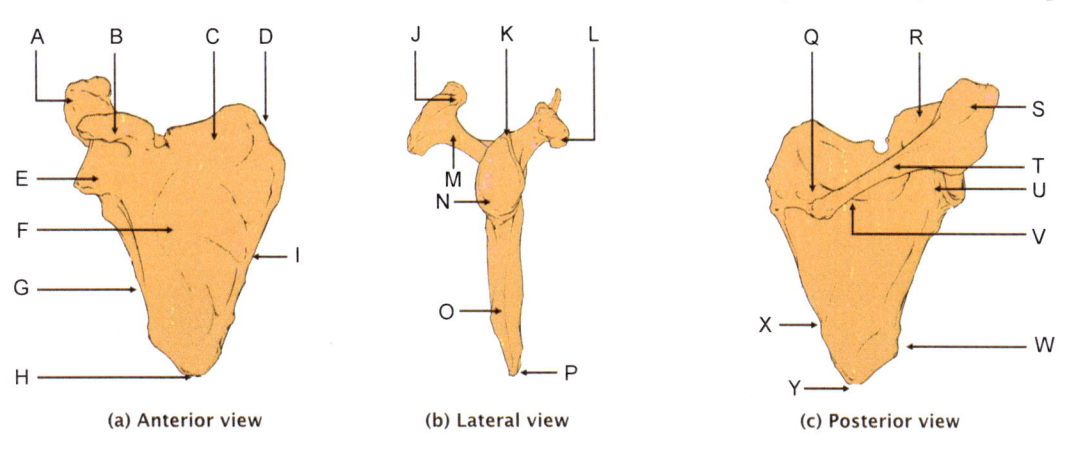

Figure 11-3. The scapulae

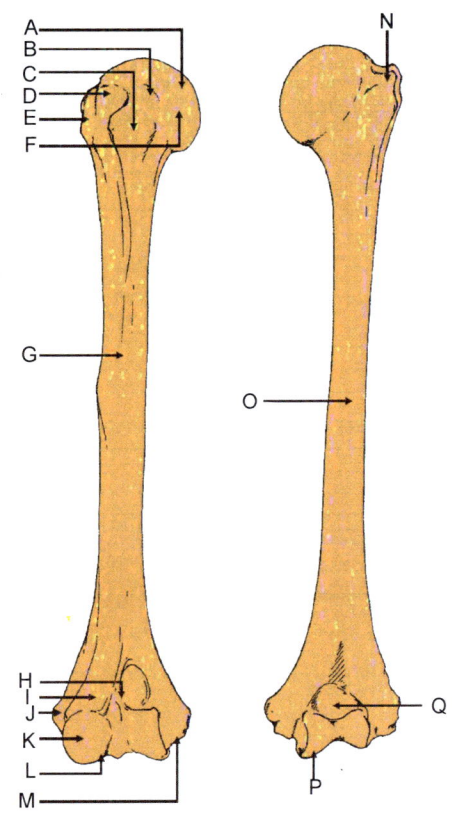

Figure 11-4. The humerus

The part of the humerus where the head meets the rougher surface of the epiphysis is the **anatomical neck**. Lateral to the anatomical neck on the superior end of the humerus is the **greater tubercle**, and slightly inferior and medial to this tubercle is the smaller **lesser tubercle**; both tubercles are attachment sites for skeletal muscles that move the arm. An **intertubercular groove** separates both tubercles and supports a muscle tendon. Inferior to the lesser tubercle, the humerus begins to narrow in a region called the **surgical neck**. This name suggests the medical significance of this region of the humerus, for it is a common site of fractures. More importantly, the surgical neck marks the position of the *epiphyseal plate* of a growing humerus.

There are two notable landmarks on the shaft of the humerus. About halfway along the shaft's lateral side is a roughened region called the **deltoid tuberosity**, so named because the large deltoid muscle attaches to it. A major nerve leading to the forearm passes along a shallow, longitudinal depression, the **radial groove**, on the posterior surface of the shaft.

The distal epiphysis of the humerus is the location of the **condyle of the humerus**, which consists of a set of articular surfaces and their adjacent fossae. The most prominent articular surface on the medial, anterior, distal epiphysis is the **trochlea** (TRŌK-lē-a). This condyle gets its name (*trochle-*, pulley) because part of the ulna (a forearm bone), glides over the trochlea like a rope moving over the grooved wheel of a pulley. Next to the trochlea on the lateral, anterior surface of the epiphysis is the **capitulum** (ka-PIT-ū-lum; *capit-*, head), named for its resemblance to a tiny, baldhead. The head of the radius (another forearm bone) articulates with the capitulum.

The condyle of the humerus also contains fossae that make room for the proximal ends of the forearm bones when the elbow joint bends or straightens. When you bend your forearm, the **coronoid fossa**, immediately superior to the trochlea, receives the coronoid process of the ulna. At the same time, the **radial fossa**, immediately superior to the capitulum, receives the head of the radius. On the posterior side of the distal epiphysis is the large **olecranon fossa** (ō-LEK-ra-non), which receives the ulna's helmet-shaped olecranon process (*-cranon*, helmet-like) when the elbow is straight.

To either side of the condyle of the humerus, two very prominent epicondyles (*epi-*, along side of) serve as attachment points for a variety of muscles that move the upper limb. The **medial epicondyle** is a rounded knob located medially and slightly superiorly to the trochlea. You can easily feel this epicondyle projecting from the medial surface of your elbow. Between the medial epicondyle and trochlea is a sulcus (groove) through which the ulnar nerve passes; you probably know this nerve as your "funnybone," because hitting it causes a sharp tingling sensation. The **lateral epicondyle** is lateral and slightly superior to the capitulum.

ULNA

The forearm contains two long bones, the *radius* and the *ulna*, and both of these articulate with the humerus proximally, and with *carpals* (wrist bones) distally. The radius and ulna are parallel to one another when the forearm is in anatomical position (Figure 11-5).

The **ulna** (UL-na; "elbow") is the larger, medial bone in your forearm. It extends from the elbow to the

THE APPENDICULAR SKELETON

medial, proximal part of the wrist (the little finger-side). You can feel your ulna along its entire length using your finger, beginning past the medial epicondyle and moving distally.

> **Note**: The letter "L" in "ulna" can help you recall this bone's position. The u**L**na runs media**L**ly along your forearm, between the troch**L**ea of the humerus and the **L**ittle finger.

The ulna is widest at its proximal end, where it displays two processes. The larger **olecranon process** forms the point of your elbow posteriorly. The olecranon process fits into the olecranon fossa on the posterior, distal end of the humerus when the elbow is straight. Distal to the olecranon process on the anterior side of the ulna is the pointed **coronoid process**. Like the coronoid process of the mandible, the coronoid process of the ulna gets its name because it looks like a bird's beak. The coronoid process fits into the coronoid fossa on the anterior, distal end of the humerus when the elbow is bent.

The ulna has two distinct notches at its proximal end. Between the olecranon and coronoid processes is the deep, U shaped **trochlear notch**, which articulates with the trochlea of the humerus. A much smaller and shallow **radial notch** on the lateral side of the coronoid process receives the head of the radius.

The distal end of the ulna is much narrower than its proximal end. The **ulnar head** is the knob-like projection that you can feel and sometimes see just superior to the wrist on the medial, posterior side of your forearm. A short, pointed **styloid process** projects distally from the ulnar head's posterior side, but it is not an attachment point for muscles or ligaments. Instead, a disc of fibrocartilage covers the styloid process and prevents it from rubbing against the carpal bones of the wrist.

RADIUS

The radius (RĀ-dē-us; "ray") is the smaller lateral bone in the forearm. In a way, the radius is sort of like an upside-down ulna: the ulna is widest at its proximal end, whereas the radius is widest at its distal end. The narrow proximal end of the radius has a wheel-like **radial head** that articulates with the capitulum of the humerus and the radial notch of the ulna. Like a wheel, the radial head can "spin" against the capitulum and radial notch, allowing the radius to rotate along its length. Inferior to the radial head, the radius narrows to form the **radial neck**. Immediately inferior and medial to this neck is the **radial tuberosity**, a rough prominence to which a large muscle from the arm attaches.

The diameter of the radial shaft (diaphysis) gradually increases toward its distal end. Like the ulna, the radius has a pointed **styloid process** at the distal end, but it is on the lateral side instead of the medial side. The **ulnar notch** on the lateral, distal end of the radius receives the head of the ulna.

CARPALS

Besides helping you to manipulate your environment, your hands are exquisitely expressive tools of communication. In most cultures, people wave, chop, flutter, curl, clench, and clap their hands to intensify the emotion behind their speech. And of course, the deaf unfold a beautiful and richly expressive language solely through hand motions. Although only three bones (the humerus, radius, and ulna) compromise three-quarters of the upper limb's total length, the

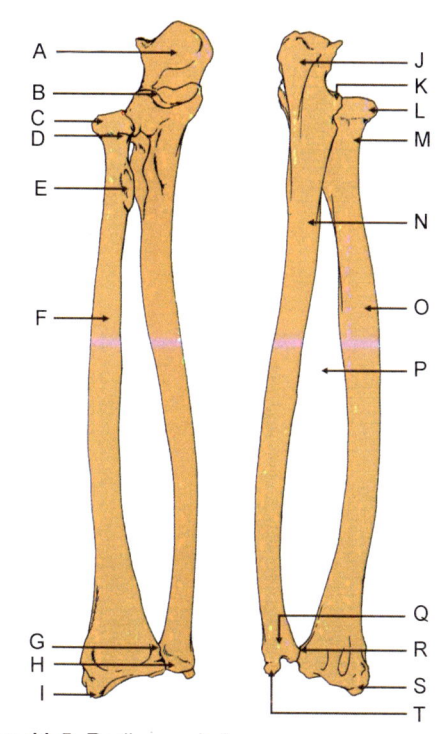

Figure 11-5. Radius and ulna

majority of bones in the upper limb are found in the hands. Each hand contains 26 bones: 8 *carpal bones* (wrist bones), 5 *metacarpal bones* (palm bones), and 14 *phalanges* (finger bones) (Figure 11-6).

The **carpal bones** (KAR-pal; "wrist"), or simply **carpals**, are tiny, short bones that form the joint between the hand and the forearm, and that allow the hand to bend at the wrist. The carpals are arranged in two irregular rows, including four carpals in the proximal row and four carpals in the distal row. The proximal row of carpals, from lateral to medial, includes the *scaphoid, lunate, triquetrum,* and the *pisiform*. The distal row of carpals articulates with the metacarpal bones, and from lateral to medial includes the *trapezium, trapezoid, capitate,* and the *hamate*.

In the proximal row of carpals, the **scaphoid** (SKAF-oyd) is the largest carpal. It is boat-shaped (*scaph-*, boat) and articulates with the distal end (including the styloid process) of the radius. Medial to the scaphoid is the **lunate** (LOO-nāt; "moon"), so-named because it looks like a crescent moon. The lunate articulates with the radius. Medial to the lunate is the **triquetrum** (trī-KWĒ-trum; "three-cornered"), a three-sided bone that articulates with a pad of fibrocartilage located at the distal end of the ulna. Lateral to the triquetrum is the **pisiform** (PIS-i-form), the smallest carpal, so named because it looks like a small pea (*pisi-*, pea). You can feel your pisiform bone as a small knob on the medial, proximal corner of your hand's anterior surface.

In the distal row of carpals, the **trapezium** (tra-PĒ-zē-um) is the most lateral in position. Its name suggests that this bone looks like a small, four-sided table (*trapez-*, table). You can remember the trapezium as the carpal closest to the thumb because trapez<u>ium</u> rhymes with th<u>umb</u>. The trapezium's proximal side articulates with the scaphoid.

Medial to the trapezium is the **trapezoid** (TRAP-a-zoyd), another carpal that looks like a four sided table. Medial to the trapezoid is the **capitate** (KAP-i-tāt), the longest carpal bone. This carpal is so-named (*capit*, head) because its smooth, rounded proximal end looks like a tiny head. Medial to the capitate is the **hamate** (HAM-āt; hook), named for a hook-like projection on its anterior surface.

Your hand is able to move at the wrist because carpal bones can slide over one another. A small degree of wrist movement is due to skeletal muscles pulling directly on some of the carpals. Most wrist movement, however, results when skeletal muscles in the forearm pull on metacarpals inferior to the carpals.

> **Note**: The carpals are "low" (inferior) on the upper limb, so you can remember their names (starting with the scaphoid and ending with the hamate) using the first letters of the phrase: **S**wing **L**ow **T**o **P**lace **T**he **T**iny **C**arpals **H**ere.

Posterior View

Anterior View

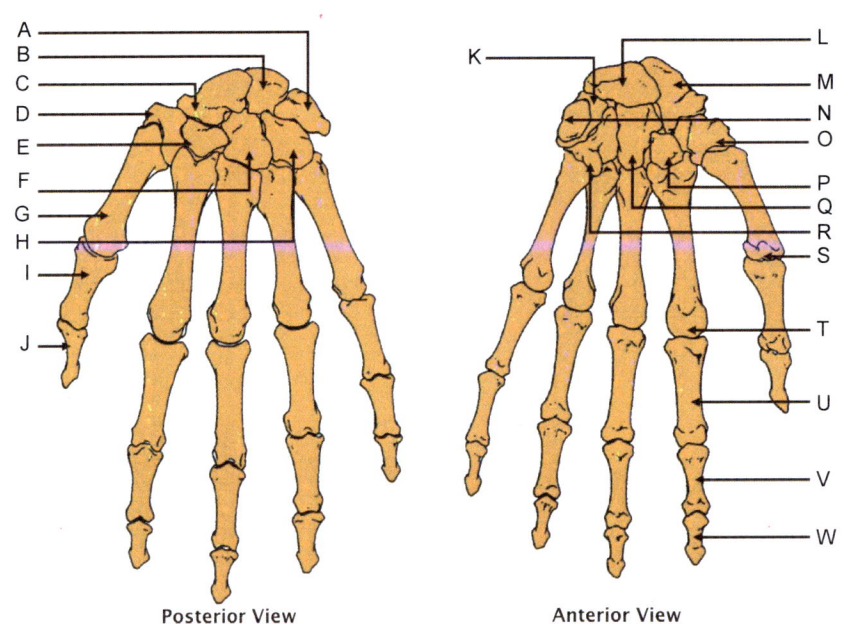

Figure 11-6. Bones of the hand

THE APPENDICULAR SKELETON

METACARPALS

Five **metacarpal bones** (MET-a-kar-pal; *meta-*, beyond) extend distally from the carpals to form the palm of the hand. These tiny long bones are numbered 1 (the most lateral) through 5 (the most medial). The proximal end of a metacarpal is its **base**, which articulates with a distal carpal bone. The bases of adjacent metacarpals also articulate with each other. A metacarpal's rounded, distal end, the **head**, is larger than its base and articulates with the proximal bone of a *digit* (finger). When you make a fist, the head of each metacarpal forms one of the knuckles (revealing how the word "knucklehead" came about). The region between the base and the head is the **body** of the metacarpal.

Tendons of skeletal muscles in the forearm attach to the heads of metacarpals, allowing the hand to bend at the wrist when the muscles contract. Other skeletal muscles connect the metacarpals to bones in the digits. Contracting different groups of these muscles enable you to spread your fingers apart or pull them together.

PHALANGES

The five slender, distal extensions of your upper limbs are called **digits** (DIJ-its), or fingers. The hand's digits are numbered in the same manner as the metacarpals. Digit 1, the **pollex** (POL-eks), or the thumb, is the most lateral, and digit 5, the little finger, is the most medial. The bones that support each finger are called **phalanges** (fa-LAN-jēz; "lines of soldiers"); each bone in a finger is a **phalanx** (FĀ-lānks). The pollex has two bones, a **proximal phalanx** and a **distal phalanx**. All other digits have three phalanges, including a **middle phalanx** between the proximal and distal phalanx.

> **Note**: Recall that the palm faces forward and the hand's dorsal surface faces backward in anatomical position. Accordingly, anatomists describe the anterior view of the hand as the *palmar view* and the posterior view of the hand as the *dorsal view*.

THE PELVIS AND PELVIC GIRDLE

Whereas the pectoral girdle joins the upper limbs to the axial skeleton, the **pelvic girdle** (PEL-vik) joins the lower limbs to the axial skeleton. The pelvic girdle lies between the sacrum and the femurs (thighbones), and consists of two **hipbones**, or **coxal bones** (KOK-sal; *coxa-*, hip).

Each hipbone lies on opposite sides of the body's midline and articulates with the opposite hipbone, anteriorly, at a joint called the *pubic symphysis*. Each hipbone articulates with the sacrum, posteriorly. The pelvic girdle is not synonymous with the *bony pelvis*, but is a significant part of it. The **bony pelvis** is the massive bowl-shaped ring of bone that includes the pelvic girdle, sacrum and coccyx.

> **Note**: The bones of the pelvic girdle are sometimes called **innominate bones** (i-NOM-i-nāt; *in-*, without; *nomin*, name); or literally, bones with no name!

By this point, you may have noticed that the pelvic girdle looks massive and rigid compared to the shoulder girdle. Why is this so? Consider that when you lift one leg off the ground as you walk, the pelvic bone on the opposite side temporarily bears all the body's weight above the sacrum *plus* the weight of the raised leg. Hence, a pelvic bone needs to be strong, and it needs a rigid articulation with the sacrum to transmit weight to the lower limb. The bones of the shoulder girdle, on the other hand, bear relatively little weight. They are loosely attached to the thoracic cage, permitting the wide range of shoulder motion that's needed for you to make full use of your upper limbs. In short, the pelvic girdle emphasizes strength over flexibility, while the shoulder girdle emphasizes flexibility over strength.

Bones of the Pelvic Girdle

Each hipbone of the pelvic girdle forms from the fusion of three bones: the large *ilium*, the medium-size *ischium*, and the slightly smaller *pubis*. The united bones form two of the pelvic girdle's most conspicuous features. A portion of the all three bones forms a large, cup-shaped socket, the **acetabulum** (as-i-TAB-ū-lum), on the lateral side of a hipbone. The acetabulum articulates with the ball-shaped proximal end of the femur (thighbone).

> **Note**: "Acetabulum" (*aceta-*, vinegar) literally means "vinegar cup," because it looks like the small bowl that was set on dinner tables during Roman and medieval times. The cup was filled with vinegar to clean grease from the fingers following a meal.

Immediately inferior to the acetabulum, curved extensions of the ischium and pubis unite to form a large opening, the **obturator foramen** (OB-too-rā-tor). This foramen is so named (*obtur-*, stop up) because it is covered over by a thick web of ligaments. The pectoral girdle is shown in Figure 11-7.

ILIUM

The **ilium** (IL-ē-um; "the flank") is the largest part of a hipbone, forming its entire superior half. The ilium has two main regions: the *wing* and the *body*. The first feature of the ilium that you probably notice is its large **wing**, or **ala** (Ā-la, "wing"). When you look at the pelvis, the paired alae (Ā-lē) looks like the outstretched wings of a butterfly. The wing of the ilium has several prominent features marking sites where skeletal muscles attach. The **iliac crest** is a thick ridge running along the superior and lateral edge of the wing. You can feel your iliac crests by pressing on the sides of your abdomen slightly inferior to the level of your navel. The anterior, medial surface of the ilium forms a large depression, the **iliac fossa**, which serves as a point of attachment for a skeletal muscle that moves the thigh.

The ilium has four *spines* that serve as attachment sites for skeletal muscles, and they serve as important landmarks during physical exams and pelvic surgeries. The names of the spines describe their location on the ilium. The **anterior superior iliac spine** is the most anterior projection on the hipbone, and marks the anterior end of the iliac crest. Inferior and slightly medial to this spine is the **anterior inferior iliac spine**, which is slightly superior and anterior to the acetabulum. The **posterior superior iliac spine** is the most posterior projection on the hipbone, and marks the posterior end of the iliac crest. Slightly inferior and anterior to this spine is the **posterior inferior iliac spine**. Immediately inferior to the posterior inferior iliac spine is the deep **greater sciatic notch** (sī-A-tik; "hip"). The body's largest nerve (the sciatic nerve) passes through this notch.

ISCHIUM

The **ischium** (ISH-ē-um or IS-kē-um; "hip") is the second largest bone to become part of a hipbone, forming its posterior, inferior half. The ischium has three main regions: the *body*, the *ischial tuberosity*, and the *ramus*. If we compare the lateral view of the ischium to an elephant head and trunk, the ischium looks like the elephant's head. The superior end of the ischial body joins with the ilium, while the anterior end joins with the pubis. Laterally, a portion of the ischial body forms another third of the acetabulum. A sharp **ischial spine** projects from the posterior rim of the ischial body. A thick ligament connects the ischial spine to the sacrum, helping to support the internal organs within the pelvic cavity.

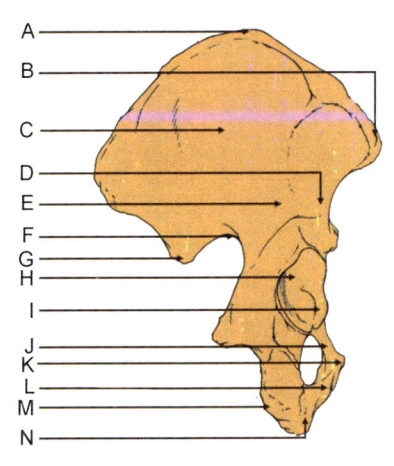

Right OS Coxae, Lateral View

Right OS Coxae, Medial View

Figure 11-7. The pelvic girdle

THE APPENDICULAR SKELETON

The **ischial tuberosity** is the ischium's most noticeable feature, and can be likened to the thickest part of an elephant's trunk. The ischial tuberosity bends at the inferior end of the ischium, and this is where hamstring muscles from the thigh attach to the hipbone. A small indentation called the **lesser sciatic notch** is located between the ischial tuberosity and the ischial spine. This notch serves as a passageway for nerves and blood vessels. By the way, if you are sitting while reading this sentence, you are sitting on your ischial tuberosities.

The **ramus** of the ischium (ischial ramus) is like the tapering, distal end of the elephant's trunk. It extends anteriorly from the ischial tuberosity to connect to the pubis. The ischial ramus and the body form the border for the posterior half of the obturator foramen.

PUBIS

The **pubis** (PŪ-bis), or **pubic bone**, is the smallest part of a hipbone, forming its anterior, inferior half.

> **Note**: The pubis derives its name from the *pubes* (Pū-bēz), the hairs that grow around the region of the external genitalia following *puberty*, the onset of sexual maturity.

From a lateral view, the pubis looks like a smaller, mirror image of the ischium. The right and left pubic bones articulate at the pubic symphysis. The angle formed by the right and left pubic bones at the pubic symphysis is called the **pubic arch**.

TRUE PELVIS AND FALSE PELVIS

The bony pelvis has a complex three-dimensional structure, so it may seem hard to visualize the spaces in the body that the pelvis surrounds. To simplify matters, anatomists make a distinction between the *false pelvis* and the *true pelvis*. The wide-but-shallow **false pelvis** is the abdominal cavity space superior to the **pelvic brim** and inferior to the wings of the alae. You can follow the pelvic brim by tracing a line from the sacral promontory, along the inner margin of either ilium, and continuing along the superior edge of either pubis to the superior margin of the pubic symphysis. The narrower-but-deeper **true pelvis** is the pelvic cavity space inferior to the pelvic brim.

To be sure that you understand that the true and false pelves (PEL-vēz) represent *spaces*, it may help to visualize the bony pelvis as two stacked and tilted bowls. The space inside the rim of the upper bowl is analogous to the false pelvis; in the body, parts of the small and large intestines occupy this space. On the other hand, the space inside the rim of the lower bowl is analogous to the true pelvis; the urinary bladder and parts of the reproductive system occupy this space.

The true pelvis has an inlet and an outlet, which suggests the route in the female pelvis through which the fetus passes during birth. The larger, superior opening of the true pelvis is the **pelvic inlet**, which is formed by the pelvic brim. The **pelvic outlet** is the smaller, inferior opening of the true pelvis. You can outline the border of the pelvic outlet by tracing anteriorly from the tip of the coccyx, to either of the ischial spines and ischial tuberosities; then continue anteriorly along either of the inferior pubic margins to the inferior margin of the pubic symphysis.

There are notable differences between the pelvis of a male and the pelvis of a female. Some of these differences relate to differences in body size; however, a number of differences relate to the female's childbearing capability.

Table 11-1 lists the characteristics of the male and female pelves and Figure 11-8 illustrates them.

THE LOWER LIMB

Genetic traits influence the size and shape of the lower limb bones, but the mechanical stress these bones receive every day ultimately determines their strength. Recall that mechanical stress triggers bone remodeling, a process that can make bones stronger. The body's weight compresses the bones of the lower limbs whenever a person stands, a situation that is analogous to resting the head of a hammer on top of a nail head. But striking forces, such as those that occur when a person jogs, multiply many times over the weight-bearing force on the lower limb bones, a situation that is analogous to striking the same nail head with a hammer. It should come as no surprise, therefore, that the lower limb bones grow many times stronger than the upper limb bones as a person matures.

Table L7-5: Comparison of Male and Female Pelvis

Feature	Female	Male
Acetabula	Smaller, farther apart	Larger, closer together
Bone texture	Smoother	More prominent markings
Bone thickness	Thinner, lighter	Thicker, heavier
Coccyx	Straighter, more flexible	More curved, less flexible
Greater sciatic notch	Larger, wider	Smaller, narrower
Iliac crest	Less arch superiorly Less curve anteriorly	More arch superiorly More curve anteriorly
Iliac fossa	Shallower	Deeper
Ilium	Broader wings	Narrower wings
Ischial spines	Farther apart	Closer together
Ischial tuberosities	Longer	Shorter
Obturator foramen	more triangular	more heart-shaped
Pelvic inlet	Wider, more oval	Narrower, more triangular
Pelvic outlet	Wider	Narrower
Pubic arch	Greater than 90°	Less than 90°
Sacrum	Wider, shorter, straighter	Narrower, longer, more curved

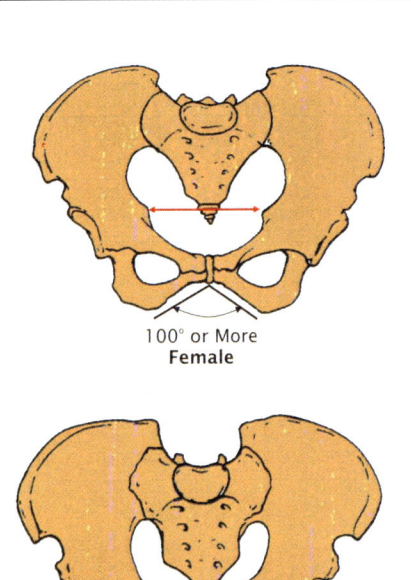

100° or More
Female

90° or Less
Male

Figure 11-8. Differences in the male and female pelvis

Apart from the differences in thickness and strength, the arrangement of different-size bones in the lower limb is similar to that in the upper limb. The largest bones are proximal to the axial skeleton, while the smallest bones are distal to the axial skeleton. In addition, each lower limb consists of 30 bones, the same quantity as in each upper limb. Each lower limb consists of 1 bone in the thigh, 2 bones in the leg, 1 large sesamoid bone in the knee, and 25 bones in the foot (which includes the ankle). Notice that the foot contains one less bone than the hand; however, the sesamoid bone in the knee makes up the difference in number.

FEMUR

The **femur** (FĒ-mur; "thigh") is the longest and thickest bone in the body, and it is the only bone in the thigh (Figure 11-9).

The femur articulates with the hipbone proximally and with the tibia (shinbone) distally. The **head** is ball-shaped and projects medially and superiorly from the

THE APPENDICULAR SKELETON

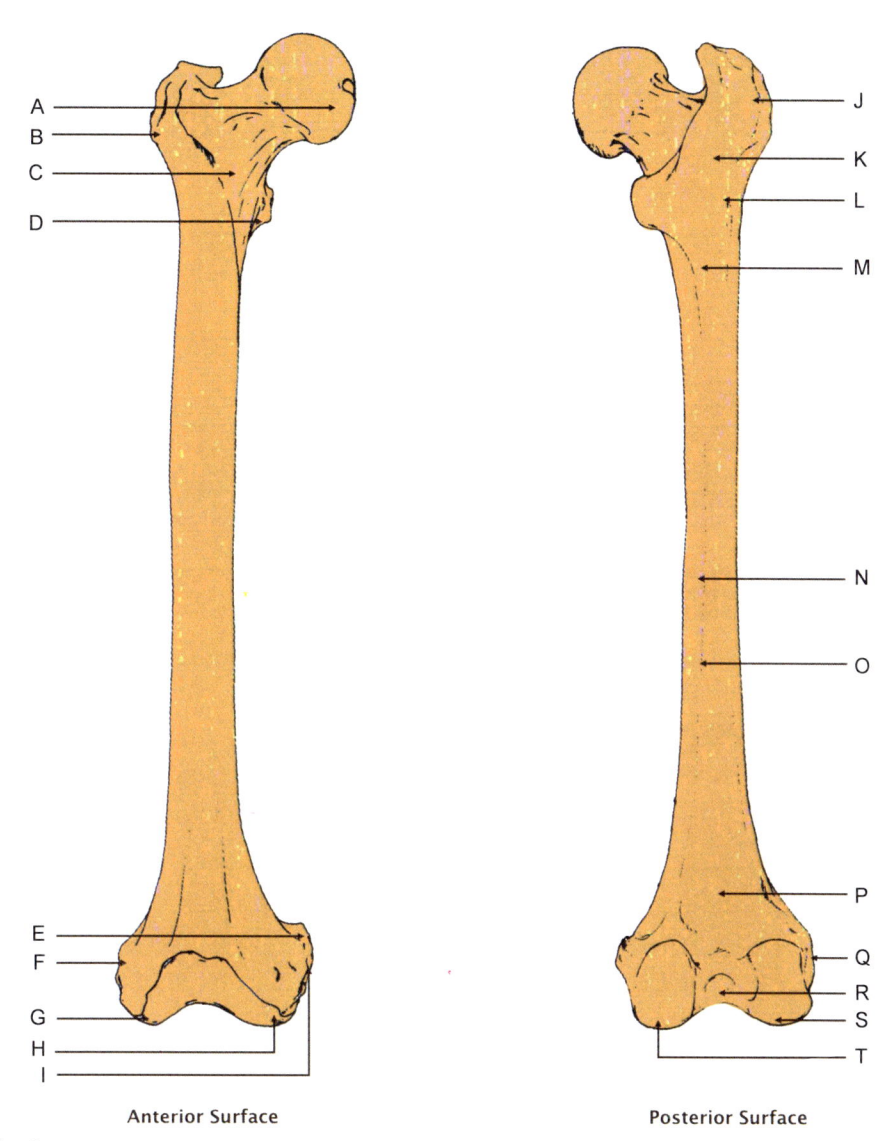

Figure 11-9. The femur

proximal epiphysis. The femoral head fits snuggly into the acetabulum of the pelvic girdle. The **fovea capitis** (FŌ-vē-a KA-pi-tis; *fov-*, pit) is a small pit in the medial part of the femoral head. A short ligament extends from the fovea capitis that anchors the femoral head to the acetabulum.

Continuing distally along the femur, the **neck** is a constricted region connecting the femoral head to the remainder of the proximal epiphysis. Lateral and superior to the neck is a large process called the **greater trochanter** (trō-KAN-ter). You can feel the greater trochanter on the lateral side of your thigh, about a hand's length inferior to the iliac crest. The **lesser trochanter** is a smaller process on the medial side of the epiphysis, inferior to the femoral neck. Both trochanters serve as attachment points for various hip and thigh muscles.

The **shaft** (diaphysis) extends medially at an oblique angle from the proximal epiphysis to end distally at the knee joint. As a result, both femurs converge toward the knees so that most of the body's weight balances on a relatively narrow base directly over the feet. This arrangement facilitates walking and running. For example, stand in anatomical position and then start jogging in place naturally and you'll notice your head and torso bob up and down along your body's midline. Then try jogging with your knees spread one foot apart, and you'll notice your body shifting in an awkward side-to-side motion. This would not be an efficient way to run.

The anterior surface of the femoral shaft is relatively smooth compared to its posterior surface. A roughened line, the **gluteal tuberosity**, on the superior, posterior surface of the shaft marks the attachment site for a large hip muscle. A long ridge, the **linea aspera** (LIN-ē-a, "line"; AS-per-a, "rough"), extends distally from the gluteal tuberosity and marks the attachment site for large hip muscles.

The most prominent features at the distal end of the femur are the two large condyles that articulate with a large bone in the leg (inferior to the knee). The **lateral condyle** of the femur aligns with the greater trochanter superiorly, while the **medial condyle** aligns with the femoral head. The outer edges of the lateral condyle and the medial condyle form rounded processes, the **lateral epicondyle** and the **medial epicondyle**, respectively.

A deep **intercondylar fossa** exists between the condyles on the posterior side and holds ligaments that stabilize the knee joint. A smooth, shallow **patellar surface** unites between the condyles on the anterior side, and marks the site where the patella (kneecap) articulates with the femur. The patellar surface can help you decide from which side of the body an individual femur originated. The femoral head always faces medially, so if you hold the patellar surface toward you and the femoral head faces to your right, you are looking at a right femur.

PATELLA

The **patella** (pa-TEL-a; "little dish"), or *knee cap*, is a large, triangular sesamoid bone on the anterior side of each knee joint. In fact, the two patellae (pa-TEL-ē) are the body's largest sesamoid bones. As with most sesamoid bones, the patella develops within a muscle's tendon; in this case, the tendon extends from a large thigh muscle that straightens the knee. In addition to protecting the knee joint, the patella keeps the muscle tendon centered over the knee joint whenever the knee joint bends.

In anatomical position, the patella looks like an upside-down triangle. The anterior surface is convex (protrudes outward or anteriorly) and has a rough texture, serving as the attachment site for the thigh muscle's tendon. A thick ligament extends from the patella's apex and attaches to the proximal end of the tibia. When the knee bends during walking, this ligament pulls the patella inferiorly. When the knee straightens, the thigh muscle tendon pulls the patella superiorly over the knee joint. The patella's posterior surface has a smooth texture that reduces friction between the patella and the femur.

TIBIA

The leg (the region between the knee and the foot) contains two long bones, the *tibia* and the *fibula*. The tibia and fibula are parallel and articulate with one another. Only the tibia, however, articulates with other bones (the femur and a large bone in the foot). In anatomical position, the tibia is located medial to the fibula.

The **tibia** (TIB-ē-a) is so named (*tibi-*, flute) because its pipe-like shape was thought to resemble a flute. The tibia is the largest bone in the leg and is the only leg bone that articulates with the femur. Consequently, the tibia is the weight-bearing bone of the leg. The proximal epiphysis of the tibia exhibits two large condyles: the **lateral condyle** and the **medial condyle**. Each condyle has a smooth, concave *articular surface* on the posterior-superior side of the proximal epiphysis that articulates with a corresponding condyle on the distal end of the femur. Medial and lateral intercondylar tubercles form a double ridge called the **intercondylar eminence** that separates the tibial condyles from one another.

Slightly inferior and anterior to the tibial condyles, the rough **tibial tuberosity** marks the attachment site for the ligament leading from the patella. You can feel your tibial tuberosity as a small knob beneath the skin immediately inferior to the patella. Lateral to the tibial tuberosity and inferior to the lateral condyle, a small facet marks the site where the tibia articulates with the proximal end (head) of the fibula.

The distal epiphysis of the tibia is slightly narrower than the proximal epiphysis, and articulates with the talus bone of the foot. A large process, the **medial**

THE APPENDICULAR SKELETON

malleolus (ma-LĒ-ō-lus; "hammer") projects medially and inferiorly from the distal epiphysis. The medial malleolus is the large knob that most people mistake for the "inside part of the ankle," even though it is really part of the leg. The lateral side of the tibia's distal epiphysis is a shallow depression, the **fibular notch**, which articulates with the distal end (lateral malleolus) of the fibula. The inferior surface on the distal epiphysis articulates with the talus bone of the foot.

FIBULA

The **fibula** (FIB-ū-la) is the other bone in the leg, and unlike the tibia, it does not articulate with the femur or any foot bones. Hence, the fibula does not support any of the body's weight that is transmitted through the femur. This is why a person can still walk—albeit painfully—with a broken fibula. As its Latin root suggests (*fibul-*, fastener or clasp), the fibula resembles the clasp of a safety pin. The fibula serves as an attachment site for many of the skeletal muscles in the leg.

The **head** is the proximal epiphysis, and it articulates with a facet on the tibia's lateral condyle. Continuing distally, the fibular **shaft** completely ends at the distal epiphysis, which is about the same size as the fibular head. The medial surface of the fibula's distal epiphysis articulates with the fibular notch on the tibia's distal epiphysis. The **lateral malleolus** projects inferiorly from the distal epiphysis. Most people may mistake this large knob for the "outside of the ankle," but like the medial malleolus of the tibia, it is indeed part of the leg. See the leg bones in Figure 11-10.

The femur, tibia, and fibula make up four-fifths of the lower limb's total length. The patella doesn't contribute to the lower limb's length. Like the hand of the upper limb, however, most bones of the lower limb are found in the foot. Each foot contains 25 bones, including 7 *tarsal bones*, 5 *metatarsal bones*, and 14 *phalanges*.

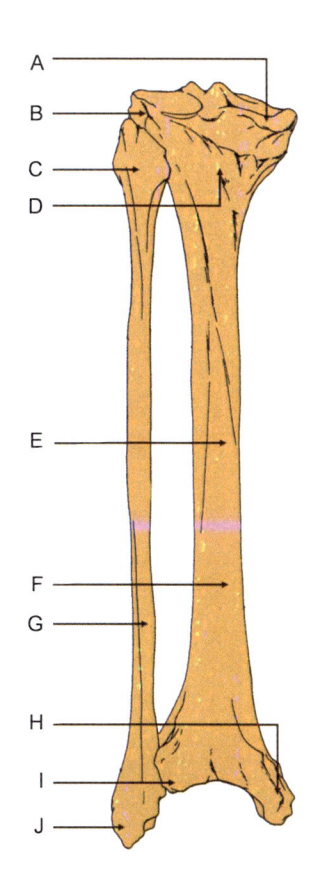

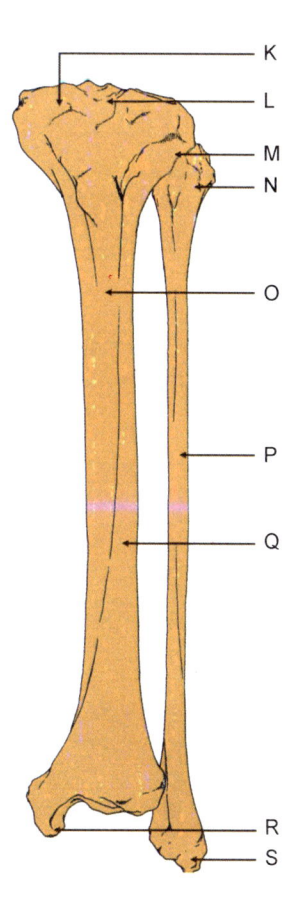

Figure 11-10. Tibia and fibula

TARSALS

The **tarsal bones** (TAR-sal; "flat surface") make up the **tarsus** (ankle). They are short bones that form the joints between the foot and the leg that allow the foot to move at the ankle. The tarsals can be grouped according to their relative sizes. The largest and most proximal tarsal bones include the *calcaneus* and *talus*. The smaller and more distal tarsals include the *navicular* and four bones that articulate with the metatarsals: the *cuboid* and the *lateral, intermediate,* and *medial cuneiforms*.

> **Note**: The following phrase may help you to remember the tarsals' names and positions (starting with the calcaneus and ending with the medial cuneiform): **C**razy **T**arsals **N**ever **C**an **L**ive **I**n **M**e.

The **calcaneus** (kal-KĀ-nē-us; "heel") is the largest and the most posterior tarsal bone. The rounded posterior and inferior projection of the calcaneus is the **calcaneal tuberosity**, the part of the foot that strikes the ground first when a person walks. The calcaneus articulates with two other tarsal bones: the talus superiorly and the cuboid bone anteriorly. A large tendon extends from the calf muscle to attach on the posterior surface of the calcaneus.

> **Note**: In anatomical position, the top of the foot (its dorsal surface) faces up while the bottom of the foot (its plantar surface) faces down. Thus, anatomists call a view looking at the top of the foot a dorsal (*not* superior) view and a view looking from below the foot a plantar (*not* inferior) view.

The **talus** (TĀ-lus; "ankle") is the second largest tarsal bone and lies on the superior surface of the calcaneus. The anterior surface of the talus articulates with the navicular bone, and the superior surface articulates with the tibia; in fact, the talus is the only tarsal bone that articulates with the tibia. For this reason, the talus bears the brunt of the body's weight and disperses it to the calcaneus and the navicular.

The **navicular** (na-VIK-ū-lar; "boat") is a curved tarsal bone that, from a plantar view, looks a bit like a canoe. The navicular's posterior surface articulates with the talus, and its anterior surface articulates with the three cuneiform bones.

Moving to the most distal tarsals, the **cuboid** (KŪ-boyd) is so-named because of its cube-like shape. The cuboid is the most lateral of the tarsal bones, and it articulates with the calcaneus posteriorly, with the lateral cuneiform and the navicular medially, and with the fourth and fifth metatarsals anteriorly.

The three **cuneiform bones** (kū-NĒ-i-form; *cunei-*, wedge; *-form*, resembles) are so named because they look like little wedges driven between the other bones of the foot. The **lateral cuneiform** articulates with the cuboid bone laterally, with the navicular bone posteriorly, with the intermediate cuneiform medially, and with the third metatarsal anteriorly. The **intermediate cuneiform** articulates with the navicular posteriorly, with the lateral cuneiform laterally, with the medial cuneiform medially, and with the second metatarsal anteriorly. The **medial cuneiform** is the most medial of the distal tarsals. It articulates with the navicular posteriorly, with the intermediate cuneiform laterally, and with the first metatarsal anteriorly. Collectively, the navicular and the cuneiform bones form the arch-shaped *instep* of the foot (Figure 11-11).

The metatarsals

Five **metatarsal bones** (MET-a-tar-sal; *meta-*, beyond) extend distally from the tarsals to form the middle portion of the foot. Like the metacarpals of the hand, the metatarsals are numbered 1 (most medial) through 5 (most lateral). The proximal end of a metatarsal is its **base**, which articulates with an anterior tarsal bone. The bases of adjacent metatarsals also articulate with each other. A metatarsal's rounded, distal end, the **head**, is larger than the base and articulates with a bone of a *digit* (toe). The region between the base and the head is called the **body** of the metatarsal.

Some metatarsals, especially the first metatarsal, often have small *sesamoid bones* on the plantar surface of their heads. The function of the sesamoid bones is unclear, but they may help reduce friction or stabilize the position of the tendons leading to the phalanges. Tendons of skeletal muscles in the leg attach to the heads of metatarsals, allowing the foot to bend at the ankle. Other skeletal muscles connect the metatarsals to bones in the digits. Contracting different groups of these muscles enable you to spread your toes apart or pull them together.

THE APPENDICULAR SKELETON

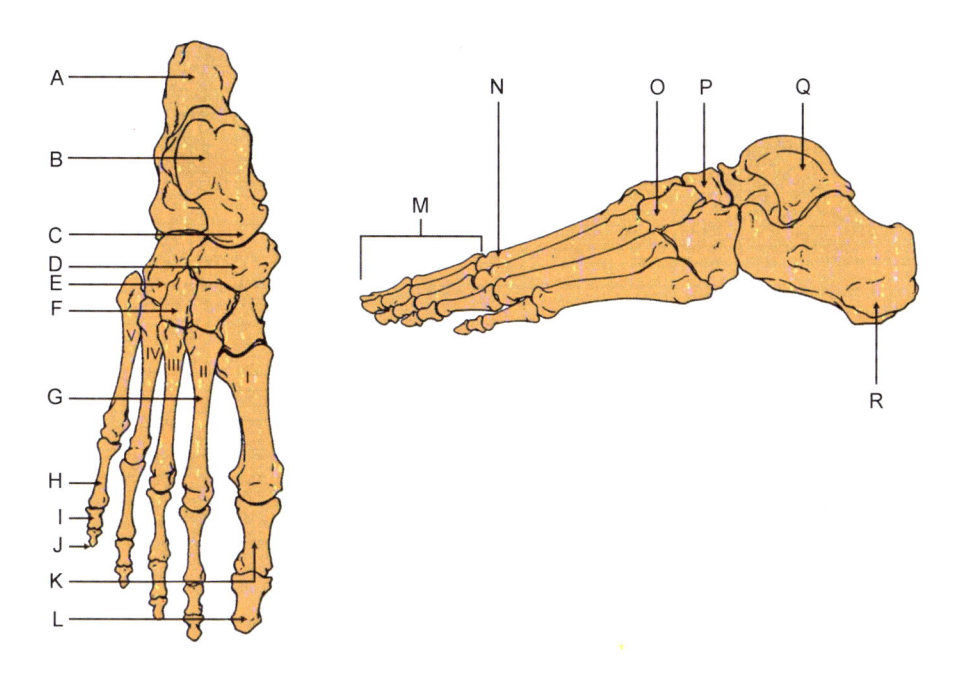

Figure 11-11. Bones of the foot

PHALANGES

The five most distal extensions of the lower limbs are called **digits** or **toes**. The foot's digits are numbered in the same order as the metatarsals. Digit 1, the **hallux** (HAL-uks) or great toe, is the most medial, and digit 5, the little toe, is the most lateral. As with the fingers of the hand, the bones that support each toe are called **phalanges**. The phalanges of the foot help a person maintain balance while standing. The hallux consists of two bones, a **proximal phalanx** and a **distal phalanx**. All the other digits of the foot consist of three phalanges, including a **middle phalanx** between the proximal and distal phalanx. Like the metatarsals, the proximal and middle phalanges have a base at the proximal end and a head at the distal end.

ARCHES OF THE FOOT

Have you ever left footprints along a sandy lakeshore, or walked along a sidewalk with bare, wet feet? If so, you probably saw that your footprints had a crescent-shaped slice missing from the medial side of each sole. You were right if you concluded that parts of your soles aren't touching the ground. Ligaments and muscle tendons in the foot pull the tarsals and metatarsals dorsally so that these bones do not align parallel to the ground. The upwardly bowed foot bones form **arches**, which are beneficial because they spread the body's weight evenly across the foot, help absorb physical impacts, and provide leverage that makes walking easier.

As a physical structure, any arch has the ability to distribute weight evenly from its center to its ends. For example, the arch of a highway bridge distributes the weight of a passing car between the bridge's ends. In the same way, because the foot has arches, the body weight bearing down on the talus spreads evenly between the calcaneus and the heads of the metatarsals. Each foot has three arches that redistribute the body's weight: two *longitudinal arches*, which run lengthwise (posterior-to-anterior), are joined together by a *transverse arch*, which runs crosswise (lateral-to-medial).

In addition to redistributing bodyweight, the arches of the foot help to put a "spring in your step" and protect soft tissues in the foot. The ligaments and various muscle tendons allow the foot's arches to remain elastic. The arches flatten slightly when a person is standing or planting the foot while walking. However, the arches spring back to their original curvature when the person sits or lifts the foot off the ground. Since the arches keep the middle portion of the foot off the ground, the anterior tarsals and the metatarsals do not compress the nerves or blood vessels in the foot.

TOPICS TO KNOW FOR CHAPTER 11 (THE APPENDICULAR SKELETON)

- acetabulum
- acromial end of clavicle
- acromion
- ala of ilium
- anatomical neck of humerus
- anterior inferior iliac spine
- anterior superior iliac spine
- appendicular skeleton
- base of metacarpal
- base of metatarsal
- body of metacarpal
- body of metatarsal
- bony pelvis
- calcaneal tuberosity
- calcaneus
- capitate
- capitulum
- carpals
- clavicles
- condyle of the humerus
- coracoid process
- coronoid fossa
- coronoid process of ulna
- coxal bones
- cuboid
- deltoid tuberosity
- digits
- distal phalanx
- false pelvis
- femoral medial condyle
- femoral medial epicondyle
- femur
- fibula
- fibular head
- fibular notch
- fibular shaft
- foot arches
- fovea capitis
- glenoid cavity
- gluteal tuberosity
- greater sciatic notch
- greater trochanter
- greater tubercle
- hallux
- hamate
- head of femur
- head of metacarpal
- head of metatarsal
- hipbones
- humeral head
- humeral lateral epicondyle
- humeral medial epicondyle
- humerus
- iliac crest
- iliac fossa
- ilium\
- infraspinous fossa
- innominate bones
- intercondylar eminence
- intercondylar fossa
- intermediate cuneiform
- intertubercular groove
- ischial spine
- ischial tuberosity
- ischium
- lateral border of scapula
- lateral condyle of femur
- lateral cuneiform
- lateral epicondyle of femur
- lateral malleolus
- lesser sciatic notch
- lesser trochanter
- lesser tubercle
- linea aspera
- longitudinal arches
- lower limb
- lunate
- medial border of scapula
- medial cuneiform
- medial malleolus
- metacarpals
- metatarsals
- middle phalanx
- navicular
- neck of femur
- obturator foramen
- olecranon fossa
- olecranon process
- patella
- patellar surface of femur
- pectoral girdle
- pelvic brim
- pelvic girdle
- pelvic inlet
- pelvic outlet
- phalanges
- phalanx
- pisiform
- posterior inferior iliac spine
- posterior superior iliac spine
- proximal phalanx
- pubic arch
- pubic bone
- pubis
- radial fossa
- radial groove
- radial head
- radial neck
- radial notch
- radial tuberosity
- radius
- ramus
- scaphoid
- scapulae
- shaft of femur
- shoulder girdle
- spine of scapula
- sternal end of clavicle
- styloid process of radius
- styloid process of ulna
- subscapular fossa
- superior border of scapula
- suprascapular notch
- supraspinous fossa
- surgical neck of humerus
- talus
- tarsals
- tarsus
- tibia
- tibial lateral condyle
- tibial medial condyle
- tibial tuberosity
- toes
- transverse arch
- trapezium
- trapezoid
- triquetrum
- trochlea
- trochlear notch
- true pelvis
- ulna
- ulnar head
- ulnar notch
- upper limb
- wing of ilium

CHAPTER 12

Joints

Try to bend your hand backwards and touch your thumb to your forearm. If you can do this, you are "double jointed." But what does that mean? Would you really have two joints where most people only have one? The answer is no. Instead, you could have really loose or stretchy ligaments holding your bones together, or you might have very shallow depressions (fossae) where bones fit into other bones. Then again, you might have a combination of these features. Being double-jointed simply means a person can move the bones at certain joints to a greater degree than most people can.

A **joint**, also called an **arthrosis** (ar-THRŌ-sis; *arthr*, joint), or **articulation** (ar-tik-ū-LĀ-shun; "fit together"), is where two or more bones come together, and the bones at a joint are said to articulate with one another. While you may have 206 bones in your skeleton, you have well over 200 joints because many of your bones articulate with more than one other bone. For example, the sphenoid bone that you learned about in the previous chapter articulates with fourteen other skull bones!

Joints serve three major purposes. First, some joints allow the skeleton to bend, making it possible to move parts of the body voluntarily. In fact, nearly everything you do voluntarily, including walking, chewing, and even turning pages in this book, requires bones to move at joints. Second, some joints allow adjacent bones to stick to one another so tightly that virtually no movement is possible. This is important in places where bones surround and protect soft internal organs. Third, some joints allow the skeleton to grow. Specifically, epiphyseal plates are special joints where growth of cartilage causes bones to grow.

While it is not practical to describe every joint in the skeleton, this chapter focuses on the structural design and functional roles of the major types of joints. Following an overview describing how joints are named and classified, we will examine each major type more closely. We will conclude by describing selected joints that play important roles in the movement of the upper and lower limbs.

NAMING AND CLASSIFYING JOINTS

Joints are injured more often than any other part of the skeleton, which make them a frequent topic of conversation in clinics and rehabilitation centers. As a result, it is beneficial for anyone, but especially those pursuing a career in the health profession, to learn the names of joints. If you learned the names of bones in the previous chapter, you will undoubtedly recognize the names of most joints, because most joints are named for their articulating bones. For example, your radioulnar joint is between the radius and ulna in your forearm, and your tibiofibular joint is between the tibia and fibula in your leg. In addition to using names of articulating bones, some joints are more commonly known by their location. For instance, your glenohumeral joint, which connects the glenoid fossa of your scapula to the head of your humerus, is better known as your shoulder joint.

A few joints have names based on guidelines other than their articulating bones or location. The *sagittal suture* (SAJ-i-tal; arrow), the joint between the two parietal bones of the skull, is named for its orientation along the body's sagittal plane. Another joint, the *lambdoidal suture* (lam-DOYD-al), which is located between the occipital bone and parietal bones, is so named because it looks like lambda (Λ), the 11th letter in the Greek alphabet.

In addition to naming joints, we can classify them according to (1) their structural design, and (2) the amount of movement possible for the articulating bones.

CLASSIFICATION OF JOINTS BY STRUCTURE

To understand how different types of joints serve different functions, we need to know about their anatomy. Two characteristics to consider when describing the general structure of a joint include (1) the presence or absence of a fluid-filled joint cavity, the *synovial cavity*, which encloses the bones articular surfaces, and (2) the type of connective tissue holding the articulating bones together. Depending on their general structure, joints are *fibrous*, *cartilaginous*, or *synovial*.

- **Fibrous joints** do not have a synovial cavity, but they are filled with dense, fibrous connective tissue. Consequently, the articulating bones united at fibrous joints do not have "free" (unbound) articular surfaces.

- **Cartilaginous joints** (kar-ti-LAJ-e-nus) lack a synovial cavity, but they are filled with cartilage connective tissue. Like at fibrous joints, the articulating bones at cartilaginous joints do not have free articular surfaces.

- **Synovial joints** (si-NŌ-vē-al) have a fluid-filled cavity between their articulating bones, meaning each bone has a free articular surface at the joint.

Over time, certain fibrous joints and cartilaginous joints ossify; that is, osseous tissue replaces the flexible connective tissue between the articulating bones. After this happens, the joint is called a **synostosis** (sen-o-STŌ-sis; *syn*, together; *osis*, condition), or **bony joint**. In short, a synostosis fuses two bones to make one bone. The cartilaginous epiphyseal plate in a developing long bone ultimately becomes a synostosis, after which time we call the joint an epiphyseal line.

CLASSIFICATION OF JOINTS BY MOVEMENT

In order for a person to perform a variety of activities, the skeleton needs different types of joints with varying degrees of mobility. A joint's **mobility** refers to how much movement the articulating bones can experience at the joint. Depending on its range of mobility, we will classify a joint as a *synarthrosis*, *amphiarthrosis*, or *diarthrosis*.

- **Synarthrosis** (sen-ar-THRŌ-sis): an *immovable* joint. In reality, no joint is completely immovable, but in synarthroses, the amount of bone movement is negligible. As the prefix "syn-" implies, the articulating bones are virtually "together." Structurally, synarthrotic joints are either fibrous or cartilaginous. In either case, connective tissue virtually fills the gap between the bones, preventing them from moving freely. In fibrous synarthroses, the collagen fibers are too short to allow much bone movement. In cartilaginous synarthroses, the binding connective tissue is hyaline cartilage, which lacks the flexibility of fibrocartilage.

- **Amphiarthrosis** (am-fē-ar-THRŌ-sis; *amphi*, both sides): *slightly movable* joint. Like synarthrotic joints, amphiarthrotic joints are filled with either fibrous or cartilaginous connective tissue. In fibrous amphiarthroses, the collagen fibers are longer and more flexible than those in fibrous synarthrotic

JOINTS

joints. In cartilaginous amphiarthroses, the binding tissue is fibrocartilage, which is more flexible than hyaline cartilage found at cartilaginous, synarthrotic joints.

- **Diarthrosis** (dī-ar-THRŌ-sis): *freely movable* joint. Unlike articulating bones at fibrous and cartilaginous joints, the articulating bones at diarthroses have a "free" articular surface. Instead of being "glued" together tightly by fibrous tissue or cartilage, the articular surfaces at diarthroses are enclosed within a fluid-filled cavity, the *synovial cavity*. In turn, the synovial cavity allows the articular surfaces of the opposing bones room to move freely. On the other hand, tight bands of connective tissue around the synovial cavity may in fact greatly restrict the ability of the articulating bones to move. Consequently, not all diarthroses are equally movable.

ANATOMY OF FIBROUS JOINTS

Fibrous joints are the simplest joints in terms of structural design and mobility. They contain dense connective tissue consisting of fibroblasts and numerous collagen fibers. The tough fibers hold the articulating bones together tightly, restricting their movement. The skeleton contains three types of fibrous joints: *sutures*, *gomphoses*, and *syndesmoses*.

Sutures

A **suture** (SŪ-chur; seam) is a type of fibrous joint found only in the skull. Sutures are so named because most of them look like zigzag seams (stitches) made with a sewing machine. The fibrous connective tissue in a suture contains short collagen fibers called *sutural ligaments*. These tiny ligaments firmly anchor the skull bones to one another, preventing them from moving; therefore, sutures are synarthrotic. Sutures allow flat cranial bones to remain in place so they can form a rigid wall of protection around the delicate brain.

Sutures form when the growing edges of skull bones meet during intramembranous ossification. The fibrous tissue within a suture is the remnant of a fibrous "membrane" that served as a model for the developing skull bones. The skull bones originate as ossification centers, and grow as osseous tissue is laid down along a leading edge. As the bones grow, the soft fibrous membrane becomes smaller. At birth, fontanels ("soft spots") are all that remains of the membranous skull model, and within a few years, even they become fibrous sutures.

Not all sutures look alike; most have jagged edges, but others have relatively straight edges. An example of a jagged suture is the *sagittal suture*, located along the sagittal plane between the right and left parietal bones. Here, the irregular edges of the parietal bones interlock, preventing them from shifting anteriorly or posteriorly. You can demonstrate this effect by clasping your hands and interlocking your fingers. It is more difficult to pull your hands apart now than it is when your hands are simply pressed together flat. An example of a relatively straight suture is the *internasal suture*, located between the right and left nasal bones.

While most sutures remain fibrous throughout life, some sutures found in children eventually become synostoses. For example, an infant has a temporary frontal (metopic; me-TOP-ik, "forehead") suture between right and left frontal bones. In early childhood, however, the frontal suture usually becomes a synostosis, after which the child has only one frontal bone.

Gomphoses

A **gomphosis** (gom-FŌ-sis; *gomph*, bolt) is a fibrous joint found only between a tooth and an alveolar socket of the maxilla or mandible. The anatomical name for this particular joint is the *dento-alveolar joint*. A gomphosis is so named because the tooth fits into the alveolar socket like a bolt fits into a hole in a piece of wood. The fibrous tissue in a gomphosis consists of extremely short collagen fibers called *periodontal ligaments*. These ligaments connect the periosteum of the jawbone to the outer covering of the tooth's root (the part beneath the gum line). Since teeth typically do not move within their sockets, gomphoses are synarthrotic.

Syndesmoses

A **syndesmosis** (sen-dez-MŌ-sis; *desmo*, bind) is a fibrous joint in which collagen fibers hold two parallel bones together. This is like holding two pencils together side by side with rubber bands. The collagen fibers in a syndesmosis are significantly longer than those in a suture or gomphosis, therefore the articulating bones in a syndesmosis are slightly movable (amphiarthrotic).

One type of syndesmosis found between the distal ends of the tibia and fibula is the cordlike *tibiofibular ligament*. The collagen fibers in this ligament are arranged in bundles, which helps the ligament to resist stretching. Consequently, very little movement is permitted at this joint. Essentially, the tibiofibular ligament allows the tibia and fibula to experience compression, tension (pulling), and torsion (twisting) forces without their distal ends separating. This is like holding the two pencils together with a single rubber band at one end.

Syndesmoses are also found between the diaphyses (shafts) of the tibia and fibula, and between the diaphyses of the radius and ulna. Here, parallel collagen fibers span the gap between the diaphyses to form an *interosseous membrane*. This membrane-like syndesmosis provides stability to the forearm and leg by preventing their long bones from separating from one another during normal activity. This is like holding the pencils together with many rubber bands along the entire length of the pencils.

ANATOMY OF CARTILAGINOUS JOINTS

Cartilaginous joints are only slightly more complex than fibrous joints, and are filled with either hyaline cartilage or fibrocartilage. The type of cartilage present determines the amount of movement possible at these joints. The skeleton has two types of cartilaginous joints: *synchondroses* and *symphyses*.

Synchondroses

A **synchondrosis** (sen-kon-DRŌ-sis) is sometimes referred to as a temporary joint, because later in life most synchondroses are replaced by bone tissue; that is, they become synostotic. In synchondroses, a layer of hyaline cartilage "glues" articulating bones together, sort of like a layer of hardened mortar holds bricks together. Like the mortar, which prevents the bricks from moving, the hyaline cartilage holds the bones together so tightly that virtually no movement occurs; for this reason, synchondroses are synarthrotic.

The most common example of a synchondrosis is an epiphyseal plate, or growth plate, located between the epiphysis and diaphysis of a developing bone. Bone growth occurs as the new cartilage is added to the epiphyseal side of the growth plate. However, ossification occurs continually along the diaphysis side of the plate, until eventually the epiphyseal plate becomes solid bone; that is, a synostosis (bony joint). The *1st sternocostal joint*, located between the first rib and the manubrium, is also a synchondrosis. This rigid joint can be compared to the joint between a coffee cup and its handle, and in the elderly, it usually becomes synostotic.

Symphyses

Symphyses (SIM-fi-sēz) contain a pad of fibrocartilage that protects articulating bones against compression forces. Fibrocartilage is extremely tough, yet it is more flexible than hyaline cartilage. Thus, a pad of fibrocartilage wedged in between two bones can work like a pillow on a chair. While the pillow can act as a shock absorber when you sit, it doesn't prevent you from changing your seating position on the chair. Likewise, a pad of fibrocartilage can cushion adjacent bones without totally restricting bone movement. The slight amount of movement at symphyses classifies these joints as **amphiarthrotic**.

Most symphyses are *intervertebral joints*, located between the bodies of **vertebrae** in the vertebral column. These joints are filled with a fibrocartilaginous pad called an *intervertebral disc*. The disc contains a soft, jelly-filled center called the *nucleus pulposus*, which is a remnant of the notochord present during embryonic development. The nucleus pulposus is surrounded by the *annulus fibrosus*, which is made of tough fibrocartilage. Intervertebral discs cushion the vertebrae against compression forces when the spine is in an upright position. This cushioning role is especially important during walking and running, when compression increases dramatically.

The only other example of a symphysis is the *pubic symphysis*, located between the right and left pubic bones in the pelvis. This joint contains a fibrocartilaginous pad called an *interpubic disc*. During walking and running,

JOINTS

the femurs send compression shockwaves through the pelvis, but the interpubic disc prevents the pubic bones from crushing each other.

ANATOMY OF SYNOVIAL JOINTS

Synovial joints are the most complex joints, but they come in an assortment of styles, making it possible for the skeleton to have a wide range of different types of movement. We will first examine the structural features that all synovial joints have in common. Features of synovial joints include *articular cartilages*, a *joint cavity*, an *articular capsule*, and *synovial fluid* (Figure 12-1).

Articular cartilage

The **articular cartilage** is a thin layer of cartilage that covers the end of an articulating bone at a synovial joint. The smooth surface of the articular cartilage helps reduce friction as the cartilages of opposing bones slide past one another. Articular cartilages are also resilient, able to spring back to their original shape after being compressed; in essence, articular cartilages can serve as springy shock absorbers. This function is especially important in the hip, knee and ankle joints, where compression forces increase then decrease repeatedly when a person walks or runs.

In most synovial joints, the articular cartilage is hyaline cartilage, but in a few joints, such as the temporomandibular joint, it is more fibrous, much like fibrocartilage. Most cartilaginous tissue in the body receives oxygen and nutrients from blood vessels in the perichondrium, a membrane on the surface of the cartilage. Articular cartilages, however, are not covered with perichondrium. Consequently, their chondrocytes rely on synovial fluid and blood vessels in the synovial membrane for their nutrients.

Joint cavity

The **joint (synovial) cavity** is a virtual space between the ends (articular cartilages) of the articulating bones. The joint cavity is a "virtual" space, because unlike a true cavity, which is empty, the joint cavity is filled with fluid, the *synovial fluid*. The fluid-filled joint cavity provides room in which the articulating bones at synovial joints can move freely. Only synovial joints have a joint cavity (recall that fibrous and cartilaginous joints are filled with connective tissue, which restricts bone movement).

Articular capsule

The **articular capsule** is a double-layered container that encloses the joint cavity. The capsule's superficial layer, or **fibrous capsule**, consists of dense irregular connective tissue that is continuous with the periosteum of each articulating bone. The tough collagen fibers within the fibrous capsule help prevent the articulating bones from pulling too far apart. The deep layer of the articular capsule is the **synovial membrane**. It consists mostly of areolar connective tissue, and its cells include fibroblasts, macrophages, mast cells, and adipocytes. The synovial membrane is thin and pink, and covers the deep surface of the fibrous capsule, but it terminates at the articular cartilages. The primary function of the synovial membrane is to secrete synovial fluid into the synovial cavity.

The articular capsule is the site where the cardiovascular and nervous systems interact with a synovial joint. An interlacing network of small blood vessels envelops the articular capsule, while smaller vessels from this network penetrate the fibrous capsule. Internally, the tiny vessels spread out between

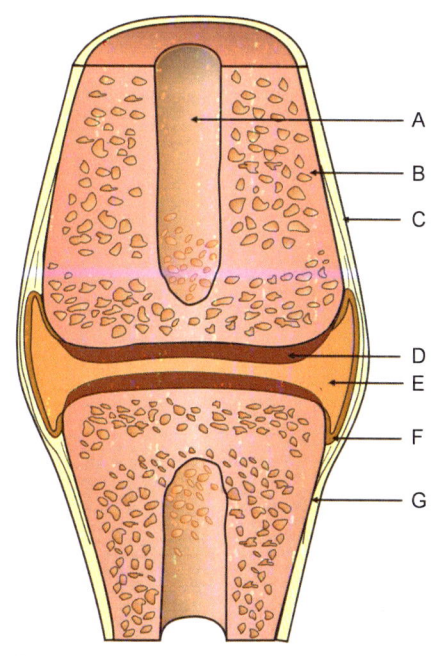

Figure 12-1.

the fibrous capsule and synovial membrane. Nerves penetrate the fibrous capsule and respond to several types of stimuli. First, tissue damage causes pain signals to be sent to the brain, which lets you know something is not right with the joint. Second, stretching a fibrous capsule initiates nerve signals that inform your brain about which joints are experiencing tension. In turn, the brain uses this information to decide which muscles need to contract to help you maintain your balance.

Synovial fluid

Synovial fluid is a clear to pale yellow fluid that fills the joint cavity. This fluid consists mostly of filtered blood plasma that leaks out of blood vessels in the synovial membrane. In fact, synovial joints are so named because its fluid looks and flows like uncooked egg white. However, the consistency of synovial fluid is negatively affected by temperature; that is, when the fluid gets warmer, it becomes less viscous. For this reason, synovial fluid circulates more freely after the articulating bones have been moving for a while and generating heat. Synovial fluid serves five important roles:

- Lubricates moving parts: Synovial fluid acts as a lubricant that reduces friction inside the joint cavity. In the same way that motor oil lubricates the gears of a car's engine, synovial fluid lubricates articular cartilages and other structures within the synovial joint. As modified blood plasma, synovial fluid is mostly water, which is, by itself, a good lubricant. In addition, however, fibroblasts in the synovial membrane add organic compounds to the fluid. The most important of these compounds is hyaluronic acid, a glycosaminoglycan, which makes the synovial fluid very slippery and reduces friction even more.

- Nourishes cartilages. Cartilages in a synovial joint are avascular, which means they must be nourished by nutrients diffusing into the cartilage from the surrounding tissues. Since synovial fluid is derived from nutrient-rich blood plasma, it can serve as an important source of nutrients for the cartilages. Articular cartilages are very porous and can act like a sponge to absorb the synovial fluid. Synovial fluid enters cartilage fastest when the cartilage is expanding after being squeezed, much as an expanding sponge absorbs water. Compression, on the other hand, squeezes synovial fluid out of the cartilage and back into the synovial cavity like wringing a sponge; this phenomenon is called **weeping lubrication**.

- Dissipates heat. Since synovial fluid is mostly water, it has a high specific heat. This means synovial fluid can absorb significant quantities of heat without a significant increase in temperature. Joints heat up as articulating bones move, but the circulating synovial fluid quickly absorbs and dissipates (radiates away) the heat. This is similar to how circulating coolant keeps a car engine from overheating. Just imagine, without synovial fluid, a marathon runner's knees might burst into flames before the end of the race! (Not really.)

- Distributes compression forces. Fluids cannot be compressed; therefore, when compression forces are exerted on synovial fluid, the forces are dispersed to all surfaces in contact with the fluid.

- Keeps the joint clean: Macrophages from the synovial membrane may enter the synovial fluid, where they phagocytize foreign particles, such as bacteria, and bits and pieces of joint structures that break free.

Accessory Structures at Synovial Joints

In addition to the structural features just described, some synovial joints have accessory structures that either stabilize the joint or cushion the bones. Accessory structures found at certain synovial joints include *ligaments, tendons, labra, menisci, articular fat pads, bursae,* and *tendon sheaths*.

Ligaments

A **ligament** is a band of dense regular connective tissue that holds articulating bones together at a joint. Ligaments work sort of like suspenders holding up a loose pair of pants. Without suspenders, the pants wouldn't stay up; without ligaments, some articulating bones wouldn't stay together.

Within the fibrous capsule of certain synovial joints, collagen fibers collect into thick bundles called

JOINTS

capsular (intrinsic) ligaments. Capsular ligaments are loose while in anatomical position, but become taut whenever the fibrous capsule stretches as the bones move. In this way, intrinsic ligaments strengthen the fibrous capsule, preventing it from splitting open. In addition, synovial joints that allow a significant amount of bone movement have *extrinsic ligaments* that are not part of the fibrous capsule. These include **extracapsular ligaments**, which are superficial to the fibrous capsule, and **intracapsular ligaments**, which are deep to the fibrous capsule. Extrinsic ligaments prevent the articulating bones from moving in awkward directions that could injure the joint.

Tendons

A **tendon** is a narrow band of dense regular connective tissue that attaches a muscle to a bone. In order for a muscle to move a bone, the muscle's tendon must cross a joint. Because they stretch over joints, tendons can also act like suspenders to keep articulating bones together.

Labra

At the two most freely movable joints, the shoulder and hip, a fibrocartilaginous lip called a **labrum** (LĀ-brum; "lip") helps hold a long bone within a deep socket. In the shoulder, the *glenoid labrum* helps hold the humeral head within the glenoid fossa of the scapula. In the hip, the *acetabular labrum* helps hold the femur's head within the deep acetabulum of the pelvis. A good analogy for the way a labrum holds the long bone's head within the socket is a button-type snap on a shirt or the small snaps on the back of an adjustable baseball cap.

Menisci and fat pads

Synovial joints that withstand intense compression may contain one or more accessory structures that cushion the articular surfaces of the bones. **Menisci** (me-NIS-sī; *meniscus*, crescent), or **articular discs**, are crescent-shaped discs of fibrocartilage that allow opposing articulating bones to fit together more evenly. The fibrocartilaginous discs are like the rubber foam insoles that make your foot and shoe fit together more evenly. Menisci reduce friction and distribute the compression forces over a greater area of the joint. Like the articular cartilages, menisci are not covered by the synovial membrane, but they are lubricated and nourished by weeping lubrication of synovial fluid. Menisci are found in the knee joints, temporomandibular joints, sternoclavicular joints, acromioclavicular joints, and the distal radioulnar joints.

In many joints, adipocytes gather around certain parts of the synovial membrane and form globules of adipose tissue called **articular fat pads**. Like menisci, fat pads act as springy cushions and help distribute compression forces across the articular surfaces. Moreover, stored triglycerides within the fat pads serve as a source of cellular energy.

Bursae and tendon sheaths

Some joints are so movable that they need accessory structures that can reduce friction and minimize the wear and tear on the bones and on the surrounding tissues. **Bursae** (BER-sē; *bursa*, purse) are flattened, fluid-filled pouches located between a bone and the overlying skin, ligament, tendon, or muscle at certain joints. Think of a bursa as a mushy, water-filled balloon you can hold between your hands. You can roll the balloon back-and-forth, deforming it in many directions, without causing much friction on either hand. Likewise, a bursa can deform in different directions to reduce friction on a bone and another structure. A bursa has a fibrous outer covering that is lined internally with a thin synovial membrane. The bursa's synovial membrane secretes fluid into the bursa cavity.

At certain joints, bursa-like structures called **tendon sheaths** reduce the friction between tendons and bones. The tendon sheath envelops the tendon, as a scabbard envelops a sword, (the word *sheath* translates "scabbard"). Whereas a bursa is flattened, a tendon sheath is more tubular, like a soda straw. Tendon sheaths are found in the wrist and ankle, where tendons and bones press tightly against one another. As a muscle contracts and relaxes, its tendon moves back-and-forth at a joint, but the tendon sheath prevents it from rubbing on bones.

JOINT STABILITY AND RANGE OF MOTION

While the shapes of articular surfaces influence the type of movement possible at a synovial joint, they also affect the joint's stability and its range of motion. **Joint stability**, or a joint's strength, refers to the joint's ability to function normally without having its articulating bones pull too far apart. A joint's **range of motion** is the maximum distance that the opposing articular surfaces can move. Considering all joints, there is generally an inverse relationship between range of motion and stability. Fibrous and cartilaginous joints are very stable, but they have limited ranges of motion. In contrast, synovial joints are less stable, but they have the greatest range of motion. Three factors affect the stability and range of motion at a synovial joint:

1. Shape of articular surfaces. Joints in which the articulating surfaces interlock are more stable than joints where bones make contact along relatively flat surfaces. For example, the rounded head of the femur and the acetabulum of the pelvis lock together, much like pieces of a jigsaw puzzle. But unlike the pieces of a puzzle, which remain rigid, the head of the femur can move freely. In fact, the ball-and-socket design of the hip joint allows the femur to move in many directions without separating from the acetabulum. Bones with flattened articular surfaces also tend to have a more restricted range of motion than bones that interlock. Flattened surfaces may slide past one another easily, but movements that cause the bones to separate will also cause associated ligaments to tighten and limit the range of motion.

2. Tension of ligaments. The stability of a joint is positively correlated with the tautness (tightness) of its accessory ligaments. Compare this to the tautness of large mooring ropes that anchor a ship to a dock. If the ropes are too loose or too stretchy, the ship can drift away from the dock. Likewise, a loose ligament may allow the articulating bones to move too far apart or move in awkward directions. Although tighter ligaments give a joint more stability, they can restrict the joint's range of motion, just like tight mooring ropes prevent a ship from moving.

3. Tension in tendons. The stability of a joint is also positively correlated with the tautness of tendons that cross the joint. When a skeletal muscle contracts, the tendon connecting it to a bone develops tension. The harder the muscle pulls on a bone, the greater the tension in the muscle's tendon. This is similar to pulling on the ship's mooring ropes in order to tighten them. Indeed, pulling on tendons hard enough causes bones to move. However, maintaining a lesser amount of tension on tendons while the bones are not moving can help hold the bones together. Even at rest, skeletal muscles are in a slight state of contraction known as **muscle tone**. In turn, muscle tone maintains tension on tendons, allowing the tendons to function like ligaments. You can increase the stability of a synovial joint by strengthening (increasing the tone of) the muscles that have tendons crossing that joint.

CLASSIFICATION OF SYNOVIAL JOINTS

While the shapes of articular surfaces influence the stability of a synovial joint, they also determine the type of bone movement possible at the joint. We can classify a synovial joint into four types, according to the number of stationary axis lines around which its articular surfaces can move.

- **Uniaxial joints** (ū-nē-AKS-sē-ul; *uni-*, single), or **monaxial joints** (mon-AKS-sē-ul; *mono-*, one), allow movement around one axis. For example, folding a piece of paper in half forms a crease that acts as a single stationary axis along which you can fold the paper back-and-forth.

- **Biaxial joints** (bī-AKS-sē-ul; *bi-*, two) allow movement around two axes. For example, fold a piece of paper lengthwise and crosswise and it forms two creases intersecting at right angles. Now you have two axes along which you can fold the paper back and forth.

- **Multiaxial joints** (*multi-*, many) allow movement around three axes; for this reason, multiaxial joints are sometimes called **triaxial joints** (trī-AKS-s-ul; *tri-*, three). Stick a pencil through the center of the paper just described and you will have a third axis around which to rotate or tilt the paper.

- **Nonaxial joints** allow a sliding motion; therefore, the movement does not revolve around an axis. Simply sliding two sheets of notebook paper past one another can be performed in several directions without being oriented around a crease ("axis").

In addition to classifying synovial joints according to the type of movement possible, we also classify them according to their basic structural design. The structural design is based on the shape of the articular surfaces. It includes *plane, hinge, pivot, condylar, saddle,* and *ball-and-socket* joints.

Plane joints

At a **plane joint**, two relatively flat articular surfaces can slide-back and-forth past one another. The sliding can be in any direction, but along one sectional plane. (Remember a sectional plane is like a piece of paper, while an axis is like a line drawn on the paper). Since there is no single axis line around which the movement occurs, we classify plane joints as nonaxial. Examples of plane joints include the intercarpal (between carpals), intertarsal (between tarsals), acromioclavicular (between the acromion process and clavicle), sternoclavicular (between the sternum and clavicle), vertebrocostal (between a vertebra and rib); and sacroiliac joints (between the sacrum and ilium).

Hinge joints

A **hinge joint** has a convex, bony process (a condyle) of one bone interacting with a concave surface (fossa) of another bone. Movement of the articulating bones is possible along one axis; therefore, hinge joints are uniaxial. Hinge joints are so named because they work like the hinge of a door. Examples include the elbow, knee, and interphalangeal joints (between phalanges).

Pivot joints

A **pivot joint** has a knobby, bony projection fitting through a "ring" formed partly by a shallow depression of another bone and partly by a ligament. The rotating movement of the knobby projection is around one axis, like the paper spinning on the pencil in our model; therefore, pivot joints are uniaxial. Examples of pivot joints include the proximal radioulnar joint and the joint between the atlas (1st cervical vertebra) and the dens (projection on the axis or 2nd cervical vertebra).

Condylar joints

A **condylar joint** (KON-di-lar; *conyl-*, knuckle), or **ellipsoidal joint** (il-IP-soy-dul) unites a convex surface with an oval-shaped depression. Movement at this joint can occur along two axes, like our paper model folded two ways; therefore, the joint is biaxial. Examples include the distal radiocarpal joint (between the radius and several carpals), the 2nd-5th metacarpophalangeal joints (between the metacarpals and proximal phalanges), and the metatarsophalangeal joints (between the metatarsals and proximal phalanges).

Saddle joints

At a **saddle joint**, two convex parts on each articulating bone fit into concave parts on the opposing bone. You can show this by forming a "U" with each hand (fingers together opposing the thumb), then interlocking the hands. In this way, each hand fits into the other hand like someone sitting in a saddle. The articulating bones at a saddle joint can move along two axes; therefore, it is biaxial. Examples of saddle joints include the carpometacarpal joint of the thumb (between the trapezium and 1st metacarpal) and the talocrural (between the talus and tibia).

Ball-and-socket joints

A **ball-and-socket joint** has a large, rounded knob (the head) of one bone fitting into a cuplike fossa of another bone. This type of joint allows the articulating surfaces to move along all three axes; therefore, it is multiaxial. The shoulder joint and the hip joint are examples of ball-and-socket joints.

BODY MOVEMENTS AT SYNOVIAL JOINTS

Knowing the names for different body movements is necessary to prevent misunderstandings when discussing the function of a joint. This is especially true for physical and occupational therapists who deal frequently with injured joints. We can classify the movement at a synovial joint into one of four major categories: *gliding, angular, rotational,* or *special* movement. Furthermore, several of these major groups include a number of more specific movements. See these movements illustrated in Figure 12-2 and read their descriptions that follow.

Gliding Movement

In gliding joints, the bones may slide in any direction (side-to-side and back-and-forth), but the angle between the articular surfaces does not change; for this reason, gliding movement is uniaxial. As a comparison, think of a hockey puck and the ice beneath it as two articulating bones. The hockey puck can slide in any direction on the ice while remaining flat and the angle between the bottom of the puck and the surface of the ice does not change. However, the puck moves in only one plane, in this case, along a horizontal surface. Gliding movements occur at intercarpal joints and intertarsal joints. These subtle movements aren't easily noticed because they occur at the same time more obvious angular movements occur at the wrist and ankle.

Angular Movement

Unlike gliding movements, angular movements may occur in one or more planes. The directional terms we use to describe angular movements are in reference to anatomical position. The major types of angular movement include *flexion, extension, hyperextension, abduction, adduction,* and *circumduction*.

Flexion, Extension, and Hyperextension

Flexion (FLEX-shun; *flex-*, to bend) occurs when the angle between articulating bones decreases in the sagittal (anterior-posterior) plane. During flexion, the nonarticulating ends of these bones move closer together. For example, if you bend your elbow joint to move your forearm anteriorly from anatomical position, you are flexing your forearm. As this occurs, the angle between your arm bone (humerus) and your forearm bones (radius and ulna) decreases. In addition, the distal ends of your forearm bones move closer to the proximal end of your humerus. Other examples of flexion include bending your fingers to make a fist, and curling your toes beneath your soles. No joints are flexed while the body is in anatomical position.

Extension (eks-TEN-shun; *exten-*, to stretch) is the opposite of flexion, and increases the angle between

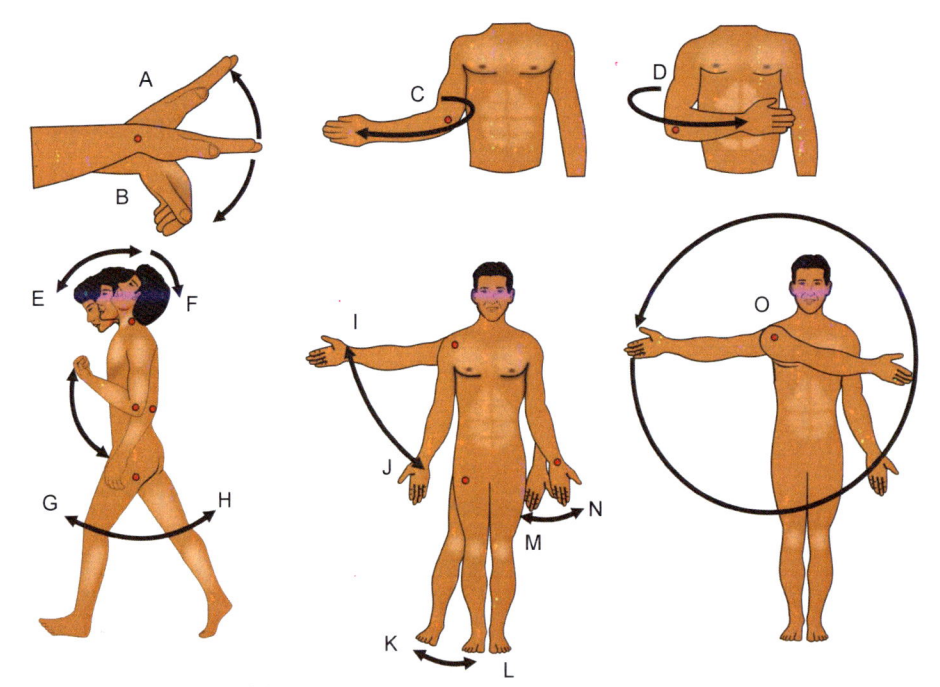

Figure 12-2. Movements at synovial joints

JOINTS

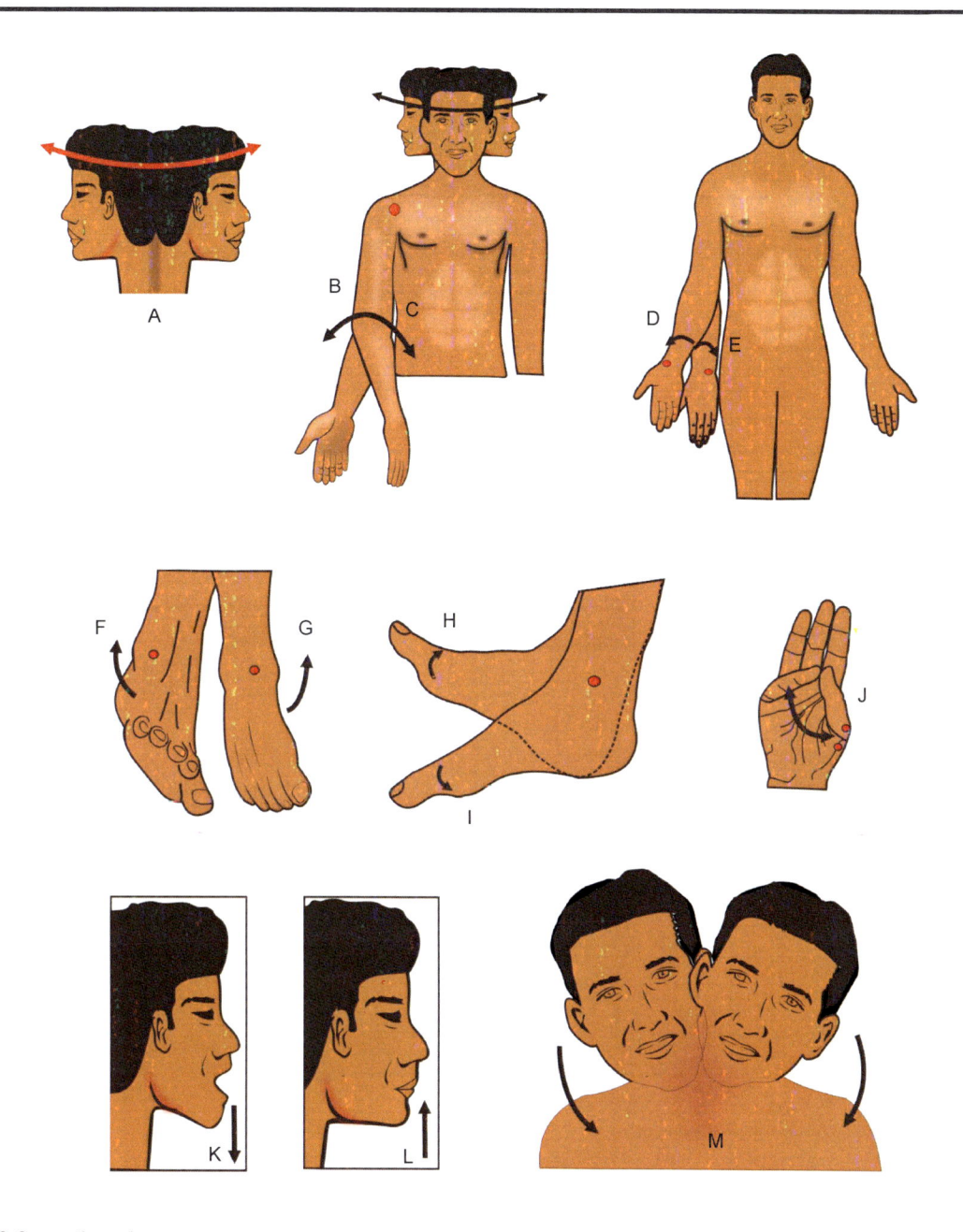

Figure 12-2. continued

articulating bones that are flexed. During extension, the nonarticulating ends of these bones move farther apart. If you straighten your elbow joint to return your forearm to anatomical position after it has been flexed, you are extending your forearm. While this happens, the distal ends of your forearm bones move farther away from the proximal end of your humerus. All extendable joints are extended when the body is in anatomical position.

Hyperextension occurs when you extend a bone beyond its anatomical position. For example, flexing your neck tilts your head forward allowing you to look at your toes; extending your neck raises your head allowing you to look straight ahead (in anatomical position); hyperextending your neck tilts your head backward allowing you to look straight up. While it is a normal movement at some joints, hyperextension at other joints is beyond the normal extension limit. For example, hyperextension is the most common cause of damage to the elbow and knee joints.

Abduction and Adduction

Abduction (ab-DUKT-shun; *abduct-*, take away) occurs when a bone moves away from its midline along a coronal (frontal) plane. Abducting the humerus raises the arm laterally. Spreading your fingers also involves abduction. In this case, digits 1 and 2 (thumb and index finger, respectively) move laterally, while digits 4 and 5 (ring finger and pinky) move medially.

Adduction (ad-DUKT-shun; *adduct-*, bring toward) is the opposite of abduction, and moves a bone toward its midline along a coronal plane. In other words, adduction moves the bone back to its anatomical position after abduction. Lowering your arm back to your side or pulling your spread fingers back together are examples of adduction.

Circumduction

Circumduction (sir-kum-DUC-shun; *circ-*, circle) occurs when the distal end of an appendage moves in a circular manner. If you move your arm like a spinning propeller, you are circumducting your humerus. Circumduction combines flexion, abduction, extension and possibly hyperextension, and adduction.

Rotational Movement

This is similar to turning a key in a lock. Rotation (rō-TA-shun; "to revolve") of the limbs may occur toward the body's midline or away from the midline. The anterior surface of the bone serves as a starting point of reference. For example, if you twist the anterior side of your right arm to the right (laterally), you are performing **lateral rotation** of your right humerus. If you twist the anterior side of your left arm to the right (medially), you are performing **medial rotation** of your left humerus. Turning your head or trunk involves **right rotation** and **left rotation**, depending on which direction the face or chest turns from anatomical position.

Special Movements

Special movements include those that do not easily fit into the descriptions of joint movements described earlier. We will describe opposite movements together.

Depression and Elevation

Depression (dē-PRESH-un; "push down") occurs when a bone moves inferiorly, such as when you lower your mandible to open your mouth. You depress your scapulae when lowering your shoulders. **Elevation** (el-e-VĀ-shun; "lift up") is the opposite of depression and occurs when a bone moves superiorly. You elevate your mandible to close your mouth, and you elevate your scapulae when shrugging your shoulders.

Protraction and Retraction

Protraction (prō-TRAK-shun: "draw forth") occurs when a bone moves anteriorly along a transverse plane. You protract your mandible when you stick out your lower jaw, and you protract your scapulae (shoulderblades) when you reach out to hug someone. **Retraction** (rē-TRAK-shun; "draw back") is the opposite of protraction, and occurs when a bone moves posteriorly along a transverse plane. Retraction returns a protracted bone to its anatomical position.

Excursion

Excursion (eks-KUR-shun; "run out") is a side-to-side movement of the mandible. *Lateral excursion* occurs when the mandible moves laterally; *medial excursion* occurs when the mandible moves medially to return to anatomical position. Protraction, retraction, and excursive movements of the mandible are common movements when chewing.

Pronation and Supination

Pronation (prō-NĀ-shun; "bending forward") occurs only when the forearm twists so that the palm faces posteriorly. Pronation causes the shaft of the radius to cross over the shaft of the ulna. **Supination** (sū-pi-NĀ-shun; "turning backward") is the opposite of pronation and occurs when the forearm twists to make the palm face anteriorly. The forearm is supinated in anatomical position, and the radius and ulna are parallel to one another. If the elbow is flexed, pronation turns the palm down, and supination turns the palm up. Remember supination allows you to hold soup in your palm (the first three letters in SUP-ination are pronounced like "soup").

JOINTS

Lateral flexion

Lateral flexion is a bending of a segment of the vertebral column in a coronal plane away from the body's midline. Tilting your head laterally to bring your ear closer to your shoulder is an example of lateral flexion.

Inversion and Eversion

Inversion (in-VER-shun; "turn inward") is a foot movement, and occurs when bending the ankle joint turns the sole in a medial direction, toward the body's midline. In effect, inversion is adduction of the foot. Excessive inversion is the cause of most ankle sprains. **Eversion** (ē-VER-shun; "turn outward") is the opposite of inversion and occurs when your sole turns laterally, away from the midline. In effect, eversion is abduction of the foot.

Dorsiflexion and Plantar flexion

Dorsiflexion (dor-si-FLEK-shun; "bend upward") is a foot movement, and occurs when bending the ankle elevates the anterior aspect of the foot. This action causes you to stand on your heels. **Plantar flexion** is the opposite of dorsiflexion and occurs when bending the ankle elevates the heel; that is, when you stand on your toes.

Opposition and Reposition

Opposition (op-ō-ZISH-un; "go against") is a thumb movement in which the thumb moves anteriorly and medially to touch the ends of the other digits on the same hand. Recall that all primates, including humans, have an opposable thumb that allows the hand to grasp and hold objects more effectively. **Reposition** (rē-pō-ZISH-un; "replace") is the movement of the thumb to its anatomical position following opposition.

CHARACTERISTICS OF SELECTED JOINTS

We conclude our study of the skeletal system by integrating information about different types of joints with information from lecture. Table 2 summarizes the classification of major joints by structure and movement, beginning at the head and ending at the foot. In addition, we will look more closely at the structure of the six complex joints that are responsible for movements of the upper and lower limbs.

THE SHOULDER JOINT

Of all the joints, the **shoulder joint**, or **glenohumeral joint**, is the most movable, but with this freedom of movement comes less stability (Figure 12-3).

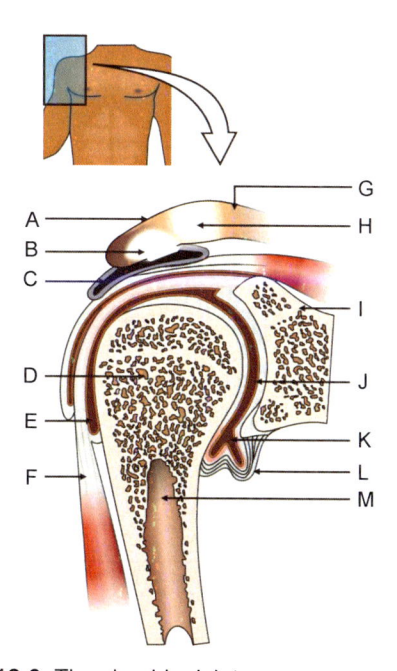

The shoulder joint is multiaxial, allowing flexion, extension, abduction, adduction, rotation, and circumduction of the arm (humerus). However, to allow for such diverse movements, the supporting ligaments around the shoulder joint must remain reasonably loose. Consequently, the articulating bones at the shoulder joint may pull apart (dislocate) more easily than bones at other, more stable joints. Dislocation injuries are especially prevalent in contact sports such as football and rugby. In addition, ligaments and tendons are frequently strained or torn in sports such as baseball and tennis, which involve frequent throwing or swinging motions.

Most superficially, we see that four capsular ligaments help hold the humeral head within the glenoid cavity. The **coracohumeral ligament** (KOR-uh-kō-HŪ-mer-ul) is the strongest of the four and is

Figure 12-3. The shoulder joint

found on the superior aspect of the articular capsule. It extends between the coracoid process of the scapula to the greater tubercle of the humerus. Due to its superior position, the coracohumeral ligament supports much of the weight of the upper limb. Three less conspicuous **glenohumeral ligaments** (GLE-nō-HŪ-mer-ul) (superior, middle, and inferior) are found on the anterior aspect of the articular capsule. They extend from the rim of the glenoid cavity to the lesser tubercle and neck of the humerus. An important extracapsular ligament at the shoulder joint is the **coracoacromial ligament** (KOR-uh-kō-a-KRŌ-mē-ul), extending between the coracoid and acromial processes of the scapula. This ligament, along with the two bony processes it connects, prevents the humeral head from being pushed superiorly out of the glenoid cavity.

While the articular capsule and capsular ligaments provide some support, muscle tendons provide most of the stability for the shoulder joint. Four tendons, collectively called the **rotator cuff**, extend from shoulder muscles on the scapula to the greater and lesser tubercles of the humerus. One of these, the tendon of the *subscapularis muscle*, can be seen extending across the anterior surface of the joint. Muscle tone maintains tension on these tendons, helping to hold the humeral head securely in the glenoid cavity. A tendon from the long head of the *biceps brachii* muscle, located on the anterior portion of the arm, also helps stabilize the shoulder joint. It extends through the joint cavity and attaches immediately superior to the glenoid labrum. The shoulder joint is weakest on its inferior aspect, since no tendons cross over at that point.

Also located superficially, we see a number of fluid-filled accessory structures that reduce friction between the articulating bones and surrounding tissues at the shoulder joint. A tendon sheath protects the biceps brachii tendon where it passes through the joint. In addition, four bursae reduce friction between the bones and the muscles at the shoulder joint.

As we remove the superficial layers of tissue, we see that the shoulder joint is a synovial, diarthrotic, ball-and-socket joint. The "ball" is the head of the humerus, and it fits into the shallow glenoid cavity (the "socket") of the scapula. The surfaces of the humeral head and the glenoid fossa are covered with smooth hyaline cartilage (articular cartilages), which reduce friction. An articular capsule extends from the rim of the glenoid cavity to the head and neck of the humerus, and encloses the fluid-filled synovial cavity. The capsule has a loose fit around the joint, allowing the humerus to move freely without overstretching the capsule. The **glenoid labrum** (LĀ-brum; "ring") is a ring of fibrocartilage extending around the rim of the glenoid cavity. The labrum slightly deepens the cavity and forms a liquid seal around about one-third of the humeral head. The moist seal functions like a small suction cup to help hold the humeral head in the glenoid cavity. Think of it as being like a moist rubber suction disc on the end of a toy arrow that holds tightly to a smooth surface.

THE ELBOW JOINT

Moving distally from the shoulder joint, the next major joint of the upper limb is the elbow joint, which allows flexion and extension of the forearm (Figure 12-4). The **elbow joint** is a compound joint, meaning it contains more than one articulation site. In this case, articulation occurs between the humerus and ulna, and between the humerus and radius.

Superficially, a thin articular capsule encloses the elbow joint and contains two capsular ligaments that help stabilize the joint. The **ulnar collateral ligament** (cō-LAT-er-ul) consists of three cordlike bands that connect the medial epicondyle of the humerus to the proximal, medial side of the ulna. This ligament prevents the ulna from bending laterally at the elbow. The triangular **radial collateral ligament** connects the lateral epicondyle of the humerus to the proximal, lateral end of the radius. This ligament prevents the radius from bending medially at the elbow. A number of tendons also provide stability to the elbow joint. These include the *biceps brachii* tendon, which crosses the anterior surface of the joint, and the *triceps brachii* tendon, which crosses the posterior surface.

A single bursa, the **olecranon bursa**, lies between the subcutaneous tissue and the olecranon process of the ulna. This bursa cushions your olecranon process when you prop your elbow on a desk. It also reduces friction between the olecranon process and the overlying subcutaneous tissue during flexion and extension of the forearm.

JOINTS
215

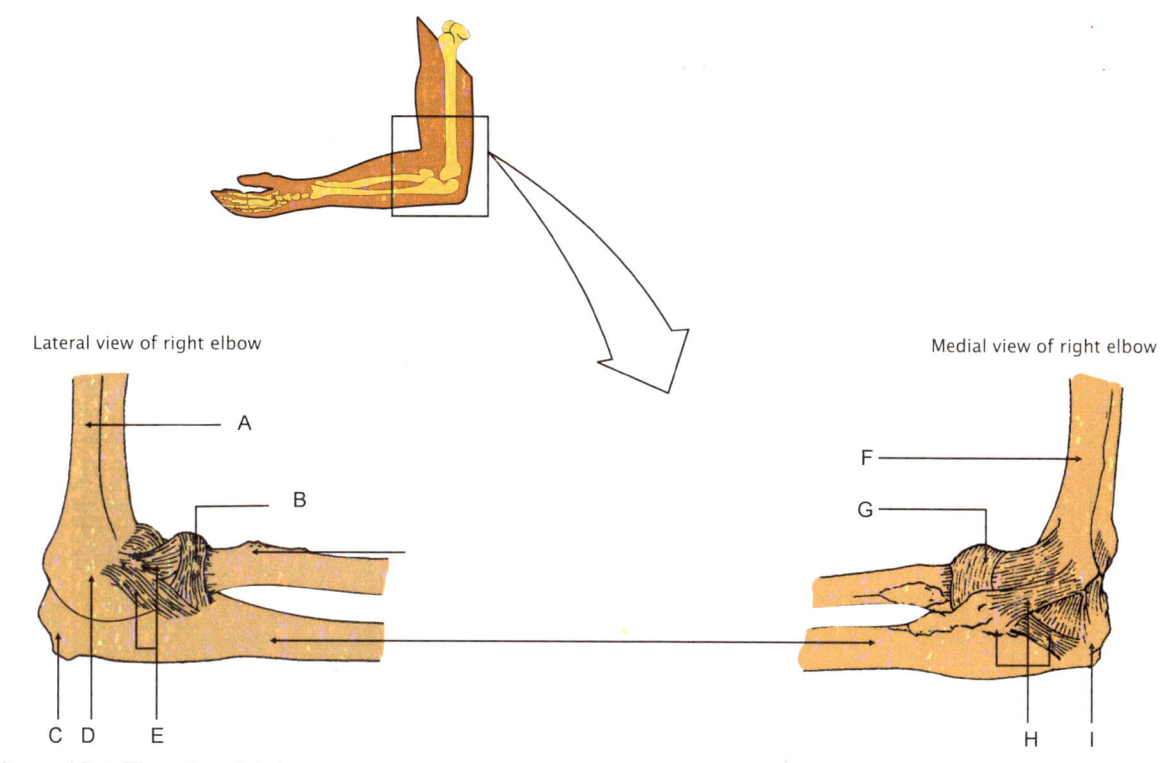

Lateral view of right elbow   Medial view of right elbow

Figure 12-4. The elbow joint

As we look deeper into the elbow joint, we see that the trochlea of the humerus articulates with the trochlear (semilunar) notch of the ulna; this is the **humeroulnar joint** (HŪ-mer-ō-UL-nar). This joint works like a hinge, allowing the ulna to swing anteriorly and posteriorly like a door. For this reason, the humeroulnar joint is a synovial, diarthrotic, uniaxial, hinge joint. Smooth articular cartilage covers the trochlea and the trochlear notch, reducing friction when the ulna moves. In anatomical position, the ulna is in full extension with its olecranon process fitting into the olecranon fossa of the humerus; this prevents hyperextension of the ulna. During full flexion, the coronoid process of the ulna fits into the coronoid fossa of the humerus.

The proximal, concave end of the radial head fits onto the rounded, convex capitulum of the humerus at the **humeroradial joint** (HŪ-mer-ō-RĀ-dē-ul). Like the humeroulnar joint, the humeroradial joint works like a hinge, allowing flexion and extension of the radius. For this reason, we classify the humeroradial joint as a synovial, diarthrotic, uniaxial, hinge joint.

Another joint, the **proximal radioulnar joint**, is so closely associated with the elbow joint that we will consider it briefly here. At this joint, the radial head articulates medially with the radial notch of the ulna. The only movement possible at this joint is rotation; therefore, the proximal radioulnar joint is a synovial, diarthrotic, uniaxial, pivot joint. Rotation of the radius allows you to pronate and supinate your forearm. The **radial annular ligament** attaches at both ends to the ulna while it arches over the head of the radius. This ligament holds the radius in place during pronation and supination of the forearm.

THE WRIST JOINT

The **wrist joint**, or **radiocarpal joint** connects the distal end of the radius to the carpal bones. This is a condylar joint with biaxial movement. The distal end of the ulna does not touch the carpal bones, but articulates with a meniscus (articular disc) that separates the ulna from the lunate and triquetral bones. Two major ligaments span the wrist joint between the radius and carpal bones; these are the **radiocarpal ligaments**.

Two ligaments prevent excessive side-to-side movement of the hand at the wrist. The **radial collateral carpal ligament** connects the radius to

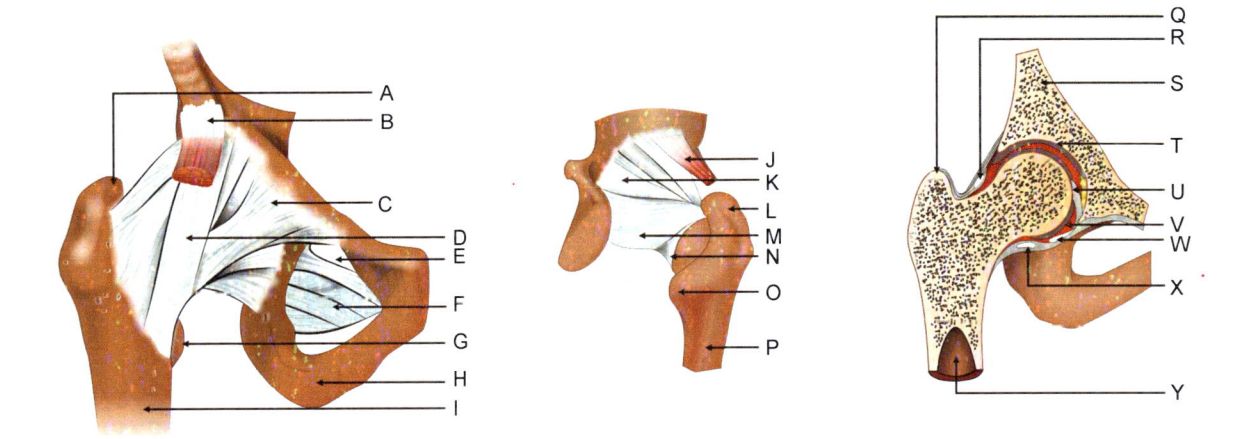

Figure 12-5. The hip joint

the scaphoid bone and prevents excessive abduction of the hand. The **ulnar collateral carpal ligament** connects the styloid process of the ulna to the triquetral and pisiform bones. This ligament prevents excessive adduction of the hand. Sometimes the word "carpal" is left off of these names, but then they can be confused with the collateral ligaments of the elbow. **Intercarpal ligaments** bridge adjacent carpal bones preventing them from pulling away from one another when the hand moves.

THE HIP JOINT

The **hip joint**, or **coxal joint**, is the joint between the head of the femur and the acetabulum (hip socket) of the pelvis (Figure 12-5). This joint is second in movability (mobility) only to the shoulder joint. Actions possible at this joint include flexion, extension, abduction, adduction, rotation, and circumduction of the thigh (femur). Although the supporting ligaments around the hip joint must remain reasonably loose to allow multiaxial movement, the hip socket is much deeper than the shoulder socket; thus, the the hip joint is much more stable than the shoulder joint.

Superficially, we see a thick articular capsule consisting of three major capsular ligaments that help hold the femoral head securely within the acetabulum. The **iliofemoral ligament** (IL-ē-ō-FEM-o-rul) extends from the anterior inferior iliac spine and rim of the acetabulum to the intertrochanteric line of the femur. This ligament prevents the femoral head from moving superiorly. The **pubofemoral ligament** (PŪ-bō-FEM-u-rul) extends from the anterior portion of the acetabular labrum to the neck of the femur, and prevents the femoral head from moving anteriorly or inferiorly. The **ischiofemoral ligament** (IS-kē-ō-FEM-u-rul) extends from the ischial portion of the acetabulum rim to the neck of the femur, and prevents the femoral head from moving posteriorly.

Looking deeper into the hip joint, we see that it is a synovial, diarthrotic, multiaxial, ball-and-socket joint. The "ball" is the head of the femur, and it fits into the deep acetabulum (the "socket") of the hipbone. Articular cartilage covers the entire surface of the femoral head, but it is lunate (C-shaped) within the acetabulum. An articular capsule extends from the rim of the acetabulum to the head and neck of the femur, and encloses a fluid-filled synovial cavity. The capsule fits loosely around the joint, allowing the femur to move freely. The **acetabular labrum** (AS-e-TAB-ū-lar) is a ring of fibrocartilage extending almost completely around the rim of the acetabulum. The labrum deepens the cavity and forms a seal around femur's neck, making it difficult to dislocate the femoral head from the acetabulum. This works like two button-type snaps fastening together on a jacket. A **transverse acetabular ligament** is a noncartilaginous band that forms the inferior rim of the labrum.

A strong intracapsular ligament called the **ligamentum teres** (lig-uh-MEN-tum TER-ēz; "round") connects the head of the femur to the acetabulum. It extends between the fovea capitis, a small

JOINTS

pit in the femoral head, to the transverse acetabular ligament to form the inferior rim of the acetabulum. This ligament does little to stabilize the hip joint, but it contains an artery that nourishes the head of the femur. Numerous hip muscles also cross the hip joint, adding stability to the already highly stable joint.

THE KNEE JOINT

Although the knee joint lacks the mobility of the shoulder or hip joints, it is the most complex joint in the body. The knee joint is largely uniaxial, allowing flexion and extension of the leg, but during these movements, it also allows slight leg rotation. Like the elbow joint, the knee joint is compound, having more than one articulation site. In the knee joint, articulation occurs between the femur and tibia, and between the femur and patella (Figure 12-6).

A thin, fibrous articular capsule is present only on the posterior and lateral aspects of the knee joint; therefore, other structures are necessary to reinforce the anterior aspect. On the anterior aspect, the *quadriceps tendon* extends inferiorly from the large, anterior thigh muscles and envelops the patella, holding it in place. This tendon extends inferiorly from the patella as the **patellar ligament**, which inserts on the tibial tuberosity.

Four extracapsular ligaments stabilize the lateral and posterior aspects of the knee joint. The **tibial collateral ligament** connects the medial condyle of the femur to the medial condyle of the tibia. This ligament prevents medial displacement of the tibia. The **fibular collateral ligament** connects the lateral condyle of the femur to the head of the fibula, and prevents lateral displacement of the tibia. Both of these ligaments are taut when the knee is in full extension (anatomical position), but become loose when the knee bends.

A number of structures cushion the knee joint, including a large joint capsule, numerous bursae, and several fat pads. The fluid-filled joint capsule at the knee joint is the largest and most elaborate in the body. It is most extensive on the anterior surface of the knee, where it extends superior to the patella to terminate as the **suprapatellar bursa**. This bursa reduces friction between the femur and *quadriceps muscle* tendon. The joint capsule attaches to the edges of the menisci and extends posteriorly to cover the femoral and tibial condyles. The **prepatellar bursa** lies between the patella and the skin, while the **infrapatellar bursa** lies between the patellar ligament and joint capsule. A

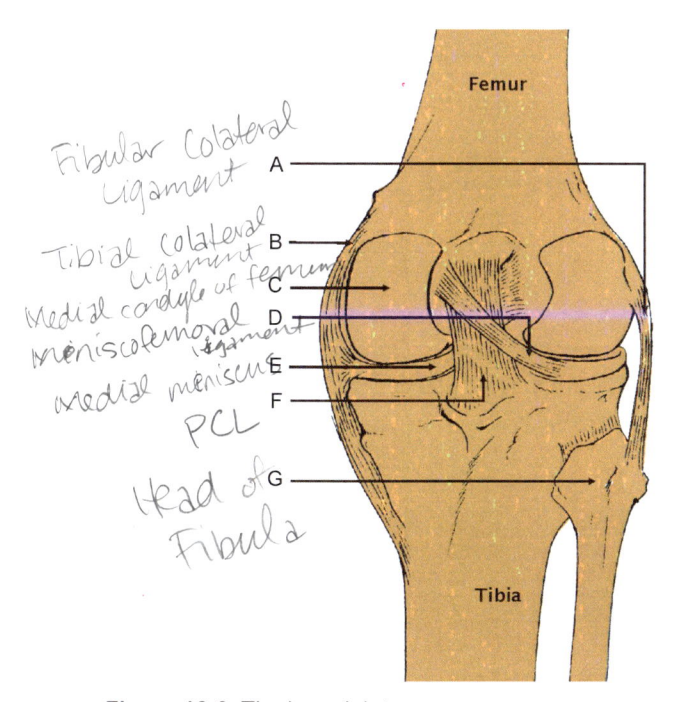

Figure 12-6. The knee joint

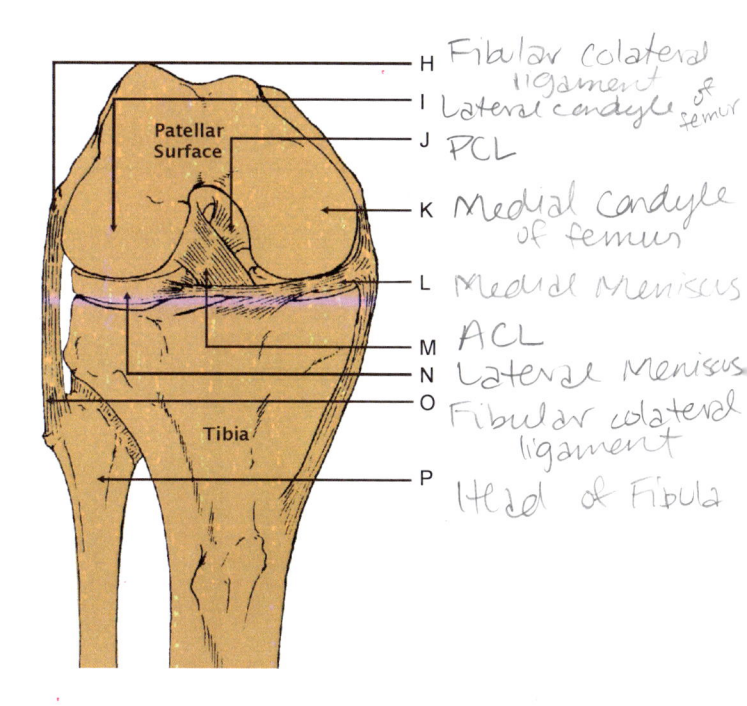

thick **infrapatellar fat pad** lies at the anterior surface of the knee joint, immediately inferior to the patella. It cushions the femoral condyles and helps prevent them from slipping anteriorly.

Two intracapsular ligaments prevent excessive anterior and posterior movements of the tibia. These ligaments are called *cruciate ligaments* (KRŪ-shē-āt; *cruci-*, cross) because they cross each other within the intercondylar notch of the femur. The **anterior cruciate ligament (ACL)** extends from the posterior-medial surface of the femur's lateral condyle to insert on the anterior portion of the tibial condyles. This ligament becomes taut when the knee is in full extension, thereby preventing the tibia from hyperextending. The **posterior cruciate ligament (PCL)** extends from the anterior-lateral side of the femur's medial condyle. This ligament prevents the tibia from sliding posteriorly and the femur from sliding anteriorly when the flexing the leg. If you could slide down a cruciate ligament, whichever side of the knee you are on when you reach the bottom is the name of the ligament. For example, after sliding down the ACL, you will be on the anterior side of the knee.

Deep to the articular capsule, we can see the weight-bearing part of the knee, the **tibiofemoral joint** (TIB-ē-ō-FEM-u-rul), which is a synovial, diarthrotic, uniaxial, condylar joint. Here, the convex lateral and medial condyles of the femur articulate with concave, fibrocartilaginous menisci (articular discs). The nearly circular **lateral meniscus** rests on the lateral condyle of the tibia, while the C-shaped **medial meniscus** rests on the medial condyle. The flexible menisci change shape as the knee bends, allowing the femoral condyles to transfer the body weight over a broader area on the tibia. Menisci cushion the femoral condyles when a person stands, and they act as shock absorbers when the person walks or runs. Smooth articular cartilage covers the surfaces of the femoral and tibial condyles, reducing friction when the knee bends. The edges of the menisci extend slightly superiorly around the edges of the femoral condyles, helping to prevent the condyles from sliding side-to-side.

Have you ever noticed that when standing for a long time, you can "lock" your knees so that your thigh muscles don't get tired. What's happening when a knee locks? When the leg is flexed (bent), each femoral condyle makes minimum contact with its corresponding meniscus; at this time, the collateral ligaments and the anterior cruciate ligaments are loose. However, because the lateral femoral condyle is smaller and less rounded than the medial condyle, it makes maximum surface contact with the lateral meniscus before leg extension is complete. As a way of making the smaller, lateral condyle "wait" on the larger medial condyle to make full contact with the medial meniscus, the femur medially rotates slightly. This action allows the leg to extend further while both menisci flatten to act like suction cups to provide maximum support for each femoral condyle. At this time, the collateral and anterior cruciate ligaments become taut and help "lock" the femur condyles in place. Before the leg can flex, the small *popliteus muscle* on the knee's posterior surface must cause the femur to rotate laterally ever so slightly, but this effectively "unlocks" the knee.

The articulation between the femur and patella is the **femoropatellar joint** (FEM-o-rō-pu-TEL-ur), which is a synovial, diarthrotic, nonaxial, plane joint. Flexing the knee joint causes the patella to glide over the patellar surface of the femur. In full flexion, the patella is anterior to the femur's intercondylar notch.

THE ANKLE JOINT

The **ankle joint**, or **talocrural joint** (tā-lō-KRU-rul; *talo*, ankle; *crur-*, leg), connects the distal end of the tibia to the talus, or second largest tarsal bone. Two major ligaments help stabilize the ankle joint, and they can be easily identified on either side of the joint. The **deltoid ligament** is a large, triangular-shaped ligament that connects the tibia's medial malleolus to the talus, calcaneus, and navicular bone. The **lateral ligaments** anchor the lateral malleolus of the fibula to the calcaneus. These ligaments are commonly stretched or torn when the ankle is "rolled" due to excessive inversion of the foot.

WHAT MAKES SYNOVIAL JOINTS "POP"?

Why do synovial joints occasionally make a "popping" sound when you pull their articulating bones apart? At first, the bones don't easily separate because synovial fluid acts like glue to hold the bones together (this is why it's difficult to lift a drinking glass off a wet table).

JOINTS

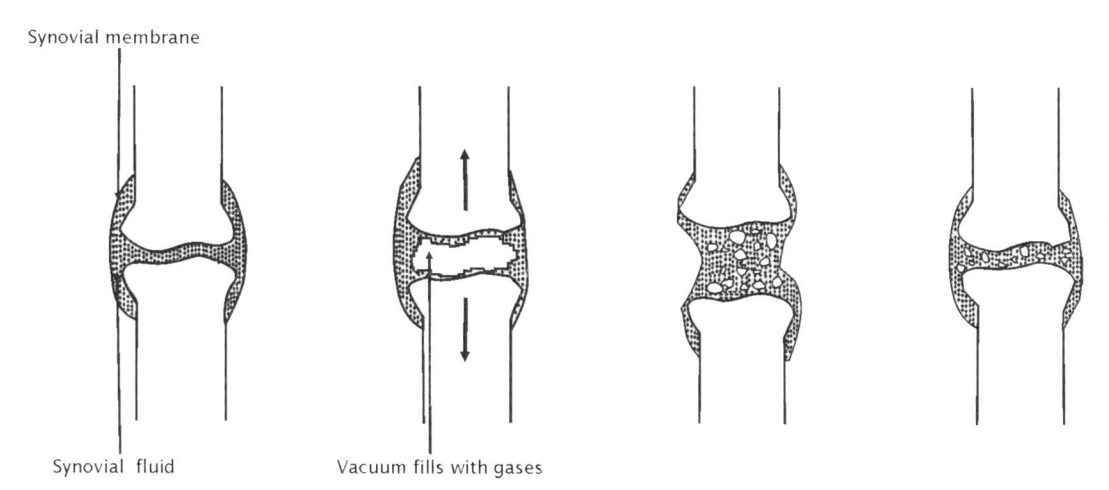

Figure 12-7. Popping a synovial joint

However, with enough force, you can separate the bones, but this stretches the synovial capsule. When the synovial cavity gets larger, the hydrostatic pressure of the synovial fluid decreases. This, in turn, causes dissolved gases (primarily CO_2) to come out of solution quickly, forming bubbles. This is why gas bubbles form in a pressurized soft drink when you remove the cap and release the pressure. The sudden formation of gas bubbles in the synovial fluid causes the "pop." This is also why removing a cork from a bottle of champagne makes a loud "pop." The pop will not occur again until the gases re-dissolve in the synovial fluid, which occurs after the synovial membrane returns to its normal size (see Figure 12-7).

The following tables summarize the different types of joints described in this chapter. You should be able to recognize these joints on models and in diagrams and be able to classify them according to structure, function, and type of movement.

Table 12-1: Classification of Joints

Classification by Structure	Classification by Range of Motion	Examples
FIBROUS JOINTS		
Suture	Synarthrosis	Coronal suture, internasal suture
Gomphosis	Synarthrosis	Dento-alveolar joints
Syndesmosis	Amphiarthrosis	Distal tibiofibular joint; interosseous membranes (tibiofibular; radioulnar)
CARTILAGINOUS JOINTS		
Synchondrosis	Synarthrosis	Epiphyseal disc; 1st sternocostal joints
Symphysis	Amphiarthrosis	Intervertebral joints; pubic symphysis
SYNOVIAL JOINTS		
Ball-and-socket	Diarthrosis	Shoulder joint; hip joint
Condylar	Diarthrosis	Radiocarpal joints
Gliding	Diarthrosis	Intercarpal; intertarsal joints
Hinge	Diarthrosis	Elbow joint; knee joint
Pivot	Diarthrosis	Atlantoaxial joint; proximal radioulnar joint
Saddle	Diarthrosis	1st carpometacarpal joint
SYNOSTOTIC JOINTS	Synarthrosis	Epiphyseal lines; metopic suture

Table 12-2. Types of Bone Movements at Synovial Joints

Movement	Description of Bone Movement
GLIDING	Bones slide along a flat surface in one plane
ANGULAR	Movement in a sagittal plane that changes the angle between articulating bones
Flexion	Decreases the angle of the articulating bones
Extension	Movement increases the angle of the articulating bones
Hyperextension	Extension beyond anatomical position
Abduction	Bone moves away from the body's midline
Adduction	Bone moves toward the body's midline
Circumduction	End of the bone moves in a circular pattern
ROTATION	Bone moves around its longitudinal axis
Lateral rotation	Anterior surface of a bone moves away from the midline
Medial rotation	Anterior surface of a bone moves toward the midline
Right rotation	Twisting the head or thorax to the right of anatomical position
Left rotation	Twisting the head or thorax to the left of anatomical position
SPECIAL	Movement occurring at only a few joints
Depression	Movement of a bone inferiorly in a vertical plane
Elevation	Movement of a bone superiorly in a vertical plane
Protraction	Movement of a bone anteriorly in a horizontal plane
Retraction	Movement of a bone posteriorly in a horizontal plane
Excursion	Moving the mandible side-to-side
Pronation	Rotating the forearm so the palm faces posteriorly or inferiorly
Supination	Rotating the forearm so the palm faces anteriorly or superiorly
Lateral flexion	Bending the vertebral column to the side
Inversion	Bending the ankle to make the sole face medially
Eversion	Bending the ankle to make the sole face laterally
Dorsiflexion	Bending the ankle to raise the toes; "standing on heel"
Plantar flexion	Bending the ankle to raise the heel; "standing on toes"
Opposition	Moving the thumb medially toward the palm
Reposition	Moving the thumb to anatomical position after opposition

Table 12-3: Classification and Actions of Selected Joints

Name of Joint	Articulating Bones	Classification by Structure	Classification by Range of Motion	Major Actions Allowed
Suture	Cranial bones	fibrous (suture)	synarthrosis	None
Temporomandibular	Temporal bone & mandible	Synovial (hinge/plane)	Diarthrosis (uniaxial)	Elevation, depression, protraction, retraction, lateral movement of mandible
Dento-alveolar	Teeth & maxilla teeth & mandible	Fibrous (gomphosis)	Synarthrosis	None
Atlanto-occipital	Atlas & occipital bone	Synovial (condylar)	Diarthrosis (uniaxial)	Flexion, extension, lateral flexion, & circumduction of head
Atlantoaxial	Atlas & axis	Synovial (pivot/plane)	Diarthrosis (uniaxial)	Rotation of head
Intervertebral	Vertebrae (bodies)	Cartilaginous (symphysis)	Amphiarthrosis	Slight flexion, extension,
	Vertebrae (processes)	Synovial (plane)	Diarthrosis (nonaxial)	Gliding of vertebrae
Vertebrocostal	Vertebrae & ribs	Synovial (plane)	Diarthrosis (nonaxial)	Gliding of ribs
Manubriosternal	Manubrium & sternum body	Cartilaginous (symphysis)	Amphiarthrosis	Slight movement
Xiphisternal	Xiphoid process & sternum body	Cartilaginous (symphysis)	Amphiarthrosis	Slight movement
Sternoclavicular	Sternum & clavicle	Synovial (saddle)	Diarthrosis (biaxial)	protraction, retraction, elevation, depression, rotation of clavicle
Sternocostal	Sternum & rib 1	Cartilaginous (synchondrosis)	Synarthrotic	None
	Sternum & ribs 2-7	Synovial (plane)	Diarthrosis (nonaxial)	Gliding of ribs
Acromioclavicular	Scapula & clavicle	Synovial (plane)	Diarthrosis (nonaxial)	Rotation of scapula
Shoulder (glenohumeral)	Scapula & humerus	Synovial (ball-and-socket)	Diarthrosis (multiaxial)	Flexion, extension, abduction, adduction rotation, circumduction of arm
Elbow (humeroulnar)	Humerus & ulna	Synovial (hinge)	Diarthrosis (uniaxial)	Flexion, extension of ulna
Elbow (humeroradial)	Humerus & radius	Synovial (hinge/pivot)	Diarthrosis (uniaxial)	Flexion, extension, rotation of radius
Radioulnar (proximal)	Radius & ulna	Synovial (pivot)	Diarthrosis (uniaxial)	Rotation of radius
Radioulnar (distal)	Radius & ulna	Synovial (pivot)	Diarthrosis (uniaxial)	Pronation, supination of hand

Name of Joint	Articulating Bones	Classification by Structure	Classification by Range of Motion	Major Actions Allowed
Wrist (radiocarpal)	Radius & proximal carpals	Synovial (condylar)	Diarthrosis (uniaxial)	Flexion, extension, abduction, adduction, circumduction of hand
Intercarpal	Carpals	Synovial (plane)	Diarthrosis (nonaxial)	Gliding of carpals
Carpometacarpal of digit 1	Trapezium & metacarpal 1	Synovial (saddle)	Diarthrosis (biaxial)	Flexion, extension, abduction, adduction, circumduction, opposition of 1st metacarpal
Carpometacarpals of digits 2-5	Distal carpals & metacarpals 2-5	Synovial (plane)	Diarthrosis (nonaxial)	Gliding of metacarpals
Metacarpophalangeal	Metacarpals & proximal phalanges	Synovial (condylar)	Diarthrosis (biaxial)	Flexion, extension, abduction, adduction, circumduction of fingers
Finger (Interphalangeal)	Phalanges	Synovial (hinge)	Diarthrosis (uniaxial)	Flexion, extension of fingers
Sacroiliac	Sacrum & ilium	Synovial (plane)	Diarthrosis (nonaxial)	Slight gliding
Pubic symphysis	Pubic bones	Cartilaginous (symphysis)	Amphiarthrosis	Slight movement
Hip (coxal)	Coxal bone & femur	Synovial (ball-and-socket)	Diarthrosis (multiaxial)	Flexion, extension, abduction, adduction, circumduction, rotation of thigh
Knee (tibiofemoral)	Femur & tibia	Synovial (condylar)	Diarthrosis (uniaxial)	Flexion, extension, slight rotation of leg
Knee (femoropatellar)	Femur & patella	Synovial (plane)	Diarthrosis (nonaxial)	Gliding of patella
Tibiofibular (proximal)	Tibia & fibula	Synovial (plane)	Diarthrosis (nonaxial)	Gliding of fibula
Tibiofibular (distal)	Tibia & fibula	Fibrous (syndesmosis)	Amphiarthrosis	Slight rotation of fibula
Ankle (talocrural)	Tibia & talus	Synovial (saddle)	Diarthrosis (uniaxial)	Dorsiflexion, plantar flexion of foot
Intertarsal	Tarsals	Synovial (plane)	Diarthrosis (nonaxial)	Inversion, eversion of foot
Tarsometatarsal	Tarsal & metatarsals	Synovial (plane)	Diarthrosis (nonaxial)	Gliding metatarsals
Metatarso-phalangeal	Metatarsals & proximal phalanges	Synovial (condylar)	Diarthrosis (biaxial)	Flexion, extension, abduction, adduction of toes
Toe (Interphalangeal)	phalanges	Synovial (hinge)	Diarthrosis (uniaxial)	Flexion, extension of toes

JOINTS

TOPICS TO KNOW FOR CHAPTER 12 (JOINTS)

1st sternocostal joint
abduction
acetabular labrum
ACL
acromioclavicular joint
adduction
amphiarthrosis
angular movement
ankle joint
annulus fibrosus
anterior cruciate ligament
arthrosis
articular capsule
articular cartilage
articular disc
articular fat pad
articulation
atlantoaxial joint
atlanto-occipital joint
ball-and-socket joint
biaxial joint
bony joint
bursa
capsular ligament
carpometacarpal joint
cartilaginous joint
circumduction
classification of joints by movement
classification of joints by structure
condylar joint
coracoacromial ligament
coracohumeral ligament
coxal joint
deltoid ligament
dento-alveolar joint
depression
diarthrosis
distal tibiofibular joint
dorsiflexion
elbow joint
elevation
ellipsoidal joint
epiphyseal plate
eversion
excursion
extension
extracapsular ligament
extrinsic ligament
femoropatellar joint
fibrous capsule
fibrous joint
fibular collateral ligament
flexion
glenohumeral joint
glenohumeral ligament

glenoid labrum
gliding movement
gomphosis
hinge joint
hip joint
humeroradial joint
humeroulnar joint
hyaluronic acid
hyperextension
iliofemoral ligament
infrapatellar bursa
infrapatellar fat pad
intercarpal joint
intercarpal ligament
interosseous membrane
interphalangeal joint
interpubic disc
intertarsal joint
intervertebral disc
intervertebral joint
intracapsular ligament
intrinsic ligament
inversion
ischiofemoral ligament
joint
joint cavity
joint mobility
joint stability
knee joint
labrum
lateral flexion
lateral ligament
lateral meniscus
lateral rotation
left rotation
ligament
ligamentum teres
manubriosternal joint
medial meniscus
medial rotation
meniscus
metacarpophalangeal
metatarsophalangeal joint
monaxial joint
multiaxial joint
nonaxial joint
olecranon bursa
opposition
patellar ligament
PCL
periodontal ligament
pivot joint
plane joint
plantar flexion
popping a joint

posterior cruciate ligament
prepatellar bursa
pronation
protraction
proximal radioulnar joint
proximal tibiofibular joint
pubic symphysis
pubic symphysis
pubofemoral ligament
radial annular ligament
radial collateral carpal ligament
radial collateral ligament
radiocarpal joint
radiocarpal ligament
range of motion
reposition
retraction
right rotation
rotational movement
sacroiliac iliac
saddle joint
shoulder joint
sternoclavicular joint
sternocostal joint
supination
suprapatellar bursa
sutural ligaments
suture
symphyses
synarthrosis
synchondroses
syndesmosis
synostosis
synovial cavity
synovial fluid
synovial joint
synovial membrane
talocrural joint
tarsometatarsal joint
temporomandibular joint
tendon
tendon sheaths
tibial collateral ligament
tibiofemoral joint
tibiofibular ligament
transverse acetabular ligament
triaxial joint
ulnar collateral carpal ligament
ulnar collateral ligament
uniaxial joint
vertebrocostal joint
weeping lubrication
wrist joint
xiphisternal joint

CHAPTER 13

Membrane Potentials

MEMBRANE POTENTIAL

Electrodes placed on opposite sides of a plasma membrane reveal an electrical difference existing across the membrane. In other words, the inside (cytosolic) border of the membrane exhibits a negative charge and the outside (extracellular) border exhibits a positive charge. An *electrical difference* between two regions is called **voltage**. If charged particles, such as ions, can move freely, a **voltage** will cause them to move toward the region of opposite charge. The voltage that exists along a plasma membrane is called a **membrane potential (MP)** (Figure 13-1). When excluding the regions next to a plasma membrane, there is no electrical difference (voltage) in the extracellular fluid or cytosol; that is, the two solutions are electrically neutral. The reason is that for every positively charged particle present, there is a negatively charged particle nearby that "neutralizes" its charge effect.

A voltage develops along a plasma membrane because the membrane is semipermeable; i.e., it allows certain ions to pass through while preventing others. In short, a membrane potential develops because there is an unequal movement of cations and anions across the membrane. The value for a membrane potential refers to the electrical condition along the *inside border* of the membrane, as it compares to the electrical condition on the outside border. For example, a membrane with a MP of -70 *millivolts* (mV—each mV is 1/1000th of a volt), means that the inside border of the membrane is 70 mV more negative than the outside border. A membrane potential of +30 mV means that the inside border of the membrane is 30 mV more positive than the outside border.

Resting membranes, which are those that have a relatively stable membrane potential, experience very little ion movement and are at equilibrium with the ECF. In this state, the membrane potential is *always negative* (i.e., the inside border is negative and the outside border is positive). Therefore, we say a resting membrane exists

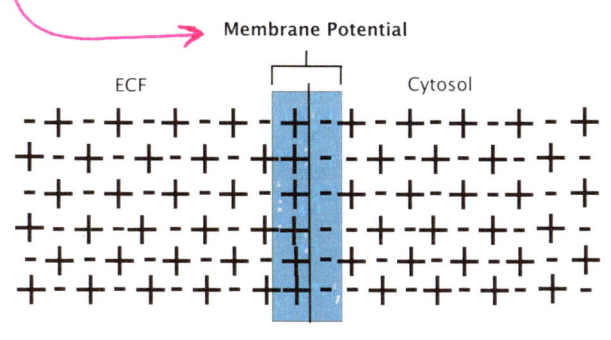

Figure 13-1. Membrane potential

in a *polarized* condition. This is much like a refrigerator magnet, car battery, or even the earth, all of which are polarized (having a positive and negative pole). All cells have a membrane potential anywhere from -5 to -100 mV.

If the plasma membrane suddenly allows a particular ion to pass through the membrane, then the membrane potential will change. If the potential becomes less negative (i.e., the value moves toward zero), the phenomenon is **depolarization** (*de*, away from). If a depolarized membrane's potential moves back toward the RMP (i.e., the value becomes more negative), the phenomenon is **repolarization** (*re*, again). If the potential becomes more negative than the RMP, the phenomenon is **hyperpolarization** (*hyper*, over). In order to understand how membrane potentials develop and how they can change, we must first understand the factors that affect the movement of ions.

FACTORS AFFECTING ION MOVEMENT

When allowed to pass through a membrane, there will be a net movement of ions from a region of higher energy to a region of lower energy. The force that drives the movement of ions is the **electrochemical gradient,** which includes the following:

1. Concentration gradient: The difference in the concentration of a substance at two locations (*grad*, step) will cause ions to move from the region of higher concentration to the region of lower concentration; i.e., they move *down* or *along* their concentration gradient (Figure 13-2).

2. Electrical gradient: The difference in the electrical potential, or *voltage*, at two locations will cause ions to move into regions having an opposite electrical potential. Cations tend to move into regions of negative potential, whereas, anions (negatively charged ions) tend to move into regions of positive potential. Likewise, regions of positive potential tend to repel cations, while regions of negative potential tend to repel anions. Furthermore, the greater the electrical difference at the two locations, the stronger the pulling and/or repelling forces (see Figure 13-3).

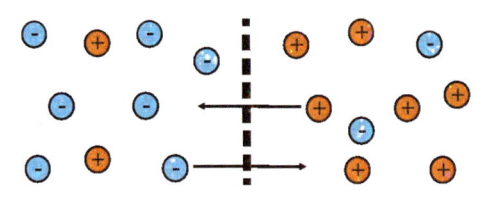

Figure 13-2. Movement along a concentration gradient

Since there are two forces acting on the movement of ions, how can you know which direction the ions will move? If the concentration gradient (or *chemical driving force*) and the electrical difference (or *electrical driving force*) act in opposite directions, there will be a net movement of ions in the direction of whichever force is greater. Notice in figure 13-3 that the cations are moving along their electrical gradient but *against* their concentration gradient, while the anions are moving along both their electrical and concentration gradients. In this course, we will not consider the mathematical calculations needed to determine which force is greater. Suffice it to say, however, that knowledge of both driving forces will help you understand how membrane potentials develop in the first place and how they can change.

MAJOR IONS AFFECTING POTENTIALS

When discussing membrane potentials, five types of ions usually pop up in the conversation: *sodium, potassium, calcium, chloride,* and *organic anions*.

Sodium ions (Na$^+$) are about 15 times more concentrated in the ECF than in the cytosol; thus, the concentration gradient tends to drive Na$^+$ *into* the cell. Na$^+$/K$^+$ pumps in the membrane transport Na$^+$ ions back into the ECF.

Potassium ions (K$^+$) are about 30 times more concentrated in the cytosol than in the ECF; thus, the concentration gradient tends to drive K$^+$ *out of* the cell. Na$^+$/K$^+$ pumps transport K$^+$ ions back into the cytosol.

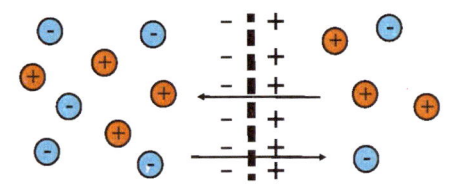

Figure 13-3. Movement along an electrical gradient

MEMBRANE POTENTIALS

Chloride ions (Cl⁻) are about 25 times more concentrated in the ECF than in the cytosol; thus, the concentration gradient tends to drive Cl⁻ into the cell. Chloride pumps in the membrane transport the Cl⁻ back into the ECF.

Calcium ions (Ca^{2+}) are about 5 times more concentrated in the ECF than in the cytosol; thus, the concentration gradient tends to drive Ca^{2+} into the cell. Calcium pumps in the membrane transport Ca^{2+} ions back into the ECF.

Organic anions (A⁻) are primarily negatively charged proteins inside the cell that are too large to pass through the membrane. Since these anions remain in the cytosol they contribute to a more negative condition on the inside border of the membrane.

DEVELOPMENT OF A MEMBRANE POTENTIAL

When excluding the region around the plasma membrane, the ECF and cytosol as a whole are electrically neutral. This is because the abundance of Na⁺ ions in the ECF is neutralized by an abundance of oppositely charged Cl⁻ ions. Likewise, the abundance of K⁺ ions in the cytosol is neutralized by an abundance of negatively charged organic ions (A⁻). So, how does a membrane potential develop? It develops primarily due to two factors:

1. Unequal diffusion of Na⁺ and K⁺: Both Na⁺ and K⁺ ions can diffuse freely through certain protein channels (pores), called **leak channels**, which are always open. However, under normal conditions, more K⁺ ions diffuse out of the cell than Na⁺ ions diffuse into the cell. This unequal diffusion of cations helps create a more negative condition on the inside border of the membrane.

2. Unequal pumping of Na⁺ and K⁺: The membrane's Na⁺/K⁺ pumps transport three Na⁺ ions out of the cell for every two K⁺ ions they transport into the cell. Thus, the unequal pumping of cations causes the inside border of the membrane to be more negative than the outside.

A resting membrane potential (RMP) is a relatively stable potential that exists only when there is very little movement of ions through the membrane. The RMP exists when all gated channels in the membrane are closed and ion concentrations approach relatively stable values on opposite sides of the membrane. To say that Na⁺ or K⁺ has reached RMP values does not mean that the concentration of the particular ion is the same on both sides of the membrane. Instead, the RMP simply means that the existing concentrations for a particular ion on opposite sides of the membrane are unchanging. So what prevents the Na⁺ and K⁺ ions from diffusing to the point that their concentration gradients become nonexistent? Let's take a closer look at the factors that maintain the concentration gradients for these ions.

Maintaining the concentration gradient for Na⁺

Generally, the plasma membrane is not very permeable to Na⁺, but still these ions find their way into the cell through leak channels. However, the rate at which the Na⁺ enters the cell under "resting" conditions are equaled by the rate at which the Na⁺/K⁺ pumps transport Na⁺ ions out of the cell. Under resting conditions, whenever three Na⁺ ions leak into the cell, the Na⁺/K⁺ pumps transport three Na⁺ ions out of the cell. However, the concentration of Na⁺ in the ECF is still much higher than in the cytosol. If a gated Na⁺ channel were to open during the RMP, Na⁺ would flow rapidly into the cell along its electrochemical gradient causing depolarization. In this case, Na⁺ would be moving along its concentration gradient *and* along the electrical gradient—toward a negatively charged region.

Maintaining the concentration gradient for K⁺

While the resting plasma membrane is not very leaky to Na⁺, it is very leaky to K⁺. However, as more K⁺ leaves the cell, the inside border of the membrane becomes more negatively charged. As a result, the negatively charged inside border begins to attract the K⁺ ions causing fewer of them to leave the cell. This means that in order to move out of the cell, K⁺ ions have to move against the electrical gradient—into a positively charged region. Even so, K⁺ will continue to leak out of the cell along its concentration gradient, but this rate is equaled by the rate at which the Na⁺/K⁺ pumps transport K⁺ ions back into the cell. Under

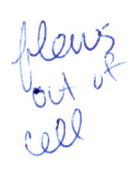

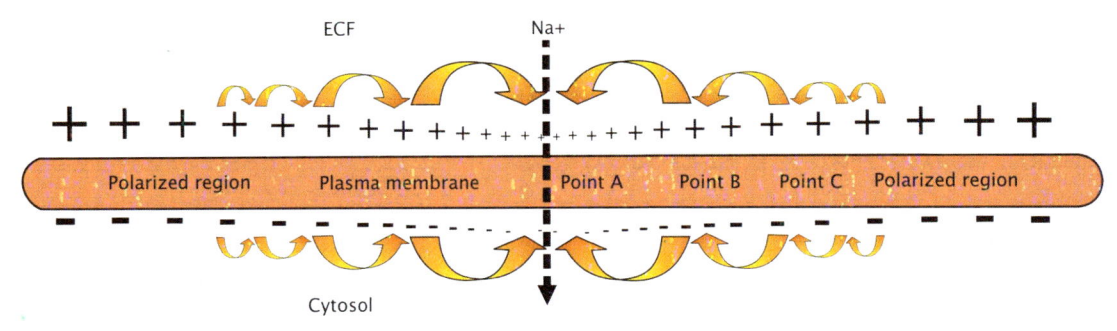

Figure 13-4. Graded potential

resting conditions, whenever two K+ ions leak out of the cell, the Na+/K+ pumps transport two K+ ions back into the cell. If a gated K+ channel were to open during the RMP, more K+ would flow out of the cell causing hyperpolarization.

When the membrane's permeability changes due to the opening of gated ion channels, the electrical conditions along the membrane change and the term *resting* potential no longer applies. Membrane potentials that are changing include *graded* potentials and *action* potentials.

GRADED POTENTIAL

A **graded potential** is a "wave" of electrical change that moves along a membrane where the magnitude of the electrical change decreases as the wave moves farther along the membrane (Figure 13-4). Graded potentials may occur in response to opening certain types of gated channels. A **ligand-gated channel** opens when a chemical, generally called a *ligand* (pronounced LĪ-gand or LIG-and; "to bind"), attaches to a receptor on the membrane. The receptor itself may function as a channel and open in response to the ligand attachment. Or the receptor may trigger reactions inside the cell that cause a channel located elsewhere in the membrane to open. A graded potential may involve either depolarization or hyperpolarization.

To illustrate how a graded potential works, let's say that a particular chemical opens a ligand-gated Na+ channel at point A on the plasma membrane. As a result, Na+ ions diffuse into the cell causing the outside border of the membrane to become less positive at point A. In turn, the inside border at point A becomes less negative. Cations in the ECF at point B quickly move toward point A to replace the cations lost from that area. Likewise, cations move from point C to point B. In addition, anions in the cytosol at point B move toward the cations entering at point A, and anions at point C move toward point B. As the figure shows, the inner border of the membrane at point B becomes slightly less negative than before. Point C also becomes less negative, but does not change as much as point B. As you can see, the depolarization "fizzles out" as it moves farther along the membrane. Points far away from point A would not depolarize at all in response to point A's depolarization.

ACTION POTENTIALS

An **action potential** is a rapid reversal in polarity in which the inside border of the cell membrane becomes positively charged and the outside border becomes negatively charged (Figure 13-5). Almost immediately after this happens, the membrane potential reverts to the original condition (becomes positive on the outside and negative on the inside). An **impulse** is a series of action potentials occurring one after another at successive locations along a membrane. Thus, an impulse moves like a wave along the membrane, but unlike a graded potential, the magnitude of electrical change generated by an impulse does not diminish as it moves farther along the membrane. Impulses occur only along membranes that contain **voltage-gated channels**. Since only neurons and muscle cells possess voltage-gated channels, these are the only types of cells along which impulses can occur.

An action potential begins when a stimulus causes either voltage-gated Na+ channels or voltage-gated Ca^{2+} channels to open. The voltage that causes a voltage-gated channel to open is called **threshold voltage**. When this happens, enough cations (Na+ and/or Ca^{2+})

MEMBRANE POTENTIALS

diffuse *into* the cell causing the inside border of the membrane to become positively charged. The region of depolarization around the voltage-gated channel covers about one square millimeter of the plasma membrane. Other voltage-gated Na^+ and/or Ca^{2+} channels in this depolarized region open and cause adjacent segments of the membrane to depolarize. In turn, more voltage-gated channels farther along the membrane open and the process continues until the impulse reaches the end of the cell.

Almost immediately after the inside border of the membrane becomes positively charged, the voltage-gated Na^+ and/or Ca^{2+} channels close and voltage-gated K^+ channels open. As K^+ ions diffuse *out* of the cell, the inside border of the cell membrane repolarizes (becomes negative again). During the time of depolarization, when the inside border of the membrane is positive, the membrane will not respond to another stimulus. This period is the **refractory period**. The membrane must repolarize before another stimulus can cause the voltage-gated Na^+ and/or Ca^{2+} channels to open. Figure 13-6 shows the involvement of different membrane channels during an action potential.

> **Note:** A perfume bottle with a pump-type sprayer also has a *refractory period*. When you depress ("depolarize") the nozzle, you get a puff of perfume ("action potential"); however, if you want another puff, you must allow the nozzle to return to its original position ("repolarize").

When threshold is reached, voltage-gated Na^+ or Ca^{2+} channels open to initiate an action potential

K^+ and/or Cl^- channels open and allow K^+ ions to leave the cell and/or Cl^- ions to enter the cell; the result is hyperpolarization; after these channels close, "pumps" move K^+ back into the cell and Cl^- back into the ECF.

Na^+ and/or Ca^{2+} channels open and allow influx of cations to cause depolarization, but threshold is not reached (ligand may be decomposed too quickly and/or not enough ligand is available); "pumps" move these ions back into the ECF to cause repolarization

Na^+ and/or Ca^{2+} channels open and allow influx of cations to cause depolarization to threshold causing voltage-gated channels to open

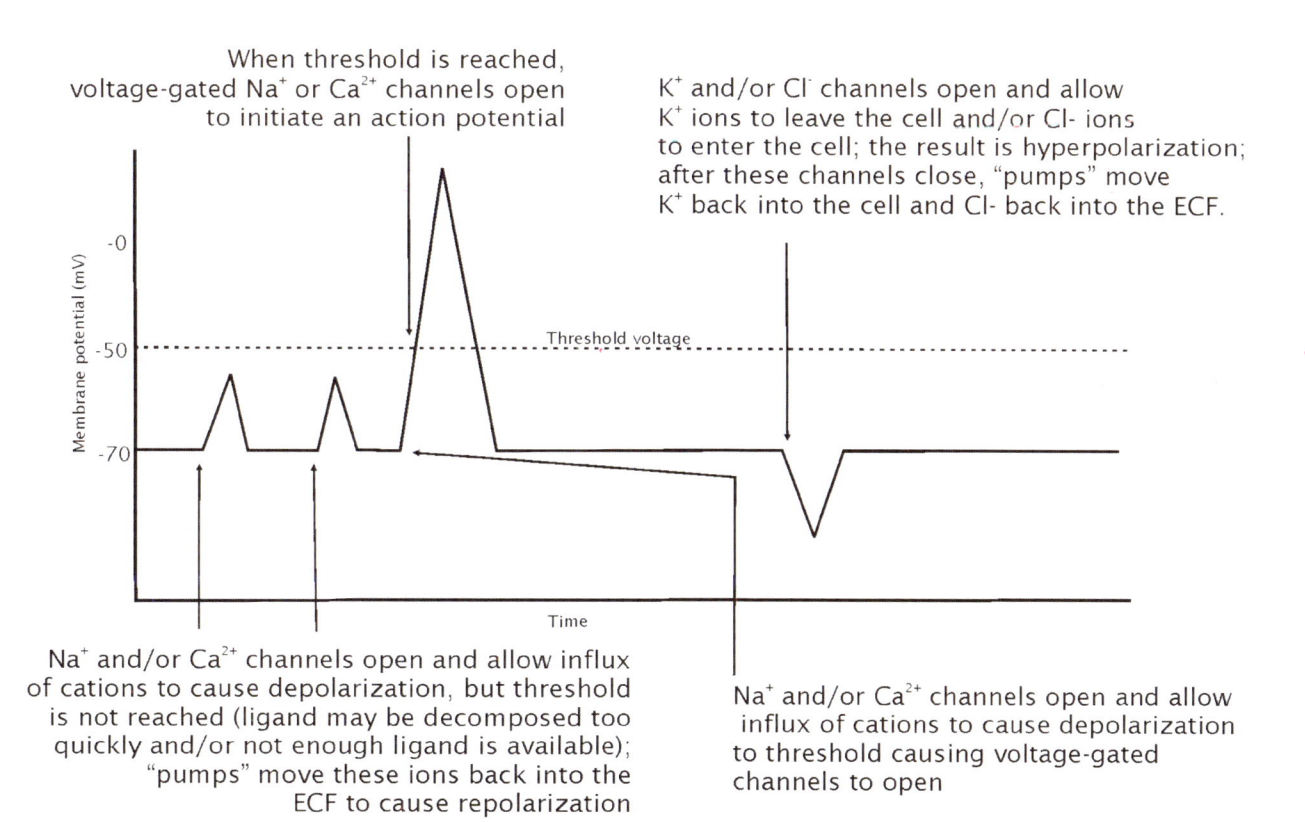

Figure 13-5. Action potential and other changes in membrane potential

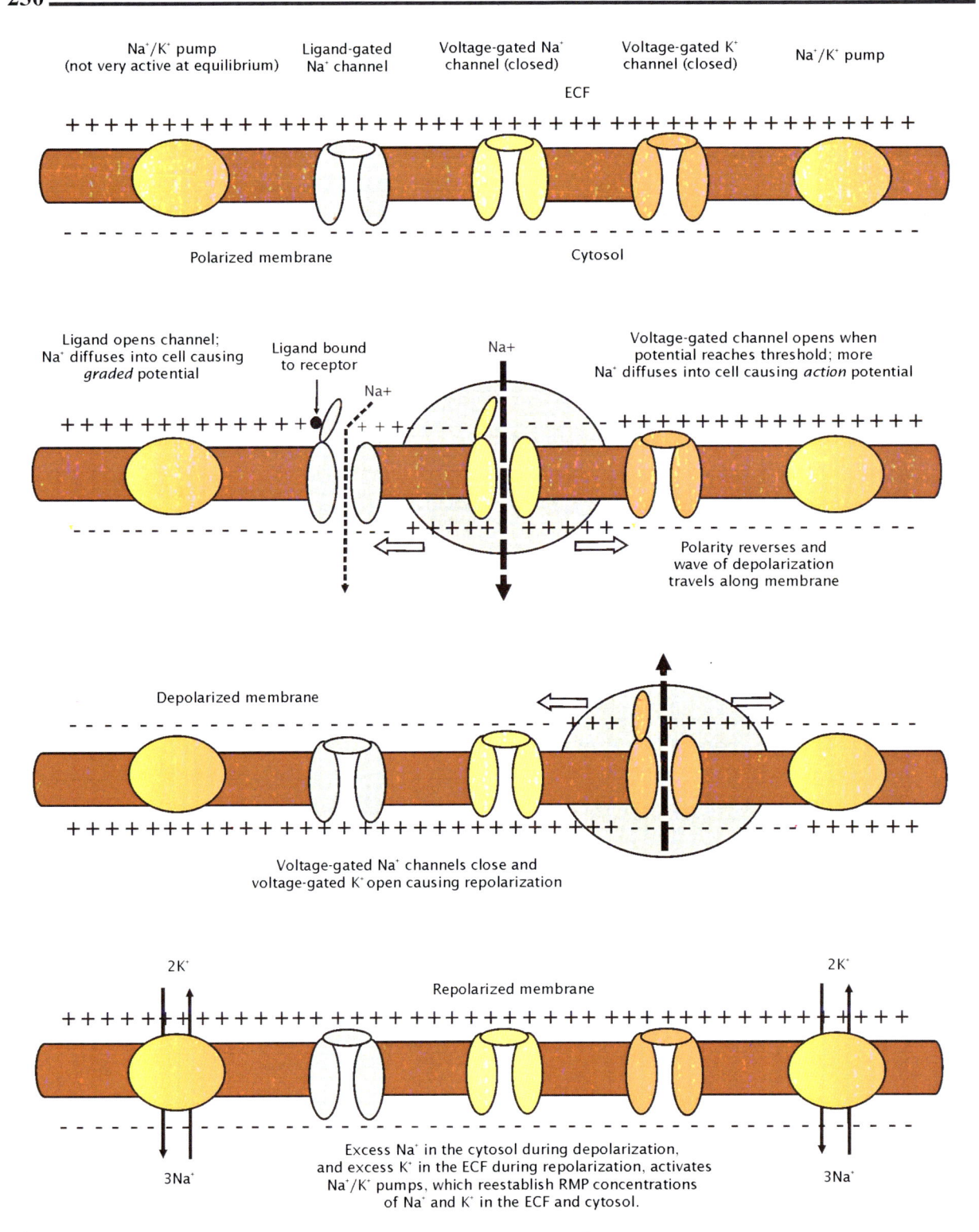

Figure 13-6. Involvement of membrane channels during an action potential

MEMBRANE POTENTIALS

TOPICS TO KNOW FOR CHAPTER 13 (MEMBRANE POTENTIALS)

- action potential
- calcium ions (Ca2+)
- chemical driving force
- chloride ions (Cl-)
- concentration gradient
- depolarization
- development of a membrane potential
- electrical driving force
- electrical gradient
- electrochemical gradient
- factors affecting ion movement
- graded potential
- hyperpolarization
- impulse
- leak channels
- ligand
- ligand-gated channel
- maintaining the concentration gradient for K+
- maintaining the concentration gradient for Na+
- major ions affecting potentials
- membrane potential (MP)
- Na+/K+ pumps
- organic anions (A-)
- potassium ions (K+)
- refractory period
- repolarization
- resting membrane potential (RMP)
- sodium ions (Na+)
- voltage
- voltage-gated channels

CHAPTER 14

Muscle Tissue

With the finish line in sight, Billy knew the end of a grueling cross-country race was near, so he mustered the last bit of energy left and began to sprint. But at that moment, he felt a sharp pain in his right hamstring muscles. Billy had just experienced a "charleyhorse" or pulled hamstring. He had torn a tendon that connected one of his hamstring muscles to the ischial tuberosity in his pelvis. As a result, the muscle was unable to help extend the thigh, so running became extremely difficult and the pain was excruciating. With perseverance, Billy finished the race with the help of his other hamstring muscles (there are actually three in each thigh).

Billy's story is not that unusual for competitive athletes, but it points out an important function of muscles; that is, movement. In fact, movement would probably have been the first thing to come to mind if you were asked, "What do muscles do?" We even nickname automobiles "muscle" cars if they can demonstrate fast movement. We often do not realize just how important muscles are to movement until we can no longer use them. While most of us probably do not run cross-country, we use muscles to walk, talk, chew, and even breathe. Muscles also move things through our bodies, such as blood and food, and they perform other vital functions.

Probably the most amazing fact about muscles is their ability to generate different levels of **tension or pulling force.** Simply by thinking, Billy was able to call upon his hamstring muscles to speed up their movements, to go from a slow pace to a sprint. This is an important trait because not all muscle tasks are the same; for example, you don't need the same amount of tension to turn this page as you do to lift a bowling ball. In this chapter, we will provide an overview of the different types of muscle tissue, and will present more detail about several types. In the end, you should be familiar with the anatomy of muscle tissue and know what makes muscles "run."

OVERVIEW OF MUSCLE TISSUES

A **muscle** is an organ consisting mostly of **muscle tissue** made up of cells called **muscle fibers**, also called **myofibers**, or simply, **muscle cells**. Muscle fibers have the unique ability to generate tension or pulling force through a process called *contraction*. This process was so named because it often causes the muscle to shorten (*contract*, draw together). However, a contracting muscle may not always shorten, but it will *always* generate tension. Then again, a muscle will shorten if its contraction force exceeds the load or force that is preventing the muscle from shortening. When a contracting muscle lessens its tension, the process is called *relaxation* ("to loosen").

TYPES OF MUSCLE TISSUES

The body contains three types of muscle tissue, each differing in location, microscopic structure, function, and control.

Skeletal muscle tissue is the most abundant type of muscle tissue, so named because most of it is bound indirectly, by way of tendons, to bones of the skeletal system. Skeletal muscle fibers are long and cylindrical and have *striations*—alternating light and dark stripes. Each end of a skeletal muscle fiber is attached to fibrous connective tissue, which is bound to another organ, usually a bone. On average, skeletal muscle fibers are the longest muscles cells in the body.

Skeletal muscle fibers are the only muscle fibers that a person can consciously control; for this reason, they are called *voluntary* muscle fibers. Despite that, sometimes it is necessary for the nervous system to control skeletal muscle fibers involuntarily. For example, the nervous system causes rhythmic, involuntary contractions of muscles in your chest to maintain breathing while you sleep. In another case, the nervous system can cause muscles in your arm to contract involuntarily to jerk your hand away from a hot stove, thus preventing a severe burn.

Cardiac muscle tissue is found only in the heart and, like skeletal muscle fibers, is striated. However, unlike skeletal muscle fibers, which resemble single rods with ends attached to connective tissue, cardiac muscle fibers are branched and connect end-to-end with other cardiac muscle fibers. The site where two cardiac muscle fibers connect to one another is called an *intercalated disc*. Since cardiac muscle is not under conscious control, we say it is *involuntary* muscle. A small group of specialized cardiac muscle fibers, called *pacemaker cells*, transmits electrical signals, called APs, to other cardiac muscle fibers causing them to contract. The rate at which pacemaker cells send out these signals is influenced by the nervous system and by chemicals, such as hormones, in the blood.

Smooth muscle tissue is abundant in the walls of soft, hollow organs, such as the stomach, intestines, urinary bladder, and blood vessels. Smooth muscle fibers are arranged together in sheets and are tapered on each end. They lack the striations seen in skeletal and cardiac muscle fibers; hence, the name "smooth" is appropriate. Some smooth muscle fibers connect to and affect adjacent smooth muscle fibers through gap junctions. Like cardiac muscle tissue, smooth muscle tissue is under *involuntary* control.

FUNCTIONS OF MUSCLE TISSUE

While each type of muscle tissue has a limited number of functions, altogether muscle tissue performs six important roles in the body:

- **Movement** is probably the first function that comes to mind when most people hear the word "muscle." Skeletal muscles are responsible for virtually all bone movement (an exception is in the ear where tiny bones vibrate in response to sound). Without the ability to move bones, a person would be unable to walk, chew, swim, or grasp and move external objects. While most skeletal muscles cause bone movement, others cause movement of soft organs. For example, muscles pulling on the skin of the face produce facial expressions such as smiling and frowning. Even at this moment, small skeletal muscles are tugging on your eyeballs to make them move so you can read this sentence.

   Movement is the most vital function of cardiac and smooth muscle. Rhythmic contractions of cardiac muscle squeeze blood out of the heart and into blood vessels where it delivers nutrients and oxygen to all of your cells and removes their wastes. Rhythmic contractions of smooth muscle moves food through the digestive system, urine through the urinary system, and gametes (sex cells) through the reproductive system. Even birth results when smooth muscle contracts in the walls of the mother's uterus and pushes a baby through the birth canal. Furthermore, smooth muscle tissue in arrector pili muscles pulls on hair follicles, causing them to push up the epidermis and form goose bumps.

- **Maintaining posture**, including the ability to sit in a chair and hold your head steady while reading, is possible because contracting skeletal

MUSCLE TISSUE

muscles can *prevent* movement of your neck and back. Maintaining posture does not require your undivided attention. You were probably not aware of your posture before reading the previous sentence, but now you are thinking about it and could voluntarily change your posture. This ability demonstrates that your brain can control skeletal muscles both voluntarily (consciously) and involuntarily.

- **Stabilizing joints** is a major function of skeletal muscles. Although ligaments are primarily responsible for holding bones together at joints, contracting skeletal muscles can help stabilize the joint. When a skeletal muscle's tendon crosses a joint, contracting the muscle can pull the articulating bones closer together and prevent their separation.

- **Regulating movement of food and liquids** is an important homeostatic function of smooth and cardiac muscle. While muscle tissue can force material through hollow organs, it can also restrict such movement. At specific sites in the digestive and urinary systems, rings of muscle tissue form *sphincters* that encircle short segments of a soft tubular organ. Contracting a sphincter can squeeze the tube so tightly that materials can no longer move through the tube. This is like squeezing your hand around a water hose to stop the flow of water. Relaxing a sphincter causes the tubular organ to expand allowing materials to pass freely through it. Some sphincters contain smooth muscle, while others contain skeletal muscle. The latter type allows a person to control urination (expelling urine from the urinary system) and defecation (expelling feces from the digestive system) voluntarily.

In addition to forming sphincters, muscle tissue also regulates the movement of blood through blood vessels. The walls of blood vessels contain smooth muscle that can respond to chemicals in the blood or signals from the nervous system. Contraction or relaxation of this smooth muscle changes the diameter of the vessels, thereby regulating the amount of blood moving into or out of certain organs.

- **Protection and support of visceral organs** is an important function of skeletal muscle tissue. Skeletal muscles form the walls and floor of the abdominopelvic cavity, and protect and support visceral organs within that cavity. The abdominal muscles offer even more protection when they contract, because contraction makes the muscles become firm. With this in mind, a boxer will contract his abdominal muscles to withstand the hard belly punches thrown by an opponent.

- **Generating body heat** is a significant function of skeletal muscles. For the same reason that a car engine generates heat as it releases energy from gasoline, muscles generate heat when they release energy from food molecules. Some of this heat is lost to the external environment, but some of it helps the body maintain a warm, stable internal temperature. When the external environment is cold, the nervous system stimulates skeletal muscles to *shiver*, or contract and relax in a vibrating pattern. Shivering generates extra heat that warms the blood and can help prevent a drop in the internal body temperature.

CHARACTERISTICS OF MUSCLE TISSUE

Muscle tissue can perform the functions just described because of the following four functional characteristics:

- **Excitability**, or **irritability**, is the ability of a muscle fiber to respond to a stimulus by generating APs that propagate (move) along its cell membrane. The APs, in turn, initiate chemical reactions inside the muscle fiber that cause the fiber to contract. Chemicals released from the nervous and endocrine systems are the major stimuli that cause muscle fibers to generate APs.

- **Contractility** is the ability of a muscle fiber to generate tension. Under normal conditions, a muscle fiber contracts only in response to stimuli that generates APs. A contracting muscle fiber generates tension (a pulling force) on the structure to which it is attached. Whereas a skeletal muscle fiber may generate tension on a tendon, cardiac

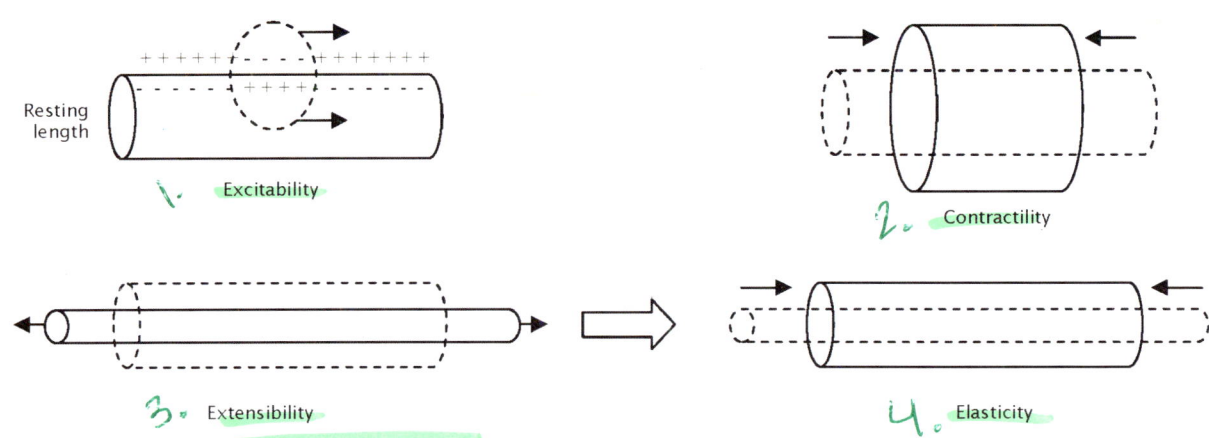

Figure 14-1. Characteristics of a muscle fiber

1. Excitability
2. Contractility
3. Extensibility
4. Elasticity

and smooth muscle fibers exert tension on neighboring muscle fibers. Contractility is unique to muscle fibers.

- **Extensibility** is the ability of a muscle fiber to stretch beyond a normal length without tearing. In this respect, a muscle fiber is like a rubber band. In many cases, one skeletal muscle stretches when another skeletal muscle shortens. For example, if you contract (shorten) the muscle on the anterior part of your upper arm, your elbow bends and stretches the muscle on the posterior side of your arm. Cardiac and smooth muscle fibers are also extensible. Blood filling the heart stretches cardiac muscle in the heart's walls, while blood coursing through blood vessels may stretch smooth muscle in the vessels' walls. Moreover, food filling the stomach and urine filling the urinary bladder stretches smooth muscle tissue in the walls of these organs.

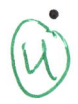

- **Elasticity** is the ability of a stretched muscle fiber to recoil (spring back) to its resting length. Elasticity is a passive process, one that does not require energy input, such as the recoil of a rubber band after it has been stretched. In essence, muscle fibers demonstrate their elasticity *after* they demonstrate their extensibility. See a muscle fiber's characteristics in Figure 14-1.

ANATOMY OF A SKELETAL MUSCLE

A skeletal muscle is a complex organ consisting of skeletal muscle tissue and connective tissue. In addition, a skeletal muscle contains organs of other body systems; these organs include blood vessels (cardiovascular system), lymphatic vessels (lymphatic system), and nerves (nervous system). Skeletal muscles come in a variety of shapes and sizes. The size of a muscle depends primarily on the number of skeletal muscle fibers present. Small skeletal muscles in the face, hands, and feet may contain only a few hundred muscle fibers. Large skeletal muscles in the chest, back, and thigh may contain many thousands of muscle fibers. In this section, we will describe the organization of a "typical" skeletal muscle, beginning with its association with connective tissue. Figure 14-2 shows the levels of organization in a skeletal muscle.

Connective tissue coverings

Layers of connective tissue serve five important functions for the muscular system. They (1) separate the muscular system from other organ systems; (2) separate, protect, and insulate individual muscles; (3) divide individual muscles into several levels of organization; (4) provide passageways for nerves and blood vessels entering and leaving the muscles; and (5) contribute to a muscle's elasticity. We will now examine the specific layers of connective tissue that are responsible for these functions.

- **Superficial fascia** (also called **subcutaneous tissue** or **hypodermis**) is a combination of adipose and areolar connective tissue that separates the dermis of the skin from the underlying skeletal muscles. The superficial

MUSCLE TISSUE

237

fascia is so named because it lies closest to the body's outer surface (*superficial*, surface). Adipose tissue in the superficial fascia acts like an insulating blanket to keep the muscles warm, and it provides the muscles with triglycerides for energy. The superficial fascia also supports blood vessels and nerves that enter and leave the outermost skeletal muscles.

- **Deep fascia** is a sheath of dense irregular connective tissue that lies deep to the superficial fascia and separates individual muscles from one another. For example, deep fascia separates five muscles in the brachial region of the upper limb. If you gently separate skeletal muscles in the lab, you can see deep fascia appearing much like strands of cotton spanning the gap between the muscles.

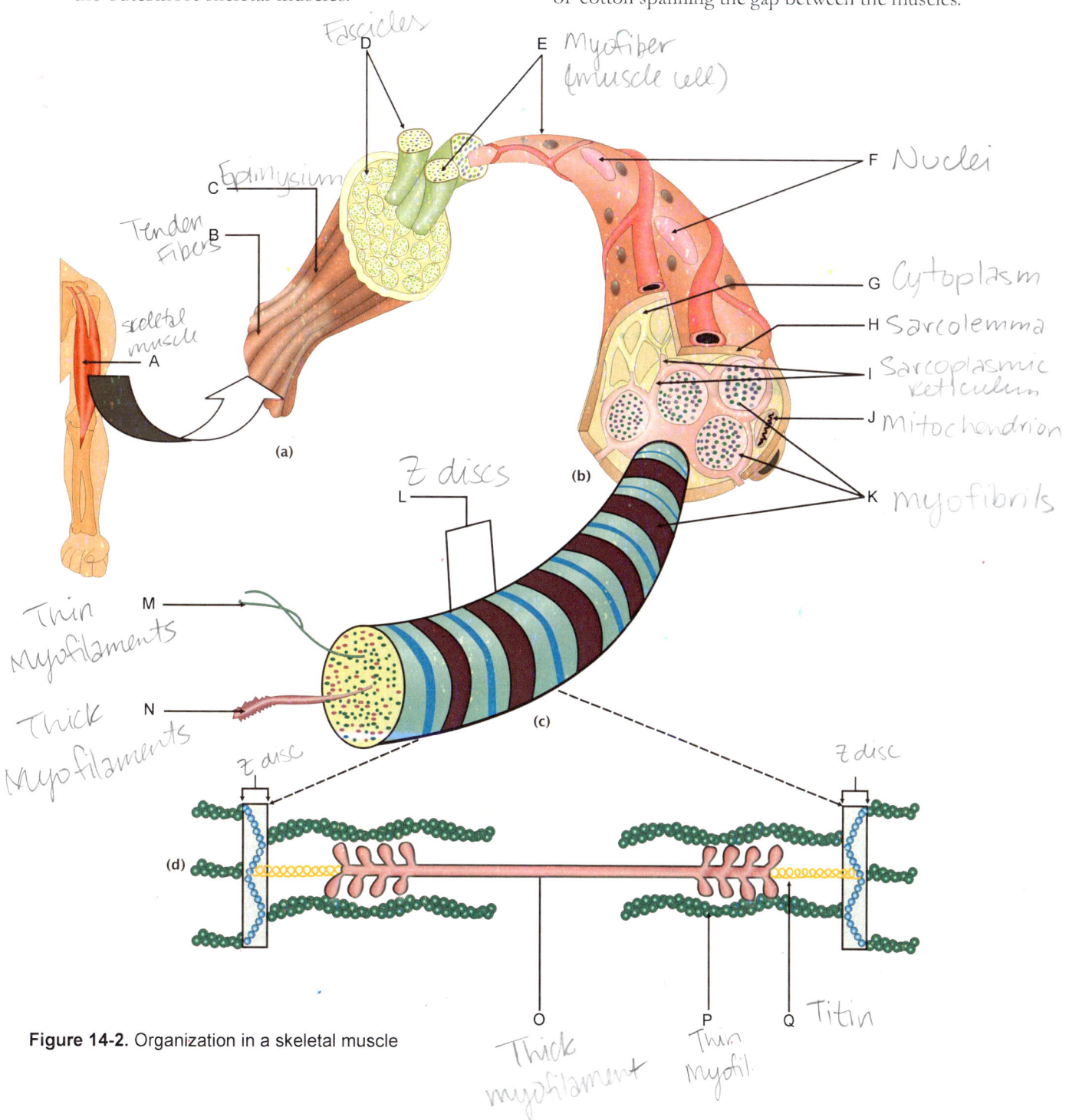

Figure 14-2. Organization in a skeletal muscle

Labels:
- A — skeletal muscle
- B — Tendon Fibers
- C — Epimysium
- D — Fascicles
- E — Myofiber (muscle cell)
- F — Nuclei
- G — Cytoplasm
- H — Sarcolemma
- I — Sarcoplasmic Reticulum
- J — Mitochondrion
- K — Myofibrils
- L — Z discs
- M — Thin Myofilaments
- N — Thick Myofilaments
- O — Thick myofilament
- P — Thin myofil.
- Q — Titin

Blood vessels and nerves course through the deep fascia where they split into smaller branches that enter the muscles.

- **Epimysium** (ep-i-MIS-ē-um; *epi*, upon; *mys*, muscle) is a sheath of dense irregular connective tissue below the deep fascia and covering individual muscles. When deep fascia is scraped away, the epimysium appears as a glistening membrane on the muscle's surface. You might compare epimysium to the clear plastic wrap that adheres tightly to a piece of meat at the grocery store. Epimysium acts like a girdle to hold muscle fibers together as a group within a skeletal muscle. If a contracting muscle becomes shorter and thicker, the epimysium helps prevent it from tearing. In addition, the natural elasticity of dense irregular tissue helps the muscle spring back to its resting length after stretching.

- **Perimysium** (per-i-MIS-ē-um; *peri*, around) is a continuation of the epimysium and extends deep into a skeletal muscle to bundle muscle fibers into groups called **fascicles**. The fascicles within a skeletal muscle are responsible for the "grain" of a meat, like the thin slivers of meat in a roast beef sandwich. If you have access to "muscle" models in the lab, look for fascicles as small parallel ridges on the surfaces of the skeletal muscles. The perimysium supports small blood vessels and nerves leading into and out of the fascicles.

- **Endomysium** (en-dō-MIS-ē-um; *endo*, inside) is mostly areolar connective tissue that extends from the perimysium to surround individual muscle fibers within the fascicles. The endomysium insulates the muscle fibers as a thin rubber coating insulates electrical wires. In this way, APs can spread along one muscle fiber without "jumping" over to stimulate an adjacent fiber. The endomysium supports tiny blood vessels and nerves that lie between the muscle fibers. In addition, elastic fibers within the endomysium help muscle fibers recoil after they are stretched.

Tendons and Aponeuroses

The connective tissues that surround and penetrate skeletal muscles also extend from the muscles as thick bands or broad sheets. These structures, which anchor the ends of skeletal muscles to other organs, include *tendons* and *aponeuroses*.

- **Tendons** are thick, cordlike bands of dense regular connective tissue that anchor a skeletal muscle to a bone. You can easily feel the calcaneal, or *Achilles*, tendon extending from your calf muscle to your calcaneus (heel bone).

- **Aponeuroses** (ap-ō-nū-RŌ-sez; *apo*, from; *neuro*, tendon) are broad, sheet-like tendons that attach a flat skeletal muscle to a bone or to another skeletal muscle. An example is the *epicranial aponeurosis* that covers the top of the skull like a helmet. Contracting and relaxing certain scalp muscles moves this aponeurosis, causing the scalp to move back and forth.

Nerve Supply

Under normal circumstances, a skeletal muscle contracts only in response to APs from the nervous system. In most cases, these APs reach the muscle through a single nerve. The nerve penetrates the epimysium near the center of the muscle then divides extensively, much like branches of a tree. The branches of the nerve course through the perimysium between the muscle's fascicles.

The nerve that penetrates a skeletal muscle not only conducts APs *into* the muscle, it also conducts APs *out* of the muscle. These "sensory" signals that exit the muscle may result from muscle stretching, cell damage, or accumulation of cellular wastes. After interpreting these signals, the brain can adjust the amount of stimulation it sends to the muscle. In this way, you can jerk your foot off a piece of broken glass without having to think about doing it.

Blood Supply

Maintaining homeostasis requires that muscle fibers have a steady supply of oxygen and nutrients, and constant removal of wastes, including excess heat. In most cases, only a single artery delivers blood rich in oxygen and nutrients to the skeletal muscle. Inside the muscle, the artery branches into many small arteries that course through the perimysium. The small arteries feed the smallest vessels, called *capillaries*, which run

MUSCLE TISSUE

alongside each muscle fiber. Oxygen and nutrients diffuse out of the capillaries and into the muscle fiber, while cellular wastes diffuse out of the fiber and into the capillaries. The capillaries also absorb heat that the fibers generate during metabolism. Numerous capillaries unite to form *veins*, which transports the blood out of the muscle.

ANATOMY OF A SKELETAL MUSCLE FIBER

We will now describe the anatomy of a skeletal muscle fiber in order to provide a firm foundation on which to explain muscle fiber physiology in later sections. We will begin this section by describing the muscle fiber's most obvious anatomical features (see Figure 14-3).

Fiber shape and size

At first glance, the two most striking differences between a skeletal muscle fiber and a "typical" body cell are cell shape and size. Whereas a typical body cell is extremely small and cube-shaped, the typical skeletal muscle fiber is a thick, cylindrical cell. Some skeletal muscle fibers are about ten times wider and hundreds of times longer than the typical body cell. Most skeletal muscle fibers normally extend the entire length of the muscle in which they are found.

> **Note:** Skeletal muscle fibers range in thickness from 10-100 um (about the same as a scalp hair) and may exceed lengths of 60 cm (24 inches).

Multiple nuclei

Skeletal muscle fibers are *multinucleate*; that is, they have more than one nucleus. Each nucleus is diploid, containing *two* complete sets or 46 chromosomes (23 maternal and 23 paternal). How do skeletal muscle fibers become multinucleate? To answer, we must look back to see how a skeletal muscle fiber develops before a person is born. At that time, undifferentiated cells called **myoblasts** (MĪ-ō-blasts; *blast*, germinate), each having only one nucleus, fuse with one another. The nucleus of each myoblast persists inside the newly formed cell, which differentiates into a skeletal muscle fiber. A few

myoblasts remain as **satellite cells** between the muscle fibers and play a role in muscle fiber regeneration. The number of nuclei within a muscle fiber depends on the number of myoblasts that fuse. Some skeletal muscle fibers have more than 200 nuclei.

Does having many nuclei provide any special benefit to the cell? Being the largest cells in the body, muscle fiber must replace many more worn-out proteins than the typical body cell. Therefore, having many nuclei along the entire length of the fiber allows gene transcription to occur at many locations in the fiber simultaneously. In turn, messenger RNA molecules are readily available for translation at ribosomes that are dispersed throughout the fiber.

Sarcolemma, Sarcoplasm, and T tubules

The cell membrane and cytoplasm of a muscle fiber have enough unique qualities that cell biologists give them special names. The cell (plasma) membrane of a muscle fiber is called the **sarcolemma** (sar-kō-LEM a;

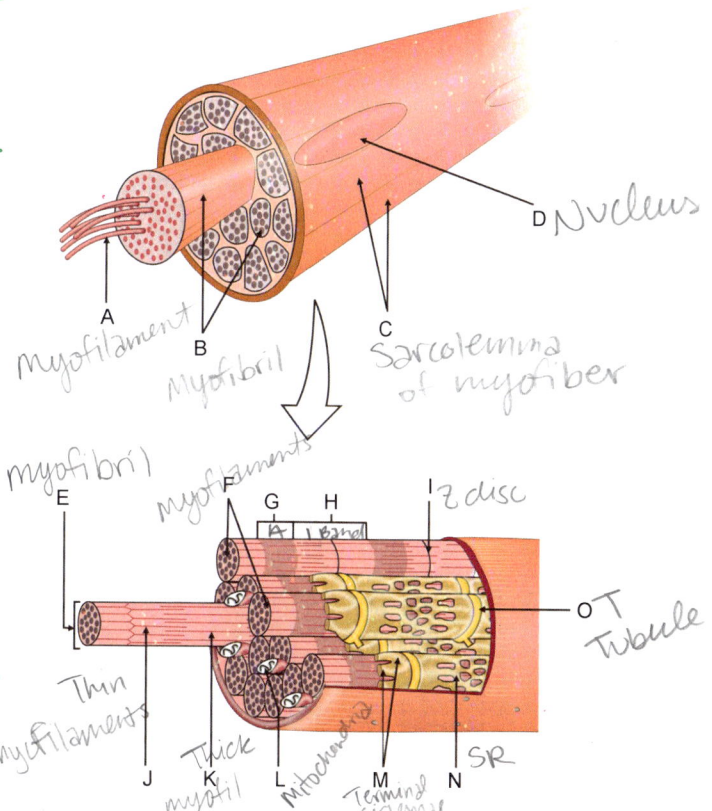

Figure 14-3. Anatomy of a skeletal muscle fiber

sarco, flesh; *lemma*, husk). Like other cell membranes, the sarcolemma consists of a phospholipid bilayer containing integral and peripheral proteins. However, the sarcolemma contains special channels that allow certain ions to pass into or out of the fiber at a rapid pace. The movement of these ions changes the electrical condition of the membrane and ultimately leads to contraction of the fiber.

The sarcolemma surrounds the muscle fiber's cytoplasm, which is called **sarcoplasm** (SAR-kō-plazm; *plasm*, something formed). In addition to having the usual organelles, skeletal and cardiac muscle fibers have some unique organelles called *myofibrils*. Myofibrils fill most of the sarcoplasm, leaving little room for other organelles and the cytosol (liquid surrounding all organelles). Muscle fibers also contain several inclusions, including *glycogen* and *myoglobin*. Glucose enters a muscle fiber through facilitated diffusion and may be stored as glycogen. Later, glycogen releases the glucose molecules that can provide energy for ATP synthesis. Myoglobin is a red-colored pigment that binds oxygen molecules. When needed, oxygen detaches from myoglobin and can enter the mitochondria to participate in ATP synthesis.

Before a skeletal muscle fiber can contract, APs must pass into the interior of the fiber. Tiny invaginations, called **T (transverse) tubules**, in the sarcolemma provide a pathway for this to happen. We can make model T tubules by pressing our fingers into a water-filled balloon. Notice that the lining of the indentations made by the fingers is continuous with the remainder of the balloon. In the same way, the linings of T tubules are continuous with the rest of the sarcolemma. The openings to thousands of T tubules dot the entire length of the skeletal muscle at regular intervals. Extracellular fluid fills the T tubules but does not mix with the cytosol.

The Sarcoplasmic Reticulum

Each T tubule runs deep into the sarcoplasm and connects with a system of fluid-filled tubes and sacs called the **sarcoplasmic reticulum (SR)**. On both sides and running parallel to a T tubule, the SR expands to form sacs called **terminal cisternae** (sis-TER-nā; reservoir for storing water). Each T tubule and its two adjoining terminal cisternae collectively form a **triad** (TRĪ-ad; three).

For the most part, the thin tubular parts of the SR that run parallel to the myofibril's long axis function like the smooth endoplasmic reticulum in other cells. However, the bulging terminal cisternae function as reservoirs for storing calcium ions (Ca^{2+}), which play a vital role in contraction. Integral **calcium pumps** located in the terminal cisternae actively transport Ca^{2+} ions from the cytosol into the lumen (internal space) of the SR. Inside the SR, Ca^{2+} ions may bind with a calcium-binding protein called **calsequestrin** (kal-se-KWES-trin), allowing the SR to take in (sequester) even more Ca^{2+} ions and store them. As a result, the concentration of Ca^{2+} in the terminal cisternae is about 40,000 times higher than in the cytosol. Prior to contraction, the terminal cisternae release Ca^{2+} ions that play an important role in the contraction process.

Myofibrils

The SR surrounds hundreds to thousands of cylindrical organelles called **myofibrils** (mī-ō-FĪ-brilz; *fibril*, little fiber), which are responsible for the muscle fiber's contractility. If we liken myofibrils to fingers, the SR would fit like a loosely woven glove around each finger. Altogether, myofibrils occupy about 80% of the sarcoplasm and run parallel to one another along the length of the muscle fiber. The ends of each myofibril are bound to the inner surface of the sarcolemma. Organelles and inclusions occupy the limited space between the myofibrils.

Each myofibril consists of repeating subunits called **sarcomeres** (SAR-kō-mērz; *mere*, part) which represent the basic contractile units of *striated* muscle (skeletal and cardiac muscle) (see Figure 14-4).

The cylindrical sarcomeres connect to one another similar to soft drink cans placed end-to-end. A sarcomere extends between two thin, dark lines called **Z discs**, or **Z lines**. (The "Z" stands for *zwischen*, a German word meaning "between.") Each Z disc consists of intertwining proteins called *actinin* that form a net-like pattern extending across the myofibril. The actinins also extend between adjacent myofibrils all the way across the muscle fiber. This interconnection between Z discs helps keep the sarcomeres of adjacent myofibrils "in line" with one another.

MUSCLE TISSUE

A sarcomere contains an assortment of proteins that group together to form **thick** and **thin myofilaments**, named according to their relative thicknesses. The two types of myofilaments run parallel along the sarcomere's long axis and interact to shorten the sarcomere during contraction. The arrangement of the thick and thin myofilaments causes the myofibrils to display alternating light and dark bands, or **striations** (strī-Ā-shunz; *stria*, stripe). The different colored striations are called *A bands and I bands*.

> Note: A simple way to remember the myofibril's striations: *A* bands are d**A**rk; *I* bands are l**I**ght).

A bands: dark striations along a myofibril. The "A" stands for *anisotropic* (an-ī-sō-TRŌ-pik), a term that means this region scatters light unevenly. The A band occupies the central portion of the sarcomere and contains both thick and thin myofilaments. The A band is further divided into three regions: *M line*, *H zone*, and *zones of overlap*.

1. The **M line** is a thin line located in the center of the A band. The "M" stands for *mittel*, a German word meaning "middle." The M line contains proteins called *myomesin* that extend across the width of the myofibril and keep the thick myofilaments in line. These proteins keep the thick myofilaments an equal distance apart within the sarcomere.

2. The **H zone** is a narrow, pale region on either side of the M line. The "H" stands for *helle*, a German word meaning "clear." The H zone contains only thick myofilaments.

3. The **zones of overlap** are two dark regions extending from either side of the H zone to the edge of the A band. These zones contain overlapping thick and thin myofilaments. Six thin myofilaments surround each thick myofilament, while three thick myofilaments surround each thin myofilament. A triad (one T tubule and two terminal cisternae) covers each zone of overlap; hence, two triads cover each sarcomere.

I bands: the light-colored striations along a myofibril. The "I" stands for *isotropic* (ī-sō-TRŌ-pik), implying that this region reflects light evenly. Each I band extends between the A bands of connected sarcomeres, with a Z line in the middle. For this reason, two sarcomeres share *half* of one I band. The I bands contain thin myofilaments, but no thick myofilaments.

MYOFILAMENTS

Before we can understand how myofilaments interact to generate tension in a muscle, we must first be familiar with their composition and structure (Figure 14-5).

Thick myofilaments have a larger diameter than thin myofilaments and are primarily responsible for muscle movement during contraction. Each thick myofilament contains about 250 contractile proteins called **myosin** (MĪ-ō-sin) and an elastic, structural protein called **titin** (TĪ-tin; *titan*, large). Up close, a thick myofilament looks something like a stem covered with teardrop-shaped leaves with a bare zone in the middle. The titin extends through the core of the thick myofilament and attaches to proteins in the Z disc. Thus, titin anchors the thick myofilament to a Z disc much like a mooring rope secures a boat to a pier. Additionally, if an external force stretches a sarcomere, the titin will stretch as well. Removing the external force

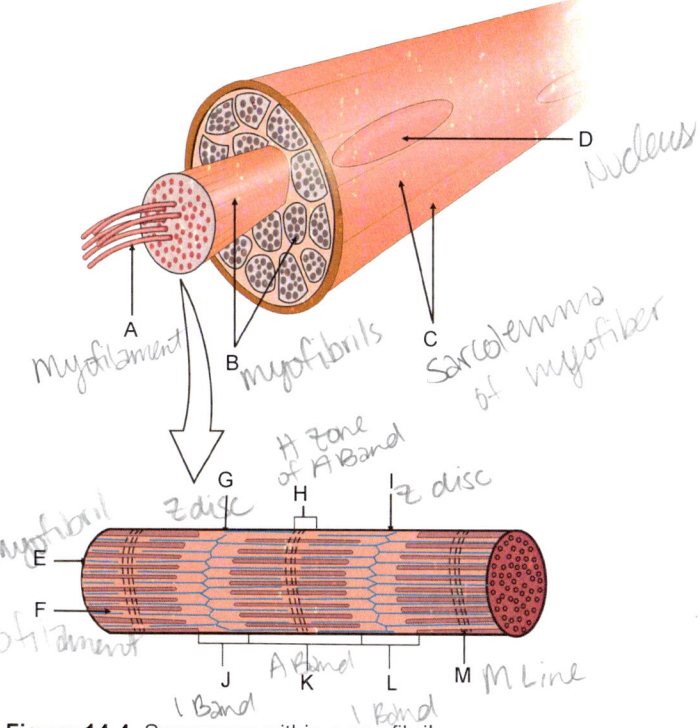

Figure 14-4. Sarcomere within a myofibril

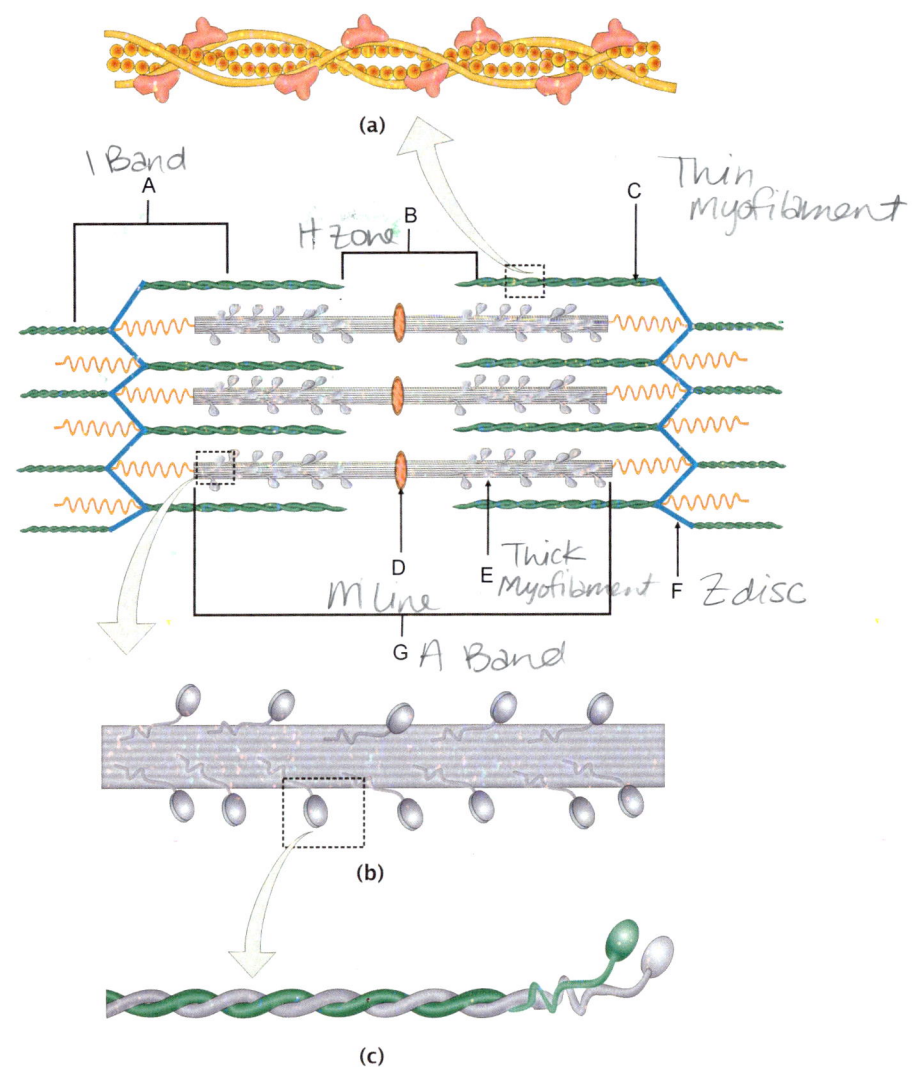

Figure 14-5. Structure of myofilaments

allows the titin to recoil and pull the Z discs closer together. As this happens, the sarcomere returns to its resting length.

> **Note:** Titin is named for its large ("titanic") size; with over 25,000 amino acids, it is the body's largest protein.

Each myosin molecule within a thick myofilament consists of two subunits resembling golf clubs. The long portions of these subunits intertwine to form a double helix. All in all, a complete myosin molecule looks like a two-headed golf club with a twisted shaft. Moreover, two myosin molecules bind to one another at the tips of their tails. The shaft of the myosin is the **tail**, and all myosin tails within a thick myofilament point toward the sarcomere's M line. The two protruding knobs at one end of each myosin molecule are the **myosin heads**. During contraction, the two heads bind to the thin myofilament, forming a "cross over" or "bridge" with the thin myofilament. For this reason, we will refer to the two heads on each myosin molecule collectively as a **myosin crossbridge**, or simply crossbridge.

The myosin crossbridge contains two sites that are important to the myosin's functional role in contraction. The **actin-binding site** is capable of binding to an actin molecule, one of the proteins in a thin myofilament. The **ATPase site** hydrolyzes an ATP to form ADP +

MUSCLE TISSUE

P$_i$ (the P$_i$ is an inorganic phosphate ion), which provides the energy for contraction. The central portion of a thick myofilament in skeletal and cardiac muscle fibers is relatively smooth because it lacks crossbridges.

A thick myofilament produces movement when it bends at two "hinge" sites. One hinge site bends the myosin tail like an arm bends at the elbow, while the other hinge site bends the crossbridge like a hand bends at the wrist. When both sites are bent, the myosin is said to be in its *low-energy position*. When the ATPase site hydrolyzes ATP, the myosin becomes cocked in a straight, *high-energy position*. In this position, the ADP and P$_i$ remain attached to the crossbridge. This is like pressing down the bar of a mousetrap and then keeping your finger on the bar. If you release the spring-loaded bar, it quickly snaps to the "sprung" position. Likewise, removing the ADP and P$_i$ from the crossbridge causes the crossbridge to "spring" back to the low-energy position.

Thin myofilaments have a smaller diameter than thick myofilaments, and they are pulled by myosin crossbridges to generate tension during a contraction. Each thin myofilament resembles two pearl necklaces that are twisted together. Each "pearl" in the chain is a globular protein called **G actin** ("G" stands for globular), while the double chain of G actin molecules is called **F actin** ("F" stands for *filamentous*). A filamentous protein called *nebulin* holds the two strands of G actin molecules together in the F actin. Each G actin contains a myosin-binding site to which a myosin crossbridge can attach.

Two regulatory proteins, *tropomyosin* and *troponin*, are found on the thin myofilament, and they control when the myosin crossbridges can attach to G actin. **Tropomyosin** (trō-pō-MĪ-ō-sin; *tropo*, turning) is a double stranded, filamentous protein that spirals through F actin. When the muscle fiber is relaxed, tropomyosin covers the myosin-binding sites on actin, preventing the crossbridges to actin. **Troponin** (TRŌ-po-nin) is a protein consisting of three polypeptide chains. One of the polypeptides holds the troponin to the actin. The second polypeptide holds the troponin to tropomyosin to form a *troponin-tropomyosin* complex. Calcium ions can bind with the remaining polypeptide, causing it to change shape and move tropomyosin away from the myosin-binding sites. Exposing the myosin-binding sites allows myosin crossbridges to bind with actin.

CONTRACTION AND RELAXATION OF SKELETAL MUSCLE FIBERS

At this point, you should be familiar with the organization and chemical composition of a skeletal muscle fiber; this information is crucial to understanding muscle fiber contraction. Now we will describe how myofilaments interact to cause contraction, and what prevents myofilaments from interacting to cause relaxation.

Sliding Filament Theory

A muscle fiber contracts (generates tension) when myosin crossbridges on the thick myofilaments attach to and pull the thin myofilaments. During this time, the thin myofilaments "slide" past the thick myofilaments, which remain stationary, but the lengths of the myofilaments do not change. This explanation of contraction is the **sliding filament theory**. Contraction according to the sliding filament theory has the following effects on sarcomeres (see Figure 14-6):

1. Z discs move closer together. Since thin myofilaments connect directly to Z discs, pulling the thin myofilaments toward the center of the sarcomere pulls the Z discs in the same direction. As a result, the sarcomere shortens during contraction.

2. I bands become narrower. Recall that one-half of an I band extends from a Z disc to the thick myofilaments. Since the Z discs of a shortening sarcomere are moving toward the thick myofilaments, the width of the I band becomes narrower.

3. Zones of overlap become wider. As the thick myofilaments pull the thin myofilaments toward the center of the sarcomere, the two types of myofilaments overlap to a greater degree.

4. H zone becomes narrower. The "free" ends of the thin myofilaments (the ends not attached to Z discs) mark the outer boundaries of the H zone. Consequently, pulling the thin myofilaments toward the center of the sarcomere causes their

free ends to move toward the M line, making the H zone narrower.

5. **Width of A bands remains constant.** Recall that the length of the thick myofilaments determines the width of the A bands; therefore, contraction does not change the width of the A bands.

Crossbridge cycling

Now that you know the effects of myofilament interaction on sarcomere length, we will describe *how* the myofilaments interact. The sequence of events by which a myosin crossbridge binds to actin, generates tension, then detaches from actin is called a **crossbridge cycle**. Even during the shortest contraction episode, a crossbridge must repeat the crossbridge cycle many times; this is called **crossbridge cycling** (Figure 14-7).

Before a crossbridge cycle begins, the crossbridge holds an ADP and Pi on its ATPase site and is "spring-loaded" in the high-energy position (explained earlier). In this position, the crossbridge attempts to bind with actin but tropomyosin prevents it by blocking the myosin-binding sites. However, Ca^{2+} ions bind to troponin and cause it to move the tropomyosin off the binding sites, thereby allowing a crossbridge cycle to begin. A crossbridge cycle involves four major stages:

1. Attachment of myosin to actin: Once tropomyosin moves off the myosin-binding site on actin, a myosin crossbridge (with its bound ADP and P_i) is able to bend at its tail hinge site and quickly

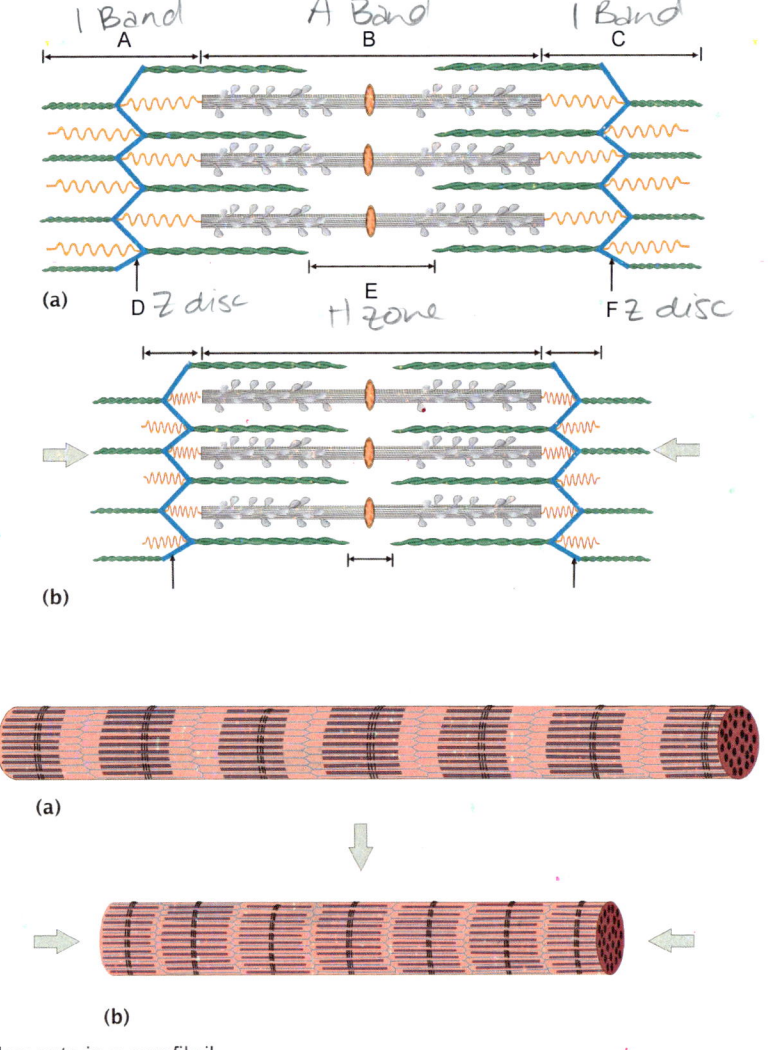

Figure 14-6. Sliding filaments in a myofibril

MUSCLE TISSUE

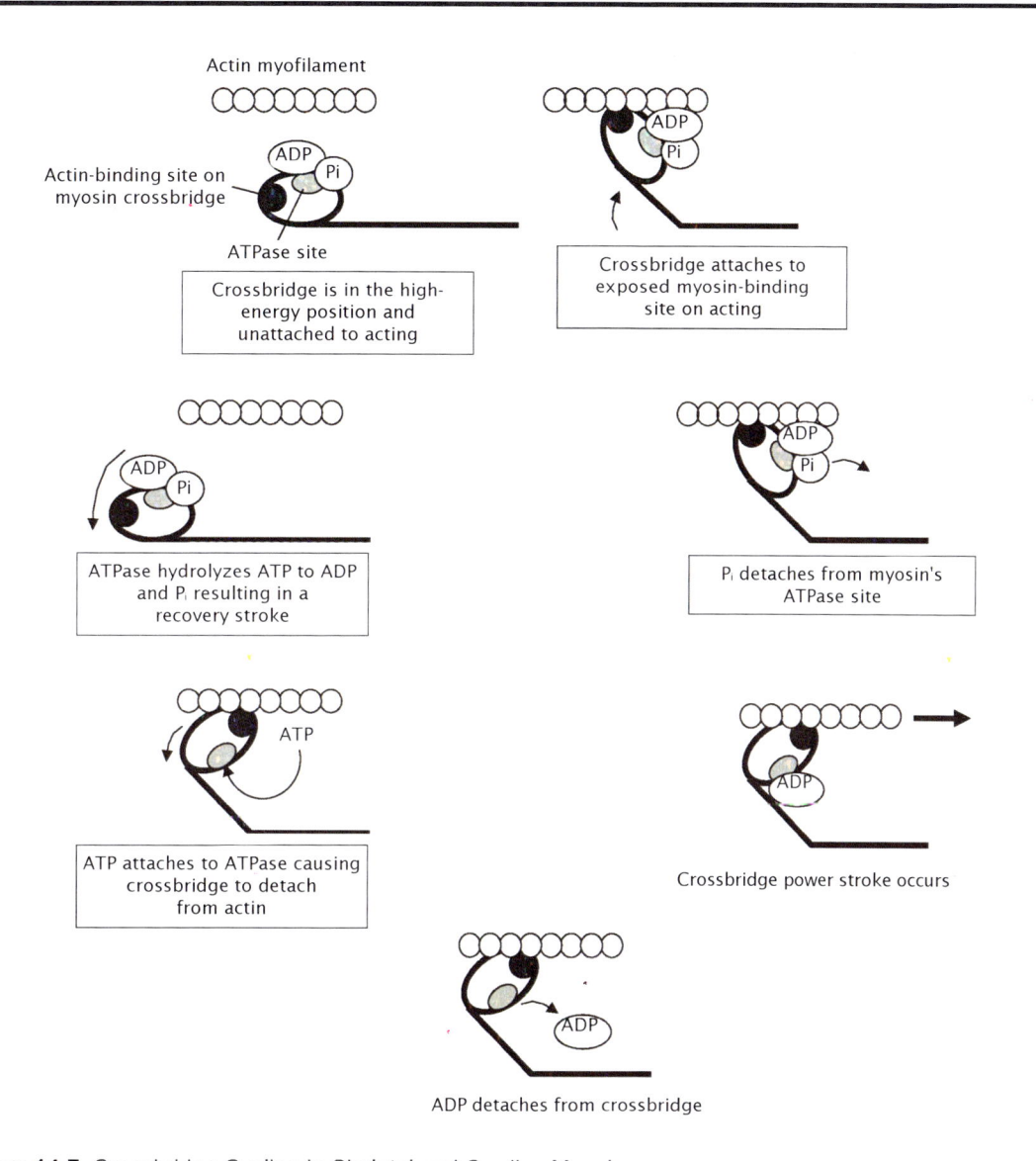

Figure 14-7. Crossbridge Cycling in Skeletal and Cardiac Muscle

attach to the actin. This action is like lowering an oar (the crossbridge) into the water (the actin) in preparation to row a boat.

2. **Crossbridge power stroke:** After binding to actin, the crossbridge releases its bound P_i. This action causes the crossbridge to bend at its own hinge site and perform a **power stroke**. During the power stroke, the crossbridge is pulling (exerting tension on) the thin myofilament. At the end of the power stroke, the crossbridge releases the ADP, creating a rigid condition known as *rigor*, meaning "stiffness." In rowing, a power stroke is when a rower pulls an oar through the water. At the end of the power stroke, the crossbridge is in its low-energy position and releases its ADP.

3. **Detachment of myosin from actin:** Rigor persists for only a short moment until ATP attaches to the ATPase site on the crossbridge. When this happens, the crossbridge changes shape and detaches from the actin. In rowing, this is similar to lifting the oar out of the water.

4. **Crossbridge recovery stroke:** After detaching from actin, the crossbridge hydrolyzes the ATP into ADP + P_i. This reaction releases energy

that enables the crossbridge to bend back to its high-energy ("straight") position; this maneuver is called a **recovery stroke**. The motion is similar to a recovery stroke in rowing, where the person re-positions an oar to prepare for another power stroke. The ADP + P$_i$ remain bound to the crossbridge in the high-energy position.

> **Note**: After death a person no longer produces ATP, and a lack of ATP prevents crossbridges from detaching from actin resulting in a stiffening of the body called **rigor mortis** (RIG-or MOR-tis; *rigor*, stiffness; *mortis*, death).

Crossbridge cycling repeats as long as the myosin-binding sites remain exposed and ATP is available to cause crossbridge detachment and recovery strokes. But what prevents the loss of tension when the crossbridge detaches from actin? During contraction, not all crossbridges are in the same stage of crossbridge cycling. Some crossbridges are performing power strokes while others are performing recovery strokes. This action is similar to a tug-of-war team pulling a rope hand over hand. While some hands are pulling the rope, other hands are releasing it, and still others are grabbing hold of the rope as it moves by.

In skeletal muscle fibers, myosin crossbridges on opposite sides of the M line pull the thin myofilaments toward the M line, causing the sarcomere to shorten. Each crossbridge performs about five crossbridge cycles per second. Considering that each thick myofilament has several hundred crossbridges, a single muscle can have millions of crossbridge cycles occurring at any moment. Astonishingly, it takes less than a tenth of a second for a skeletal muscle to shorten to its fullest extent, or about 35% less than its resting length. Now that we've seen how a muscle fiber contracts, we need to see how it relaxes.

Relaxation of a skeletal muscle fiber

Situations that can halt crossbridge cycling include: (1) A lack of ATP, which prevents crossbridges from detaching from actin at the end of the power stroke, and (2) an inability of the crossbridges to attach to actin. The first situation was described in the previous section. Under normal conditions, the second situation is most responsible for causing muscle fibers to relax.

While Ca^{2+} ions are bound to troponin, the troponin keeps tropomyosin off the myosin-binding sites on actin. When Ca^{2+} ions detach from troponin, the troponin changes shape and moves tropomyosin over the myosin-binding sites. When this happens, a crossbridge is unable to reattach to actin and remains in the high-energy position at the end of a recovery stroke. When tropomyosin covers all binding sites, thick myofilaments cannot generate any tension on the thin myofilaments. The muscle fiber then loses tension as the thin myofilaments "slide" back to their resting position, returning the sarcomeres to their resting length. During relaxation, Ca-pumps actively transport Ca^{2+} ions back into the terminal cisternae.

REGULATION OF MUSCLE CONTRACTION

In order to regulate muscle fiber contraction and relaxation, the nervous system regulates the availability of Ca^{2+} ions inside the sarcomere. To understand how this happens, we must first examine the site where a nervous system cell, a *neuron*, stimulates the muscle fiber.

The Neuromuscular Junction

A skeletal muscle fiber contracts in response to stimulation from a nervous system cell called a **motor neuron**. The word "motor" means that the neuron stimulates movement in other cells. A motor neuron has a long, fiber-like extension, the **axon** (AKS-on; axle), which courses through a nerve. Inside a skeletal muscle, the axon branches into many fine strands called **telodendria** (tel-ō-DEN-drē-a; *telo*, end; *dendr*, tree) that have small, bulb-like endings called **axon terminals**.

An axon terminal lies very close to the sarcolemma of a muscle fiber but does not touch it. The narrow space between the axon terminal and sarcolemma is the **synaptic cleft**. The region of the sarcolemma that borders the synaptic cleft is called the **motor end plate**. Finally, the site where an axon terminal and a motor end plate meet at the synaptic cleft is called the **neuromuscular junction**. Each skeletal muscle fiber has one neuromuscular junction.

MUSCLE TISSUE

When the nervous system is ready to stimulate a muscle fiber, it sends an AP along the motor neuron's axon to the neuromuscular junction. The AP causes the neuron to release a chemical, **acetylcholine** (**Ach**; as-e-til-KŌ-lēn), from its axon terminals. Ach is a type of *neurotransmitter*, a chemical that "transmits" an electrical signal from a neuron to another cell. Ach binds to receptors in the skeletal muscle fiber's motor end plate where it triggers an AP. The AP propagates (travels) along the sarcolemma and into the sarcoplasm where it initiates contraction. Before explaining how Ach triggers an AP, we must describe the electrical conditions that exist along the sarcolemma.

Membrane Potentials of Muscle fibers

In the previous chapter, you learned about membrane potentials. We can illustrate the RMP of a resting muscle fiber on an **electromyogram** (**EMG**; e-lek-trō-MĪ-ō-gram; *gram*, drawing) (see Figure 14-8a). The plotted line or *tracing* on the EMG depicts the relative electrical condition of the inside of the muscle fiber compared to the outside. The RMP of a resting skeletal muscle fiber is about -85 mV, which means the inside border of the sarcolemma is 85 mV more negative than the outside border. While the RMP of a skeletal muscle fiber is a stable value, various factors can cause the membrane potential to become less negative or more negative.

End-Plate Potential

Acetylcholine (Ach) initiates a slight electrical change in the sarcolemma of skeletal muscle fibers by opening specific types of membrane channels. The receptors to which Ach binds on the motor end plate are actually *ligand-gated* Na^+ channels. Since the ligand in this case is Ach, we will refer to these channels as **Ach-gated Na^+ channels**. The channels open when Ach binds to them and allows Na^+ ions to diffuse into the cytosol from the ECF. Consequently, the membrane potential of the motor end plate becomes less negative; this local depolarization is called an **end-plate potential (EPP)**.

While Ach-gated Na^+ channels can generate an EPP, they do not allow enough Na^+ ions into the cytosol to reverse the membrane's polarity (that is, make the inside of the fiber become positively charged). The reason is that Ach-gated channels remain open for only a brief period. Shortly after binding to the channel, Ach is broken down by an enzyme called **acetycholinesterase** (**AchE**; as-e-til-kō-lin-ES-ter-ās) located in the synaptic cleft. This event causes the Ach-gated channel to close, preventing further diffusion of Na^+ ions through the channel. If not for the opening of another type of Na^+ channel nearby (described shortly), closing the Ach-gated Na^+ channels would halt depolarization and the voltage line on the EMG would stop moving toward zero.

While an EPP in a skeletal muscle fiber is a depolarization, an EPP in other types of muscle fibers may be a depolarization or a hyperpolarization. The "direction" of the voltage change depends on the type of ligand-gated channel causing the change. Opening ligand-gated Na^+ or Ca^{2+} channels allow Na^+ or Ca^{2+} to diffuse into the cytosol, resulting in depolarization. Opening ligand-gated K^+ channels allow K^+ ions to diffuse out of the cytosol, resulting in hyperpolarization. Likewise, opening ligand-gated chloride (Cl^-) channels allow Cl^- ions to diffuse into the cytosol, resulting in hyperpolarization.

Action Potential in Skeletal Muscle fibers

Recall that an **action potential (AP)** is a dramatic reversal of the membrane potential that propagates as an electrical signal along the sarcolemma. Under normal conditions, a skeletal muscle fiber will not contract unless an AP passes into the sarcoplasm. APs differ from EPPs in three major ways: (1) EPPs can vary in intensity, but APs are always the same intensity. (2) EPPs always remain negative, but APs reverse the membrane potential twice (the inside of the muscle fiber becomes positive then reverts to the RMP). (3) EPPs result from ions passing through ligand-gated channels, while APs result from ions passing through *voltage-gated* channels.

The sarcolemma of a skeletal muscle fiber contains two types of voltage-gated channels: **voltage-gated Na^+ channels** and **voltage-gated K^+ channels**. These channels are located near the edge of the motor end plate and all along the remainder of the sarcolemma, including the T tubules. These channels open in response to a certain level of change in the membrane potential. The voltage that causes a particular type of voltage-gated channel to open is the channel's **threshold voltage (TV)**. An AP has two phases: a *depolarizing phase* and a *repolarizing phase* (Figure 14-8b).

Depolarizing phase: Normally, an EPP will reach the threshold voltage for nearby voltage-gated Na^+ channels in the sarcolemma. When this happens, the voltage-gated Na^+ channels open and allow a large number of Na^+ ions to diffuse into the cytosol. As a result, the cytosol next to the sarcolemma becomes positive and the ECF next to the sarcolemma becomes negative. This event is the **depolarizing phase** of the AP and causes the voltage line on the EMG to cross over to the positive side of the graph.

Opening a voltage-gated Na^+ channel will cause more voltage-gated Na^+ channels to open. This happens as the depolarization that occurs around a voltage-gated channel reaches threshold for other voltage-gated channels within a 1-millimeter radius. Therefore, depolarization at one site on the sarcolemma initiates depolarization at an adjacent site. The effect is like dominoes falling against one another. The result is a "wave" of depolarization that propagates along the sarcolemma like a wave traveling on the surface of a pond.

Repolarizing phase: When the membrane potential reaches about +30 mV, the voltage-gated Na^+ channels close. However, this positive membrane potential allows voltage-gated K^+ channels to open. When these channels open, a large number of positive K^+ ions diffuse *out of* the cytosol, causing the voltage to return to the resting membrane potential (about -85 mV). This event is the **repolarizing phase** of the AP. Since repolarization always follows depolarization, a "wave" of repolarization follows immediately behind the wave of depolarization. After repolarization, Na/K pumps transport Na^+ ions out of the cell and K^+ ions into the cell, thereby maintaining their steep concentration gradients across the sarcolemma.

Muscle fibers normally abide by an **all-or-nothing principle** in regard to APs. In other words, an AP occurs at full strength or it does not occur at all. EPPs, however, can vary in strength. To help you remember these facts, let's compare an EPP to a match and an AP to sparks traveling along a burning fuse of a firecracker. You can use a lighted match (stimulus) to make the fuse hot (generate an EPP), but if the match goes out too quickly (the EPP does not reach threshold voltage), the fuse will not ignite (an AP will not occur). However, once you ignite the fuse (generate an AP), it will travel along the fuse to cause the firecracker to explode (the AP ultimately causes muscle fiber contraction).

When an AP is at a specific site on the sarcolemma, that site will not respond to another stimulus until the repolarizing phase is complete. This period of unresponsiveness is called the **refractory period** (rē-FRAK-to-rē; to break up). In other words, voltage-gated Na^+ channels cannot re-open until the region around them repolarizes. To understand this, think of a voltage-gated channel as being like a perfume bottle with a spray nozzle. Depolarizing the membrane to threshold voltage to generate an AP is like depressing

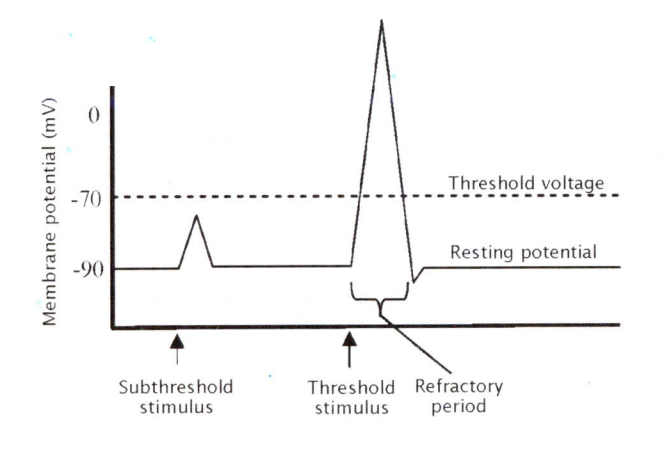

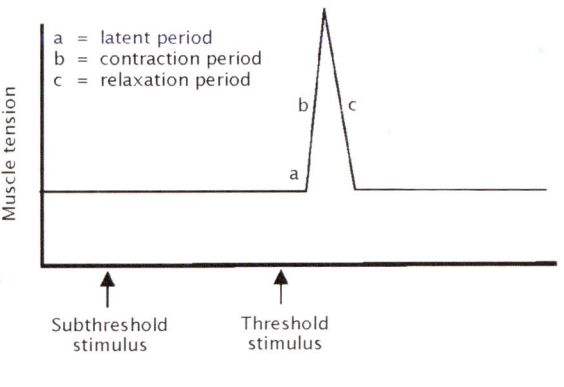

(a) Electromyogram

(b) Myogram

Figure 14-8. The EMG and myogram

MUSCLE TISSUE

the nozzle on the perfume bottle to emit a puff of perfume. Before you can get another puff of perfume, you must release the nozzle so it can return to its original "resting" position. Likewise, before another AP can occur at a specific site, that site must repolarize to the resting membrane potential.

EXCITATION-CONTRACTION COUPLING

Recall that a muscle fiber is "excitable," which means it can respond to stimulation by generating *electrical* signals (APs) along its sarcolemma. These electrical signals ultimately cause contraction, which is a *mechanical* event. Hence, the sequence of events leading from the stimulation of a muscle fiber to the resulting contraction of that fiber is called **excitation-contraction coupling**.

In skeletal muscle fibers, excitation-contraction coupling involves four major steps. Relaxation of the fiber then follows in two major steps:

1. Generation of the EPP: An AP traveling along a motor neuron's axon causes the axon terminals to release Ach into the synaptic cleft at the neuromuscular junction. The Ach binds to Ach-gated Na^+ channels located on the muscle fiber's motor end plate. These channels open in response to the binding with Ach and allow Na^+ ions to diffuse into the muscle fiber, thereby generating the EPP. The Ach-gated Na^+ channels close when acetycholinesterase removes Ach from the channel's receptor.

2. Generation of the AP: The EPP reaches threshold voltage to open the voltage-gated Na^+ channels at the edge of the motor end plate. Diffusion of Na^+ ions into the cytosol through these channels causes the depolarizing phase of the AP. The positive membrane potential closes the voltage-gated Na^+ channels and opens voltage-gated K^+ channels. The outflow of K^+ ions from the cytosol through these channels causes the repolarizing phase of the AP. Following the all-or-nothing principle, an AP propagates along the sarcolemma and enters the T tubules.

3. Release of Ca^{2+} from terminal cisternae: The AP enters the T tubules where it stimulates voltage-sensing receptors in the walls of the T tubules. The AP causes these receptors to open **Ca^{2+} release channels** in the membrane of the terminal cisternae. In response, Ca^{2+} ions quickly diffuse out of the terminal cisternae and into the cytosol.

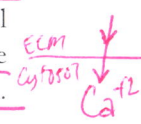

4. Crossbridge cycling and development of tension: After entering the cytosol, the Ca^{2+} ions diffuse through the myofibrils where they bind to troponin on the thin myofilaments. In response, the troponin changes shape and moves tropomyosin off of the myosin-binding sites on actin. The myosin crossbridges quickly attach to the actin and crossbridge cycling begins. Tension develops as the Z discs move toward the center of the sarcomere.

5. Removal of Ca^{2+} ions: When a motor neuron stops stimulating the muscle fiber, no APs pass into the T tubules, so the Ca^{2+} release channels in the terminal cisternae close. At the same time, Ca-pumps actively transport Ca^{2+} ions from the cytosol back into the terminal cisternae. As the Ca^{2+} concentration in the cytosol drops, Ca^{2+} ions diffuse off of troponin.

6. Relaxation of muscle fiber: Losing its bound Ca^{2+} ions causes the troponin to change shape and move tropomyosin back over the myosin-binding sites on the actin. Covering the binding sites prevents the crossbridges from reattaching to actin after performing recovery strokes and, thus, the muscle fiber relaxes.

Effect of stimulus intensity

In addition to stimulation by a motor neuron, an outside electric current applied anywhere along the sarcolemma can stimulate the muscle fiber to contract. However, the electric current must be of sufficient magnitude to depolarize the sarcolemma to threshold voltage in order to generate an AP. Any stimulus that causes the membrane potential to reach threshold voltage and generate an AP is a **threshold stimulus**. In contrast, a **subthreshold stimulus** depolarizes the sarcolemma but the membrane potential does not reach threshold voltage. Both types of stimulation are detectable on an electromyogram. Normally, each stimulus applied to a resting skeletal muscle fiber by a motor neuron is a threshold stimulus.

TENSION IN SKELETAL MUSCLE FIBERS

The amount of tension that a skeletal muscle fiber can exert at any one time depends on three factors: (1) the availability of Ca^{2+} ions in the myofibrils; (2) the length of the sarcomeres; and (3) the diameter of the muscle fiber. Before elaborating on each of these factors, we will describe the way that a muscle fiber develops tension in response to a single AP.

Muscle fiber twitch

When a motor neuron stimulates a skeletal muscle fiber with one AP, the muscle fiber responds by initiating a series of crossbridge cycles. A **muscle fiber twitch** is the amount of tension that develops within a muscle fiber during a single excitation-contraction episode. Twitches in skeletal muscle fibers may last between 10-100 milliseconds (msec). Measuring a fiber's tension from the moment a motor neuron stimulates it until the time the fiber relaxes, we can identify three distinct periods: the *latent period*, the *contraction period*, and the *relaxation period*. These periods are shown on a graph called a **myogram** (MĪ-ō-gram).

> **Note**: A muscle twitch is a spastic jerk of a muscle when some or all of its muscle fibers experience a single excitation-contraction event; a muscle twitch is responsible for blinking.

The latent period (LĀ-tent; hidden): a short delay, about 1-2 milliseconds (msec), between initiation of an AP on the sarcolemma and the beginning of crossbridge cycling. This period is so-named because the events occurring during this time do not produce any deflection on the myogram. The following is a review of events that occur during the relatively short latent period:

- Ach attaches to Ach-gated Na^+ channels on the motor end plate, causing these channels to open
- Na^+ ions diffuse into the muscle fiber and generate an end-plate potential (EPP)
- The EPP reaches threshold voltage and causes nearby voltage-gated Na^+ channels to open
- More Na^+ ions diffuse into the muscle fiber and generates an AP
- The AP in one region of the sarcolemma causes voltage-gated Na^+ channels in adjacent regions to open; thus, an impulse ("wave" of APs) propagates along the sarcolemma and into the T tubules
- The AP causes Ca^{2+}-release channels in the terminal cisternae to open
- Ca^{2+} ions diffuse out of the terminal cisternae and into the sarcoplasm where they bind to troponin on the thin myofilaments
- The Ca-troponin complex changes shape and moves tropomyosin off the myosin-binding sites on actin
- Myosin crossbridges attach to the actin and crossbridge cycling begins

Contraction period: lasts 4-40 msec when the muscle fiber steadily increases tension, which causes an upward sloping line on the myogram. During this period, tension develops as myosin crossbridges pull the thin myofilaments toward the central portion of the sarcomere. As this continues, the thin myofilaments overlap the thick myofilaments even more, allowing more crossbridges to bind with actin. This is like having more people grabbing hold of a tug-of-war rope and pulling it. The tension reaches a maximum height on the myogram when no more crossbridges can bind to actin during this excitation-contraction episode. This is primarily due to the limited number of Ca^{2+} ions that enter the cytosol in response to a single AP.

Not all skeletal muscle fibers contract at the same speed. For example, muscle fibers that move your eyeball allowing you to look in different directions very quickly have contraction periods of about 5 msec. Fibers within the *gastrocnemius* muscle on the posterior side of the lower leg have contraction periods of 15 msec. Furthermore, the *soleus* muscle just deep to the gastrocnemius has fibers with contraction periods of 40 msec. The reason for these differences is that myosin crossbridges in some muscle fibers can perform crossbridge cycling faster than others do.

MUSCLE TISSUE

Relaxation period: lasts 5-60 msec when the muscle fiber steadily loses tension causing a downward sloping line on the myogram. There is a positive correlation between contraction period and relaxation period; that is, fibers with the long contraction periods have long relaxation periods, while fibers with short contraction periods have short relaxation periods. Relaxation results when Ca^{2+} ions detach from the crossbridges and move back into the terminal cisternae. When Ca^{2+} ions are no longer available to bind with troponin, the tropomyosin covers the myosin-binding sites so the crossbridges are unable to bind to actin. Consequently, the tension that was generated during the contraction period is lost as thin myofilaments slide back to their "resting" positions and the sarcomeres lengthen.

> **Note**: The **refractory period** is an **e**lectrical event recorded on an **e**lectromyogram; the **relaxation period** is a **m**echanical event that is recorded on a **m**yogram.

Since Ca^{2+} ions are important in uncovering myosin-binding sites on actin, the amount of tension that a muscle fiber generates is directly proportional to the amount of Ca^{2+} ions within its sarcomeres. Two situations that increase the availability of Ca^{2+} ions within a sarcomere are *treppe* and *wave summation*.

Treppe

If a skeletal muscle fiber contracts and completely relaxes, then quickly receives a second stimulation, the second contraction generates slightly more tension than the first contraction. If the fiber completely relaxes again then quickly receives a third stimulation, the third contraction generates slightly more tension than the second contraction. This pattern may repeat for up to 50 stimulations before the tension of each subsequent contraction remains constant. This gradual increase in tension resulting from successive stimulations is called **treppe** (TREP; "staircase") (Figure 14-9), and may be caused by:

- An inability of Ca-pumps to transport all the Ca^{2+} ions back into the terminal cisternae before the next stimulation occurs. The next stimulation causes the terminal cisternae to release more Ca^{2+} ions, adding to those remaining in the sarcomere from the first stimulation. The result is that more Ca^{2+} ions are available to bind with more troponin molecules, freeing up more myosin-binding sites for crossbridge cycling.

- Higher temperature resulting from contraction causes Ca^{2+} ions to diffuse more rapidly, thereby allowing crossbridge cycling to occur at a faster pace. This is one of the advantages of performing "warm up" exercises before an athletic event, because warm muscles contract more efficiently than "cold" muscles.

Wave Summation

Up to a maximum level, the amount of tension that a skeletal muscle fiber exerts is positively correlated to the *rate* of stimulation. Let's first consider how a single twitch affects tension. As a single AP propagates along the sarcolemma, only the *depolarized* regions will have Ca^{2+} ions moving into the cytosol from the terminal cisternae. Therefore, only the sarcomeres in the depolarized regions will be experiencing crossbridge cycling to generate tension. The terminal cisternae in the polarized regions "ahead" of the AP are not releasing Ca^{2+} ions because the AP has not yet arrived. Moreover, Ca^{2+} ions in the repolarized regions "behind" the AP would be moving back into the terminal cisternae. This, in turn, would cause crossbridge cycling in the repolarized regions to slow down and cease.

Now imagine that crossbridge cycling in the depolarized region creates a small "bulge" that moves along the muscle fiber like a wave following the AP. This single contraction bulge would generate the same amount of tension at any location along the fiber. You can demonstrate this with a rope. Tie a knot near one end of the rope then pull the rope tight. Measure the

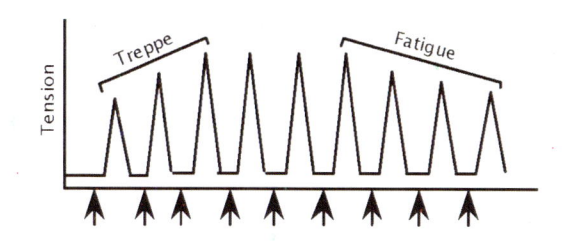

Figure 14-9. Treppe

distance between the ends of the rope. Now untie the knot and repeat the exercise by tying the knot in the middle of the rope. Regardless of where you tie the knot, the rope shortens the same amount as before. Furthermore, the rope lengthens when you untie the knot. Likewise, when the AP and contraction bulge reach the end of the muscle fiber, that region repolarizes, crossbridge-cycling ceases, the contraction bulge disappears, and the fiber relaxes.

Now consider what happens if we stimulate a muscle fiber two times in rapid succession. While the sarcolemma must respect the refractory period, responding to stimulation *only* after repolarization occurs, relaxation need not occur. If we apply a second stimulus before the first contraction bulge disappears, the muscle fiber will develop a "wave of contraction." At this time, the second contraction bulge "adds" to the tension generated by the first contraction bulge. For this reason, the effect of successive stimulations on muscle fiber tension is **wave summation** (Figure 14-10).

You can demonstrate wave summation by tying knots in a rope. As you would see, multiple knots cause the rope to shorten more than one knot. Figure 14-11 illustrates this idea and the figure's explanation follows.

In reality, a muscle fiber experiencing wave summation does not look exactly like a knotted rope with similar size knots (contraction bulges) following one after another. Instead, each successive AP initiates a contraction wave that is larger (generating more tension) than the previous wave. This is due to having additional Ca²⁺ ions entering the cytosol before all of those released during a previous AP can be pumped back into the terminal cisternae. More Ca²⁺ ions in the cytosol at any one time allow more crossbridges to attach to actin, so successive stimulations cause more forceful contractions than the first.

If we stimulate a muscle fiber so frequently that complete relaxation cannot occur between stimulations, then the fiber remains in a state of contraction known as **tetanus** (TET-a-nus; convulsive tension). If the stimulation rate allows at least *partial* relaxation between contractions, the condition is **incomplete (unfused) tetanus**. If the stimulation rate is so rapid that no relaxation occurs between stimulations, the condition is **complete (fused) tetanus**. If you are sitting while reading this page, some of the muscle fibers in your neck and back muscles are experiencing tetanus. This allows you to maintain your posture and to keep your head in an upright position.

Length-tension relationship

The amount of tension that a skeletal muscle fiber generates is positively correlated to the number of myosin crossbridges that are bound to actin. More tension develops when there is optimum overlap between thick and thin myofilaments; that is, when the free ends of the thin myofilaments extend to the edge of the H zone. The normal working length of sarcomeres in a contracting muscle fiber is usually ± 20% of this optimum length (Figure 14-12).

Reducing the length of a muscle fiber can reduce the tension that the muscle fiber can generate. There are two reasons why this happens. (1) The thin myofilaments from opposite sides of the sarcomere begin to overlap one another and interfere with crossbridge binding to actin. (2) Further shortening of the sarcomere can cause the thick myofilaments to collide with the Z lines. In this case, the Z lines are unable to move any closer toward the center of the sarcomere so no tension can develop.

Stretching a skeletal muscle fiber pulls the Z lines farther apart, narrowing the zones of overlap between the thick and thin myofilaments. Consequently, fewer crossbridges can grab hold of the actin and the muscle fiber is unable to generate maximum tension. If a skeletal muscle fiber stretches 70% longer than its optimum length, there is no overlap between the thick and thin myofilaments. At this length, the muscle fiber is unable to contract. However, tension can still exist within the muscle fiber due to the elasticity of the titin filaments within the sarcomeres.

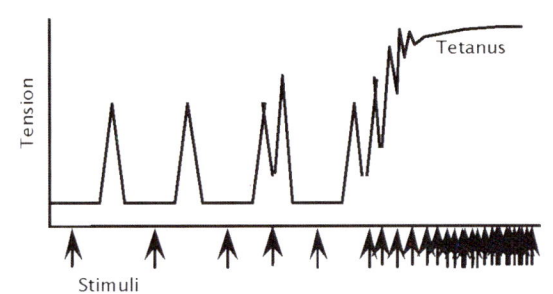

Figure 14-10. Wave summation

MUSCLE TISSUE

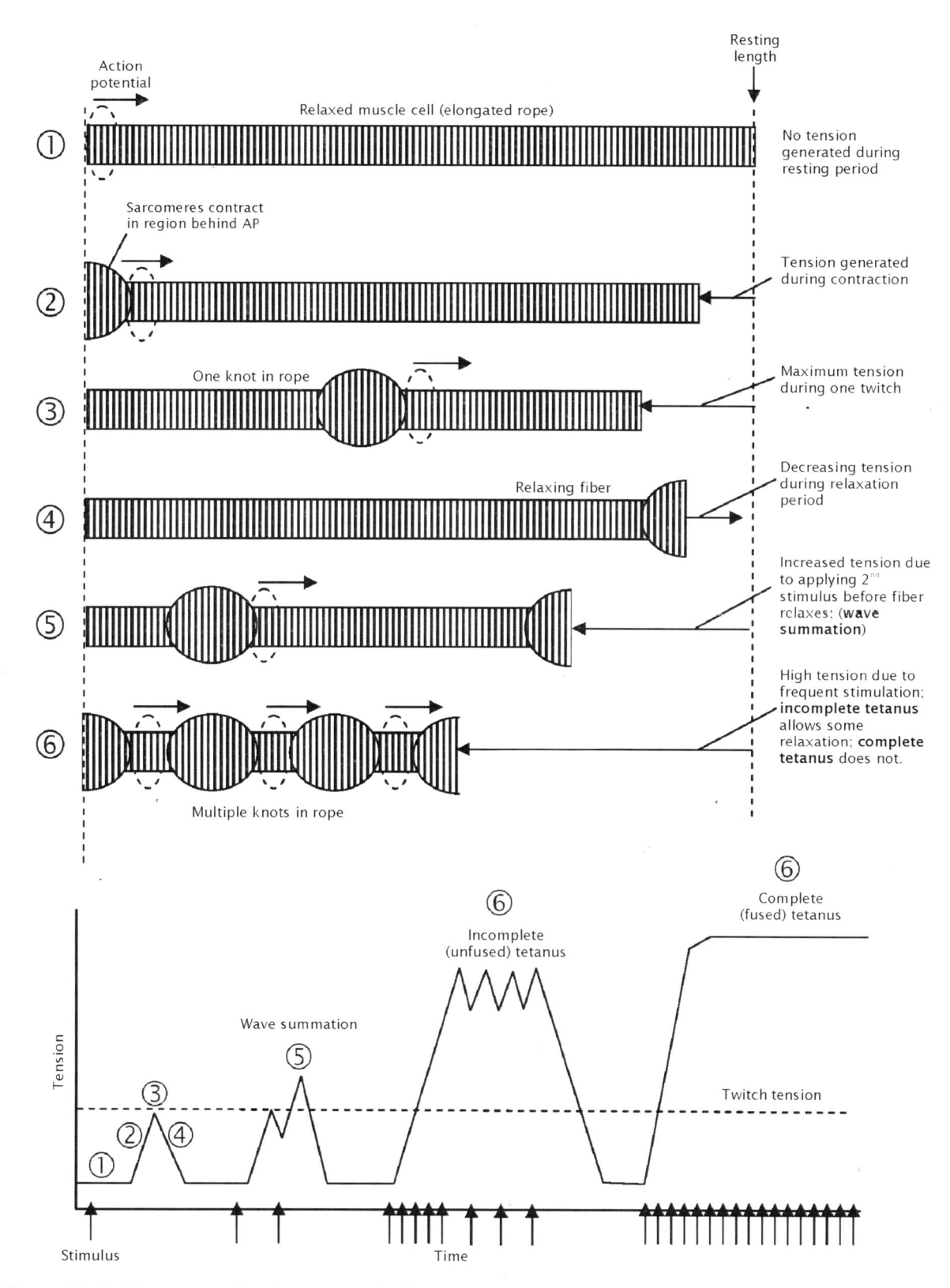

Figure 14-11. Wave summation demonstrated with a rope

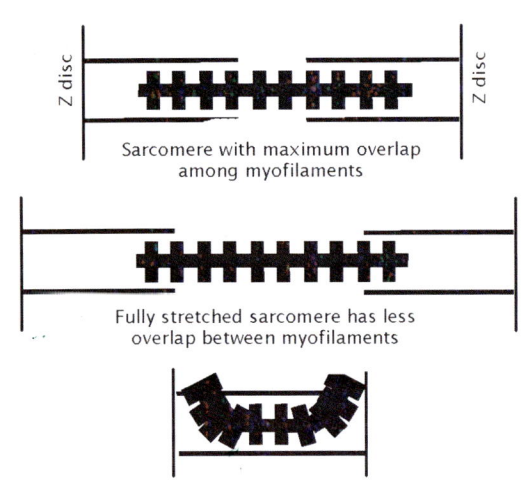

Figure 14-12. Length-tension relationship

There are situations where a person might notice differences in muscle strength due to changes in muscle length, such as when performing a chin-up by starting with the arms straight versus starting with the elbows bent. With straight arms, the *biceps* muscles, which bend the elbows, are "stretched" and have less overlap among their myofilaments. From this position, beginning the chin-up may be more difficult. With elbows bent, the biceps muscles are shorter and have more overlap among their myofilaments. From this position, the muscles can exert more tension and it is easier to complete the chin up.

Under normal circumstances, titin filaments, elastic tissues in the muscle and tendons, and the position of bones limit the distance that muscles can stretch. Thus, even in a muscle that seems to be "stretched," there is still almost optimum overlap between the myofilaments.

Diameter-tension relationship

Earlier, you read that muscle fiber tension depends on the number of crossbridges that attach to actin. Therefore, it stands to reason that the maximum tension that a fiber can generate is directly proportional to the number of sarcomeres in the fiber. However, it is not simply the total number of sarcomeres lying end-to-end that is important in determining the maximum tension possible, but rather the number of sarcomeres lying side-by-side. In other words, a muscle fiber that has more myofibrils can exert a greater maximum tension than a fiber with fewer myofibrils. To make the diameter-tension relationship easy to remember, think about muscle fibers as steel rods. A thick steel rod is stronger than a thin steel rod.

ENERGY FOR CONTRACTION

ATP is the *only* molecule that a muscle fiber can use directly as a source of energy to power its crossbridge cycling and operate its Ca-pumps and Na-K pumps. This section provides an overview of ATP synthesis in muscle fibers, and describes the effects that various activities have on muscle fiber performance.

In order to continue functioning, a muscle fiber must continually replenish its supply of ATP. At any moment, there are very few ATP molecules inside a muscle fiber (we will call this supply "stored" ATP, although it is simply dispersed in the cytosol). On the other hand, there is usually an ample supply of its building substrates, ADP and P_i. Enzymes within the muscle fiber can combine these substrates to form ATP. Adding P_i to a substrate is *phosphorylation*, and in this reaction, the ADP becomes phosphorylated. Phosphorylation of ADP is an endergonic reaction, or one that requires energy:

$$ADP + P_i + energy \rightarrow ATP$$

As a muscle fiber works harder, its available ATP falls and its concentration of ADP rises. In response, the fiber begins making ATP at a faster rate. Muscle fibers utilize three energy "systems" (chemical processes) to convert ADP to ATP: the *creatine phosphate-creatine system*, the *glycogen-lactic acid system*, and *aerobic respiration*.

Creatine Phosphate System

At the onset of contraction, all three energy systems may be converting ADP to ATP; however, the glycogen-lactic acid and aerobic respiration systems require a few seconds to "gear up" to speed. During this time, **creatine phosphate system** (KRĒ-a-tēn or KRĒ-a-tin) serves as the primary energy system for converting ADP to ATP.

In a fully rested skeletal muscle fiber, there is only enough stored ATP available to generate about eight twitches, or to sustain maximum contraction for about four seconds. The muscle fibers in the legs of a world-

MUSCLE TISSUE

class sprinter would deplete this source of ATP during the first 40 meters of a 100-meter sprint. To continue contracting with full force to reach the finish line, these muscle fibers need a "quick" way to convert ADP to ATP. The quickest way to do this is by reacting ADP with a compound called **creatine phosphate (CP)** or **phosphocreatine** (fos-fō-KRĒ-a-ten) An enzyme called *creatine kinase* catalyzes this reaction, transferring an inorganic phosphate ion (P_i) from CP to ADP. In this reaction, ADP becomes ATP and CP becomes creatine.

Creatine kinase transfers P_i from CP to ADP so rapidly that new ATP molecules are available almost instantaneously after the muscle fiber depletes its stored ATP. Beyond this time, CP provides phosphate ions to generate enough ATP for an additional 6-8 seconds of maximum contraction. Altogether, stored ATP plus CP makes up the muscle fiber's **phosphagen system** (FOS-fa-jen), and can provide enough ATP for about 10-15 seconds of maximum contraction. This is roughly the amount of ATP needed by a sprinter to run a 100-meter dash.

If a muscle fiber uses CP to generate ATP, how does a muscle fiber replenish its CP? Ironically, regenerating CP requires ATP. A resting muscle fiber produces a surplus of ATP molecules primarily through the other two energy systems. An enzyme transfers P_i from some of these extra ATPs to creatine molecules. In the process, ATP becomes ADP, and creatine becomes CP. Thus, CP serves as a temporary storage site for P_i. When needed, the CP "gives back" the P_i to an ADP.

Glycogen-Lactic Acid System

The fact that some people run marathons, although not at a sprinter's pace, indicates that muscle fibers can continue to regenerate ATP long after depleting their stores of CP. After the creatine/CP system, the second fastest system for generating ATP is the **glycogen-lactic acid system**. This system is so-named because it utilizes *glycogen* as a primary source of glucose, which it breaks down to release energy, and eventually produces a compound called *lactic acid*. Glucose enters the muscle fiber through facilitated diffusion and is stored as glycogen during times of rest. When needed, enzymes cleave glucose molecules from the glycogen, making them available for breakdown.

Glucose breakdown begins in a process called **glycolysis** (glī-KOL-i-sis), a series of ten chemical reactions that converts one glucose molecule into two molecules of pyruvic acid. Glycolysis represents only the *initial* stages of glucose breakdown, and converts the glucose to a variety of compounds before finally forming pyruvic acid. Glycolysis is important to a muscle fiber in three ways:

- **It generates ATP.** Glycolysis releases only a small percentage of the total chemical energy stored in a glucose molecule, but enzymes use some of the released energy to convert ADP to ATP. Glycolysis makes only *two* ATPs for each glucose molecule that it breaks down, but this happens very rapidly. For this reason, after about 4 seconds of maximum contraction, glycolysis takes over for CP as the primary synthesizer of ATP.

- **It supplies substrates and energy to mitochondria.** After glycolysis, most of the stored energy in glucose exists in the chemical bonds of two pyruvic acid molecules. When oxygen is present, the pyruvic acids enter the mitochondria, where they provide energy for the synthesis of many more ATPs.

- **It occurs with or without oxygen.** Aerobic respiration must have oxygen in order to utilize the pyruvic acids from glycolysis, but 10-12 seconds of maximum contraction can deplete the muscle fiber's oxygen supply. Glycolysis, on the other hand, is an *anaerobic* process, meaning that it does not require oxygen. Thus, glycolysis allows a muscle fiber to continue making ATP even when oxygen is not available. With ample glucose, glycolysis can provide enough ATP to sustain maximum contractions for up to a minute or so after aerobic respiration can no longer meet the demand for ATP.

Although glycolysis generates ATP anaerobically, a muscle fiber's ability to contract diminishes after a minute or so under anaerobic conditions. Why does this happen? Under anaerobic conditions, enzymes convert the pyruvic acid into **lactic acid**. As lactic acid accumulates, it lowers the pH of the cytosol, and the acidic conditions begin to disrupt metabolic reactions. Lactic acid diffuses into the blood and eventually reaches the liver, heart, or kidneys. These organs convert the lactic acid back to pyruvic acid, which can enter their own mitochondria to provide energy for aerobic respiration.

Aerobic Respiration

The slowest method for converting ADP to ATP is through a series of chemical reactions called **aerobic (cellular) respiration** or **oxidative phosphorylation**. This process is so-named because it proceeds only when oxygen (O_2) is available. Aerobic respiration occurs inside the mitochondria and represents the *final* stages of glucose breakdown. In addition, aerobic respiration also breaks down fatty acids (from triglycerides) and amino acids (from proteins). All of these substrates release energy for ATP synthesis but, again, this occurs only when oxygen is present. Altogether, aerobic respiration releases enough energy from food molecules to make 36 ATP molecules. While this means that aerobic respiration produces about 95% more ATP molecules than glycolysis, it is a much slower process.

Muscle fibers have two sources of O_2 that can support aerobic respiration. One source is the blood. Red blood cells contain a substance called *hemoglobin*, which binds O_2 in the lungs. As blood flows through capillaries around the muscle fibers, the hemoglobin releases the O_2, which diffuses through the sarcolemma. Inside the sarcoplasm, some of the O_2 enters the mitochondria, while "extra" O_2 may bind with **myoglobin** (MĪ-ō-glō-bin). When needed for aerobic respiration, the myoglobin releases the O_2 allowing it to diffuse into the mitochondria.

Nutrient utilization and levels of activity

The nutrient that a skeletal muscle fiber uses as a primary source of energy for ATP synthesis depends on a fiber's activity level. Resting skeletal muscle fibers usually have plenty of O_2 available for aerobic respiration, and primarily utilize fatty acids as a source of energy for this process. Fatty acids pass freely through the phospholipid bilayer sarcolemma and into the mitochondria. The breakdown of fatty acids is a relatively slow process compared to the breakdown of glucose. But a resting muscle fiber needs only a *steady* supply of ATP, not necessarily a quick source of ATP.

A resting skeletal muscle fiber, therefore, stores most of its glucose in glycogen. The surplus ATP made during aerobic respiration using fatty acids helps to replenish the phosphagen system and to synthesize glycogen.

Nutrient utilization within the muscle fiber changes when contraction begins. During the first few seconds of contraction, the phosphagen system supplies most of the muscle fiber's ATP. Moreover, the phosphagen system provides virtually all the ATP for contractions lasting less than about 10 seconds. Examples include throwing a baseball, sprinting to first base, and jumping out of the path of an oncoming truck. Utilizing the quicker phosphagen system during this time allows glycolysis and aerobic respiration time to pick up their pace to meet the rising demand for ATP.

After a few seconds of contraction, glycolysis replaces the phosphagen system as the major source of ATP. Glycolysis is most important for activities involving short bursts of near maximum effort lasting between 10-20 seconds; for example, tennis, football, and the 100-meter sprint. Between these short bursts of activity, the pyruvic acid from glycolysis can enter the mitochondria to undergo aerobic respiration. During the next burst of activity, aerobic respiration is too slow-paced to meet the muscle fiber's high demand for ATP. Once again, glycolysis comes to the rescue, being able to "power up" more quickly than aerobic respiration and synthesize ATP rapidly. The muscle fiber first utilizes glycogen as a source of glucose, but thirty minutes of moderate exercise can deplete the glycogen supply. Thereafter, the muscle fiber must rely on the blood for glucose.

During long periods of activity, when glycogen is no longer available, glucose becomes less important and fatty acids become more important as a source of energy for ATP synthesis. (But remember, this requires O_2.) By the end of a marathon race, aerobic respiration of fatty acids is providing almost all of a muscle fiber's ATP. If a muscle fiber does not have any glucose or fatty acids, it will use amino acids as a source of energy for ATP synthesis. Since amino acids come from the breakdown of proteins, which form most of the structural components of the fiber, this source of energy is usually a last resort. Figure 14-13 shows the sources of ATP for skeletal muscles and Table 14-1 lists different athletic activities and their primary sources of ATP.

MUSCLE TISSUE

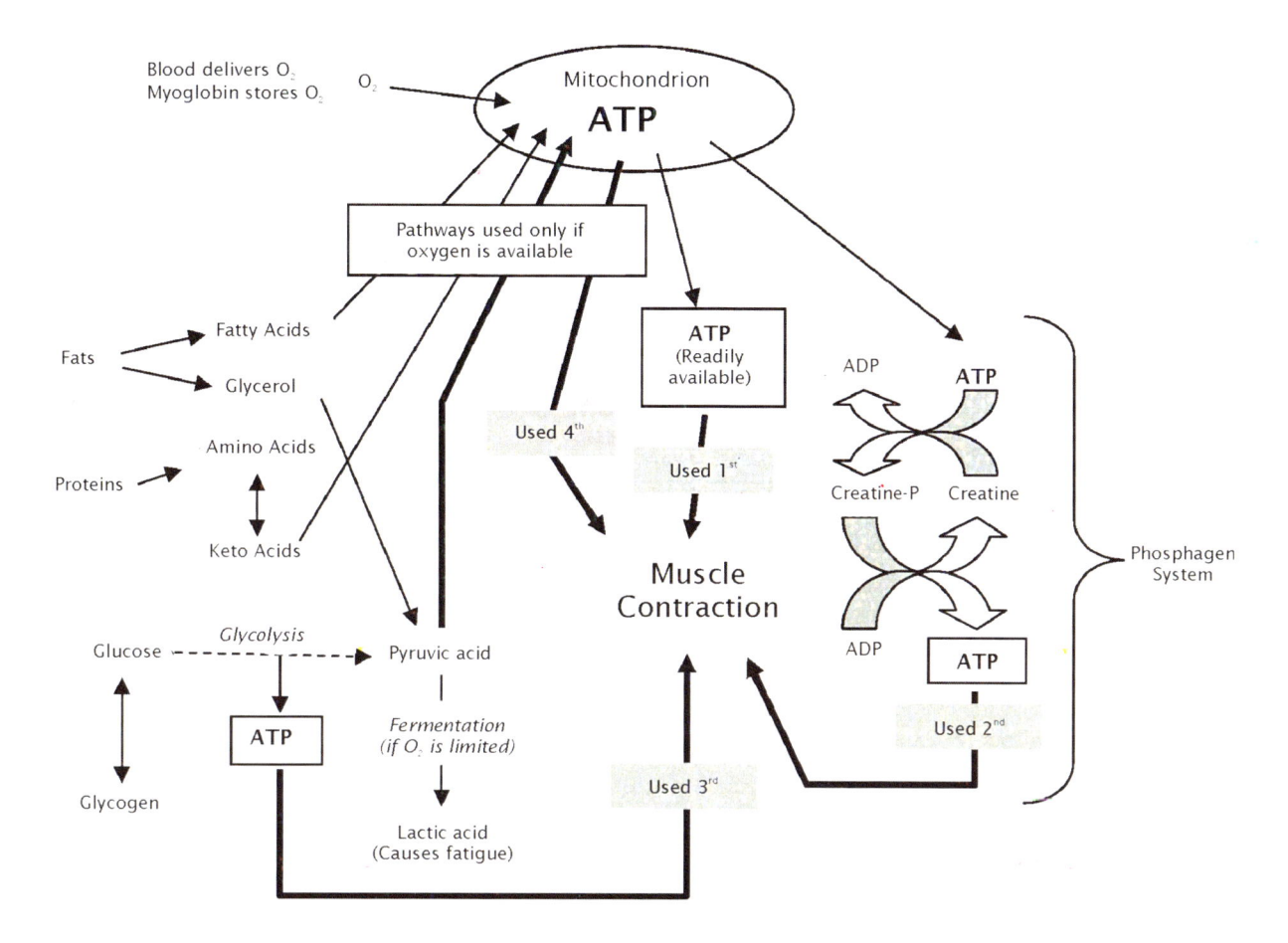

Figure 14-13. Sources of ATP for muscle contraction

MUSCLE FATIGUE

Prolonged contractions may result in a physiological condition that inhibits contraction, a condition called **muscle fatigue**, or **physiological fatigue**. This differs from *psychological fatigue*, which is a "state of mind," where a person feels tired but the muscles are still able to contract with full force. Psychological fatigue (in the brain) likely relates to sensory signals from the muscles and changes in blood pH due to a buildup of lactic acid.

Muscle fatigue may result from continual contractions without relaxation, such as in the hand and arm muscles while pulling hard on a tug-of-war rope. Muscle fatigue can also result from repeated contraction and relaxation, such as in the same muscles while rowing a boat. Muscle fatigue has number of causes:

Table 14-1. Energy systems used for various sporting activities

Phosphagen System	Phosphagen System & Anaerobic Respiration	Anaerobic Respiration	Anaerobic & Aerobic Respiration	Aerobic Respiration
100 meter run Weight lifting Diving Jumping	200 meter run Basketball Hockey	400 meter run 100 meter swim Tennis Soccer	800 meter run 200 meter swim Boxing	Marathon Cross-country run Skiing

- **Lack of nutrients**: Prolonged activity will eventually diminish the supply of glucose and fatty acids in the muscle fiber. Without an adequate supply of these nutrients, the muscle fiber lacks the sources of energy needed to synthesize adequate amounts of ATP. A deficiency of ATP decreases the number of crossbridge cycles possible, resulting in weaker contractions. A deficiency of ATP can also prevent Na/K pumps and Ca-pumps from maintaining steep concentration gradients for ions across membranes. Consequently, the membrane potential may be disrupted, resulting in erratic depolarization or repolarization. The length of time that a muscle fiber can contract before succumbing to a lack of nutrients depends on the amount of stored glycogen and the availability of glucose and fatty acids in the blood.

- **Buildup of lactic acid**: If prolonged activity depletes the muscle fiber's O_2 supply, glycolysis will have to continue without ample aerobic respiration, resulting in a buildup of lactic acid. As mentioned earlier, accumulation of lactic acid lowers the pH of the cytosol and interferes with enzyme activity and overall muscle metabolism. Lactic acid makes your muscles feel tired and "burn" after you exercise vigorously for too long.

- **Muscle fiber damage**: Prolonged activity may result in physical damage to the neuromuscular junction or other parts of the sarcolemma, myofibrils, or other cellular components. As a result, the muscle fiber may be less responsive to stimulation or may perform less crossbridge cycling within its sarcomeres.

Oxygen debt

Have you ever wondered why a person breathes heavily during vigorous exercise? Prolonging contractions depletes oxygen (O_2) from myoglobin, so more O_2 must diffuse into the muscle fiber from the blood. As a result, the concentration of O_2 in the blood drops. Eventually, the blood is unable to supply enough O_2 to the muscle fibers to sustain aerobic respiration at a rate adequate to meet the high demands for ATP. During these anaerobic conditions, the muscle fibers rely on glycolysis for ATP, but they also produce lactic acid. Lactic acid accumulates in the blood and is a major stimulus causing the brain to speed up a person's breathing rate.

After exercising stops, why does the breathing rate remain fast for some time? During this time, the body must take in extra oxygen to reestablish aerobic respiration and restore the cells to their resting or pre-exercise condition. This extra amount of oxygen that a person must breathe into the body after exercise is the **oxygen debt**, or *excess post-exercise oxygen consumption (EPOC)*. As an example, assume that a certain activity requires 5 liters of O_2 to maintain aerobic respiration, but the body takes in only 2 liters of O_2 during the activity. The body would have an oxygen debt of 3 liters of O_2. The fast breathing at the end of the activity is the body's way of repaying the oxygen debt. Completely repaying the oxygen debt involves the following:

- Reestablishing aerobic respiration to pre-exercise rates in all cells that have mitochondria

- Re-synthesizing the phosphagen system (CP and stored ATP) to pre-exercise levels in muscle fibers

- Replacing oxygen in the myoglobin of muscle fibers to pre-exercise levels

- Removing all lactic acid and converting it to pyruvic acid (occurs mostly in the liver)

- Replenishing all glycogen stores to pre-exercise levels

While all skeletal muscle fiber can build up an oxygen debt, certain fibers are able to contract forcefully for a longer period. In other words, not all skeletal muscle fibers are the same. In the next section, we will describe the three types of muscle fibers that make up skeletal muscles.

TYPES OF SKELETAL MUSCLE FIBERS

If you are in the mood to eat chicken skeletal muscles at a restaurant, you may order either "white" or "dark" meat. Your skeletal muscles are not as color-defined as skeletal muscles in a chicken, but like a chicken, you have different types of skeletal muscle fibers. These muscle fibers differ in both anatomy and physiology.

MUSCLE TISSUE

Human skeletal muscles are a composite of three types of muscle fibers: (1) *slow oxidative fibers*, (2) *fast glycolytic fibers*, and (3) *fast oxidative fibers*.

The terms "slow" and "fast" refer to the relative speed of contraction, which is directly proportional to the rate of ATPase activity on the myosin crossbridges. Slow fibers hydrolyze ATP slower than fast fibers and, therefore, have fewer crossbridge cycles in a set amount of time. The terms "oxidative" and "glycolytic" refer to the muscle fiber's primary energy system for producing ATP. Oxidative fibers rely mostly on oxidative phosphorylation of ADP (aerobic respiration), whereas, glycolytic fibers rely mostly on the glycogen-lactic acid system.

Slow oxidative fibers

When a person orders "dark" chicken meat at a restaurant, they are really asking for slow oxidative skeletal muscle tissue. **Slow oxidative fibers** (also called **red fibers, slow-twitch fibers,** or **type I fibers**) appear dark red because they have a high concentration of myoglobin. They have a relatively thin diameter due, in part, to relatively small glycogen reserves. As their name implies, slow oxidative fibers generate ATP primarily through aerobic respiration. This is evident by the large number of mitochondria in their sarcoplasm.

Since aerobic respiration strips all of the available energy from a glucose molecule, the slow oxidative fiber can function efficiently with fewer stored glucose molecules. Think about it this way: A slow oxidative fiber is like a person who lives on candy, and when he eats a piece of candy none of it goes to waste. By extracting all of the available energy from each piece of candy (glucose), the person (slow fiber) does not need many pieces of candy in the house (sarcoplasm). Slow oxidative fibers also rely heavily on aerobic respiration of fatty acids.

Slow oxidative fibers are important for endurance activities, such as marathons and jogging, because they can utilize aerobic respiration extensively for ATP synthesis. There are four reasons for this:

- Numerous mitochondria serve as sites for the oxidation of fatty acids. Having many mitochondria enable slow fibers to oxidize fatty acids very efficiently, without having to rely on a steady supply of pyruvic acid from glycolysis to function.

- Many capillaries surround the fibers and increase the amount of oxygen available through diffusion from the blood. This provides more oxygen to the fiber, allowing aerobic respiration to continue longer during maximum exertion.

- Abundant supply of myoglobin allows slow fibers to remain in an aerobic condition longer, thereby, prolonging aerobic respiration. As a result of this storage, slow fibers can rely less on O_2 diffusing from the blood at the time of contraction.

- A higher surface area: volume ratio, due to being narrower than large-diameter fibers, means that slow fibers have a relatively larger percentage of their total mass exposed to the ECF. This high surface area to volume ratio allows slow fibers to more easily absorb adequate quantities of O_2 from the blood to meet the O_2 demands of the mitochondria.

Fast glycolytic fibers

If you were to order "white" chicken meat at a restaurant, you are really asking for fast glycolytic skeletal muscle tissue. **Fast glycolytic fibers** (also called **white fibers, fast-twitch fibers,** or **type II-B fibers**) appear white due to a low concentration of myoglobin. These fibers are "faster" than slow fibers in two ways: (1) a twitch *begins* faster because the myosin ATPase hydrolyzes ATP faster; (2) a twitch *ends* faster because Ca-pumps in the terminal cisternae of the sarcoplasmic reticulum remove Ca^{2+} ions from the cytosol faster.

Fast glycolytic fibers may be twice as thick as slow fibers due, in part, to large glycogen reserves. They primarily use glycolysis to make ATP, but remember that glycolysis strips only a small percentage of the available energy from each glucose molecule. Therefore, to continue contracting for an extended period, there must be an abundance of glucose molecules available. Indeed, fast glycolytic fibers store large amounts of glucose in glycogen. In the candy bar analogy, a fast glycolytic fiber is like a person who takes one bite out of a candy bar and throws away the rest of the bar. Because this person is "wasteful" with the nutrient, there needs to be an ample supply of nutrients. Fast glycolytic fibers can prolong their ATP production through glycolysis by having an ample supply of glycogen.

Another reason why fast glycolytic fibers are thicker than slow fibers is that they contain more side-by-side sarcomeres. As a result, fast glycolytic fibers can generate more tension than the thinner, slow oxidative fibers. For this reason, fast glycolytic fibers are important in activities requiring strength and/or speed, such as weight lifting and sprinting. However, fast glycolytic fibers fatigue more rapidly than slow fibers because they produce lactic acid quickly. Having the following four anatomical features explain why fast glycolytic fibers rely more on glycolysis and less on aerobic respiration to generate their ATP:

- Few mitochondria
- Few capillaries surround the fibers means less O_2 available from the blood to support aerobic respiration.
- Limited supply of myoglobin means less O_2 available; thus, fast glycolytic fibers become anaerobic sooner than slow fibers during maximum exertion.
- A lower surface area: volume ratio, due to being thicker than smaller-diameter fibers, means that fast fibers have less of their total mass exposed to the ECF. A low surface area to volume ratio prevents fast glycolytic fibers from absorbing adequate quantities of O_2 from the blood to maintain aerobic respiration during maximum contractions.

Fast oxidative fibers

A third type of skeletal muscle fiber has characteristics of both slow oxidative and fast glycolytic fibers. These *intermediate fibers* are **fast oxidative fibers** (or **type II-A fibers**). Like slow oxidative fibers, fast oxidative fibers appear red due to a significant amount of myoglobin, but not as much as in slow fibers. With myoglobin and numerous capillaries to maintain a high oxygen supply, fast oxidative fibers make a significant amount of ATP through aerobic respiration. In addition, fast oxidative fibers contain much more glycogen than slow fibers; therefore, they make a considerable amount of ATP rapidly through glycolysis. By utilizing both glycolysis and aerobic respiration, fast oxidative fibers are like mid-size cars; they are powerful but also get good gas mileage.

As a comparison, a fast glycolytic fiber is like a powerful "muscle" car; one that is very quick off the starting line in a race (has fast twitches). However, it gets terrible mileage (mainly uses glycolysis) and must have a large gas tank (much glycogen) to go very far. In contrast, a slow oxidative fiber is like a small economy car. It's not very quick or powerful (has slow twitches), but it gets great gas mileage (mainly uses aerobic respiration) and can go very far even with a small gas tank (not much glycogen). Lastly, a fast oxidative fiber is like a mid-size car; one that is reasonably powerful and gets reasonable gas mileage. Table 14-2 compares the different fibers.

DISTRIBUTION OF MUSCLE FIBERS

Genetics is the primary factor that determines the relative percentages of different muscle fiber in a particular skeletal muscle; however, certain types of physical activity can modify existing fibers. Muscles used primarily for endurance activities, such as maintaining posture, have a higher percentage of slow oxidative fibers. Muscles used primarily for performing tasks that require strength, such as lifting and pushing, have a higher percentage of fast glycolytic fibers. Muscles used for tasks requiring a combination of endurance and strength have a higher percentage of slow and fast oxidative fibers.

REGENERATION OF MUSCLE FIBERS

After myoblasts fuse to form a particular type of skeletal muscle fiber, they lose their ability to perform mitosis and cytokinesis. Consequently, the muscle fiber cannot undergo normal cell division to form new muscle fibers. However, the satellite cells remain active between the muscle fibers of adult skeletal muscles. In the event of injury to muscle fibers, **satellite cells** can (1) fuse to form new muscle fibers, or (2) fuse

MUSCLE TISSUE

with damaged muscle fibers; thus, enlarging the fibers. However, satellite cells can offer skeletal muscles only a limited ability to regenerate.

CONTRACTION OF WHOLE SKELETAL MUSCLES

In previous sections, we examined factors that affect the amount of tension that a single muscle fiber can generate but now we turn our attention to whole muscles. The amount of tension that a skeletal muscle generates at any one time depends on two major factors: (1) the tension generated by each contracting muscle fiber, and (2) the number of muscle fibers that are contracting. Recall that a muscle will shorten only if its contraction can generate enough tension to exceed the load on the muscle (force preventing the muscle from shortening). In this section, we will distinguish the different types of skeletal muscle contractions and describe how the nervous system influences the strength of a contraction.

Types of muscle contractions

Muscles can perform useful functions when they contract, whether the contractions cause movement or not. Since not all contractions produce movement, we can classify them into two functional categories: *isotonic* and *isometric* contractions.

Isotonic contractions

Many people who lift weights for exercise prefer repetitious movements, lifting a weight up-and-down or back-and-forth a certain number of times. These movements result from **isotonic contractions** (ī-sō-TON-ik; *iso*, same; *tonic*, strength), during which time the muscle's length changes. Isotonic contractions are

Table 14-2. Characteristics of different types of skeletal muscle fibers

	Slow Oxidative Fibers (I)	**Fast Glycolytic Fibers (II-B)**	**Fast Oxidative Fibers (II-A)**
Anatomical Features			
Density of capillaries	High	Low	High
Color	Red	Pale	Red
Diameter	Small	Large	Intermediate
Glycogen content	Low	High	Intermediate
Density of mitochondria	High	Low	High
Myoglobin content	High	Low	Intermediate
Metabolic Features			
Ca^{2+} ATPase activity	Slow	Fast	Fast
Level of "power"	Low	High	Intermediate
Oxygen consumption	High	Low	High
Glycolysis capacity	Low	High	Intermediate
Myosin ATPase activity	Slow	Fast	Fast
Primary energy source	Lipids	Carbohydrates	Carbohydrates
Resistance to fatigue	High	Low	Intermediate
Twitch duration	Long	Short	Short
Activities	posture, marathons	weight lifting, sprinting	Walking

so named because once the muscle generates sufficient tension to overcome a load, the tension can remain constant throughout the range of movement. In other words, the tension within a muscle can remain the same whether the muscle is moving a 10-kg weight 5 cm or moving it 10 cm.

Isotonic contractions are classified in two ways according to how the muscle changes length. During a **concentric isotonic contraction** (kon SEN-trik; around the center) the muscle *shortens* while it is contracting. For example, lifting a book off a table requires the biceps muscle in the arm to shorten in order to pull the forearm and hand toward the chest. During an **eccentric isotonic contraction** (ē-SEN-trik; away from center), the muscle *lengthens* while it is contracting. Slowly lowering the book onto the table requires the biceps muscle in the arm to become longer but still maintain tension to prevent dropping the book.

Interestingly, eccentric contractions are about twice as powerful as concentric contractions. You can notice this difference when performing push-ups. Pushing yourself off the floor requires that you straighten your arms. You can do this by shortening the *triceps muscles* on the posterior side of your upper arms. Slowly lowering yourself to the floor requires bending your arms while maintaining tension in the triceps muscles. You'll find that it is much easier to lower yourself to the floor (perform an eccentric contraction with the triceps muscle) than it is to raise yourself off the floor (perform a concentric contraction).

Isometric contractions

Some people prefer exercises that force muscles to push against immovable objects. An **isometric contraction** (ī-sō-MET-rik; *metric*, measure) generates muscle tension but the muscle's length remains the same. Contracting a muscle to try moving an immovable object that prevents the muscle from shortening is an example of an isometric contraction. The triceps muscles also perform isometric contractions during different stages of a push-up. If a person struggles to perform a last push-up (or maybe, the first) but can hold a position only halfway through the motion, at that point the triceps muscles are performing an isometric contraction. An interesting fact about isometric contractions is that although they do not involve shortening of muscle fibers, they *do* involve shortening of sarcomeres. The explanation for this relates to the difference between a muscle's *internal* and *external* tension.

Internal and external tension

Tension that develops within muscle fibers must generate tension within a muscle's connective tissues before bones or other body parts will move. Sarcomeres represent a skeletal muscle's **contractile components**, because they are directly responsible for the muscle fiber's ability to generate tension. When sarcomeres contract, they actively generate tension *within* muscle fibers, and for this reason, it is called **internal tension**. Internal tension alone, however, cannot move bones or other body parts because the ends of the muscle fibers do not connect directly to these movable structures. Therefore, the muscle must be able to transmit internal tension to tendons or aponeuroses that *do* connect directly to the movable structures.

Some of a skeletal muscle's noncontractile components *passively* transmit tension from the ends of muscle fibers to a tendon or aponeurosis. These noncontractile components, listed in order leading away from a muscle fiber include the endomysium, perimysium, and epimysium. Because these components are stretchable (elastic), and because tension passes through them one after the other (in series), they are called the muscle's **series elastic components**. Since the passive tension that develops within the series elastic component exists *outside* the muscle fibers, it is **external tension**.

In order to move another structure, a skeletal muscle must shorten. For this to happen, the muscle's internal tension must generate external tension that overcomes the load. The initial stages of contraction, however, do not cause the muscle to shorten. Although sarcomeres are becoming shorter, the series elastic components are stretching. Before the muscle can shorten, the contractile components must generate enough internal tension to make the series elastic components become taut. Only then can the series elastic components generate external tension to overcome the load. A single twitch may not allow enough time to tighten the series elastic components, but tetanic contractions do provide time to generate external tension. However, if the external tension does not overcome the load, the muscle will not shorten.

MUSCLE TISSUE

To understand how series elastic components generate external tension to overcome a load, consider the following demonstration: Break a rubber band and tie it around the handle of a coffee cup. Place the cup on a table then slowly pull the end of the rubber band to lift the cup. You will notice that the rubber band must stretch tight (become taut) before the cup rises off the table. In this analogy, your moving arm is the internal tension; the rubber band is the series elastic component; the tension in the rubber band is external tension; and the weight of the cup is the load.

The external tension generated by a whole muscle at any one time depends on the *number* of muscle fibers contracting and the types of muscle fibers contracting. The nervous system controls these factors through a process called *recruitment*.

Motor unit recruitment

Imagine how jerky your movements would be if you lifted a pencil with the same force as lifting a bowling ball? Obviously, lifting a heavy weight requires more muscle tension than lifting a lighter weight. One way that the nervous system can vary the amount of tension in a skeletal muscle is by stimulating more or fewer muscle fibers. Each axon within a nerve has multiple axon terminals, and each terminal stimulates a single muscle fiber. Therefore, one motor neuron can stimulate more than one muscle fiber. But remember, a single skeletal muscle fiber receives stimulation from only one motor neuron. One motor neuron plus all the skeletal muscle fibers that it stimulates is a **motor unit**. A skeletal muscle has multiple motor units.

An AP propagating along a motor neuron's axon stimulates every muscle fiber in that neuron's motor unit. In response, all muscle fibers within the same motor unit contract simultaneously. By stimulating (activating) more or fewer motor units, the nervous system alters a skeletal muscle's tension to perform a specific task. Activating more motor units to increase a skeletal muscle's tension is called **recruitment**, because the nervous system is "recruiting" (stimulating) more muscle fibers to contract.

For the sake of illustration, consider a simplified example of motor unit recruitment. A particular muscle contains three motor units; one has 3 muscle fibers, a second has 6 muscle fibers, and a third has 9 fibers. By stimulating different combinations of motor units, the nervous system can stimulate 3, 6, 9, 12, 15, or 18 muscle fibers, depending on the task at hand (Figure 14-13).

Types of motor units

While all motor units contain only one neuron, they may differ in three ways. First, they may have different numbers of muscle fibers. "Small" motor units may contain as few as three muscle fibers per motor neuron, while the largest motor units may contain several thousand muscle fibers. The average motor unit in the body contains about 150 muscle fibers.

Skeletal muscles that perform fine motor movements, such as moving your eyeballs in many directions, have relatively small motor units. The nervous system can control these precise eyeball movements by stimulating only a few muscle fibers at a time. In contrast, skeletal muscles used for gross motor movements, such as moving the thighs and legs during walking, have large motor units. In general, large motor units are in muscles that exert tension against relatively large loads.

A second difference between motor units is that they do not all contain the same types of skeletal muscle fibers. On the other hand, all muscle fibers within a single motor unit are the same type. Depending on the task, the nervous system can alter a skeletal muscle's tension by switching stimulation between "slow," "medium," and "fast" motor units. For most activities, the nervous system recruits slow oxidative fibers first; fast oxidative fibers second; and fast glycolytic fibers last. In this way, fibers that are more suited for endurance will contribute longer to a muscle's tension.

A third difference between motor units is that they may have muscle fibers of different size (diameter). Then again, all muscle fibers within a motor unit are approximately the same size. Large motor units generally have large muscle fibers, while smaller motor units generally have smaller muscle fibers. The nervous system can alter a skeletal muscle's tension by switching stimulation between large-fiber motor units and small-fiber motor units.

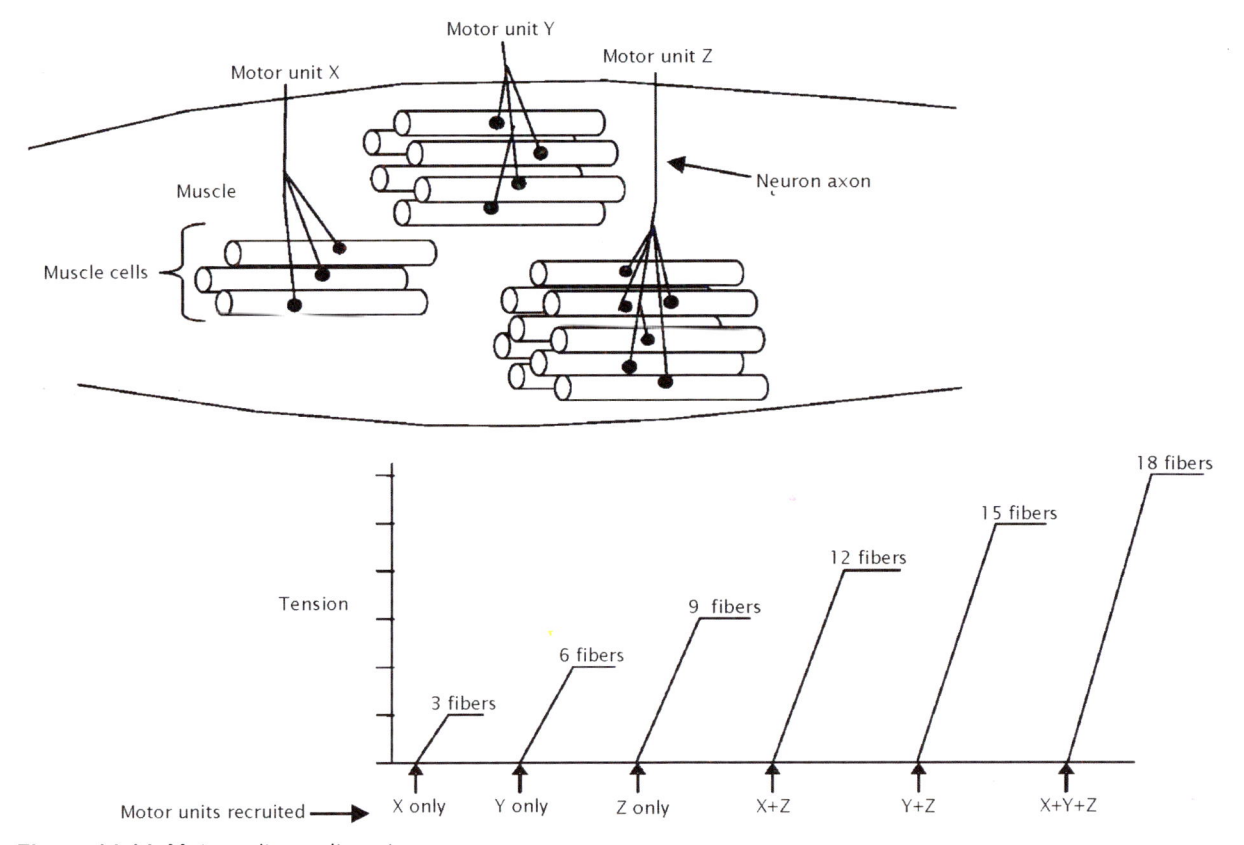

Figure 14-14. Motor unit recruitment

Note: The *gastrocnemius muscle*, which forms the bulk of your calf, has extremely large motor units, each consisting of about 2000 muscle fibers.

The size principle

The order of recruitment of different size motor units is directly proportional to the amount of force required to perform a particular muscle activity. In other words, to generate a small amount of tension to move a small load, the nervous system first recruits small motor units. As the load increases, the nervous system recruits larger and larger motor units. The relationship between the size of a motor unit and its order of recruitment is called the **size principle**. In our previous example, the nervous system would recruit motor unit X first, motor unit Y second and motor unit Z last.

The size principle is very important to precise motor control of skeletal muscles. For example, making subtle muscle movements is usually more important when the load is relatively small. In these cases, recruiting small motor units can generate enough tension to perform the subtle movements. Usually when the load increases, subtle movements become less important. Therefore, the nervous system can recruit larger motor units to perform the more gross (greater) movements.

Muscle tone

Some people may say they lift weights to "tone up" their arms or legs, but what does that mean? It simply means that they want their muscles to be firm, even at rest. The nervous system continually stimulates small numbers of motor units in skeletal muscles, even though the muscle as a whole is "relaxed," or not generating external tension. These few active motor units sustain a low level of internal tension known as **muscle tone**. If a nerve leading to a muscle is cut, the muscle loses its tone and become flaccid (limp).

Muscle tone does not generate enough external tension to cause the muscle to shorten; therefore, muscle tone does not move other structures. However,

MUSCLE TISSUE

muscle tone can be useful in *preventing* movement. For example, maintaining posture relies on muscle tone in muscles of the torso and neck to prevent movement of the spine and head. But would maintaining posture over a long period of time cause muscle fibers to fatigue? This would be likely if the same motor units had to remain active indefinitely. The nervous system avoids fatiguing its motor units by constantly switching its stimulation to different motor units. As a result, motor units get a chance to rest while the amount of muscle tone remains fairly constant.

Regular exercise can increase muscle tone, and this allows muscle's tension to either increase or decrease in order to make adjustments in body position, posture, and movement. Also, if the muscles are in a slight state of contraction, there is more overlap between the thick and thin myofilaments in the sarcomeres. When called upon to contract, these sarcomeres can generate greater force. Increasing a muscle's tone with regular exercise also increases the muscle's metabolic activity at rest. The reason for this increased metabolic activity is that more motor units are consuming more ATP.

Load-velocity relationship

In previous sections, we described factors that influence the *amount* of tension that a muscle can generate. Now we will consider how a load affects the *speed* at which a muscle contracts. If you have ever lifted weights, you know that muscles can move small loads faster than they can move large loads. Earlier, we compared the speed at which different types of muscle fibers contract, but we were not considering their loads. When lifting the same size load, fast fibers contract faster than slow fibers. When moving different size loads, the speed of contraction is *inversely* correlated with the load.

Since muscles contain different types of muscle fibers that can be recruited at different times, a muscle's contraction speed at any one time depends on three factors: (1) the number of muscle fibers contracting; (2) the types of muscle fibers contracting; and (3) the load being moved. If the first two factors remain constant, the speed with which a whole muscle contracts is inversely correlated to the load being moved. In other words, greater loads slow the rate of contraction. This is because it takes longer to stretch the muscle's series elastic components. Furthermore, the amount of shortening that a muscle experiences is inversely proportional to the load; that is, the greater the load, the less shortening will occur.

You can appreciate the load-velocity relationship if you have tried to lift an object that at first seemed too heavy to lift, but with a little more effort, you were able to lift it. At first, some of your "slower" muscle fibers are performing isometric contractions; therefore, the muscle does not shorten and the load does not move. By recruiting faster motor units, the muscle was able to experience isotonic contraction, thereby lifting the object. However, even if the nervous system recruits all of a muscle's motor units, the speed at which it will contract is still inversely correlated to the load.

Response of Skeletal Muscles to Exercise

Research has shown that a reasonable amount of exercise can provide tremendous health benefits, including increased muscle strength and endurance. In sports, the type of exercise that offers the most benefits depends on whether an athlete is training to increase muscle strength, increase endurance, or both. Exercise does not change the type of myosin within the fibers; therefore, no type of exercise is able to convert fast fibers to slow fibers or slow fibers to fast fibers. However, some exercises may effectively convert fast glycolytic fibers to fast oxidative fibers, or fast oxidative fibers to fast glycolytic fibers. With this in mind, exercise-training regimens may fall into three groups: *endurance training*, *resistance training*, and *cross training*.

Endurance training

Jogging, swimming, long distance running and cross-country (alpine) skiing are examples of sports that require endurance, where muscles must contract repeatedly for long periods. To do this, muscles rely more on slow oxidative muscle fibers, which primarily use aerobic respiration to generate ATP. For this reason, activities relying more on endurance, rather than strength, are called *endurance* or *aerobic* activities. In turn, the training regimen that increases muscle endurance is called **endurance training**.

Endurance training requires muscles to exert tension against relatively small loads for long periods. For example, lifting a lightweight dumbbell numerous times helps increase endurance in the arm's biceps muscles. Jogging at a comfortable pace for longer and longer distances helps increase the endurance of the thigh and leg muscles. Endurance training does very little for increasing the size or strength of a muscle, but it does result in a number of changes within the muscle:

- Increased number of mitochondria
- Increased amount of myoglobin
- Increased number of capillaries
- Increased aerobic respiration (fast glycolytic fibers may become fast oxidative fibers)

Resistance training

Weight lifting, bodybuilding, and sprinting are examples of sports that require strength and short bursts of power. To do this, muscles rely more on fast glycolytic fibers, which are capable of making ATP very quickly. Fast glycolytic fibers produce ATP primarily using CP and glycolysis, neither of which requires oxygen. For this reason, activities relying more on muscle strength, rather than endurance, are called *anaerobic* activities. To have an adequate supply of glucose to oxidize in glycolysis, the muscle fibers must store large quantities of glycogen. The training regimen of exercises that increases muscle strength and quickness is called **resistance training**.

Resistance training requires muscles to exert tension against large loads for short periods. In response, muscle fibers produce more parallel myofibrils and store more glycogen, resulting in greater muscle size and strength. Resistance training may be either isotonic or isometric, but isometric contractions seem to be more effective. For example, raising and lowering a heavy dumbbell five times in 10 seconds will increase the strength and size of the biceps muscles. But forcing the biceps to use maximum force for 10 seconds against an *immovable* load causes more rapid increase in muscle strength and size. Sprinting at maximum pace for short distances helps increase the strength and quickness of the thigh and leg muscles. Resistance training does very little for muscle endurance, but it can result in a number of changes within the muscle:

- Increased amount of glycogen
- Increased number of myofibrils
- Increased glycolysis (fast oxidative fibers become fast glycolytic fibers)

Note that resistance training increases muscle size due to an increase in myofibrils and stored glycogen, not an increase in muscle fibers. However, resistance training may cause some muscle fibers to "split." Although this splitting process does not represent true cell division, the resulting fibers may grow more or less independently, much like daughter cells following mitosis and cytokinesis.

Cross training

A variety of sports, including tennis, soccer, boxing, and basketball rely on a combination of muscle endurance and quickness. For these activities, muscles rely more on fast oxidative fibers, which utilize glycolysis and aerobic respiration for ATP synthesis. The training regimen of exercises that increases muscle endurance and quickness is called **cross training**, because it incorporates both endurance and resistance training. This includes jogging intermediate distances to increase endurance, and lifting weights to increase strength and quickness.

CARDIAC MUSCLE CELLS

The only organ in the body that contains cardiac muscle cells is the heart, which will be studied in detail in the next anatomy & physiology course. Here we will only present a brief overview of the anatomy and physiology of cardiac muscle cells.

At first glance, cardiac muscle cells look like skeletal muscle cells. Both types of muscle cells are striated and wrapped in connective tissue coverings called endomysium. But a close look at cardiac muscle cell reveals their unique structure. Each cardiac muscle cell has one nucleus and a cell body with many branches. Cardiac muscle cells join to one another at special junctions called **intercalated discs** (in-TER-ka-lā-ted, "inserted between"), wavy borders that look like tiny interlocking fingers. Cardiac muscle cells don't rip apart from each other as the heart beats because desmosomes "spot weld" the discs together. What is more, gap

MUSCLE TISSUE

junctions tunnel across the intercalated discs and allow ions to diffuse from one cardiac muscle cell to another.

The organelles in a cardiac muscle cell differ somewhat in structure and number from those in a skeletal muscle cell. The limited SR that folds around each myofibril is a clue that a cardiac muscle cell doesn't rely on the SR for all the Ca^{2+} ions it needs to contract. The mitochondria in cardiac muscle cells are larger and more numerous than those in skeletal muscle cells, a fact suggesting how important a generous supply of ATP is to a beating heart. And while the myofilaments within skeletal muscle cells are packed tightly, the number of sliding filaments in a cardiac muscle cell can vary from thousands to only a few, depending on the exact role the cell plays in the heart.

In terms of how they work, cardiac muscle cells differ from skeletal muscle cells in how they depolarize and where they get the Ca^{2+} ions they need to contract. Skeletal muscle cells only depolarize when motor neurons stimulate a neuromuscular junction, but *some cardiac muscle cells can depolarize automatically* and then stimulate other cardiac muscle cells to depolarize. This self-triggering property in the heart is called **automaticity** (aw-tō-ma-TIS-i-tē). After an AP fires in a cardiac muscle cell, about 80 percent of the Ca^{2+} ions that cause the sliding filaments to move come from the SR. The remaining 20 percent diffuse into the cardiac muscle cell from extracellular fluid in T tubules or across gap junctions between neighboring cardiac muscle cells.

SMOOTH MUSCLE TISSUE

Probably the most obvious and unique anatomical feature of smooth muscle fibers is their shape. Unlike cylindrical skeletal and cardiac muscle fibers, smooth muscle fibers are tapered on each end (Figure 14-15). A single oval-shaped nucleus resides in the center of the sarcoplasm. Smooth muscle fibers secrete their own endomysium, consisting of fine collagen fibers and glycoproteins. (Recall that connective tissue cells called fibroblasts form the endomysium around skeletal and cardiac muscle fibers). The endomysium supports blood vessels and nerves.

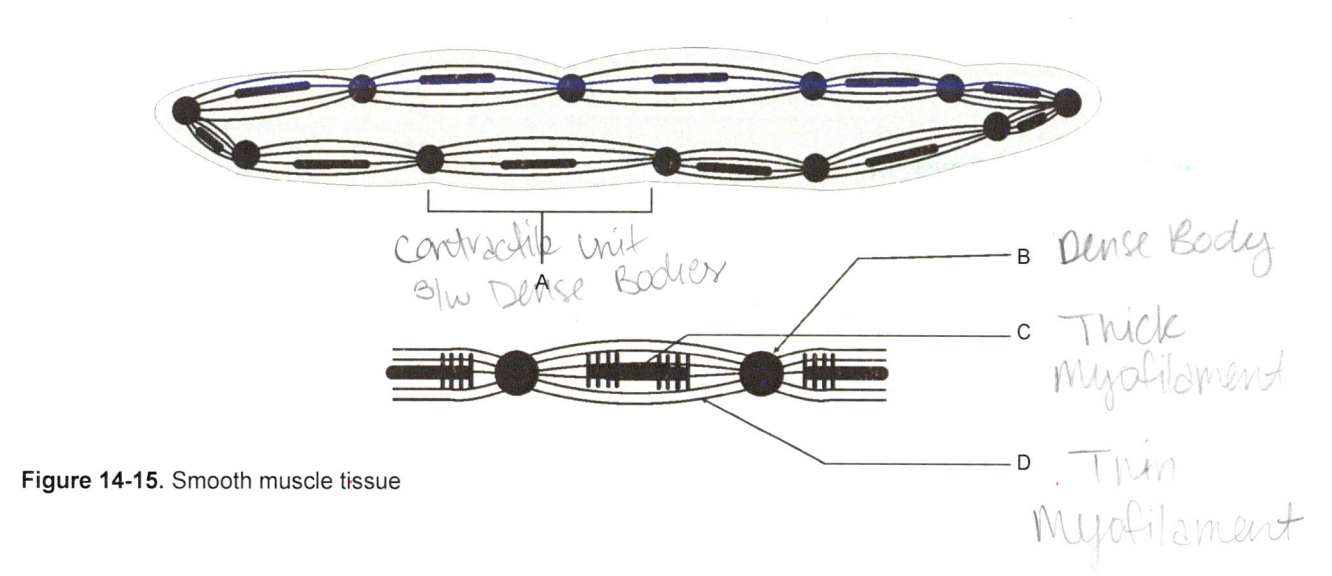

Types of Smooth Muscle

Unlike skeletal muscle fibers, smooth muscle fibers lack motor end plates to which neurotransmitters can bind. Instead, receptors that bind neurotransmitters may be found all along the sarcolemma. Furthermore, a motor neuron that stimulates smooth muscle fibers does not release neurotransmitter primarily from axon terminals. Instead, it releases most of the neurotransmitter molecules from bulb-like regions called **varicosities** (var-i-KOS-i-tēz; "dilated vessel") located along the axon. Depending on whether a neuron stimulates the muscle fibers individually or relies on gap junctions between fibers to transmit APs, smooth muscle tissue is classified as either *single-unit* or *multiunit* (Figure 14-16).

Single-unit smooth muscle is so named because groups of muscle fibers contract together as one unit. Single-unit muscle is also called **visceral muscle** (VIS-er-al; internal organ) because it forms the walls of

Figure 14-15. Smooth muscle tissue

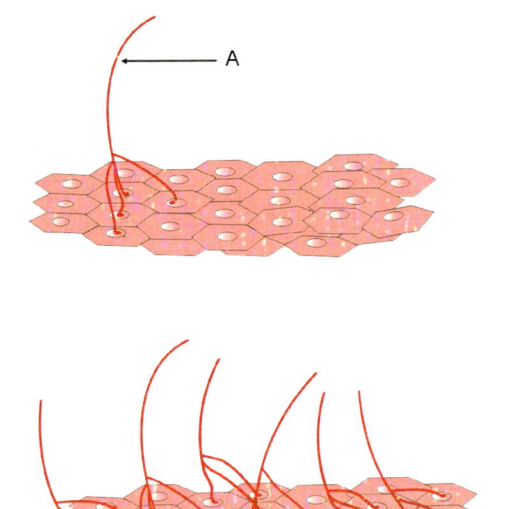

Figure 14-16. Types of smooth muscle

hollow visceral organs such as the stomach, intestine, and blood vessels. The muscle fibers are organized into sheets and each fiber is linked to its neighboring fiber through gap junctions.

Neurotransmitters bind to only a few muscle fibers within single-unit muscle tissue. If the neurotransmitter is excitatory, it initiates APs, which quickly pass to nearby muscle fibers through the gap junctions. In this way, every muscle fiber in the tissue reacts to the simulation almost simultaneously, as a "single unit." Some single-unit muscle fibers in the body can depolarize without any external stimulation, because they contain "leaky" channels that allow enough Ca^{2+} ions to diffuse into the cytosol to initiate contraction. These fibers, called **pacemaker cells**, are found in the stomach and other parts of the digestive tract. They are so named because they "set the pace" for how often the tissue will contract.

Multiunit smooth muscle is not as common as single-unit muscle, and each muscle fiber lies next to a varicosity or an axon terminal of a motor neuron. Moreover, there are very few gap junctions in this tissue. This feature allows the brain to have much more control over tension in multiunit smooth muscle. The brain may choose to stimulate only a few or many muscle fibers, depending on the amount of tension needed.

Multiunit smooth muscle is found inside the eyeballs (where it controls pupil diameter and aids in the focusing of light), arrector pili muscles in the skin, and the walls of tubular passageways in the lungs, large blood vessels and the uterus. During pregnancy, however, the muscle fibers in the uterus develop gap junctions and effectively function as single-unit muscle. During childbirth, this "single-unit" uterine muscle is better able to squeeze a baby through the birth canal.

Anatomy of Smooth Muscle Fibers

The second most striking feature of a smooth muscle fiber is its "smooth" appearance or lack of striations due to a lack of sarcomeres. Instead of connecting to Z lines, the myofilaments within smooth muscle fibers attach to **dense bodies** (look back at Figure 14-15). Dense bodies consist of filamentous actinin proteins, the same proteins found in Z discs of skeletal and cardiac muscle fibers. In fact, dense bodies serve the same purpose as Z discs, anchoring the thin myofilaments in place. A *contractile unit* of a smooth muscle fiber consists of two dense bodies and the myofilaments extending in between them. **Intermediate filaments**, which are noncontractile proteins of the cytoskeleton, also extend from one dense body to the next and help the muscle fiber resist overstretching.

The sarcoplasmic reticulum (SR) in smooth muscle fibers is not well developed; consequently, it does not serve a major role in supplying Ca^{2+} ions for contraction. The sarcolemma lacks T tubules, but it contains numerous pocket-like indentations called **caveolae** (ka-VĒ-ō-lē; vesicles) that contain extracellular fluid. The ECF within a caveola has a higher-than-normal concentration of Ca^{2+} ions due to the action of calcium pumps within the caveola's membrane. For this reason, caveolae serve as important Ca^{2+} ion-storing structures that are important in the contraction process.

The thin myofilaments within smooth muscle fibers consist of intertwining actin and tropomyosin, but they lack troponin. Moreover, the tropomyosin never covers the myosin-binding sites on actin and probably serves more for structural support than to regulate contraction. Instead of running parallel to the length of the fiber, the myofilaments in smooth muscle fibers run diagonally, forming a spiral pattern through the sarcoplasm. As a result, contraction causes the fiber to become globular.

MUSCLE TISSUE

Smooth muscle fibers contain many more thin myofilaments than thick myofilaments. Whereas, the ratio of thin to thick myofilaments in skeletal and cardiac muscle fibers is about 3:1, the ratio in smooth muscle fibers is about 15:1. In addition, the thick myofilaments are structurally different from those in skeletal and cardiac muscle fibers in two major ways. First, they have crossbridges along their entire length, without any "bare" central regions. This feature allows smooth muscle fibers to shorten much farther than other muscle fibers. Second, the crossbridges have two sites that interact with ATP, instead of just one.

Contraction of Smooth Muscle

Like other muscle fibers, smooth muscle fibers require Ca^{2+} ions and energy from ATP for contraction. However, the crossbridges in smooth muscle fibers must first interact with a special enzyme before crossbridge cycling can occur. The steps leading up to and including crossbridge cycling are as follows (see Figure 14-17):

1. Formation of Ca^{2+}-calmodulin complex: When Ca^{2+} ions become available in the cytosol, they bind to a protein called **calmodulin** (**CaM**; kal-MOD-ū-lin), forming a *Ca^{2+}-CaM complex*.

2. Activation of myosin kinase: The Ca^{2+}-CaM activates an enzyme called **myosin light-chain kinase (MLCK)**.

3. Phosphorylation of light-chain region of crossbridge: The activated MLCK transfers a phosphate ion (Pi) from ATP to a special site on the crossbridge, called the *myosin light-chain (MLC) region*. Phosphorylation of the MLC must occur before the ATPase site (on a different part of the crossbridge) can use ATP to perform repeated crossbridge cycles.

4. Binding of ATP to ATPase site: ATP binds to the myosin's ATPase site (not the same ATP that was used at the light-chain region)

5. ATPase activity: The myosin ATPase site hydrolyzes the ATP to form ADP + Pi, causing the crossbridge to become "cocked" in the high-energy position.

6. Binding of crossbridge to actin: The "spring-loaded" crossbridge binds to the actin, causing the Pi to detach from the ATPase site.

7. Crossbridge cycling: Releasing the Pi from the ATPase site causes the crossbridge power stroke. At the end of the power stroke, the ATPase releases the ADP and another ATP binds to the ATPase site, causing the crossbridge to detach from the actin. The ATPase site hydrolyzes the ATP, causing the crossbridge to perform a recovery stroke and return to its high-energy position. As long as the MLC region remains phosphorylated, crossbridge cycling continues to move the thin myofilaments farther past the thick myofilaments and pull the dense bodies closer together. Since there are no sarcomeres to run into, the thick myofilament can pull the thin myofilaments much farther than in skeletal muscle fibers. Each contraction cycle in a smooth muscle fiber is about 30 times slower than a contraction cycle in a skeletal muscle fiber. This is due to the slow activity of the myosin's ATPase site; it hydrolyzes ATP slowly. Consequently, the crossbridges attach and detach from actin more slowly than in skeletal muscle fibers. This allows a smooth muscle fiber to use only 1% as much ATP as a skeletal muscle fiber during one excitation-contraction event. Having such a low demand for ATP during contraction is especially important in blood vessels, the intestines, and the urinary bladder, where smooth muscle tissue must maintain contractions for extremely long periods.

8. Relaxation of the smooth muscle fiber: Crossbridge cycling occurs less frequently and the muscle fiber will eventually relax after an enzyme called **myosin phosphatase** (FOS-fa-tās) *dephosphorylates* the MLC.

9. After dephosphorylation of the MLC, the ATPase site becomes less active. However, relaxation is not instantaneous after myosin phosphatase does its job. For reasons not understood, the crossbridge may remain bound to the actin for some time before detaching; this is called the **latch state**. The latch state enables smooth muscle to maintain tension for long periods without the need for ATP.

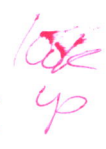

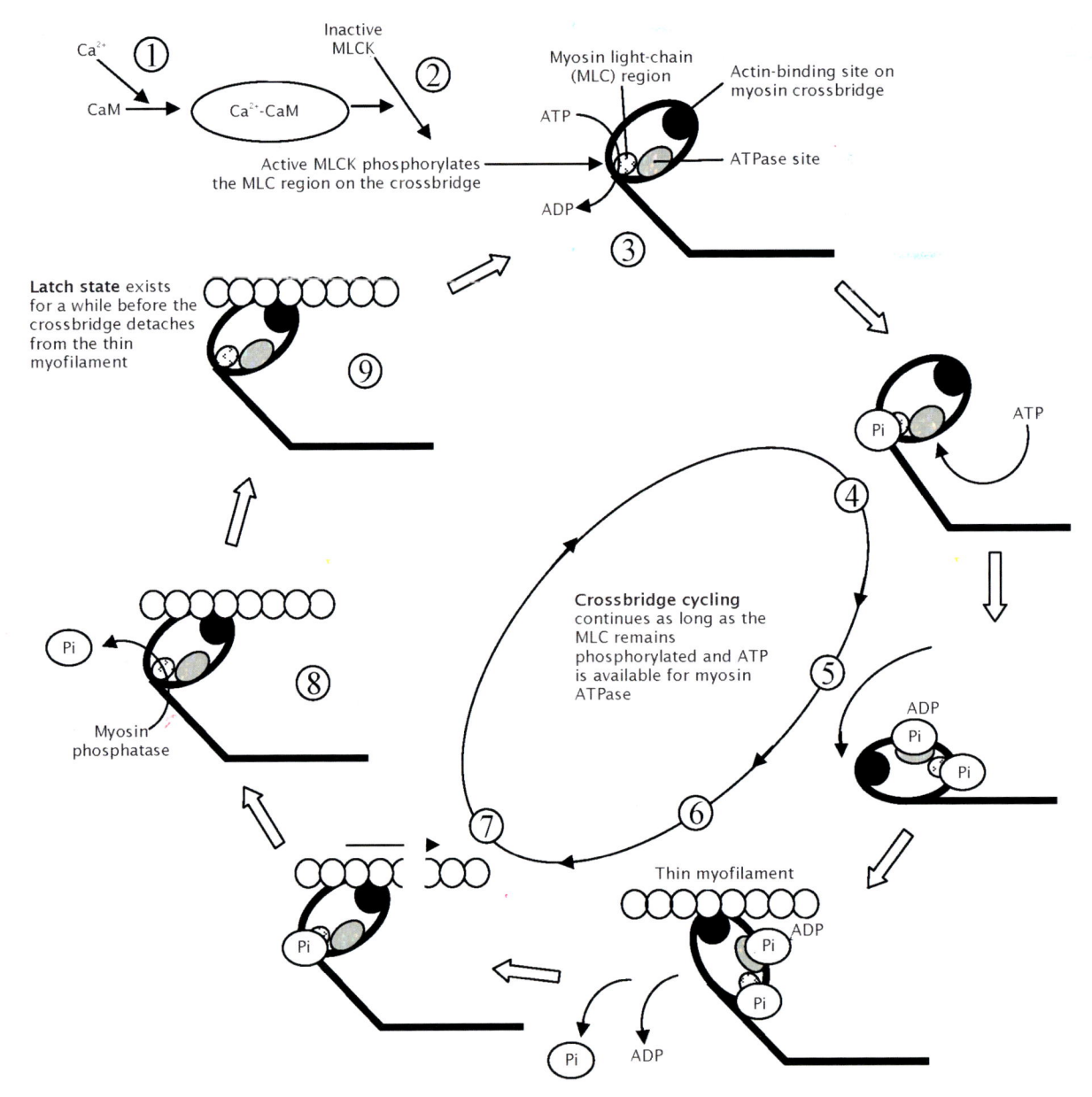

Figure 14-17. Smooth muscle contraction

Myosin phosphatase is always present and continually removing P_i from the light chain regions of the crossbridges, even during crossbridge cycling. So, how can crossbridge cycling continue for any considerable time? During stimulation, more Ca^{2+} ions enter the cytosol causing more Ca^{2+} calmodulin complexes to form, which, in turn, activate more MLCK. Eventually, the concentration of activated MLCK exceeds the concentration of myosin phosphatase. When this happens, phosphorylation of the light-chain regions occurs more often than their dephosphorylation, resulting in prolonged contractions. After stimulation ceases, Ca-pumps remove Ca^{2+} ions from the cytosol, resulting in fewer Ca^{2+} calmodulin complexes and fewer activated MLCK enzymes. At this point, myosin phosphatase is able to keep the light-chain regions dephosphorylated and relaxation occurs.

Sudden stretching of smooth muscle causes the muscle to contract, but then it slowly relaxes over the next few minutes. This phenomenon is **stress-**

MUSCLE TISSUE

relaxation, and is important in hollow visceral organs that stretch as materials pass through them. For example, when excess food enters the stomach, the stomach stretches and its internal pressure increases. The smooth muscle tissue in the stomach wall responds to the stretch (stress) by relaxing, allowing the stomach to expand and decrease its internal pressure.

Stimulation of Smooth Muscle

Whereas skeletal muscle fibers normally contract only in response to stimulation from neurons, smooth and cardiac muscle fibers respond to a number of different stimuli. These stimuli include neurotransmitters from motor neurons, hormones from endocrine glands, cellular waste products, and stretching of the sarcolemma. Moreover, stimulation of a smooth muscle fiber may be either *excitatory* or *inhibitory*. After reading about excitatory and inhibitory stimulation, review Table 14-3, which compares the different types of muscle tissue.

Excitatory stimulation: Excitatory stimulation *always* causes Ca^{2+} ions to enter the cytosol, and most of these Ca^{2+} ions come from the extracellular fluid (ECF) at the time of stimulation. Ca^{2+} ions may enter the cytosol from the ECF through *ligand*-gated and *voltage*-gated calcium channels in the sarcolemma. (In smooth muscle fibers, voltage-gated Ca^{2+} channels far outnumber voltage-gated Na^+ channels.)

Ligand-gated Ca^{2+} channels normally open in response to a ligand binding to a receptor on the sarcolemma, which, in turn, initiates chemical reactions inside the cytosol. Ultimately, these reactions produce a chemical, known as a *second messenger*, which comes back to open the Ca^{2+} channels in the sarcolemma, including the caveolae. As Ca^{2+} ions enter the cytosol through these channels, the sarcolemma depolarizes. If the membrane potential reaches threshold voltage, nearby voltage-gated calcium channels will open. An influx of Ca^{2+} ions into the cytosol through voltage-gated Ca^{2+} channels initiates an AP that propagates along the sarcolemma. Some of the inflowing Ca^{2+} ions bind to calmodulin to initiate contraction cycles.

Smooth muscle fibers usually maintain a small amount of tension even while "resting," because some of the Ca^{2+} ions remain in the cytosol and cause sporadic crossbridge cycling. A low level of tension in these fibers that is not due to external stimulation is **smooth muscle tone**. Recall that skeletal muscle tone requires a constant low level of stimulation from motor neurons.

Inhibitory stimulation: Inhibitory stimulation may cause relaxation or prevent contraction by (1) halting the movement of Ca^{2+} ions into the cytosol; (2) removing Ca^{2+} ions from the cytosol; or (3) causing hyperpolarization. The hyperpolarization can result when a ligand opens potassium (K^+) channels, allowing K^+ ions to diffuse *out* of the fiber, or opens chloride (Cl^-) channels, allowing Cl^- ions to diffuse *into* the fiber. In either case, the membrane potential increases (becomes more negative). When the sarcolemma hyperpolarizes, voltage-gated Ca^{2+} channels remain closed, preventing Ca^{2+} ions from entering the cytosol.

In some cases, an inhibitory ligand decreases the concentration of Ca^{2+} ions in the cytosol. In these situations, the ligand binds to a receptor on the sarcolemma, which, in turn, causes the formation of a second messenger (mentioned earlier). In time, the second messenger stimulates Ca^{2+} pumps in the sarcolemma and sarcoplasmic reticulum to work faster. The action of the Ca^{2+} pumps decreases the cytosol's Ca^{2+} ion concentration, and without Ca^{2+} ions to bind to calmodulin, crossbridge cycling ceases.

Table 14-3. Comparison of Skeletal, Cardiac, and Smooth Muscle Tissue

Characteristic	Skeletal Muscle	Cardiac Muscle	Smooth Muscle
Location	Most are attached to bones via tendons	Heart	Single-unit: walls of hollow visceral organs (except the heart); multiunit: intrinsic eye muscles, arrector pili muscles
Fiber appearance	Single, cylindrical, striated, and multinucleate (nuclei near sarcolemma)	Branched, cylindrical, striated and uninucleate (centrally located nucleus); connect to one another via intercalated discs	Single, tapered ends, no striations, and uninucleate (centrally located nucleus);
Connective tissues	Endomysium, perimysium, epimysium	Endomysium	Endomysium
Sarcomeres present	Yes	Yes	No
Myofilament anchoring sites	Z discs	Z discs	Dense bodies
Myofilaments associated with thick myofilaments	myosin, titin	myosin, titin	myosin, titin*
Proteins associated thin myofilaments	Actin, troponin, tropomyosin	Actin, troponin, tropomyosin	Actin, tropomyosin (no with troponin)
Actin: Myosin ratio	3:1	3:1	15:1
Sarcoplasmic reticulum	Extensive	Less extensive	sparse or absent
T tubules present	Yes	Yes	No (only caveolae)
Gap junctions	No	Yes	Single-unit: Yes Multiunit: No
Autorhythmicity	No	Yes	Single-unit: Yes Multiunit: No
Regulation of contraction	Voluntary	Involuntary	Involuntary
Source of Ca^{2+}	SR	SR and extracellular fluid	SR and extracellular fluid
Neuromuscular junctions	At each muscle fiber	Only at selected fibers	Single-unit: At selected fibers Multiunit: At every fiber
Contraction speed	Fastest	Intermediate	Slowest

*Titin in smooth muscle is slightly different than titin in skeletal and cardiac muscle and is sometimes referred to as *sm*-titin.

MUSCLE TISSUE

TOPICS TO KNOW FOR CHAPTER 14 (MUSCLE TISSUE)

A bands
acetycholinesterase (AchE)
acetylcholine (ACH)
ACH-gated Na+ channels
actin
actin-binding site
actinin
I in skeletal muscle fibers
ADP + Pi
aerobic (cellular) respiration
all-or-nothing principle
anatomy of a skeletal muscle
anatomy of a skeletal muscle fiber
aponeuroses
ATP
ATPase site
automaticity
axon
axon terminals
blood supply to muscles
Ca2+ ions
Ca2+-calmodulin complex
calcium pumps
calmodulin
calsequestrin
CaM
cardiac muscle tissue
caveolae
characteristics of muscle tissue
comparison of muscle tissues
complete (fused) tetanus
concentric isotonic contraction
contractile components
contractile unit
contractility
contraction
contraction of a skeletal myofiber
contraction of smooth muscle
contraction of whole skeletal muscles
contraction period
creatine phosphate (CP)
creatine phosphate system
cross training
crossbridge cycle
deep fascia
dense bodies
dephosphorylation
depolarizing phase
diameter-tension relationship
distribution of muscle fibers
eccentric isotonic contraction
elasticity
electromyogram (EMG)
endomysium

end-plate potential (EPP)
endurance training
energy for contraction
energy systems for sports
epimysium
excess post-exercise oxygen consumption (EPOC)
excitability
excitation-contraction coupling
excitatory neurotransmitter
excitatory stimulation
extensibility
external tension
F actin
fast glycolytic fibers
fast oxidative fibers
fast-twitch fibers
functions of muscle tissue
G actin
glycogen-lactic acid system
glycolysis
H zone
high-energy position
hypodermis
I bands
incomplete (unfused) tetanus
inhibitory neurotransmitter
inhibitory stimulation
intercalated disc
intermediate filaments
internal tension
irritability
isometric contractions
isotonic contractions
lactic acid
latch state
latent period
length-tension relationship
ligand-gated calcium channels
ligand-gated Na+ channels
load
load-velocity relationship
low-energy position
M line
MLC
MLCK
motor end plate
motor neuron
motor unit
motor unit recruitment
multinucleate
multiunit smooth muscle
muscle cells
muscle fatigue

muscle fiber twitch
muscle fibers
muscle tissue
muscle tone
myoblasts
myofibers
myofibrils
myoglobin
myogram
myomesin
myosin
myosin crossbridge
myosin heads
myosin light-chain
myosin light-chain kinase
myosin phosphatase
myosin tail
myosin-binding site
nerve supply to muscles
neuromuscular junction
neurotransmitter
oxidative phosphorylation
oxygen debt
pacemaker cells
perimysium
phosphagen system
phosphocreatine
physiological fatigue
power stroke
psychological fatigue
recovery stroke
red fibers
refractory period
regeneration of muscle fibers
regulation of muscle contraction
relaxation of smooth muscle
relaxation period
repolarizing phase
resistance training
response of skeletal muscles to exercise
rigor mortis
sarcolemma
sarcomere
sarcoplasm
sarcoplasmic reticulum
satellite cells
second messenger
series elastic components
single-unit smooth muscle
size principle
skeletal muscle tissue
sliding filament theory
slow oxidative fibers
slow-twitch fibers

smooth muscle anatomy
smooth muscle tissue
smooth muscle tone
SR
stimulation of smooth muscle
stress-relaxation
striated muscle
striations
subcutaneous tissue
subthreshold stimulus
superficial fascia
synaptic cleft
T (transverse) tubules
tendons
tension
tension in skeletal muscle fibers
terminal cisternae
tetanus
thick myofilament
thin myofilament
threshold stimulus
threshold voltage (TV)
titin
treppe
triad
tropomyosin
troponin
troponin-tropomyosin complex
type I muscle fibers
type II-a muscle fibers
type II-b muscle fibers
types of motor units
types of skeletal muscle contractions
types of muscle tissue
types of smooth muscle
varicosities
visceral muscle
voltage-gated calcium channels
voltage-gated Na+ channels
voluntary muscle fibers
wave summation
white fibers
Z disc
Z line
zones of overlap

CHAPTER 15

The Muscular System

INTRODUCTION TO THE SKELELTAL MUSCLES

What do a ballet, a kung-fu movie, and a weight-lifting competition have in common? You might say they all feature people who enjoy performing but, almost certainly, visions of agility and strength come to mind. What is more, ballerinas, martial artists, and body builders perform their feats of dexterity and power *voluntarily*, meaning they utilize voluntary, or skeletal, muscles. Skeletal muscles are the only muscles that you can control consciously, just by thinking about it, and altogether they comprise your muscular system.

The muscular system includes approximately 700 skeletal muscles and their associated tendons. As their name implies, skeletal muscles attach directly or indirectly to bones, cartilage, or bands of connective tissue that make up the skeletal system. As you will soon see, having a working knowledge of the skeletal system will help you learn the names and locations of many skeletal muscles. In turn, learning the names, location, and actions of skeletal muscles will help you understand how the body can move in so many extraordinary ways. Furthermore, if a person suddenly becomes unable to move in a certain way, having a working knowledge of the muscular system may help pinpoint the problem.

MUSCLE INTERACTIONS

To understand how skeletal muscles produce coordinated body movements, we must first know how muscles interact with the skeletal system and with other muscles. In this section, we describe how a muscle's attachment sites to bones determine the muscle's action. Then we describe how bones function as levers for muscle action, and how muscles work together or against one another to accomplish specific movements.

Muscle-bone interaction

A skeletal muscle is able to move bones or other structures *efficiently* because one end of the muscle remains stationary during contraction. To explain, imagine using a rope to try to pull a friend across a room if both of you are standing on an oil-covered floor. With each pull, both of you would move a short distance toward one another. In the end, you and your friend would only get halfway across the room. To move your friend efficiently (get the most distance out of each pull), you would have to remain stationary. The muscle's attachment site that remains relatively motionless during contraction is the muscle's **origin**, whereas, the movable attachment site is the muscle's

insertion. The muscles for which you need to know the origin and insertion are printed in boldface within the tables shown in this chapter.

Many coordinated body movements, such as walking, involve alternating contractions between skeletal muscles that have insertion sites on the same bone. For example, to take a step, muscles on the femur's anterior surface pull the femur forward. As soon as those muscles relax, muscles on the femur's posterior surface pull the femur back. We can classify a muscle into one of four types based on its primary action, but depending on the task, a given muscle may function as any one of these types.

1. A **prime mover**, or **agonist** (AG-o-nist), is a muscle primarily responsible for a specific movement.

2. An **antagonist** (an-TAG-o-nist) is a muscle that opposes the action of an agonist, much like two athletes competing against one another in a contest (*ant-*, against; *agon-*, contest). Most often, tendons of antagonists cross on opposite sides of the joint they are moving. When an agonist for a particular action is contracting and becoming shorter (*concentric* contraction), the antagonist is stretching. The antagonist may be relaxed or it may be in a slight state of *eccentric* contraction. In the latter case, the antagonist can help control the speed and range of movement caused by the agonist.

3. A **synergist** (SIN-er-jist) is a muscle that works together (*syn-*, together; *erg-*, work) with a prime mover to produce a certain movement. Synergists serve two important roles. First, they may provide extra pulling force to help the prime mover cause movement. Second, synergists may stabilize a prime mover's origin site while the prime mover contracts. Certain muscles of the back hold the shoulder joint steady while arm muscles with origins in the shoulder area contract. In this way, the prime mover is able to produce movement more efficiently, as described earlier.

4. A **fixator** (FIK-sā-ter) is a synergist that stabilizes or "fixes" one joint (holds it steady) while a prime mover moves another joint. For example, while large superficial back muscles move the arm to row a boat, certain deep back muscles act as fixators of the vertebral column, keeping it straight.

SKELETAL MUSCLE NAMES

Skeletal muscle names may relate to a muscle's location, shape, size, orientation, relative position, or action. While some muscle names may seem complicated at first, they can actually help you learn something about the muscle. Anatomists have used seven criteria for naming muscles:

1. **Location**. If you are familiar with names for different regions of the body and the parts of the skeleton, you can determine the approximate location of many muscles simply by interpreting their names. For example, where would you expect to find the brachialis (BRĀK-ē-AL-is) muscle? If you said the arm, you are correct because *brachi-* means "arm." Where would you find the iliacus (il-ē-Ā-kus) muscle? If you said on the iliac bone, you are correct again. Sometimes the muscle's location may not be so obvious in its name. For instance, the anconeus (an-KŌN-ē-us) is located at the elbow (*ancon* is the Greek word for elbow). Other examples of names that indicate muscle location include *capitis* (head), *nasalis* (nose), *thoracis* (thorax), and *popliteus* (back of the knee).

2. **Shape**. Some muscle names contain root words referring to the muscle's shape. If you know the Greek alphabet, you can visualize the triangular shape of the deltoid muscle (named for the Greek letter delta, △). Some slender muscles in the hands and feet look like worms; hence, they get the name, *lumbrical* (LUM-bri-kal), meaning "earthworm." Other names referring to muscle shape include *quadratus* (four-sided), *serratus* (saw-toothed), *rhomboid* (diamond shaped), and *piriformis* (pear-shaped).

3. **Size**. Sometimes muscles located in the same region may have names that distinguish one another based on their relative size. For instance, the *gluteus maximus* muscle is the largest of three major muscles in the buttocks region, while the *gluteus minimus* is the smallest (*maximus*, largest; *minimus*, smallest). In the chest, the *pectoralis* major

muscle is larger than the underlying pectoralis minor (*major*, larger; *minor*, smaller). Other names indicating indicate size include *magnus* and *vastus* (both meaning "large"), *brevis* (short), and *longus* (long).

4. **Fascicle orientation**. A few skeletal muscles have names relating to fascicle orientation. The *external oblique* muscle has fascicles running in an *oblique* (diagonal) manner across the anterior abdomen, while the *transversus abdominis* has fascicles running across the long axis of the body (*transversus*, across).

5. **Number of origins**. Some muscle names refer to the number of origins, where each origin is a "head." The biceps brachii has two origins (*bi*, two; *ceps*, heads), the triceps brachii has three (*tri*, three), and the quadriceps femoris has four (*quadri*, four).

6. **Relative position**. A number of names denote a muscle's relative position on the body or its position relative to another muscle. Examples include *lateralis* (lateral), *medialis* (medial), *superficialis* (superficial), *profundus* (deep), *superioris* (superior) and *inferioris* (inferior).

7. **Action**. Some muscle names indicate a major action on a body part. For example, can you determine the action of the *abductor pollicis* (ab-DUC-tor POL-i-kis) muscle? If you said it abducts the thumb (*pollex*, thumb), you are correct. If someone identifies the *extensor digitorum* in the forearm, would you know its major action? Sure, this muscle extends the digits (fingers). Other names indicating action include *supinator* (supinates the forearm), *pronator* (pronates the palm), and *levator* (elevates or lifts a structure superiorly).

LEARNING SKELETAL MUSCLES

The remainder of this chapter presents information about the anatomy, location, attachment sites, actions, and nerve supply of the major skeletal muscles of the body. While learning all of this information is a daunting task, it will be easier to learn about muscles if you practice the following:

(1) Read about the muscle in the text and tables instead of simply trying to memorize all the muscles on a figure or model. The more you know about a muscle, the less likely you are to forget it.

(2) Practice reciting a muscle's name while you look at the muscle on a figure or model. To begin with, seeing a muscle and hearing its name at the same time will help you learn faster. Secondly, if you can say the name correctly, you are more likely to spell it correctly.

(3) Study muscles in groups that produce an action for the same body part; for example, muscles that move the arm. Then state the action of each muscle within the group. Learning anatomy from this functional standpoint is more practical, especially for the health profession, and the layout of the text and figures should simplify this task.

(4) Identify and palpate muscles on your own body. In your career, it is unlikely that you will see many muscles without skin covering them.

We begin with a brief overview of the major *superficial* muscles of the body. Take a moment to examine the anterior and posterior views of the body's musculature. These views can serve as a quick review after you have identified the muscles in more detailed figures later in the chapter. As you come across new muscles, try to determine if its name relates to location, shape and size, number of origins, relative position, or action. All names in this chapter coincide with those in *Terminologia Anatomica*, an international publication recognized as an authority on anatomical nomenclature.

In the following sections, we describe skeletal muscles in groups based on location and action. Unless stated otherwise, each muscle described has a partner with the same name but located on the opposite side of the body. Figure 15-1 provides an overview of the body's superficial muscles.

MUSCLES OF THE HEAD

If one end of every skeletal muscle must attach to a moving structure, and the head contains only seven moving bones (mandible and 6 ear ossicles), why do we have more than 50 skeletal muscles in our head? If

278   **CHAPTER ■ 15**

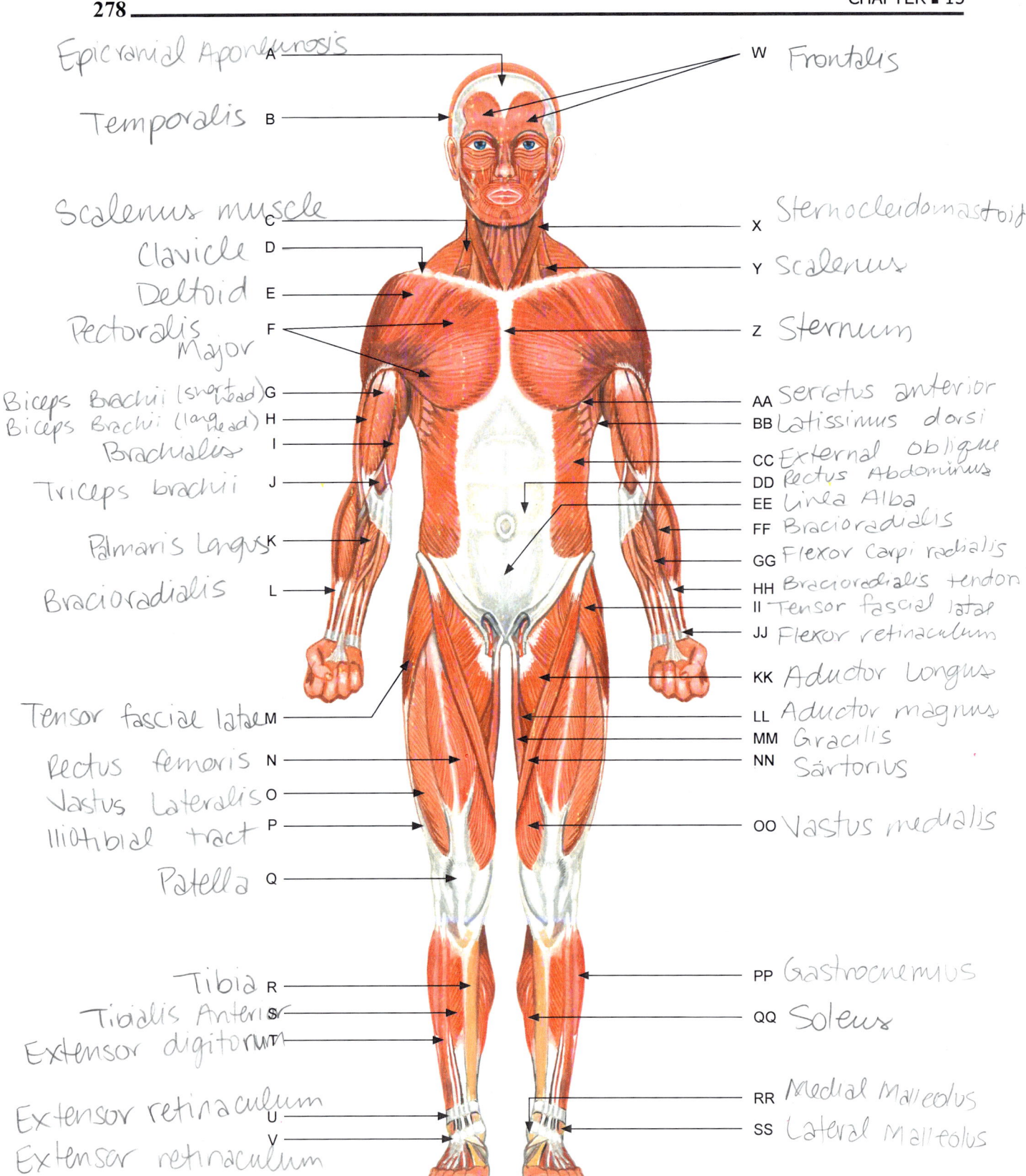

- A. Epicranial Aponeurosis
- B. Temporalis
- C. Scalenus muscle
- D. Clavicle
- E. Deltoid
- F. Pectoralis Major
- G. Biceps Brachii (short head)
- H. Biceps Brachii (long head)
- I. Brachialis
- J. Triceps brachii
- K. Palmaris Longus
- L. Bracioradialis
- M. Tensor fasciae latae
- N. Rectus femoris
- O. Vastus Lateralis
- P. Iliotibial tract
- Q. Patella
- R. Tibia
- S. Tibialis Anterior
- T. Extensor digitorum
- U. Extensor retinaculum
- V. Extensor retinaculum
- W. Frontalis
- X. Sternocleidomastoid
- Y. Scalenus
- Z. Sternum
- AA. Serratus anterior
- BB. Latissimus dorsi
- CC. External Oblique
- DD. Rectus Abdominus
- EE. Linea Alba
- FF. Bracioradialis
- GG. Flexor Carpi radialis
- HH. Bracioradialis tendon
- II. Tensor fascial latae
- JJ. Flexor retinaculum
- KK. Aductor Longus
- LL. Aductor magnus
- MM. Gracilis
- NN. Sartorius
- OO. Vastus medialis
- PP. Gastrocnemius
- QQ. Soleus
- RR. Medial Malleolus
- SS. Lateral Malleolus

Figure 15-1. Overview of the muscular system

THE MUSCULAR SYSTEM 279

- A. Occipitalis
- B. Nuchal Ligament
- C. Sternocleidomastoid
- D. Latissimus Dorsi
- E. Lumbodorsal Fascia
- F. Gluteus Maximus
- G. Gracilis
- H. Gastrocnemius
- I. Gastrocnemius
- J. Calcaneal (Achilles) Tendon
- K. Extensor Digitorum
- L. Nuchal Ligament
- M. Trapezius
- N. Deltoid
- O. Triceps Brachii
- P. Triceps Brachii
- Q. Flexor carpi Ulnaris
- R. Extensor retinaculum
- S. Intrinsic hand muscle
- T. Semitendinosis
- U. Vastus lateralis
- V. Gastrocnemius
- W. Extensor retinaculum
- X. Intrinsic Foot Muscle

Figure 15-1. Overview of the muscular system (continued)

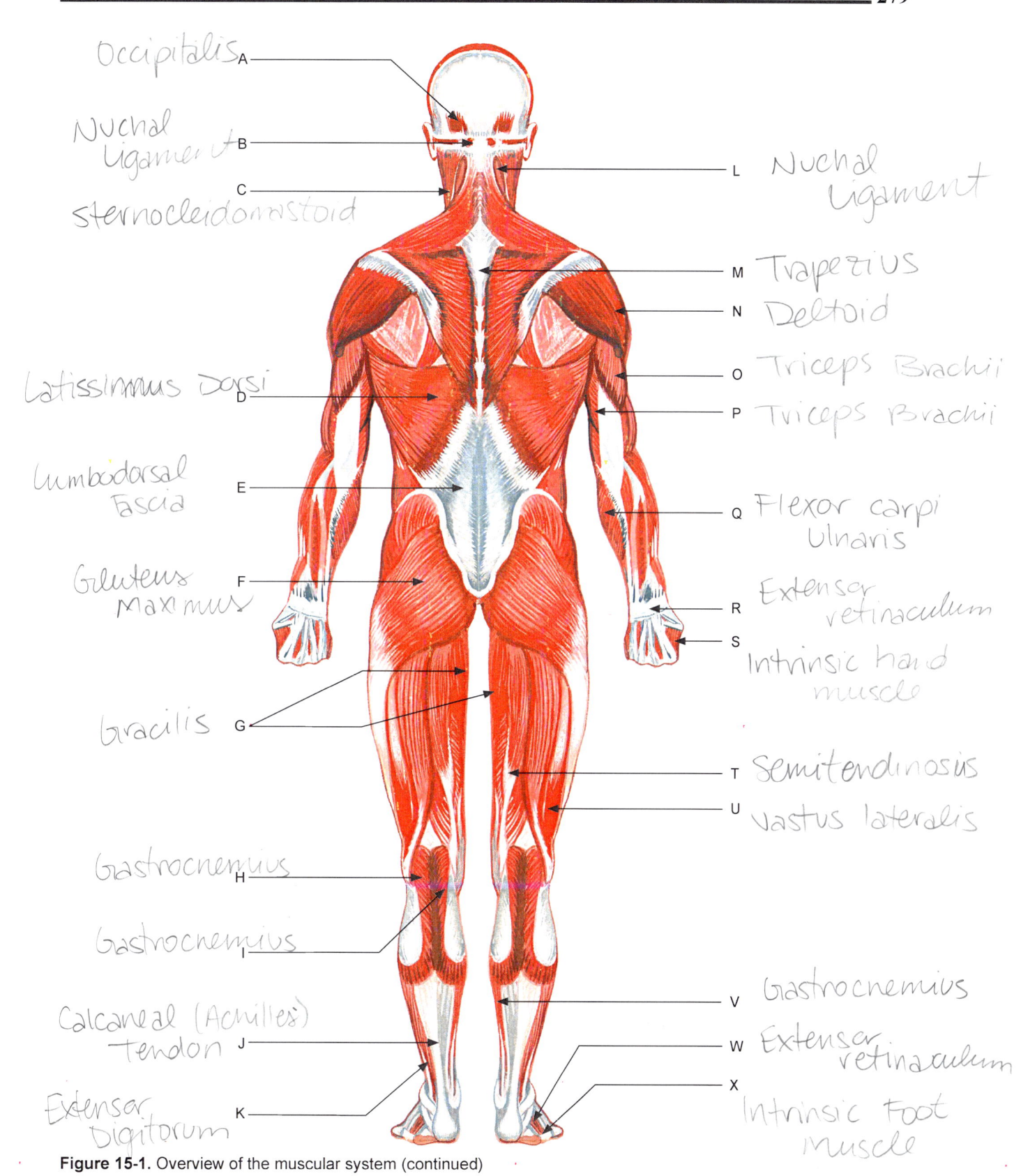

your eyes are moving while reading this sentence, and if you smiled at someone today, you have two hints about how to answer this question. Certainly, you have much soft tissue (mostly skin) on the surface of your skull, and you need skeletal muscles to move it. With one exception, muscles that move the scalp and skin of the face are located entirely within the head. The scalp muscles produce limited movement, while a multitude of facial muscles enable a person to form words and display an impressive variety of facial expressions. The muscles of the face not only produce signs of happiness, sadness, and many other emotions, they also allow a person to form words with the lips. Facial muscles are relatively small and often have fascicles that mesh with one another. There is no single muscle responsible for a given facial expression. Instead, facial muscles can work together with varying levels of effort to change your expression dramatically or ever so slightly. Facial muscles insert into the superficial fascia and pull the skin of the face. Find the muscles of the head in Figure 15-2 and Table 15 1.

Muscles That Move the Scalp

Can you "wiggle" your ears? Although you cannot move them like those of a cat, you can change their position slightly by shifting your scalp back and forth. The major muscle responsible for this action is the single **occipitofrontalis** (ok-SIP-i-tō-frun-TAL-is). It lies over the occipital and frontal bones. The **epicranial aponeurosis** (ep-ē-KRĀ-nē-al), or *scalp*, spans the superior domed portion of the skull and connects the two bellies. The occipitofrontalis raises the eyebrows and wrinkles the forehead skin horizontally, as in a look of surprise, and it pulls the scalp posteriorly.

Superficial muscles are located on each side of the scalp but they play only a minor role in scalp movement. The **temporoparietalis** (TEM-por-ō-pa-rī-e-TAL-is) is so-named for its position over the temporal and parietal bones. It tightens the scalp and pulls the ear superiorly and anteriorly. Near the insertion of the temporoparietalis are three **auricularis** muscles (aw-rik-ū-LAR-is). These tiny muscles connect to the skin around the ear and move the ear slightly. The temporoparietalis and auricularis muscles are *vestigial* (ves-TIJ-ē-al), believed to represent only a remnant (*vestige*, trace) of more developed ear muscles found in other primates.

Muscles That Move the Eyelids and Nose

Four sets of muscles move the skin around the eyes and nose. The **orbicularis oculi** (or-BIK-ū-LAR-is OK-ū-lī) is a circular muscle that surrounds the orbit. It closes the eye and produces squinting. The single **procerus** (prō-SĒ-rus) muscle is small triangular muscle located near the bridge of the nose. It draws the medial end of the eyebrow inferiorly and wrinkles the forehead skin horizontally. You might contract this muscle when you smell a bad odor. The **corrugator supercilii** (KOR-a-gā-tor SOO-per-SI-lē-ī) lies deep to the occipitofrontalis at the superior, medial corner of the orbit. It draws the eyebrow medially and wrinkles the forehead skin vertically, yielding the expression of deep thought. The **nasalis** (nā-SAL-is) covers the superior half of the nose. Different parts of the nasalis compress the superior portion of the nose, pull the tip of the nose inferiorly, and flare (widen) the nostrils.

Muscles That Move the Cheeks, Lips, and Mouth

Twelve sets of muscles move the lips, thereby comprising the largest group of facial muscles. Three of these muscles elevate the upper lip. The slender **levator labii superioris alaeque nasi** (LĒ-va-tor LĀ-bē-ī sū-PĒR-ē-OR-is al-ā-kā NA-sī) stretches along the side of the nose to attach to the upper lip. Incidentally, for such a small muscle, it has the longest name in the muscular system. The **levator labii superioris** is a thicker muscle that extends from the orbicularis oculi to meet with the alaeque nasi muscle in the upper lip. The **zygomaticus minor** crosses a small portion of the levator labii superioris and inserts into the upper lip near the nose.

Three facial muscles insert into the angle (corner) of the mouth, drawing it posteriorly and superiorly to producing the expression of smiling. The **zygomaticus major** runs parallel to the zygomaticus minor but is slightly lateral and inferior to it. The **risorius** (rī-ZOR-ē-us) is a delicate, superficial muscle lying within the superficial fascia of the cheek. Lastly, the **levator anguli** (ANG-gū-lī) lies deep to the levator labii superioris.

> **Note**: According to some experts, and contrary to popular belief, it takes more muscles to make a *genuine* smile than to make an ugly frown, but a simple *grin* requires only two risorius muscles.

THE MUSCULAR SYSTEM
281

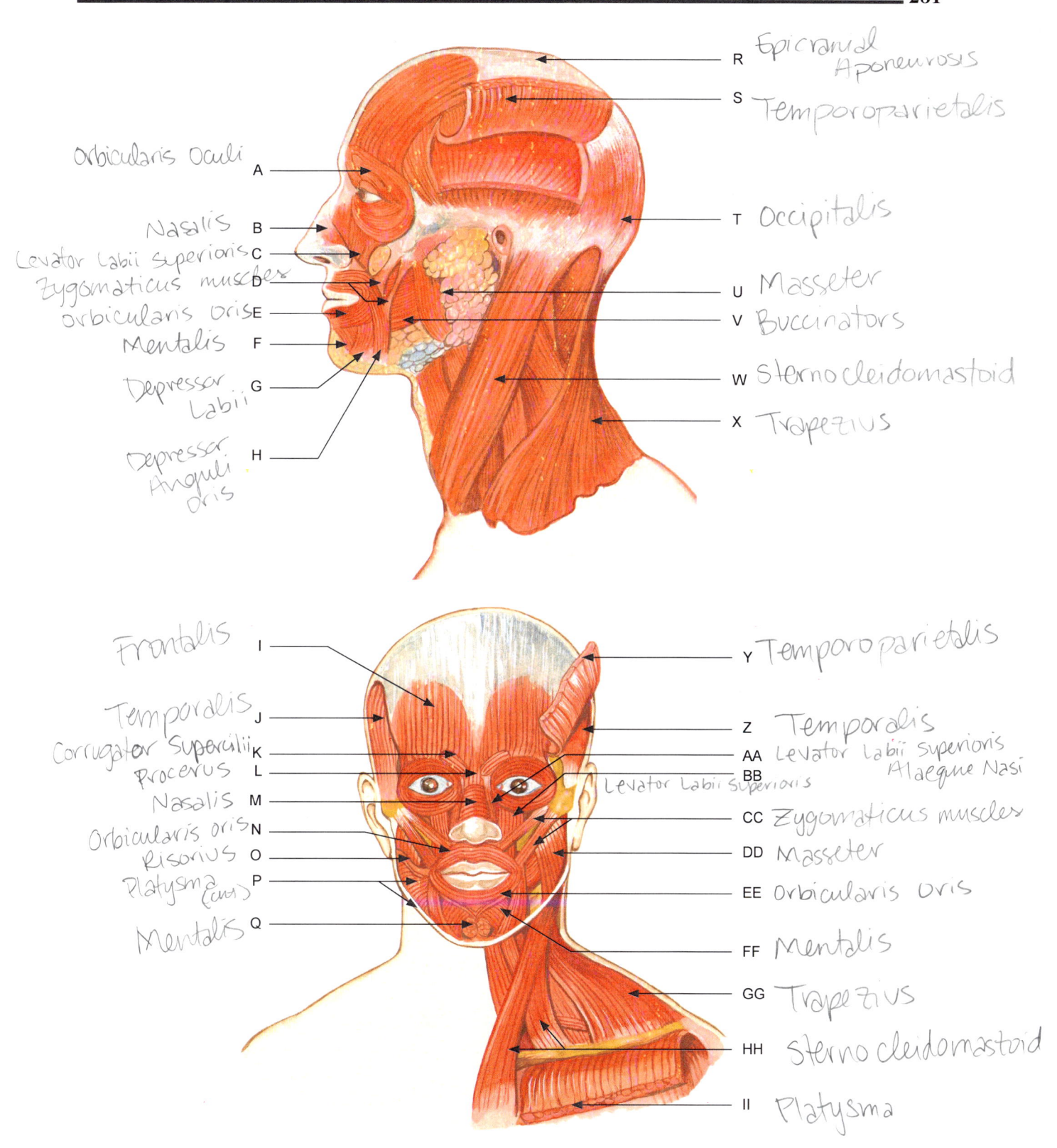

A. Orbicularis Oculi
B. Nasalis
C. Levator Labii Superioris
D. Zygomaticus muscles
E. Orbicularis Oris
F. Mentalis
G. Depressor Labii
H. Depressor Anguli Oris
I. Frontalis
J. Temporalis
K. Corrugator Supercilii
L. Procerus
M. Nasalis
N. Orbicularis Oris
O. Risorius
P. Platysma (cut)
Q. Mentalis
R. Epicranial Aponeurosis
S. Temporoparietalis
T. Occipitalis
U. Masseter
V. Buccinators
W. Sternocleidomastoid
X. Trapezius
Y. Temporoparietalis
Z. Temporalis
AA. Levator Labii Superioris
BB. Levator Labii Superioris Alaeque Nasi
CC. Zygomaticus muscles
DD. Masseter
EE. Orbicularis Oris
FF. Mentalis
GG. Trapezius
HH. Sternocleidomastoid
II. Platysma

Figure 15-2. Muscles of the head and neck

Table 15-1. Muscles of the Head

Muscle	Major Origin	Major Insertion	Major Action
Auricularis	Scalp skin	Skin around ear	Moves ear
Buccinator	Mandible, maxilla	Orbicularis oris	Compresses cheek
Corrugator supercilii	Frontal bone	Skin of brow	Wrinkles brow
Depressor anguli	Mandible	Mouth angle	Lowers mouth angle
Depressor labii	Mandible	Lower lip	Curls lower lip
Levator anguli	Maxilla	Mouth angle	Raises mouth angle
Levator labii superioris	Maxilla	Upper lip	Curls upper lip
Levator labii superioris alaeque nasi	Maxilla	Nose, upper lip	Flares nostril and raises upper lip
Levator palpebrae	Orbit	Upper eyelid	Raises eyelid
Masseter	Zygomatic arch	Mandible	Raises jaw
Mentalis	Mandible	Skin of chin	Raises lower lip; wrinkles chin
Nasalis	Maxilla	Bridge of nose	Flares nostril
Occipitofrontalis	Epicranial aponeurosis	Scalp skin	Raises eyebrows; wrinkles forehead
Orbicularis oculi	Orbit	Eyelids	Closes eye
Orbicularis oris	Muscles around mouth	Lips	Closes/protrudes lips
Platysma	Skin of chest	Mandible	Lowers jaw; tenses neck skin
Procerus	Nasal bone	Skin of nose/forehead	Lowers eyebrows; wrinkles forehead
Pterygoids	Sphenoid bone	Mandible	Raises jaw, lateral excursion
Risorius	Cheek fascia	Mouth	Pulls mouth angle
Temporalis	Temporal bone	Mandible	Raises jaw
Temporoparietalis*	Scalp skin	Epicranial aponeurosis	Tightens scalp
Zygomaticus major	Zygomatic bone	Mouth	Raises mouth angle
Zygomaticus minor	Zygomatic bone	Upper lip	Elevates upper lip

The **orbicularis oris** (OR-is) is a circular muscle that surrounds the mouth and serves as an insertion site for other muscles acting on the mouth. The orbicularis oris is the only muscle that closes the lips, and it protrudes them, which allows a person to form words and pucker the lips. The ability to protrude the lips has given this muscle the nickname, "the kissing muscle." Lying posterior to the orbicularis oris and inserting into its lateral border is the **buccinator** (BUK-si-nā-tor). While you chew, the buccinator compresses your cheeks (pulls them inward) to keep food between your teeth.

Three facial muscles are located inferior to the mouth and move the lower lip and angle of the mouth. The most superficial and lateral of these muscles is the **depressor anguli oris** (dē-PRES-or). It depresses the angle of the mouth (pulls it inferiorly) to yield the expression of a grimace. Lying medially and partially deep to the depressor anguli oris is the **depressor labii**. It curls the lower lip producing the expression of pouting. The **mentalis** (men-TA-lis) is the deepest muscle of the chin and is located adjacent to the mandibular symphysis. It also produces signs of pouting, including elevating and protruding the lower lip and wrinkling the chin.

Lastly, the largest superficial muscle that plays a role in facial expression is the **platysma** (pla-TIZ-ma). It is a flat superficial muscle covering a portion of the chest and much of the anterior neck. The platysma depresses the mandible and tightens the skin of the neck to give the expression of horror.

Muscles That Move the Mandible

Chewing, or *mastication* (mas-ti-KĀ-shun; *mastic-* to chew), involves moving the mandible in a slightly circular pattern with considerable upward force to crush food between the teeth. Two muscles that provide most of the grinding force for the mandible originate deep to the scalp and facial muscles. The largest of these is the **temporalis** (tem-por-A-lis), which covers the temporal bone and inserts on the coronoid process of the mandible. The **masseter** (MA-se-ter), considered by some to be the most powerful muscle in the body, is located anterior to the ear and extends from the zygomatic arch to the angle, ramus, and coronoid process of the mandible. You can feel the temporalis and masseter bulge if you place your hand on your temple and jaw then clench your teeth. The **pterygoid** muscles connect the sphenoid's pterygoid processes to the mandible's ramus. They raise the mandible and produce excursion (side-to-side movement) of the mandible. The platysma (described earlier) lowers the mandible. We will describe other muscles of mastication and muscles that move the tongue, pharynx (throat), hyoid bone, and larynx with the digestive and respiratory systems.

MUSCLES OF THE NECK AND SPINE

Imagine how an active person's daily routine would be affected if suddenly he or she could not turn or tilt their head, straighten up from a stooped position, or even sit up straight in a chair. All of these activities require the actions of muscles located in the neck or deep along the spine (vertebral column). In this section, you will read about muscles responsible for turning the head and maintaining posture (Figure 15-3 and Table 15-2).

Muscles Acting on the Head

When you need to move your head, muscles can do it in two ways: (1) *directly*, by having insertion sites on the head, and (2) *indirectly*, by having insertion sites on the neck. One set of muscles (right and left) that moves the head directly and is located in the anterior neck is the **sternocleidomastoid** (ster-nō-klī-dō-MAS-toyd) muscles. These muscles connect the mastoid process of the temporal bones to the sternum and clavicles, forming a distinct "V" in the neck. When both sternocleidomastoids contract together, the head flexes (tilts forward). Contracting one of these muscles causes the head to turn to the *opposite* side. In addition, these muscles elevate the sternum when a person is taking a deep breath; at that time, the sternum is the insertion.

The remaining muscles that move the head are *vertebral muscles*, having attachment sites on the vertebrae. One group of vertebral muscles that move the head indirectly and are located in the lateral part of the neck are the **scalenes** (SKĀ-lēnz), including anterior, middle, and posterior muscles. These muscles connect the upper two ribs to the transverse processes of cervical vertebrae. Contracting scalene muscles on both sides of the neck flexes the neck, causing the head to tilt forward. Contracting muscles on one side of the neck causes the neck to rotate to the opposite side.

Four sets of vertebral muscles move the head directly and are located in the posterior neck. Most of these muscles originate on the lower cervical and upper thoracic vertebrae and insert directly on the skull; for this reason, they have *capitis* (KAP-i-tis, meaning "head") in their name. The **splenius capitis** (SPLĒN-ē-us KAP-i-tus) and **longissimus capitis** (long-JIS-i-mus) groups insert on the mastoid process, while the **semispinalis capitis** (sim-ē-spī-NAL-is) inserts on the nuchal lines of the occipital bone. Contracting muscles on one side of the vertebral column may rotate or laterally flex the head to the

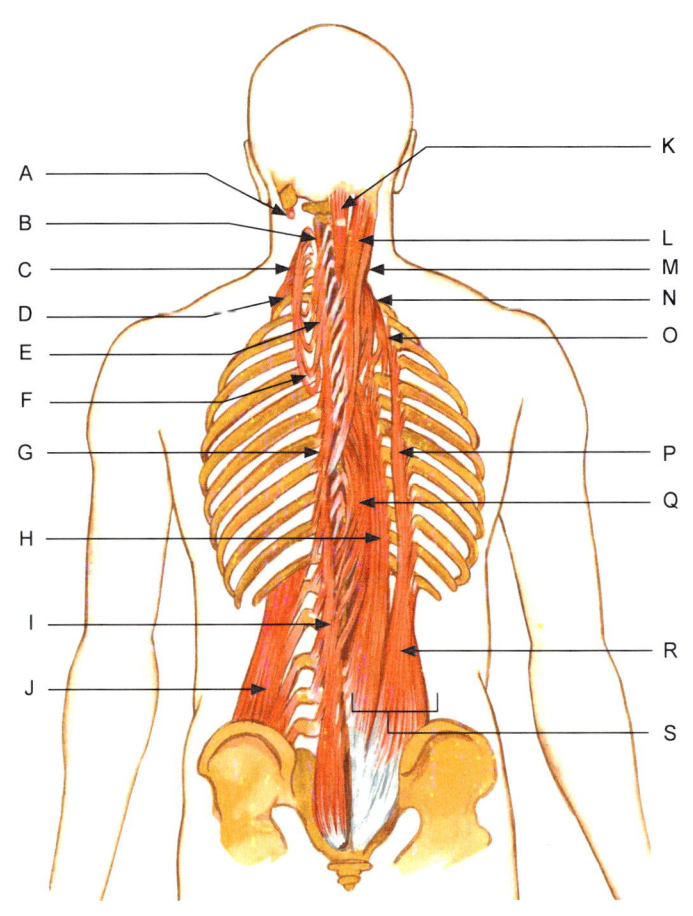

Figure 15-3. Back muscles that move the head and spine

Table 15-2. Muscles of the Neck and Spine

Muscle	Major Origin	Major Insertion	Major Action
Iliocostalis group	Ribs and ilium	Vertebrae, ribs	Flexes/extends head/back
Longissimus group	Vertebrae	Temporal bone, vertebrae, ribs	Flexes/extends head/back
Quadratus lumborum	Ilium	Vertebrae	Laterally flexes/extends spine
Scalenes	Cervical vertebrae	Ribs	Flexes/rotates neck; raises ribs
Semispinalis group	Vertebrae	Occipital bone, vertebrae	Rotates/extends head/back
Spinalis group	Vertebrae	Occipital bone, vertebrae	Extends head/back
Splenius group	Nuchal ligament, vertebrae	Temporal bone, vertebrae	Rotates/extends head
Sternocleidomastoid	Sternum, clavicle	Temporal bone	Rotates/flexes head
Trapezius	Occipital bone; nuchal ligament, vertebrae	Clavicle, scapula	Rotates/raises/lowers/abducts scapula; tilts/extends head

same side. Extending muscles on both sides of the body extends the head (tilts it back).

Five groups of muscles located on the posterior side of the neck laterally flex the neck to the same side or they extend the neck. All of these muscles have *cervicis* (SER-vi-kis, meaning "neck") in their name. The most lateral muscle within this group is the **iliocostalis cervicis** (IL-ē-ō-kos-TAL-is), and it is the only one that originates on the ribs. Immediately medial to this muscle is the **longissimus cervicis**. Slightly more medial is the **splenius cervicis**, which lies deep to the splenius capitis, and the **semispinalis cervicis**, which lies deep to the semispinalis capitis. The medial muscle in this group is the **spinalis cervicis**, which originates and inserts on spinous processes of vertebrae. These four muscle groups extend the neck and laterally flex it to the same side.

Muscles Acting on the Spine

Vertebral muscles that move the thoracic and lumbar curvatures of the spine are typically longer and more superficial than the muscles that stabilize these regions. Moving from most lateral to medial, four groups of muscles bend the thoracic curvature and have *thoracis* (thor-A-sis) in their name. These include the **iliocostalis thoracis, longissimus thoracis, semispinalis thoracis** and **spinalis thoracis**. Moving from lateral to medial in the lumbar region, three muscle groups that bend the lumbar spine and, thus, have *lumborum* in their name include the **quadratus lumborum, iliocostalis lumborum** and **longissimus lumborum**. Contracting these muscles on both sides of the spine simultaneously extends the spine. Contracting only one side tends to laterally flex or rotate the spine.

The deepest and smallest vertebral muscles function primarily as fixators or stabilizers of the spine. However, there is one exception, the **multifidus** (mul-TIF-i-dus). This extensive muscle group connects the transverse processes of each vertebra to the spinous process of the third or fourth more superior vertebra. Contracting the multifidus on one side of the vertebral column laterally flexes the column to the opposite side. Contracting all multifidus muscles extends the vertebral column. The **rotatores** (rō-tō-TŌ-rēz; this name is singular) connects the transverse process of each vertebra to the spinous process of the vertebra above it. The **intertransversarii** (in-ter-trans-vers-AR-ē-ī), as the name implies, connects the transverse processes of adjacent vertebrae. Likewise, the **interspinales** (in-ter-spī-NĀL-ēz) connects the spinous processes of adjacent vertebrae.

You may have noticed that most of the muscles just described extend the vertebral column. Why are there so many muscles that perform this action, but no vertebral muscles that flex the vertebral column anteriorly? In the torso and head, most of a person's soft-tissue weight is located anterior to the vertebrae. Since gravity tends to pull the body forward, it takes considerable effort from vertebral muscles to keep a person upright. Even so, you do have muscles that flex your upper and lower back, but these are located in the abdomen.

MUSCLES OF THE TORSO

Now we will describe the body's largest muscles, which reside in the torso and move the pectoral girdles and arms. Their coordinated efforts produce motions such as reaching, throwing, and pulling (Figure 15-4 and 15-5 and Table 15-3).

Muscles Acting on the Pectoral Girdle

Two muscles that lie deep to the pectoralis major are the *subclavius* and the *pectoralis minor*. The **subclavius**, (sub-KLĀ-vē-us), which stabilizes the pectoral girdle, is the smallest of the two muscles. As its name suggests, the subclavius is located below the clavicle, where it connects the clavicle to the first rib. The subclavius pulls the clavicle inferiorly and anteriorly. This action occurs when the arm is moving forward such as when throwing a ball. Located inferior to the subclavius is the **pectoralis minor**. It extends between the coracoid process of the scapula and ribs 2-5. Contracting the pectoralis minor with the ribs held in place protracts the scapula (pulls it forward). Contracting this muscle with the scapula held in place elevates the ribs; for this reason, the pectoralis minor has a role in inhalation.

As we move laterally around the thorax, we see the **serratus anterior** muscle. Named for its "serrated" appearance, the serratus anterior connects the medial border of the scapula to the upper nine ribs. The serratus anterior pulls the scapula anteriorly and rotates

286

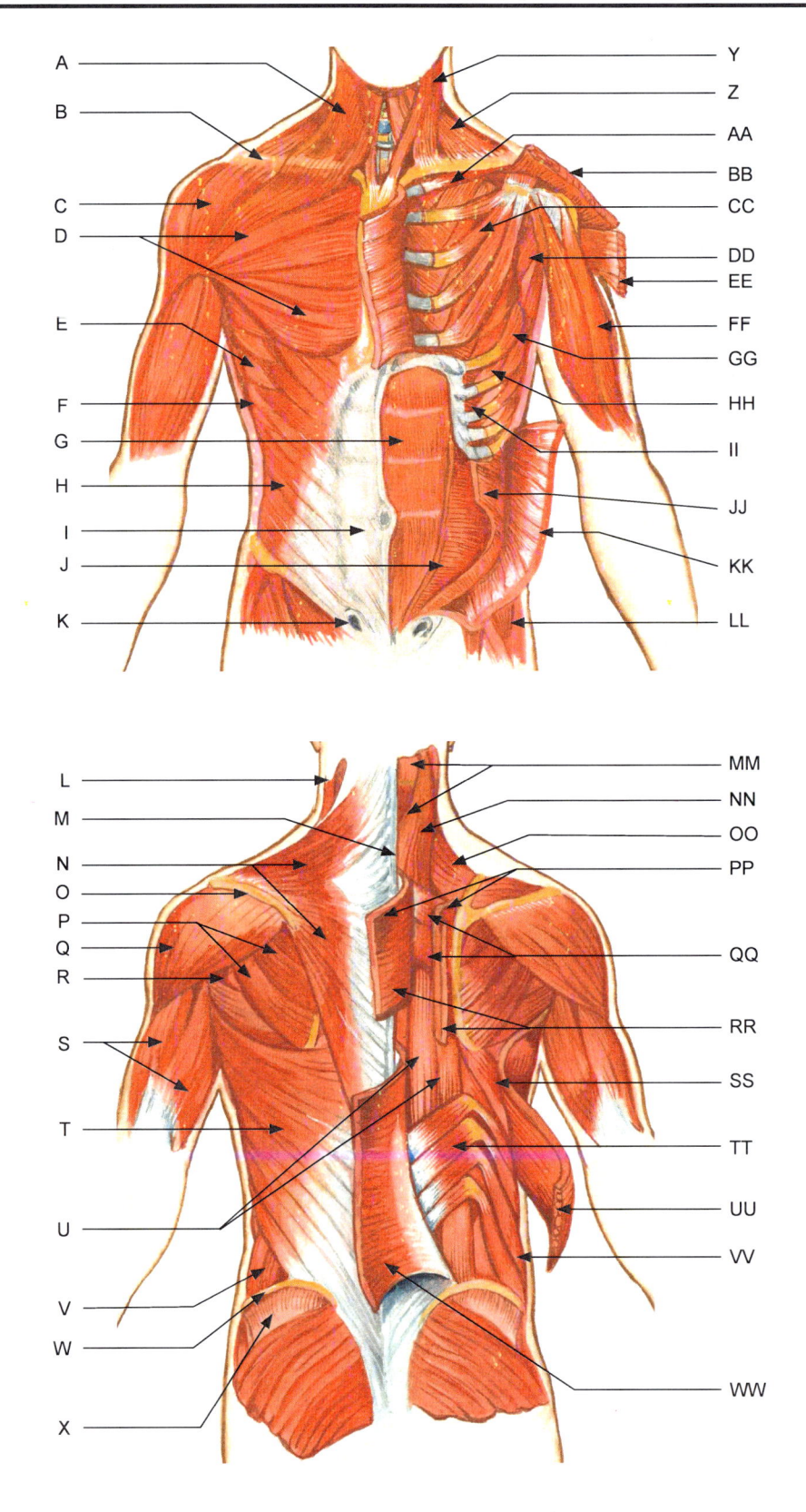

Figure 15-4. Muscles of the chest, back, and shoulders

THE MUSCULAR SYSTEM

it, holding it next to the ribs. This action is useful when pushing objects with the arm. The serratus anterior muscle is nicknamed the "boxer's muscle" because boxers use it to extend the shoulder when jabbing an opponent.

Moving posteriorly, we find four sets of muscles that act on the pectoral girdle. The largest muscle of the upper torso is the trapezoid-shaped **trapezius** (tra-PĒ-zē-us). It originates on the occipital bone and all thoracic vertebrae and inserts on the clavicle and the acromion and spine of the scapula. You use this muscle to demonstrate that you do not know the answer to a question; that is, you shrug (elevate) your shoulders. It also extends the head and pulls it laterally. Lying deep to the trapezius is the **levator scapulae** (LĒ-vā-tor SKA-pyoo-lē) and **rhomboid** (ROM-boyd) muscles. The levator suspends the scapula from the transverse processes of the upper four cervical vertebrae, and as its name suggests elevates the scapula. The rhomboid muscles (major and minor) connect the scapula to the spinous processes of T2-T5. These muscles adduct and rotate the scapula.

Muscles Acting on the Arm

Bodybuilders spend much of their time in the gym developing large muscles in the chest and back, but interestingly this development comes through exercising the arms. The reason is that the prime movers of the arm are located in the chest and lower back. The largest muscles on the chest are the **pectoralis major** (pek-tō-RAL-is) muscles, sometimes referred to in the gym as "peks." It is a broad fan-shaped muscle with origins on the clavicle, ribs, sternum, and the aponeurosis of the external oblique muscle. The pectoralis major inserts on the intertubercular groove of the humerus, and adducts and medially rotates the arm. Birds use their pectoralis majors to flap their wings. You can mimic this action by extending your arms and clapping your hands together.

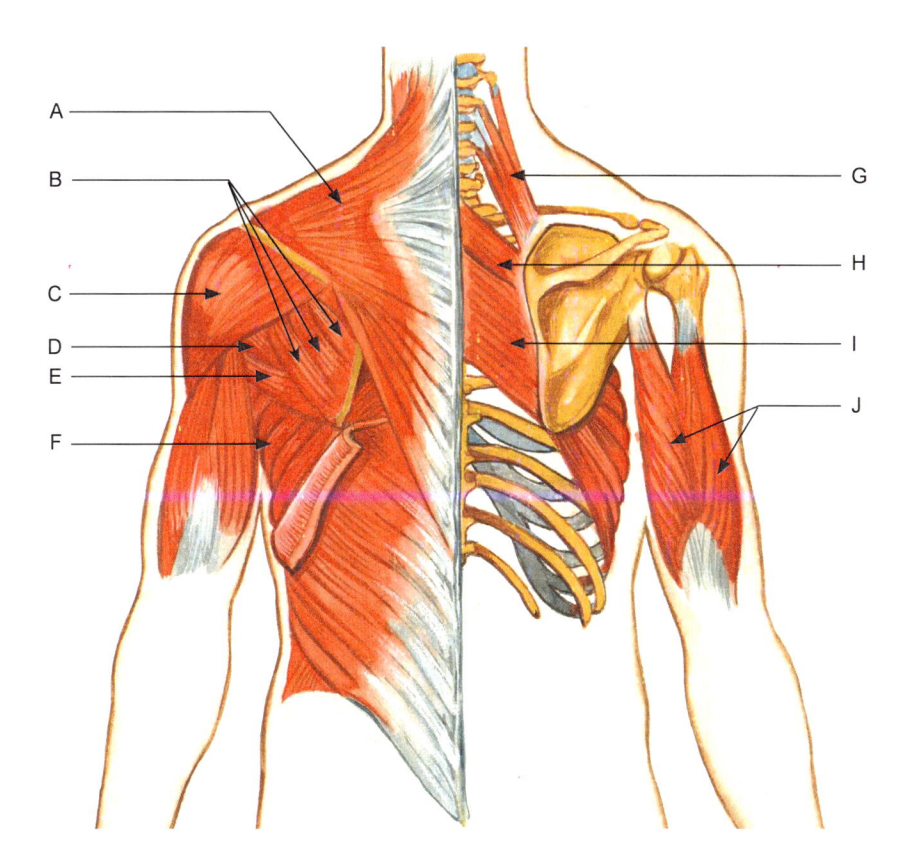

Figure 15-5. Muscles that stabilize the pectoral girdle

Table 15-3. Muscles of the Chest, Back, and Shoulder

Torso muscles that move the PECTORAL GIRDLE			
Muscle	**Major Origin**	**Major Insertion**	**Major Action**
Levator scapulae	Vertebrae	Scapula	Elevates/rotates scapula
Pectoralis minor	Scapula	Ribs	Protracts scapula; elevates ribs
Rhomboid group	Vertebrae	Scapula	Adduct/rotates scapula
Serratus anterior	Ribs	Scapula	Protracts/rotates scapula
Subclavius	1st rib	Clavicle	Depresses/protracts clavicle
Trapezius	Occipital bone; vertebrae	Scapula, clavicle, occipital bone	Rotates/elevates/depresses/retracts scapula; Elevates clavicle; Extends head
Torso muscles that move the ARM			
Coracobrachialis	Scapula	Humerus	Adducts/flexes arm
Deltoid	Clavicle and scapula	Humerus	Circumducts arm
Infraspinatus	Scapula	Humerus	Laterally rotates arm
Latissimus dorsi	Vertebrae and thoracolumbar fascia	Humerus	Extends/adducts/medially rotates arm
Pectoralis major	Sternum and clavicle	Humerus	Flexes/adducts/medially rotates arm
Subscapularis	Scapula	Humerus	Medially rotates arm
Supraspinatus	Scapula	Humerus	Abducts arm
Teres major	Scapula	Humerus	Adducts/medially rotates/extends arm
Teres minor	Scapula	Humerus	Laterally rotates/adducts arm
Torso muscles that move the ABDOMEN and BACK			
External oblique	Ribs	Ilium, linea alba	Tenses abdomen; flexes/rotates back
Internal oblique	Ilium, inguinal ligament, thoracolumbar fascia	Ribs, linea alba	Tenses abdomen; flexes/rotates back
Rectus abdominis	Pubis	Xiphoid process, ribs	Flexes trunk, compresses abdomen
Transversus abdominis	Ilium, thoracolumbar fascia, ribs	Linea alba, pubis	Tenses abdomen

The triangular **deltoid** muscle forms the rounded portion of the shoulder. It has origins on the clavicle and scapula and inserts on the deltoid tuberosity of the humerus. Because the deltoid has fascicles on the anterior, lateral, and posterior sides of the body, it can abduct, flex, and extend the arm. You use this muscle to perform arm circumduction (moving your arm like a propeller). Coursing just below the deltoid is the largest muscle on the back, the **latissimus dorsi** (la-TIS-i-mus DOR-sī). This triangular muscle has a broad origin on the thoracolumbar fascia. The latissimus dorsi converges rapidly to insert on the proximal humerus. This muscle extends, adducts, and medially rotates the arm and is *antagonistic* to the pectoralis major. The latissimus dorsi is known as the "rower's muscle" because rowers use it to pull oars back during a recovery stroke.

Four shoulder muscles originate on the scapula and have tendons that cross and, therefore, reinforce the *rotator cuff*, the fibrous capsule enclosing the shoulder joint. The **supraspinatus** (SŪ-pra-spī-NĀ-tus) and **infraspinatus** (IN-fra-spī-NĀ-tus) occupy the fossae located above and below the scapular spine and insert on the greater tubercle of the humerus. The supraspinatus abducts the arm and the infraspinatus laterally rotates it. The **subscapularis** (sub-skap-ū-LĀIR-ris) resides in the subscapular fossa of the scapula and inserts on the lesser tubercle of the humerus. It medially rotates the arm; therefore, the subscapularis is antagonistic to the infraspinatus. The **teres minor** (TAIR-ēz) extends from the lateral border of the scapula to the greater tubercle, and laterally rotates the arm, similar to the action of the infraspinatus.

Although its tendon does not cross the rotator cuff, the **teres major** runs inferior to the teres minor to insert on the lesser tubercle. It laterally rotates and adducts the arm. The slender **coracobrachialis** (KOR-a-kō-brāk-ē-AL-is) extends from the coracoid process of the scapula to insert on the medial surface of the humeral shaft. This muscle flexes and adducts the arm.

Muscles Acting on the Vertebral Column

Can you remember performing sit-ups? If so, you can appreciate having muscles that can flex your spine. Several of these "back-flexing" muscles reside in the anterior walls of the abdomen. In addition to bending the vertebral column, muscles of the abdomen compress the abdominal cavity. This action is important in defecation and forcefully exhaling air from the lungs. Figures 15-1 and 15-4 show the abdominal muscles that we will describe.

The abdominal muscles that probably attract the most attention in the gym are the **rectus abdominis** (REK-tus ab-DOM-i-nis), commonly referred to as the "Abs." These muscles lie on the anterior abdomen beneath the *rectus sheath*, a sheet of dense regular connective tissue. The rectus abdominis extends from the xiphoid process and costal cartilages of ribs 5-7 to the pubis bone. A white band of connective tissue, the *linea alba* (LIN-ē-a AL-ba; *linea*, line; *alb-*, white), runs along the midline of the abdomen to separate the right and left rectus abdominis muscles. Three horizontal bands of connective called *tendinous intersections* divide each rectus abdominis into four rectangular segments. Contracting the rectus abdominis flexes the vertebral column, and is the major muscle used when performing sit-ups. Its action also compresses the abdominal viscera, thereby aiding in the movement of materials through the intestines.

Three sheet-like muscles form the lateral walls of the abdomen. The most superficial of these is the **external oblique**. It originates on the lower 8 pairs of ribs (5-12) and inserts on the iliac crest and linea alba. A broad band of connective tissue, the *aponeurosis of the external oblique*, stretches from the external oblique to the linea alba and inguinal ligament. If placed on clock, the fascicles of the right external oblique would run in a 10:00 → 4:00 direction; fascicles of the left external oblique run in a 2:00 → 8:00 direction. Due to this pattern and having insertions inferiorly, contracting either the right or left external oblique rotates the trunk to the *opposite* side. Contracting both external oblique muscles simultaneously flexes the trunk and compresses the abdominal cavity.

The **internal oblique** lies just deep to the external oblique. It originates on the inguinal ligament, iliac crest, and *thoracolumbar fascia* (a diamond-shaped aponeurosis in the lower back) and inserts on the linea alba and ribs 9-12. The right internal oblique has fascicles running in a 2:00 → 8:00 direction; fascicles of the left internal oblique run in a 10:00 → 4:00 direction. Since the insertion sites are located superiorly, contracting one internal oblique rotates the trunk to the *same* side. Contracting both internal oblique muscles flexes the trunk and compresses the abdominal cavity.

Lying deep to the internal oblique is the **transversus abdominis** muscle (trans-VER-sus ab-DOM-in-us), which forms the wall of the abdominal cavity and so the parietal peritoneum covers its internal surface. The transversus abdominis extends from the inguinal ligament, iliac crest, thoracolumbar fascia, and costal cartilages of ribs 9-12 to the linea alba and pubis. Both right and left muscles have fascicles running in a 9:00 → 3:00 direction; consequently, they cannot flex the abdomen. On the other hand, both muscles work together like a large sphincter to squeeze the abdominal cavity.

MUSCLES OF THE ARM

Muscles of the torso are not the only muscles that can move the arm; several muscles of the arm can move the arm too (Figure 15-6 and Table 15-4).

Muscles Acting on the Arm and Forearm

The largest muscle on the anterior arm is the **biceps brachii** (BĪ-seps BRĀK-ē-ī). This muscle has two heads of origin, both on the scapula, and it inserts on the radial tuberosity of the radius. The biceps brachii flexes the arm at the shoulder, and flexes and supinates the forearm. To feel its action for arm flexion, straighten your arm and place your palm under the edge of the desk. Now lift up forcefully and use your other hand to feel the biceps muscle tighten. To see its action in forearm flexion, simply bend your elbow.

Lying deep to the biceps brachii is the **brachialis** (BRĀK-ē-AL-is) muscle. It attaches to the distal anterior surface of the humerus and to the ulnar tuberosity and coronoid process of the ulna. The brachialis has only one action: forearm flexion. You can force this muscle to work harder, and thus increase its strength, by doing chin-ups with palms pronated on the bar. The biceps brachii works harder with palms supinated.

The **triceps brachii** resides on the posterior side of the arm. It has three heads of origin, one on the scapula and two on the humerus. The only insertion is the olecranon process of the ulna. The triceps muscle can extend both the arm and the forearm. You would use this muscle to push yourself off the floor when doing pushups.

MUSCLES OF THE FOREARM

The forearm is more complex than the arm because it contains muscles responsible for a myriad of movements at the hand and fingers. In order to approach a study of forearm muscles that is more

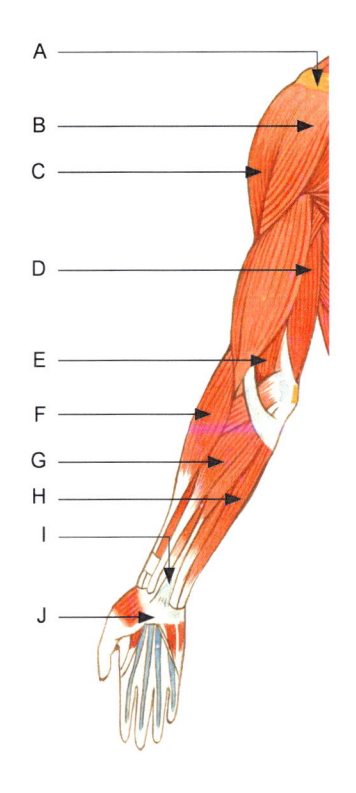

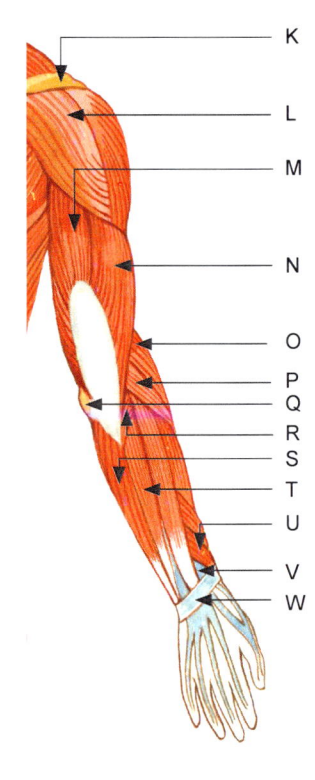

Figure 15-6. Muscles of the arm and forearm

THE MUSCULAR SYSTEM

Table 15-4. Muscles of the Arm

Muscle	Origin	Insertion	Action
Biceps brachii	Scapula	Radius	Flexes arm/forearm, supinates forearm
Brachialis	Humerus	Ulna	Flexes forearm
Triceps brachii	Scapula, humerus	Ulna	Extends arm/forearm, adducts arm

similar to studying them on a cadaver, we will divide these muscles into four groups (Figures 15-6 and 15-7 and Tables 15-5 and 15-6).

Superficial Anterior Muscles

Most superficial muscles of the anterior forearm are flexors of either the hand or fingers; however, the *brachioradialis* and *pronator teres* act on the forearm. The largest of these is the **brachioradialis** (BRĀK-ē-ō-rā-dē-AL-is), which flexes the forearm. This muscle originates on the distal, lateral end of the humerus and inserts on the styloid process of the radius. The **pronator teres** is a short muscle that originates on the medial epicondyle of the humerus and runs diagonally to insert on the radial shaft. As its name suggests, the pronator teres pronates the forearm.

All of the other superficial muscles of the forearm have origins on the medial epicondyle of the humerus and are flexors. The **flexor carpi ulnaris** (FLEK-ser KAR-pē ul-NĀR-is) and **flexor carpi radialis** are located on opposite sides of the forearm and insert in the wrist and hand. Each muscle aligns with the forearm bone for which it gets its name (either ulna or radius). When both flexor carpi muscles contract, the hand flexes at the wrist (carpus). Contracting the ulnaris muscle alone causes hand adduction; contracting the radialis muscle alone causes hand abduction.

The most centrally located superficial muscle in the forearm is the **palmaris longus** (pawl-MĀR-is). It inserts into the *palmar aponeurosis* and flexes the hand

Table 15-5. Muscles of the Forearm

Muscle	Origin	Insertion	Action
Abductor pollicis	Radius, ulna	Phalanx	Abducts thumb
Anconeus	Humerus	Ulna	Extends forearm
Brachioradialis	Humerus	Radius	Extends forearm
Extensor carpi radialis	Humerus	Metacarpals	Extends/abducts hand
Extensor carpi ulnaris	Humerus	5th metacarpal	Extends/adducts hand
Extensor digiti minimi	Humerus	Proximal phalanx	Extends finger
Extensor digitorum	Humerus	Phalanges	Extends fingers/hand
Extensor indicis	Ulna	Extensor digitorum tendon	Extends index finger
Extensor pollicis	Radius, ulna	Phalanx	Extends thumb
Flexor carpi radialis	Humerus	2nd metacarpal	Flexes/abducts hand
Flexor carpi ulnaris	Humerus, ulna	Carpals, 5th metacarpal	Flexes/adducts hand
Flexor digitorum	Humerus, radius, ulna	Phalanges	Flexes fingers
Flexor pollicis	Radius	Phalanx	Flexes thumb
Palmaris longus	Humerus	Retinaculum, palmar aponeurosis	Flexes hand
Pronator quadratus	Ulna	Radius	Pronates forearm
Pronator teres	Humerus, ulna	Radius	Pronates palm; flexes forearm
Supinator	Humerus, ulna	Radius	Supinates palm

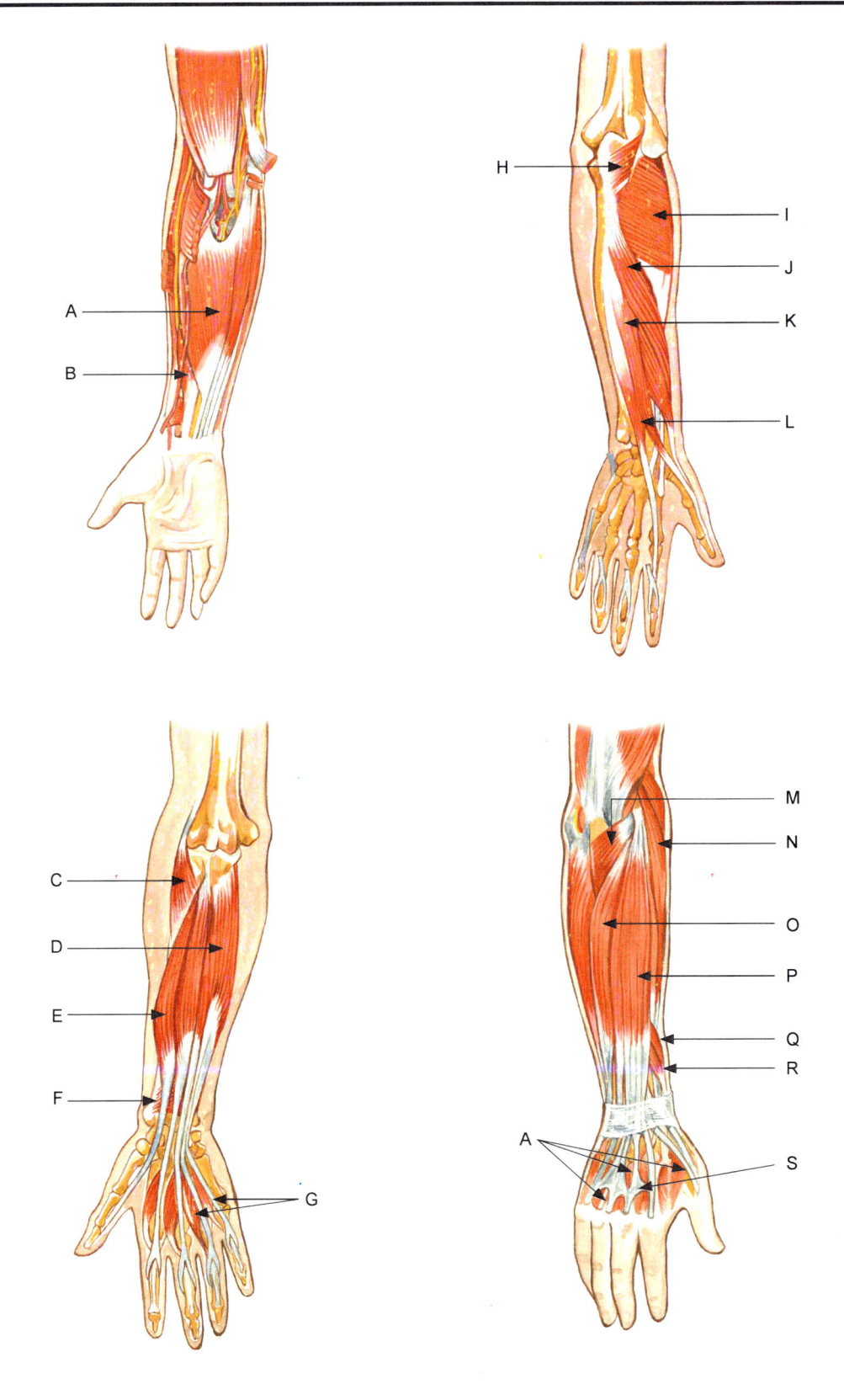

Figure 15-7. Deep muscles of the forearm

at the wrist. If you have a palmaris longus, you can see its tendon by placing your palm under the edge of the desk and lifting up while slightly flexing the hand. If you see two tendons, the smaller one belongs to the palmaris; the larger, more lateral tendon belongs to the flexor carpi radialis. If the palmaris longus is absent, the most lateral superficial flexor muscle is the **flexor digitorum superficialis**. It inserts into the middle phalanges of digits 2-5 and flexes the fingers.

> **Note:** You may not have a palmaris longus; its may be absent from one or both forearms.

In the wrist, the insertion tendons of all these superficial muscles, except that of the palmaris longus, pass deep to a connective tissue band called the *flexor retinaculum* (ret-i-NAK-ū-lum; *retin-*, to hold back). As the name suggests, this retinaculum holds the flexor tendons in place when the muscles contract.

Deep Anterior Muscles

Out of the three deep muscles in the anterior forearm, one acts on the forearm. The **pronator quadratus** (kwah-DRĀ-tus) is a rectangular muscle connecting the distal anterior surfaces of the radius and ulna. Like the pronator teres, it pronates the forearm. The **flexor digitorum profundus** (prō-FUN-dus) originates on the ulna and flexes the fingers (not the thumb); the **flexor pollicis longus** (POL-i-kis) originates on the radius and flexes the thumb.

Superficial Posterior Muscles

Most of the superficial posterior muscles of the forearm are extensors of the hand or fingers, but one acts only on the forearm. The **anconeus** (an-KŌN-ē-us) is a short muscle extending from the lateral epicondyle of the humerus to insert on the olecranon and proximal lateral side of the ulna.

The other superficial muscles of the posterior forearm originate on the lateral condyle of the humerus. The **extensor carpi radialis longus** (LON-gus) and **extensor carpi radialis brevis** (BREV-is) course along the "radius" (lateral) side of the forearm. The longus is the longer of the two and inserts on the 2nd metacarpal; the brevis is the "abbreviated" version (shorter) and inserts on the 3rd metacarpal. The **extensor carpi ulnaris** is located on the "ulnar" (medial) side of the forearm and inserts on the 5th metacarpal. Contracting the radialis and ulnaris muscles together extends the hand. Contracting the radialis muscles alone abducts the hand and contracting the ulnaris muscle alone adducts the hand.

The **extensor digitorum** is the major extensor of the fingers and stretches between the lateral condyle of the humerus to insert on the middle and distal phalanges of the fingers (excluding the thumb). In addition to finger extension, this muscle extends the hand. A forearm muscle devoted entirely to extending the little finger is the **extensor digiti minimi** (DIJ-i-tī MIN-i-mī); it inserts on the little finger's proximal phalanx.

Deep Posterior Muscles

Five muscles lie deep in the posterior forearm including one that acts on the forearm itself. The **supinator** (SOO-pi-nā-tor) is located at the proximal end of the forearm. It extends from the lateral epicondyle of the humerus to the proximal lateral surface of the radius and supinates the forearm.

Three deep posterior muscles, the **abductor pollicis longus, extensor pollicis longus**, and **extensor pollicis brevis** insert on the proximal phalanx of the thumb and have actions corresponding to their names. Each muscle originates partly on the interosseous membrane between the radius and ulna and partly on the posterior surface of the radius or ulna. The **extensor indicis** (IN-di-kus) extends from the ulna and interosseous membrane to insert on the extensor digitorum tendon leading to the index finger (digit #2). This muscle also weakly extends the hand.

> **Note**: A triangular-shaped depression, the **anatomical snuffbox**, is visible when the thumb is extended laterally; it is formed by tendons of extensor pollicis and abductor pollicis muscles.

The insertion tendons of all hand and finger extensor muscles in the forearm pass under the *extensor retinaculum*, a band of dense fibrous connective tissue located in the wrist.

> **Note**: The **carpal tunnel** is the region through which flexor tendons and the median nerve pass in the wrist; it is formed by the flexor retinaculum on the anterior side and carpal bones on the posterior side.

INTRINSIC HAND MUSCLES

The intrinsic hand muscles, those with origins and insertions located solely within the hand, enable the fingers to experience a wider range of motion than would be possible using only the forearm muscles. We will describe these muscles in three groups based on their location relative to the palm (Figure 15-8 and Table 15-6).

Thenar Group

Four muscles form the **thenar group** (THĒ-nar; "palm"), which act on the thumb and form the bulge area located just superior and lateral to the palm. Each muscle's name tells you the action of that muscle. The largest superficial thenar muscle is the **abductor pollicis**. Also superficial, but more toward the palm is the **flexor pollicis**. Lying immediately deep to the abductor muscle is the **opponens pollicis**, which causes the thumb to "oppose" the little finger. Finally, distal from the opponens muscle is the **adductor pollicis**.

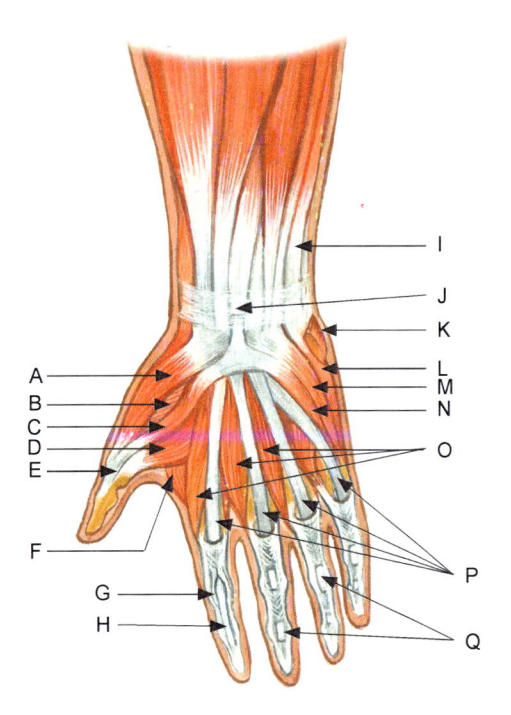

Hypothenar Group

The name **hypothenar** may be misleading since it is not "below" (hypo-) the palm; instead, it is on the opposite side of the palm from the thenar group. The hypothenar group contains three muscles, each acting solely on the little finger. The most medial muscle is the **abductor digiti minimi**. Moving laterally (toward the palm), we find the **flexor digiti minimi brevis**. The most lateral muscle in this group is the **opponens digiti minimi**, which causes the little finger to oppose the thumb.

Midpalmar Group

The **midpalmar group** contains the deepest muscles of the hand, and is located between the thenar and hypothenar groups. The most superficial, anterior muscles are four **lumbrical** (LUM-bri-kul) muscles, one between adjacent metacarpals. These muscles are so-named for their resemblance to worms (*lumbric*, earthworm) and insert on the proximal phalanges of digits 2-5. The lumbricals flex the fingers at the

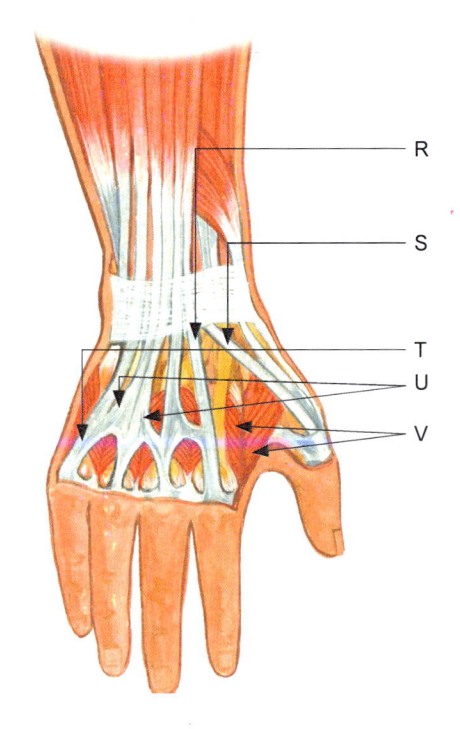

Figure 15-8. Intrinsic hand muscles

THE MUSCULAR SYSTEM

Table 15-6. Intrinsic Hand Muscles

Muscle	Origin	Insertion	Action
Thenar Group			
Abductor pollicis	Carpals, flexor retinaculum	Proximal phalanx	Abducts thumb
Adductor pollicis	Carpals, metacarpals	Proximal phalanx	Adducts thumb
Flexor pollicis	Carpals, flexor retinaculum	Proximal phalanx	Flexes thumb
Opponens pollicis	Carpals, flexor retinaculum	1st metacarpal	Opposes thumb
Hypothenar Group			
Abductor digiti minimi	Carpals, flexor carpi tendon	Proximal phalanx	Abducts little finger
Flexor digiti minimi	Carpals, flexor retinaculum	Proximal phalanx	Flexes little finger
Opponens digiti minimi	Carpals, flexor retinaculum	5th metacarpal	Opposes little finger
Midpalmar Group			
Dorsal interossei	Metacarpals	Proximal phalanges	Abducts/flexes fingers
Lumbricals	Flexor digitorum tendon	Extensor digitorum tendon	Extends/flexes fingers
Palmar interossei	Metacarpals	Proximal phalanges	Adducts/flexes fingers

metacarpophalangeal joints and extend the fingers at the interphalangeal joints. On the palm (anterior) side of the hand are three **palmar interossei** muscles, one between adjacent metacarpals 2-5. These muscles *adduct* and flex the fingers (excluding the thumb) at their metacarpophalangeal joints, and extend the fingers at their interphalangeal joints. On the dorsal (posterior) side of the hand are four **dorsal interossei** (in-ter-OS-ē-ī) muscles, one between all adjacent metacarpals. These muscles *abduct* and flex the fingers (excluding the thumb) at their metacarpophalangeal joints, and extend the fingers at their interphalangeal joints.

MUSCLES OF THE ILIAC AND GLUTEAL REGIONS

Like certain muscles of the chest, back, and pectoral girdle that move the arm, certain muscles from the iliac and gluteal regions move the thigh (Figure 15-9). We will consider these muscles separately.

Muscles of the Iliac Region

Two muscles, the **iliacus** (il-ē-Ā-kus) and **psoas major** (SŌ-as) join to function as a single **iliopsoas** (il-ē-ō-SŌ-as) muscle. The iliopsoas tendon inserts on the lesser trochanter of the femur. The iliacus originates on the iliac fossa, and the psoas major originates on the transverse processes of the twelfth thoracic through the fourth lumbar vertebrae. Contraction of the iliopsoas flexes the thigh (lifting the knee toward the chest); in fact, the iliopsoas is the prime mover for thigh flexion. A small **psoas minor** muscle originates on the bodies of vertebrae T12 and L1, and travels alongside the psoas major to insert on the pelvis. Its function is unclear, but may weakly flex the trunk.

Muscles of the Gluteal Region

The gluteal, or buttock, region contains muscles that are important to walking, running, and twisting the thigh. The most obvious muscle in this region, and the one we sit on, is the large **gluteus maximus** (GLU-tē-us MAX-i-mus) (see Figure 15-2). It originates on the posterior surface of the pelvis and inserts on the gluteal tuberosity of the femur. The gluteus maximus is the prime mover for thigh extension (pulling the thigh posteriorly) when you walk or run. Lying deep to this muscle are the **gluteus medius** and **gluteus minimus**. Both of these muscles originate on the posterior ilium and insert on the greater trochanter of the femur. They both abduct and medially rotate the

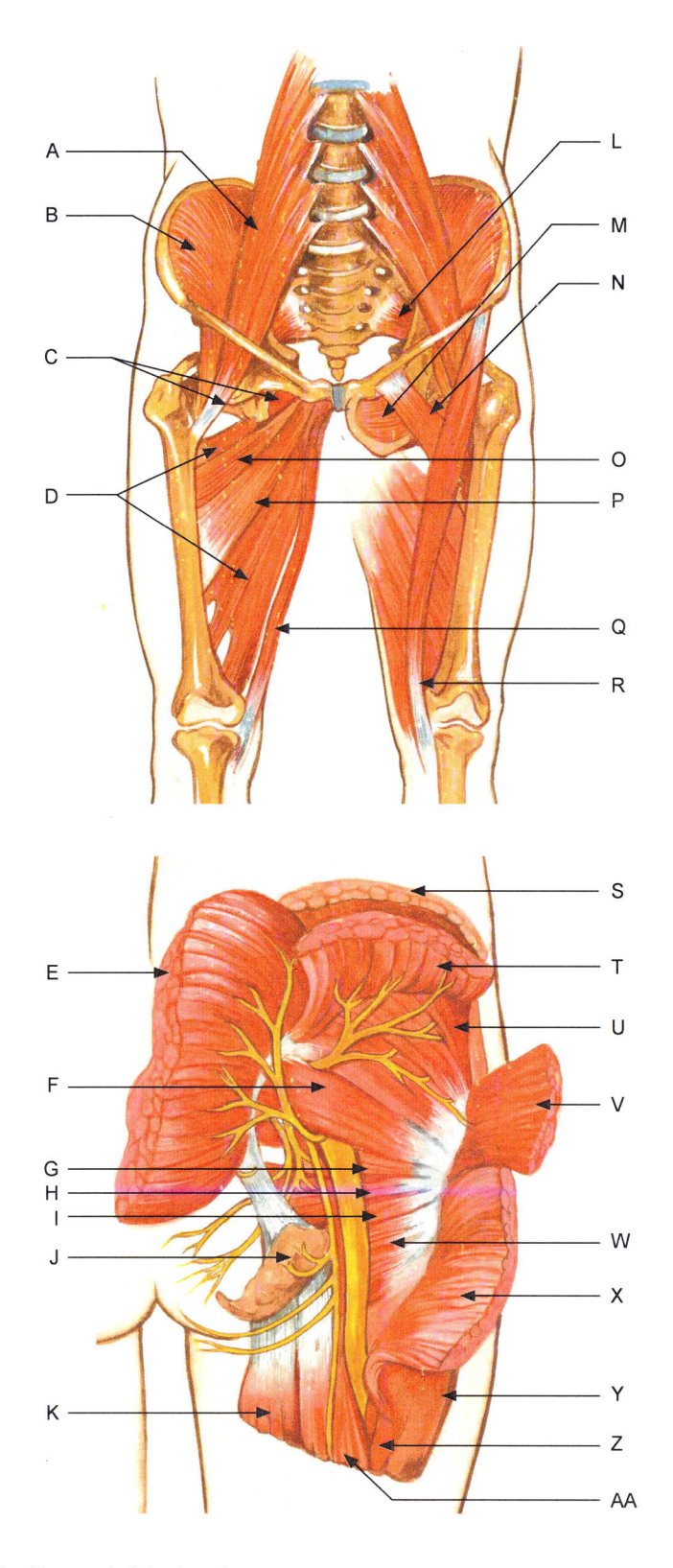

Figure 15-9. Muscles of the iliac and gluteal regions

THE MUSCULAR SYSTEM

thigh, but the gluteus medius is the prime mover for thigh abduction. Medially rotating the thigh allows you to point your foot inward, like that of a pigeon.

> **Note**: Humans have the largest gluteus maximus of any primate, and only about 60% of humans have psoas minor muscles.

Six muscles lie inferior to the gluteus minimus, and we will cover them in order from superior to inferior. Five of these insert on the greater trochanter, and they laterally rotate and abduct the thigh (allowing a person to point their foot outward, like that of a penguin). The **piriformis** (pir-i-FOR-mis) originates on the anterior surface of the sacrum. The **obturator externus** (OB-tū-rā-tor) originates on the external surface of the obturator foramen membrane, while the **obturator internus** originates on the internal surface. The **gemellus superior** (jem-EL-us) originates on the ischial spine, while the **gemellus inferior** originates on the ischial tuberosity. The last muscle, the **quadratus femoris** (FEM-or-is) originates on the ischial tuberosity and inserts on the intertrochanteric crest of the femur. Table 15-7 summarizes the muscles of the hip.

MUSCLES OF THE LOWER LIMB

You might say we are now on the last "leg" of our journey through the muscular system, so it is appropriate that we now cover the muscles that allow us to be mobile. Keep in mind that for our descriptions, "leg" refers is the region between the knee and foot.

Muscles of the Thigh

The thigh muscles are among the strongest muscles in the body, and for good reason; we use them to move most of the body's weight. We will describe them in three groups based on their location.

Anterior Group. The anterior thigh muscles primarily extend the lower leg, but some of these muscles have actions at the hip joint (Figure 15-10). The **tensor fasciae latae** (TEN-sor FA-shē-ē LĀ-

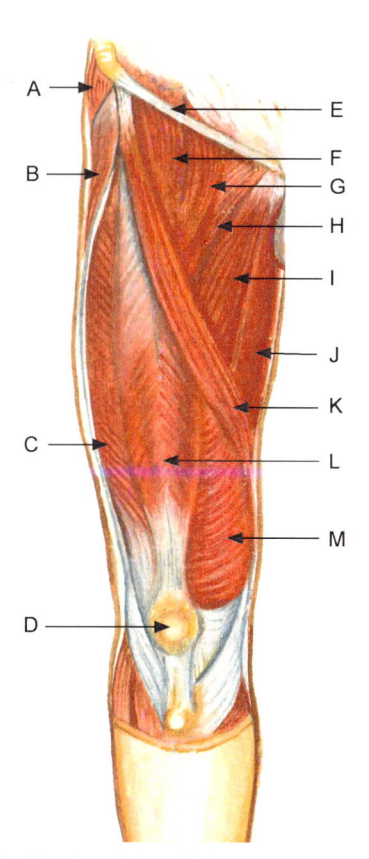

Figure 15-10. Musles of the thigh

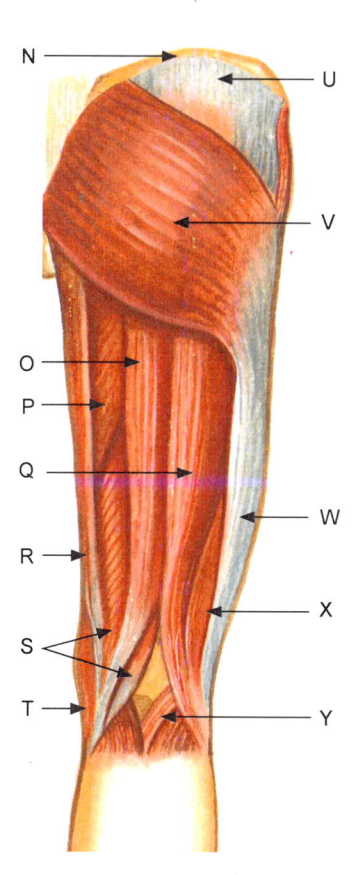

Table 15-7. Muscles of the Hip

Muscle	Origin	Insertion	Action on Thigh
Gemellus	Ischium	Femur	Laterally rotates and abducts
Gluteus maximus	Ilium, sacrum	Femur	Abducts, laterally rotates
Gluteus medius	Ilium	Femur	Extends/medially rotates
Gluteus minimus	Ilium	Femur	Abducts/medially rotates
Iliacus*	Ilium	Femur	Flexes
Obturator group	Obturator foramen	Femur	Laterally rotates/abducts
Piriformis	Sacrum	Femur	Laterally rotates/abducts
Psoas major*	Vertebrae	Femur	Flexes
Quadratus femoris	Ischium	Femur	Laterally rotates

*Part of the Iliopsoas group

tē) is a short muscle extending from the iliac crest to connect with a broad band of connective tissue called the *iliotibial tract*. The iliotibial tract is a thickened distal portion of the *fascia lata*, or deep fascia of the hip and groin region (the name refers to its width; *lat-*, wide). The tensor fasciae latae is so-named for its ability to tense (tighten) the fascia lata. By pulling on the iliotibial tract, the tensor fasciae latae extends the leg. However, this muscle can also abduct, flex, and medially rotate the thigh. The **sartorius** (sar-TOR-ē-us) muscle stretches from the anterior superior iliac spine to the distal medial surface of the tibia. It flexes, abducts, and laterally rotates the thigh and flexes the leg. The sartorius is more active when you need to flex your thigh and leg at the same time, such as when crossing your legs while seated.

> **Note:** The sartorius is the longest muscle in the body and its name means "tailor." Tailors use the sartorius to cross their legs while sitting and sewing fabric.

Four muscles on the anterior thigh work together as the **quadriceps femoris** (KWAH-dri-seps), which is the prime mover for leg extension. All four muscles insert onto the patella via the *quadriceps tendon*. The patella, in turn, connects to the tibial tuberosity via the *patellar ligament*. When the quadriceps contracts it elevates the patella, which, in turn, tightens the patellar ligament and extends the leg. The most central, superficial muscle in the quadriceps is the **rectus femoris**. It originates above the hip joint; therefore, it can flex the thigh. The **vastus lateralis** (VAS-tus), **vastus medialis** are located on the lateral and medial sides of the rectus femoris, respectively. The **vastus intermedius** lies deep to the rectus femoris.

Medial Group. Five muscles reside on the medial side of the thigh, and all of these function as thigh adductors. The most medial of all is the **gracilis** (GRAS-i-lis, "slender"). This slender muscle stretches from the pubis to the proximal medial end of the tibia. Besides adduction, the gracilis medially rotates the femur. Moving laterally from the gracilis, the next superficial muscle is the **adductor longus**. It attaches to the pubis and the linea aspera of the femur. Next to this muscle is the **pectineus** (pek-ti-NĒ-us), which attaches the pubis to the region between the lesser trochanter and linea aspera of the femur. Two muscles in the medial group lie deep to those just described. The **adductor magnus** is the largest and the **adductor brevis** is the smallest.

Posterior group. The muscles in the posterior group are nicknamed hamstrings, possibly because their long length makes them look like strings, and the fact that they are in the "ham" part of the thigh. The hamstrings are the prime movers for leg flexion. The most lateral hamstring muscle is the **biceps femoris**. It has two origins; a *long head* originates on the ischial tuberosity and a *short head* originates on the linea aspera. The biceps femoris inserts on the head of the fibula and lateral condyle of the tibia. You can easily feel its tendon on the lateral posterior side of the knee. The medial superficial hamstring is the **semitendinosus** (SEM-ē-ten-di-NŌ-sus), and just deep to it is the **semimembranosus** (SEM-ē-mem-bra-NŌ-sus). Both of these hamstrings originate on the ischial tuberosity. The semitendinosus inserts on the medial proximal surface of the tibia and the semimembranosus inserts on the tibial medial condyle. You can palpate these tendons behind your knee on the medial side.

> **Note**: Remember the biceps femoris as the lateral hamstring by thinking it is going "outside" (lateral), and you are saying "Bye" to it (for biceps).

Muscles of the Leg

While the thigh muscles focus most of their effort on moving the leg, the leg muscles focus most of their effort on moving more distal structures; namely, the foot and toes. We will divide the descriptions of leg muscles that have actions primarily on the foot and toes into four groups based on their location in the leg (Figure 15-11).

Anterior Group. Four muscles in the anterior leg have actions on the foot and all the toes (including the great toe). The prime mover for foot dorsiflexion is the **tibialis anterior** (tib-ē-Ā-lis). If you dorsiflex your foot, you can palpate this muscle as it bulges just lateral to the tibia (shin). This muscle attaches to the tibial lateral condyle and interosseous membrane between the tibia and fibula and inserts on the 1st metatarsal and medial cuneiform. You can feel its tendon on the front of the ankle during dorsiflexion. In addition to dorsiflexion, the tibialis anterior inverts the foot (turns the sole inward) and adducts the foot.

Moving laterally from the tibialis anterior you will see the **extensor digitorum longus** muscle, which is the prime mover for toe extension. You can identify this muscle on a model or figure as the muscle that has the most tendons extending into the foot. The extensor digitorum longus originates on the lateral condyle of the tibia and inserts on the proximal phalanges of toes 2-5.

Two deep muscles are part of the anterior group and originate on the interosseous membrane between the tibia and fibula. The **fibularis (peroneus) tertius** (fib-ū-LĀR-is or per-ō-NĒ-us TER-shus) inserts on the 5th metacarpal and dorsiflexes and everts the foot. The **extensor hallucis longus** (HAL-a-kis) inserts on the big toe and extends it; this muscle also dorsiflexes and everts the foot. Two connective tissue bands, the *superior* and *inferior extensor retinacula* are located on the anterior side of the ankle. These bands hold all the extensor tendons from the leg in place when the extensor muscles contract.

Lateral Group. Two muscles comprise this group and are located just lateral to the extensor digitorum. The **fibularis longus** is longer and originates on the head and lateral surface of the fibula shaft. It inserts on the 1st metacarpal and medial cuneiform bone allowing it to evert and plantar flex the foot. Lying partially deep to the fibularis longus is the **fibularis brevis**. It is much shorter than the longus, originating on the distal two-thirds of the fibula and inserting on the 5th metacarpal. It also everts and plantar flexes the foot. A *fibular retinaculum* stretches over the tendons of the lateral group in the region of the lateral malleolus.

Posterior Group. Seven muscles reside in the posterior leg (calf). The largest of these is the **gastrocnemius** (gas-trok-NĒ-mē-us) and it has two heads of origin. The *medial head* originates on the medial epicondyle of the femur; the *lateral head* originates on the lateral epicondyle of the femur. It inserts on the calcaneus via the large *calcaneal (Achilles) tendon*. Lying immediately deep to the gastrocnemius is the **soleus** (SŌ-lē-us) muscle. It originates on the proximal one-third of the fibula and shares the calcaneal tendon with the gastrocnemius to insert on the calcaneus. Together, the gastrocnemius and soleus form the **triceps surae** (*triceps*, three heads; SER-ē; *sural*, calf of leg), which acts as the prime mover for plantar flexion. Since its origins are above the knee joint, it can also flex the leg.

The **plantaris** (plan-TAR-is) is a long, slender muscle extending from the lateral condyle of the femur to insert into the calcaneal tendon. Like the gastrocnemius muscle, the plantaris plantar flexes the foot and flexes the leg. The **popliteus** (pop-LIT-ē-us) is deep and medial to the plantaris, originating on the lateral epicondyle of the femur and the lateral meniscus in the knee joint. The most important role of the popliteus is laterally rotating the femur to unlock the knee.

> **Note**: Some people have two plantaris muscles, one in each leg, and about 10% of humans do not have one at all.

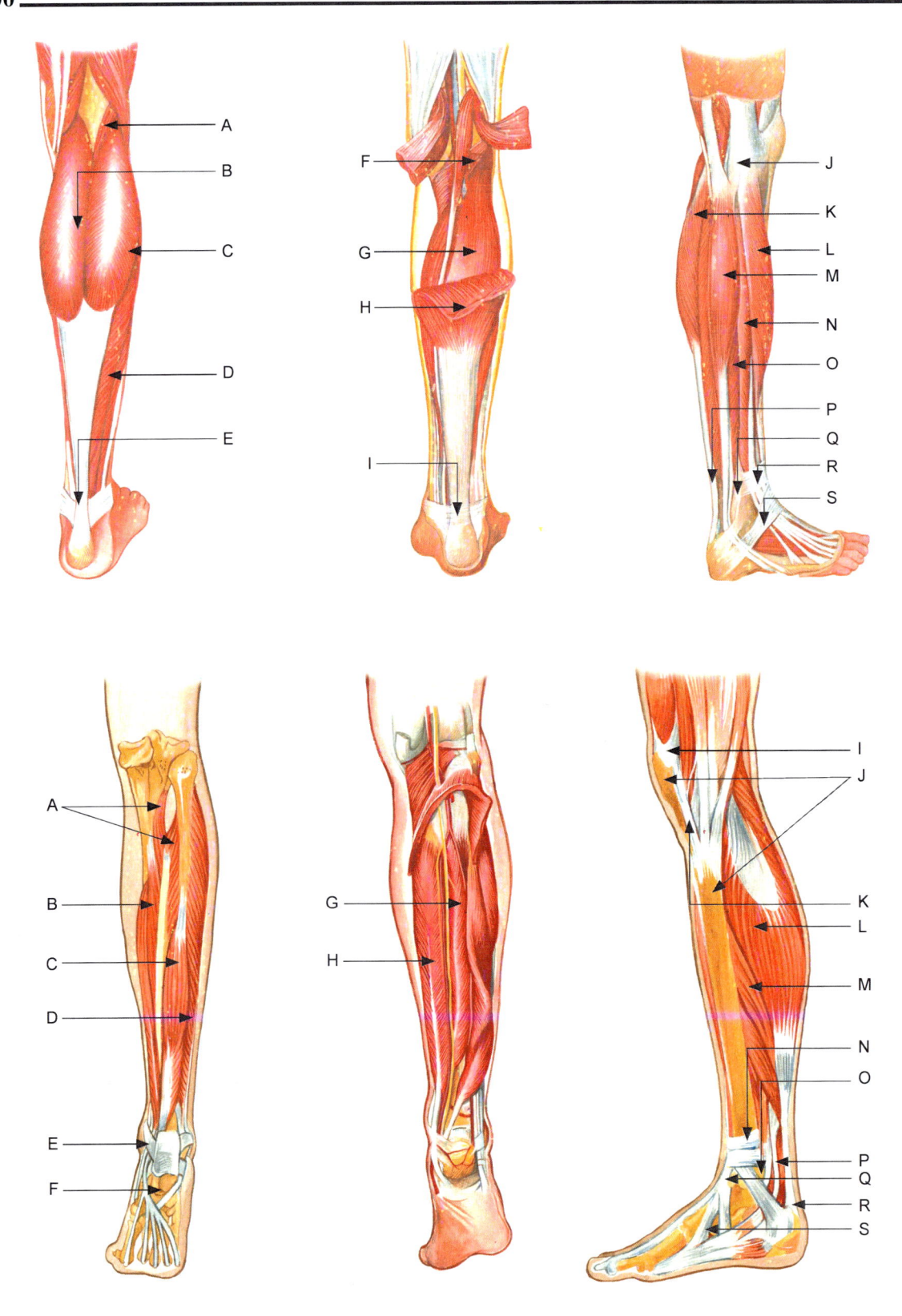

Figure 15-11. Muscles of the leg

THE MUSCULAR SYSTEM

Located deep to the soleus is the **flexor digitorum longus** and the **flexor hallucis longus**. Both muscles originate on the posterior surface of the tibia. The longus muscle inserts on the distal phalanges of toes 2-5, while the hallucis muscle inserts on the great toe. As their names suggest, these muscles flex their respective digits, but they also plantar flex the foot. A *flexor retinaculum* in the medial ankle stretches over and holds the tendons of these flexor muscles in place. The deepest muscle of the calf and running along the surface of the tibia is the **tibialis posterior**. It inserts on the navicular, all cuneiforms, cuboid, and metatarsals 2-4, and causes plantar flexion, inversion, and adduction of the foot. Table 15-8 summarizes the muscles of the thigh and leg.

Table 15-8. Muscles of the Thigh and Leg

Muscle	Origin	Insertion	Action
Adductor group*	Pubis, ischium	Femur	Adducts/flexes/extends, rotates thigh
Biceps femoris	Ischium, femur	Femur, tibia	Flexes leg; extends thigh
Extensor digitorum	Tibia, fibula	Distal phalanges	Extends toes, dorsiflexes/everts foot
Extensor hallucis	Fibula	Distal phalanx	Extends big toe
Fibularis group	Fibula	Metatarsals, tarsal	Dorsiflexes/everts/plantar flexes foot
Flexor digitorum	Tibia	Distal phalanges	Flexes toes; plantar flexes foot
Flexor hallucis	Fibula	Distal phalanx	Flexes big toe
Gastrocnemius	Femur	Calcaneus	Plantar flexes/inverts foot; flexes leg
Gluteus maximus	Ilium, sacrum	Femur	Abducts, laterally rotates thigh
Gluteus medius	Ilium	Femur	Extends/medially rotates thigh
Gluteus minimus	Ilium	Femur	Abducts/medially rotates thigh
Gracilis	Pubis	Tibia	Flexes/laterally rotates thigh
Pectineus	Pubis	Femur	Flexes/adducts/medially rotates thigh
Plantaris	Femur	Calcaneus	Flexes leg; plantar flexes foot
Popliteus	Femur	Tibia	Flexes leg; laterally rotates thigh (unlocks knee)
Rectus femoris	Ilium	Patella	Extends leg; flexes thigh
Sartorius	Ilium	Tibia	Flexes/abducts, laterally rotates thigh; flexes leg
Semimembranosus	Ischium	Tibia	Flexes leg; extends thigh
Semitendinosus	Ischium	Tibia	Flexes leg; extends thigh
Soleus	Fibula	Calcaneus	Plantar flexes foot
Tensor fascia latae	Ilium	Iliotibial tract to tibia	Abducts/flexes/medially rotates thigh
Tibialis anterior	Tibia	1st metatarsal; tarsal	Dorsiflexes/inverts/adducts foot
Tibialis posterior	Tibia, fibula	Tarsals, metatarsals	Plantar flexes/inverts/adducts foot
Vastus intermedius	Ilium	Tibia	Extends leg
Vastus lateralis	Ilium	Tibia	Extends leg
Vastus medialis	Ilium	Tibia	Extends leg

INTRINSIC FOOT MUSCLES

If you are wondering if there is a new, long list of muscles to learn here, relax. The muscles in the foot have the same or very similar-sounding names to those in the hand (Figure 15-12). Furthermore, we do not have opposable toes, so are no "opponens" muscles to identify. To make the foot muscles easier to see, we will describe them in order, from most superficial to deepest. Two muscles reside on the dorsal side of the foot. The most medial is the **extensor hallucis brevis**. It extends from the calcaneus to the proximal phalanx of the great toe. Moving laterally, you can see the **extensor digitorum brevis** muscle extending from the calcaneus to toes 2-4.

Three muscles exist in the superficial layer on the plantar side of the foot. The most superficial of these is the **flexor digitorum brevis**. It lies just deep to a connective tissue sheet, the plantar *aponeurosis*, and extends from the calcaneus to the middle phalanges of toes 2-5. The **abductor hallucis** originates on the calcaneus and inserts on the proximal phalanx of the great toe, which it abducts and flexes. The **abductor digiti minimi** extends from the calcaneus to the proximal phalanx of the little toe, which it abducts and flexes.

Two groups of muscles form a second layer just deep to the superficial layer of muscles. The **quadratus plantae** (PLANT-tē) originates on the calcaneus and inserts onto the tendons of the flexor digitorum muscle. The quadratus muscle flexes toes 2-5. The **lumbricals** stretch from the flexor digitorum longus tendons to the proximal phalanges of toes 2-5. They flex the toes at the metatarsophalangeal joints and extend the toes at the interphalangeal joints.

Three muscles form the deep layer of intrinsic foot muscles. The **flexor hallucis brevis** originates on the cuboid and lateral cuneiform, whereas, the **adductor hallucis** originates on metatarsals 2-4 and

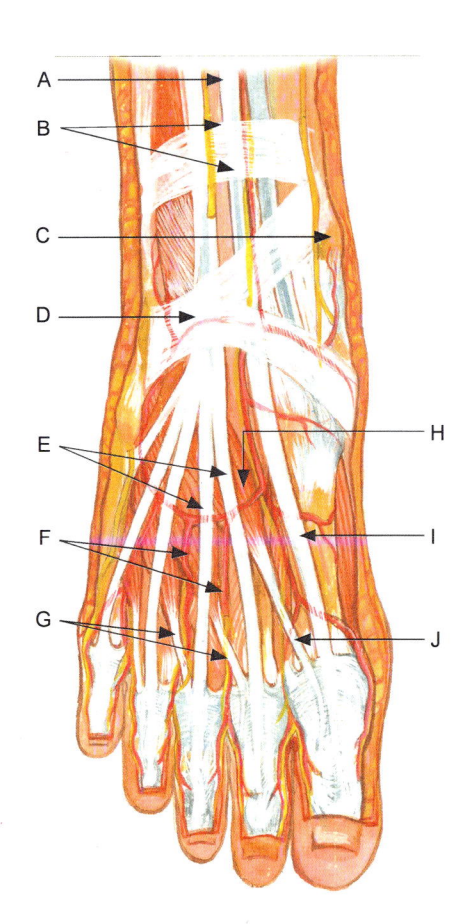

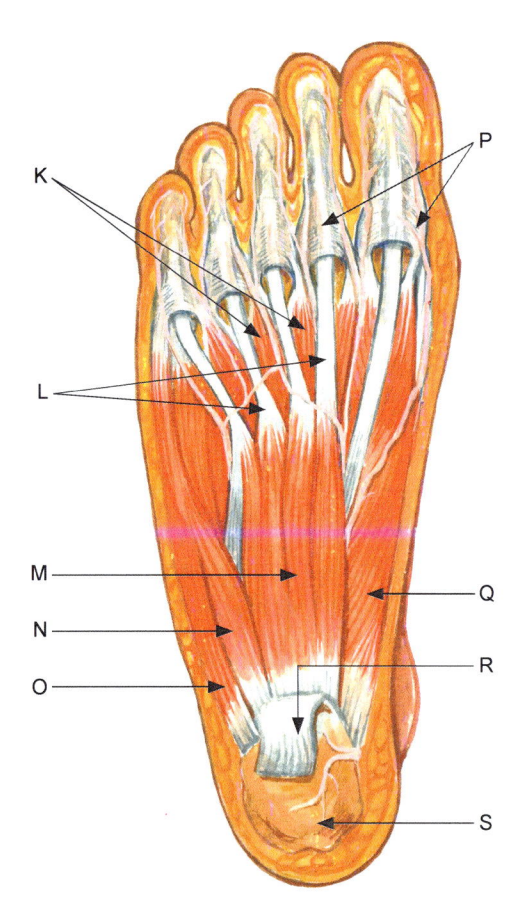

Figure 15-12. Intrinsic foot muscles

THE MUSCULAR SYSTEM

insert onto the proximal phalanx of the great toed. Two groups of muscles form the deepest intrinsic foot muscles. The **plantar interossei** originate on metatarsals 3-5 and insert on the proximal phalanges of toes 3-5. The **dorsal interossei** originate on the adjacent sides of the metatarsals and insert onto toes 2-4. Both sets of interossei muscles abduct and flex the toes at metatarsophalangeal joints and extend the toes at interphalangeal joints. Table 15-9 summarizes the intrinsic foot muscles

Table 15-9. Intrinsic Foot Muscles

Muscle	Origin	Insertion	Action
Abductor digiti minimi	Calcaneus	Proximal phalanx	Abducts/flexes toe
Abductor hallucis	Calcaneus	Proximal phalanx	Abducts/flexes toe
Adductor hallucis	Toe ligaments	Proximal phalanx	Adducts/flexes toe
Dorsal interossei	Metatarsals	Proximal phalanges	Abducts/flexes toes
Extensor digitorum	Calcaneus	Extensor digitorum tendon	Extends toes
Extensor hallucis	Calcaneus	Proximal phalanx	Extends big toe
Flexor digiti minimi	5th metatarsal	Proximal phalanx	Flexes little toe
Flexor digitorum	Calcaneus	Middle phalanx	Flexes toes
Flexor hallucis	Tarsals	Proximal phalanx	Flexes big toe
Lumbricals	Flexor digitorum	Proximal phalanx	Flexes toes
Plantar interossei	Metatarsals	Proximal phalanges	Abducts/flexes toes
Quadratus plantae*	Calcaneus	Flexor digitorum	Flexes toes

TOPICS TO KNOW FOR CHAPTER 15 (THE MUSCULAR SYSTEM)

abductor digiti minimi
adductor digiti minimi
abductor hallucis
abductor pollicis
abductor pollicis longus
adductor brevis
adductor hallucis
adductor longus
adductor magnus
adductor pollicis
agonist
anatomical snuffbox
anconeus
antagonist
aponeurosis of the external oblique
auricularis
basis of skeletal muscle names
biceps brachii
biceps femoris
brachialis
brachioradialis
buccinator

carpal tunnel
coracobrachialis
corrugator supercilii
deltoid
depressor anguli
depressor labii
dorsal interossei (hand)
dorsal interossei (foot)
epicranial aponeurosis
extensor carpi radialis brevis
extensor carpi radialis longus
extensor carpi ulnaris
extensor digiti minimi
extensor digitorum (forearm)
extensor digitorum brevis (leg)
extensor digitorum longus (leg)
extensor hallucis brevis
extensor hallucis longus
extensor indicis
extensor pollicis brevis
extensor pollicis longus
external oblique

fascia lata
fibular retinaculum
fibularis (peroneus) tertius
fibularis brevis
fibularis longus
fixator
flexor carpi radialis
flexor carpi ulnaris
flexor digiti minimi brevis
flexor digitorum brevis
flexor digitorum longus
flexor digitorum profundus
flexor digitorum superficialis
flexor hallucis brevis
flexor hallucis longus
flexor pollicis
flexor pollicis longus
flexor retinaculum (wrist)
flexor retinaculum (ankle)
gastrocnemius
gemellus inferior
gemellus superior

gluteus maximus
gluteus medius
gluteus minimus
gracilis
hypothenar group
iliacus
iliocostalis cervicis
iliocostalis lumborum
iliocostalis thoracis
iliopsoas
iliotibial tract
inferior extensor retinaculum
infraspinatus
internal oblique
interspinales
intertransversarii
intrinsic foot muscles
latissimus dorsi
levator anguli
levator labii superioris
levator labii superioris alaeque nasi
levator scapulae

linea alba
longissimus capitis
longissimus cervicis
longissimus lumborum
longissimus thoracis
lumbricals (hand)
lumbricals (foot)
masseter
mentalis
midpalmar group
multifidus
muscle insertion
muscle origin
nasalis
obturator externus
obturator internus
occipitofrontalis
opponens digiti minimi
opponens pollicis
orbicularis oculi
orbicularis oris
palmar aponeurosis

palmar interossei
palmaris longus
patellar ligament
pectineus
pectoralis major
pectoralis minor
piriformis
plantar aponeurosis
plantar interossei
plantaris
platysma
popliteus
prime mover
procerus
pronator quadratus
pronator teres
psoas major
psoas minor
pterygoid muscles
quadratus femoris
quadratus lumborum
quadratus plantae

CHAPTER 16

Introduction to the Nervous System

REGULATORY SYSTEMS

Your body has two **regulatory systems**, which are systems that affect other systems and, in doing so, help you maintain homeostasis. Your two regulatory systems are the nervous and endocrine systems. The endocrine system sends out messages in the form of blood-borne chemicals, called *hormones*; we will deal with this system in a later chapter. The nervous system communicates with other systems through *impulses* (action potentials) that travel along specialized cells called **neurons**. The cells that respond directly to the signals of a regulatory system are *targets*, or *effectors*, of that system. In this chapter, you will read about the organization of the nervous system and its cells. **Neurology** (nu-ROL-ō-jē) is the study of this system.

The nervous system constantly monitors the body's internal environment (e.g., blood chemistry, muscle tension, temperature, etc) and its external environment (outside temperature, light, etc.). Any change in these environments that the nervous system can detect is a **stimulus** ("to goad"). The body contains a variety of **receptors**, which are specialized structures at the ends of neurons that detect specific types of stimuli. When stimulated by a stimulus, the receptor sends *afferent* impulses to an *integration center*, which determines the appropriate response. The integration center then sends *efferent* impulses to **effectors**, such as muscles and glands.

OVERVIEW OF THE NERVOUS SYSTEM

Due to the complexity of the nervous system, it is beneficial to break down its hierarchy and look at each major component in separate chapters. In this chapter, we will first provide an overview of the nervous system's hierarchy and then describe nervous tissue in detail. The nervous system includes two main divisions: the *central* and *peripheral* nervous systems.

Central Nervous System

The **central nervous system (CNS)** is the body's main integration center and includes the brain and spinal cord, both of which occupy the body's dorsal cavity.

More specifically, the brain is located in the cranial cavity of the skull, whereas, the spinal cord resides in the vertebral cavity. You will read about the specific parts and functions of the brain and spinal cord in the next chapter.

Peripheral Nervous System

The **peripheral nervous system (PNS)** includes all nervous system structures that are not part of the CNS. The PNS communicates with the CNS through the *sensory* and *motor* divisions.

- **Sensory (afferent) division**: detects stimuli in the PNS and sends afferent information from its receptors to neurons in the CNS. The sensory division includes two subdivisions: the *somatic* and *visceral* divisions:
  - **Somatic sensory division**: conducts impulses from receptors in the skin, skeletal muscles, and joints to the CNS.
  - **Visceral sensory division**: conducts impulses from smooth muscle and cardiac muscle to the CNS.
- **Motor (efferent) division**: conducts impulses from the CNS to effectors (muscles and glands) in the PNS. Like the sensory division, the motor division includes two divisions: the *somatic* and *autonomic* nervous systems:
  - **Somatic nervous system**: includes somatic motor neurons that conduct impulses from the CNS to skeletal muscles. Since you can consciously control skeletal muscles, this division is also called the *voluntary motor* division.
  - **Autonomic nervous system** (aw-tō-NOM-ik): includes visceral motor neurons that conduct impulses from the CNS to smooth muscle, cardiac muscle, and glands. Since you have no voluntary control over these effectors, this division is sometimes called the *involuntary nervous system*. Furthermore, this system includes two subdivisions: the *sympathetic* and *parasympathetic* divisions. When the sympathetic division is more active, the parasympathetic division is less active, and when the sympathetic division is less active, the parasympathetic division is more active.

- **Sympathetic division**: controls cardiac muscle, smooth muscle, and certain glands during times of fear, anger, and other forms of stress, including exercise. For this reason, physiologists call it the *"fight-or-flight"* division. Since neurons of this division exit the dorsal cavity only in the thoracic and lumbar regions, neurologists also call it *thoracolumbar* division.

- **Parasympathetic division**: controls many of the same effectors that are controlled by the sympathetic division. However, where the sympathetic division may have an excitatory effect, the parasympathetic division has an inhibitory effect, and where the sympathetic division has an inhibitory effect, the parasympathetic division has an excitatory effect. Since the parasympathetic division is more active during less stressful times, neurologists call it the *"rest-and-digest"* division. Since its neurons exit the dorsal cavity in the head and sacral regions, neurologists also call it *craniosacral* division.

As a system, the nervous system includes a variety of organs, which in turn consist of a variety of tissues. The major tissue comprising the nervous system is nervous *tissue*, which includes two major types of cells: *glial cells* and *neurons*.

GLIAL CELLS

Glial cells (GLĒ-al; glue) are part of the nervous system, but unlike neurons, cannot conduct impulses; instead, they support and protect neurons. Many brain tumors are *gliomas* (glē-Ō-muz), consisting of glial cells dividing uncontrollably. Glial cells in the CNS include *astrocytes, ependymal cells, microglia,* and *oligodendrocytes,* whereas glial cells in the PNS include *Schwann* cells and *satellite cells* (Figure 16-1).

- **Astrocytes** (AS-trō-sīts; *astro*, star) are the most abundant type of glial cell and help maintain

INTRODUCTION TO THE NERVOUS SYSTEM

homeostasis in the ECF around neurons. They have many branches and resemble a star. They surround capillaries and regulate the movement of materials between the blood and neurons. Astrocytes are found only in the CNS.

- **Ependymal cells** (e-PEN-de-mal; "upper garment") contain cilia and exist within cavities of the brain and spinal cord (i.e., they are found only in the CNS). They secrete and circulate a clear *cerebrospinal fluid* that circulates through the central nervous system.

- **Microglia** (mī-krō-GLĒ-uh) display many pseudopodia (extensions of the plasma membrane) that engulf foreign particles; thus, microglia are phagocytic and clean the ECF around neurons.

Microglia are the least abundant glial cells, existing only in the CNS.

- **Oligodendrocytes** (ol-i-gō-DEN-drō-sīts; *oligo*, few; *dendro*, tree-like) are octopus-shaped cells that form protective wrappings called *myelin sheaths* (MĪ-e-lin) around axons in the CNS. Myelin is a lipoproteinaceous material (LĪ-po-prō-tēn-Ā-shus; lipid + protein) that insulates the axon and increases the rate at which it conducts impulses.

- **Schwann cells** form myelin sheaths around axons in the PNS. Schwann cells are also called neurolemmocytes (ner-ō-LEM-ō-sīts; *lemma*, husk).

- **Satellite cells** form protective coverings around neuron cell bodies in the PNS. Their function in the PNS is similar to that of astrocytes in the CNS.

NEUROGLIA

Peripheral Nervous system		Central Nervous System			
Satellite cells	Schwann cells	Oligodendrocytes	Astrocytes	Microglia	Ependymal cell

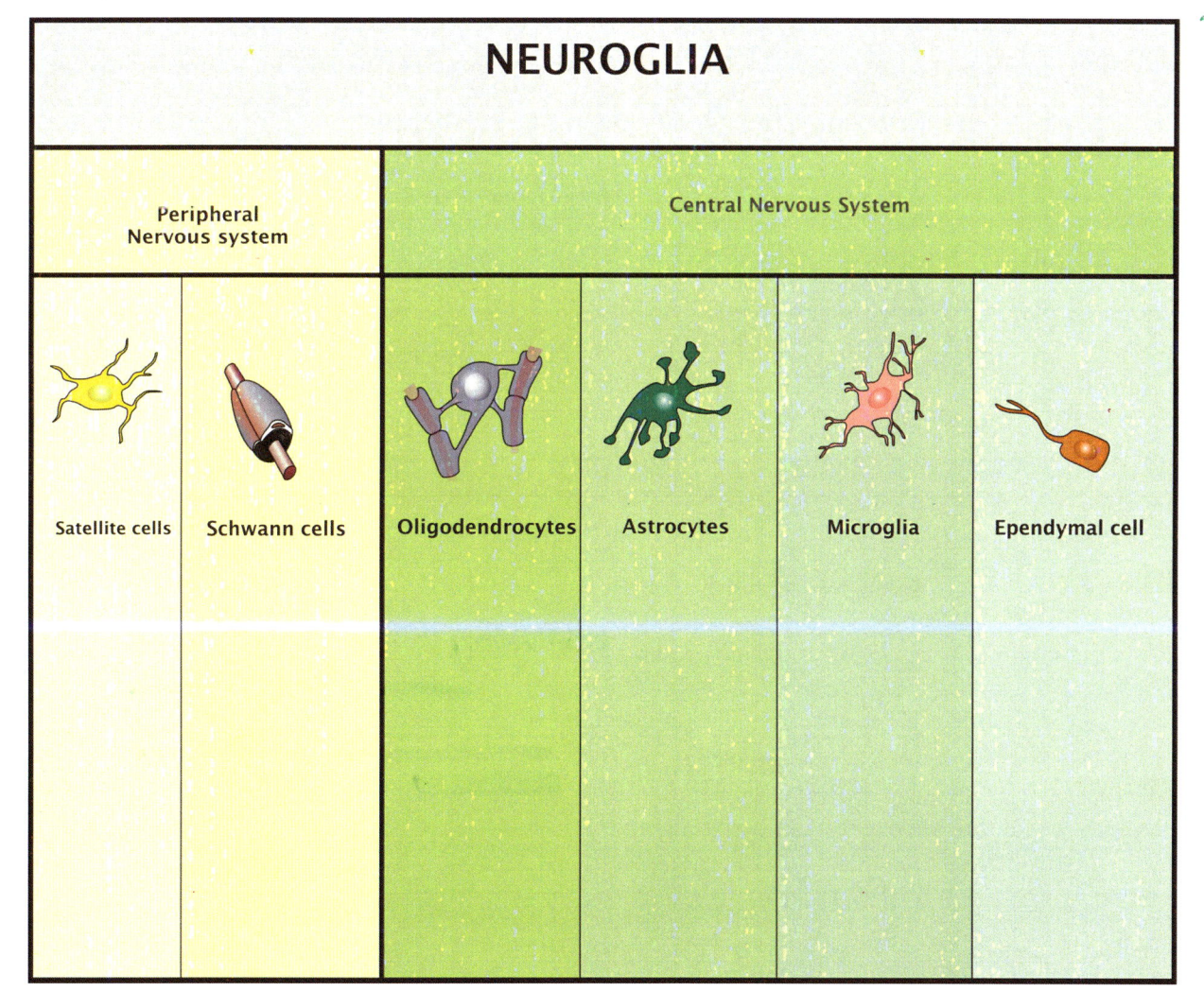

Figure 16-1. Glial cells

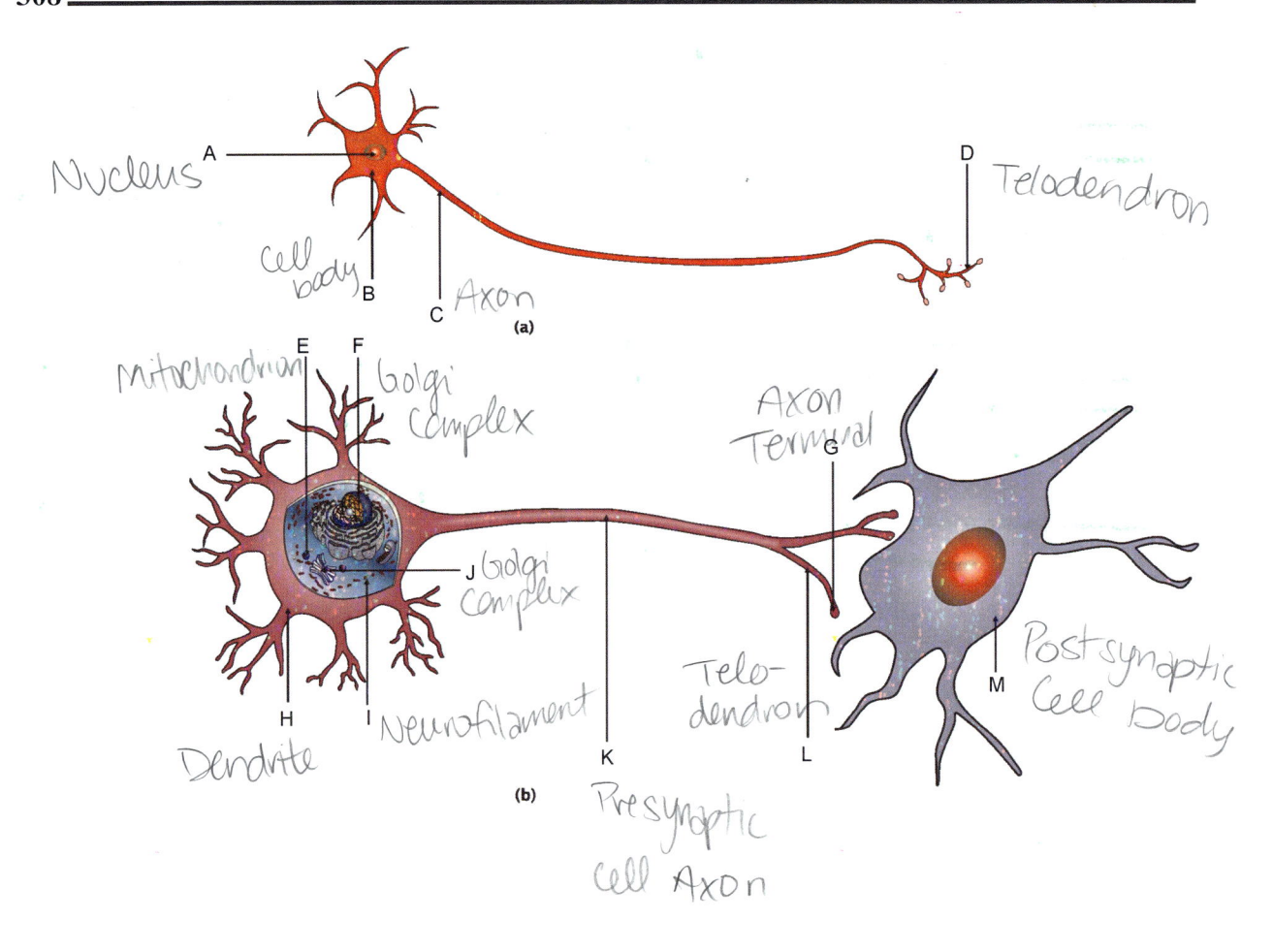

Figure 16-2. Structure of a neuron

NEURONS

Neurons are capable of conducting impulses along certain regions of their plasma membrane and are able to transmit these electrical signals to other cells; therefore, neurons function sort of like electrical wires in a house. Although the body cannot function without neurons, most of these cells are *amitotic* (unable to divide). However, some neurons in the peripheral nervous system can regenerate certain cellular components if they suffer damage. In addition, a few specialized cells in the nasal cavity can differentiate into neurons to replace those that are damaged or worn-out. In order to understand how neurons work, it is necessary to understand their structure. A neuron contains three major parts: the *cell body*, *dendrites*, and *axon* (Figure 16-2).

Cell Body

A neuron's **cell body** (also called the **soma**, "body") contains the nucleus and most of the cell's organelles. The cytoplasm that surrounds the nucleus is called the **perikaryon** (per-i-KAIR-ē-on; *peri*, around; *karyon*, nucleus). Like other cells, RNA synthesis (transcription) occurs in the nucleus and protein synthesis (translation) occurs in the cytosol at ribosomes. Protein synthesis maintains the neuron's supply of enzymes and the proteins that function as channels and pumps in the cell membrane, or become part of other intracellular structures.

INTRODUCTION TO THE NERVOUS SYSTEM

The neuron's nucleus is diploid (2n), with 46 chromosomes (23 maternal and 23 paternal), but mitosis does not usually occur after embryonic development. Consequently, neurons in the adult do not usually divide. However, in a few locations, special cells develop into neurons to replace those that are damaged or worn out. For example, these cells periodically replace *olfactory neurons* that function in smelling.

The cytoskeleton of a neuron is similar to that of other cells, but the names of the components are specific for neurons. For example, the neuron's microfilaments are **neurofilaments** and the microtubules are called **neurotubules**. The cell body is supported by bundles of microfilaments and microtubules called **neurofibrils**, which appear visible under the light microscope.

A neuron's rough endoplasmic reticulum (RER) stains readily in histological preparations and appears as dark regions called **Nissl bodies** (NIS-sul). These bodies are responsible for the "gray" appearance of gray matter.

Dendrites

The **dendrites** (DEN-drītz; *dendr*, tree) of a neuron are short branches that conduct *graded potentials* directly to either the cell body or an axon. Since dendrites lack voltage-gated channels, they cannot conduct impulses. In *sensory* neurons, dendrites display specialized structures called *sensory receptors* that respond to various stimuli. For example, you have sensory receptors in your skin that respond to touch. Upon stimulation, these receptors transmit graded potentials to the axon, which in turn, transmits an impulse to the CNS for interpretation. In some neurons, a dendrite may have multiple branches at its distal ends (end farthest away from the cell body).

Axon

The **axon** (AKS-on; "axle"), or **nerve fiber**, of a neuron is a filamentous extension that contains voltage-gated channels, enabling it to conduct impulses along its entire length. The axon's plasma membrane is the **axolemma** (aks-sō-LEM-a; *lemma*, husk) and the cytoplasm inside the axon is the **axoplasm** (AK-sō-plazm). A raised area, called the **axon hillock** (HIL-ok; "small hill") connects the axon to the cell body.

Some axons possess side branches called **axon collaterals**, allowing the axon to conduct impulses to more than one cell. The distal end of the axon (not connected to the cell body) and any axon collaterals display tiny branches called **telodendria** (tel-o-DEN-drē-a; *telo*, end). The end of each telodendron (tel-o-DEN-dron) contains a tiny knoblike structure called an **axon terminal** or **synaptic knob**. Axon terminals release chemicals called *neurotransmitters* at sites called *synapses* (sin-NAP-sez). For this reason, axon terminals are sometimes called *synaptic terminals*.

Synapses

A **synapse** (SEN-aps; "to clasp") is the site where two cells communicate with one another. It includes two cells and a narrow, slit-like space, called the *synaptic cleft*, located between the two cells. Neurotransmitters released from one of the cells diffuse across the synaptic cleft and attach to receptors on the adjacent cell. The cell that releases the neurotransmitter is the **presynaptic cell**, and the cell that receives the neurotransmitter is the **postsynaptic cell**.

MYELINATION OF AXONS

A **myelin sheath** (MĪ-e-lin) is an insulating covering around segments of certain axons and consists of phospholipids and proteins. An axon that has a myelin sheath is a *myelinated* axon. The myelin sheath forms when certain glial cells wrap tightly around the axon. As they wrap repeatedly around the axon, the glial cell's cytoplasm squeezes away from the axon. To visualize this, think about wrapping a tube of toothpaste around a pencil. If you begin by wrapping the bottom of the tube tightly around the pencil, the paste squeezes toward the cap. When you finish, the multiple wrappings near the pencil no longer have much toothpaste left in them and is much like the myelin sheath. Two different types of glial cells form myelin sheaths around axons: *Schwann cells* and *oligodendrocytes*. (See figure 16-3).

Myelination in the PNS

Schwann cells, or **neurolemmocytes** (nu-rō-LEM-ō-sīts), form the myelin sheaths around axons in the peripheral nervous system. It takes many Schwann cells to myelinate one axon because each cell wraps itself around only a short segment of the axon. Adjacent Schwann cells do not touch each other, so small gaps remain where the axon contacts the ECF. The tiny gaps between the Schwann cells are **neurofibril nodes** (nu-rō-FĪ-bril), or **nodes of Ranvier** (ron-vē-Ā). A myelinated axon in the PNS looks somewhat like a pearl necklace. The pearls (Schwann cells) wrap around the string (axon) with gaps (nodes) between the pearls. The **neurilemma** (or **sheath of Schwann**) is external to the myelin sheath and is the outer, cytoplasmic part of the Schwann cells. In the toothpaste tube analogy, the sheath of Schwann is the part of the tube near the cap that contains toothpaste.

Myelination in the CNS

Oligodendrocytes form myelin sheaths in the CNS. Unlike a single Schwann cell that attaches to only one myelinated axon, a single oligodendrocyte can help form myelin sheaths around many axons. This is like two people wrapping their hands around two broomsticks, each person holding both sticks. The hands are close together but not touching. The broomstick represents

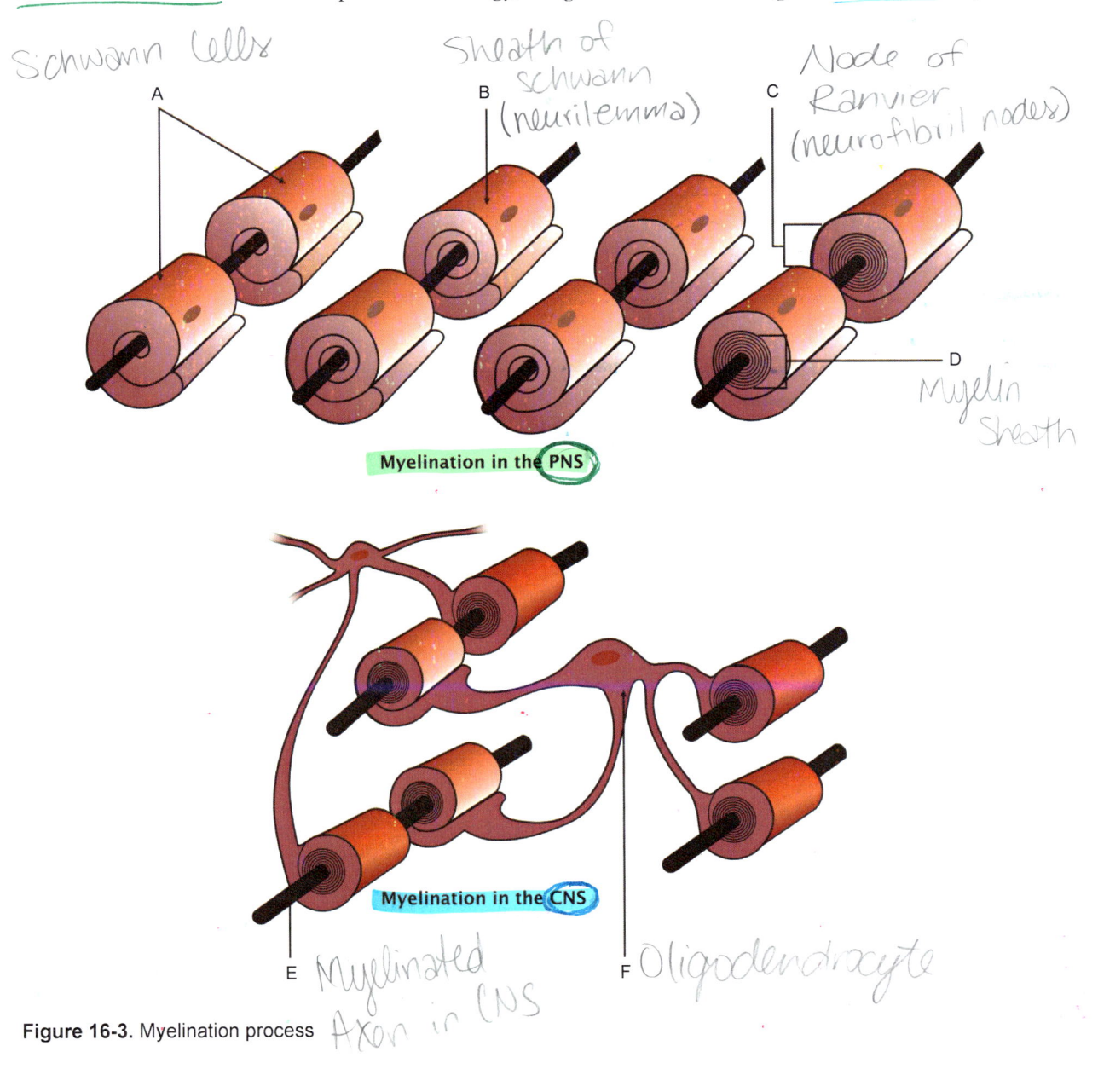

Figure 16-3. Myelination process

INTRODUCTION TO THE NERVOUS SYSTEM

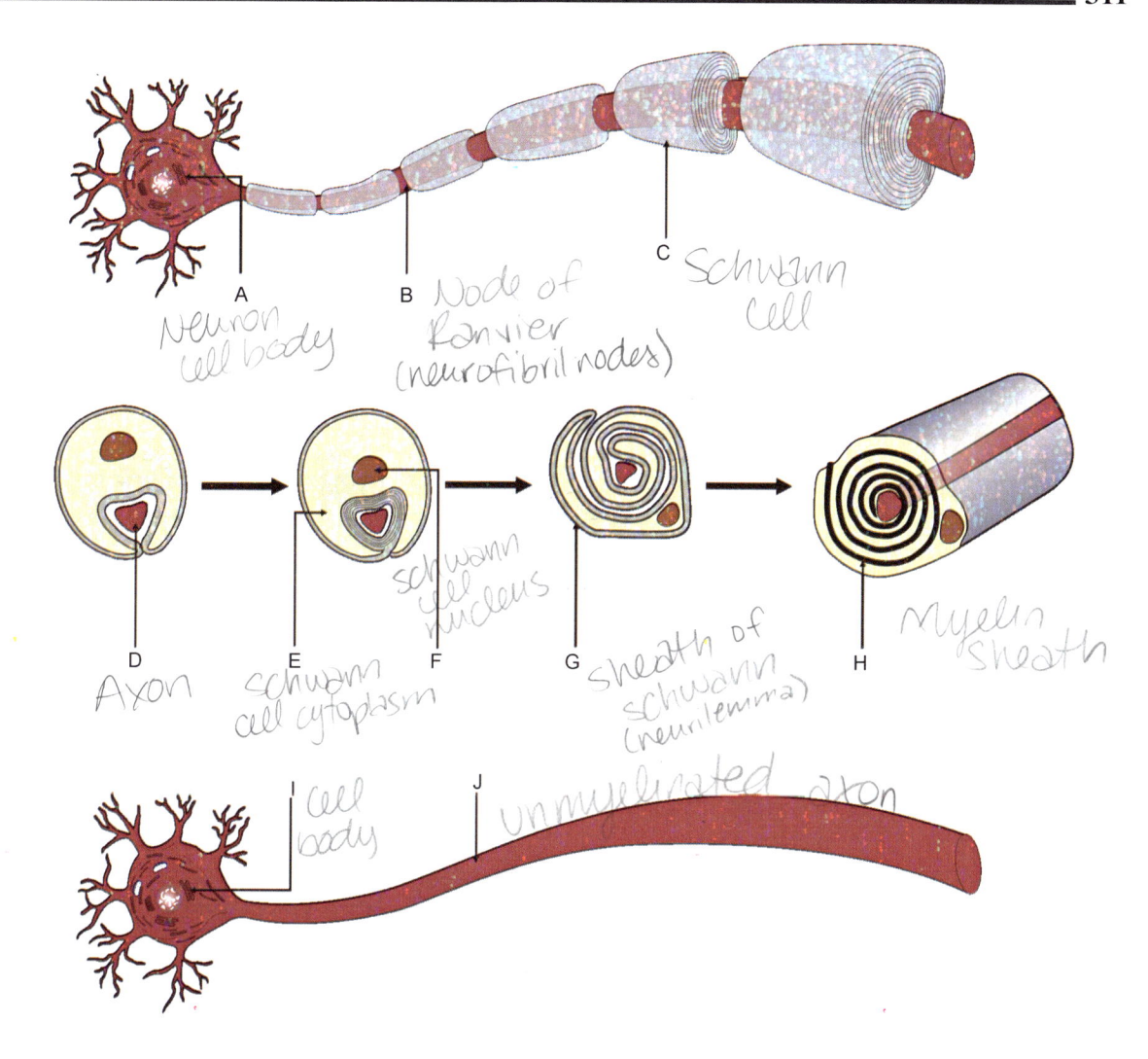

Figure 16-4. Myelinated and unmyelinated axons

an axon; the arms and hands represent the extensions of two different oligodendrocytes; and the spaces between the hands represent nodes of Ranvier.

UNMYELINATED AXONS

Axons that do not contain myelin sheaths are *unmyelinated* axons. Instead, these axons "embed" themselves within Schwann cells or oligodendrocytes. This might look similar to several pencils pressed longitudinally into a cylindrical roll of clay. Since unmyelinated axons lack nodes of Ranvier, they have contact with the ECF along their entire length. Every PNS axon associates with multiple Schwann cells, and every CNS axon associates with multiple oligodendrocytes. One Schwann cell may associate with *only* one myelinated axon, or it may associate with many *unmyelinated* axons. One oligodendrocyte may be associated with many myelinated or unmyelinated axons.

GRAY MATTER AND WHITE MATTER

The nervous system is packed with neurons and glial cells, but this system is not homogeneous regarding the distribution of neuron structures. Regions where neuron cell bodies are abundant appear darker and make up the system's **gray matter**. Depending on their location, concentrations of gray matter have a variety of names. The **cerebral cortex** is a thin layer of gray matter occupying the outermost region of the cerebrum, the largest part of the brain. A region of gray matter lying deep within the brain or spinal cord is a **nucleus** (plural is *nuclei*). A **horn** is a projection of gray matter extending outward from a nucleus in the spinal cord. A collection of neuron cell bodies in the PNS is a gray matter structure called a **ganglion** (GANG-lē-on; plural is *ganglia*).

Regions containing bundles of neuron axons appear lighter in color than gray matter due to the presence of myelin. These light-colored regions comprise the nervous system's **white matter**. White matter in the CNS contains bundles of axons called **tracts**, whereas, white matter in the PNS is found mainly within **nerves** (there are no "nerves" in the CNS). Within the spinal cord, white matter is divided into regions called **columns**, which surround the cord's nuclei and horns.

CLASSIFICATION OF NEURONS

Neurologists classify neurons based on their shape and function. The nervous system contains four major shapes of neurons: *anaxonic, multipolar, unipolar,* or *bipolar*.

- **Anaxonic neurons** lack an axon and are not very abundant in the body. They are found in the brain and in the eyeball.

- **Multipolar neurons** have many dendrites and a single axon attached to the cell body. These are the most abundant neurons in the nervous system, and conduct most impulses in the CNS. They also conduct impulses from the CNS to effectors in the peripheral nervous system. The axons of most multipolar neurons in the adult are myelinated.

- **Unipolar neurons** have an axon extending from one side of the cell body, and dendrites attached to the axon. These neurons are found primarily in the peripheral nervous system where they conduct impulses from sensory receptors to the CNS. In the adult, the axons of unipolar neurons are myelinated.

- **Bipolar neurons** have one axon and one dendrite, each of which attaches directly to the cell body. The dendrite may have multiple branches and is not myelinated. The axon may or may not be myelinated. Bipolar neurons are the least abundant of all neurons and are found in special sensory structures of the eye, nose, and ear.

Based on function, neurologists classify neurons as *sensory, motor,* or *interneurons*.

- **Sensory (afferent) neurons** have dendrites with specialized endings called *receptors* that respond to a stimulus. Different receptors respond to different stimuli (e.g., temperature, touch, stretch, chemicals in the blood, light, etc.), but each sensory neuron has only one type of receptor. Most sensory neurons are unipolar. In the adult, the axons of sensory neurons are myelinated.

- **Interneurons** are multipolar in shape and relay impulses from one neuron to another. Interneurons are the most abundant neurons in the nervous system and are found mostly in the CNS. Other names for interneurons include *association* neurons, *connector* neurons, and *internuncial* neurons (en-ter-NUN-sē-al; "messenger").

- **Motor (efferent) neurons** are multipolar and conduct impulses from the CNS to effectors, such as muscles and glands. In the somatic nervous system, a motor neuron's cell body and dendrites exist only within the CNS, but most of its axon is in the PNS. In the autonomic nervous system, certain motor neurons exist partly in the CNS and partly in the PNS, while other motor neurons exist entirely within the PNS.

REPAIR OF DAMAGED AXONS

Neurons in the PNS have a limited ability to repair damaged axons, but the same is not necessarily true of neurons in the CNS. It is important to remember, however, that neurons do not undergo cell division. The steps in the repair process for a severed or damaged axon in the PNS are as follows (Figure 16-5):

INTRODUCTION TO THE NERVOUS SYSTEM

1. The entire portion of the axon and myelin sheath that is distal to the injured site disintegrates.

2. Surviving Schwann cells in the damaged region multiply and form a line of cells that will guide the re-growing axon to the original axon's destination site. The Schwann cells also secrete chemicals that stimulate the axon's growth.

3. As the axon elongates and encounters new Schwann cells, the Schwann cells wrap repeatedly around the axon to form a new myelin sheath.

It is possible for a person with limited nerve damage to regain sensitivity and motor function after the axons heal. (A *nerve* is a collection of axons in the PNS.) However, the chance of this happening diminishes if the part of the nerve that is distal to the site of damage is no longer aligned with the proximal end of the nerve.

If axon damage occurs in the CNS, regeneration does not usually occur. There are several possible reasons why axons in the CNS do not regenerate. (1) Oligodendrocytes may release chemicals that inhibit their growth. (2) Scar tissue in the damaged brain or spinal cord may impede their growth. (3) There may be a lack of growth-stimulating chemicals in the CNS; therefore, the axons do not receive adequate chemical signals to regenerate.

NEUROTRANSMITTERS

Now we will take a closer look at how axons release neurotransmitters and what effect the neurotransmitter has on the postsynaptic cell. When an impulse reaches an axon terminal, voltage-gated Ca^{2+} channels in the terminal open and allow Ca^{2+} ions to diffuse into the terminal. The Ca^{2+} influx causes vesicles in the axon terminal to unite with the plasma membrane and release **neurotransmitter** molecules via exocytosis into the synapse. The neurotransmitter is a *ligand* that diffuses across the synapse and attaches to a receptor on the postsynaptic cell's membrane. The effect of the neurotransmitter can be either *direct* or *indirect* (Figure 16-6).

Direct Effect of Neurotransmitters

A neurotransmitter can *directly* affect a cell by binding to a receptor functioning as an ion channel. In this

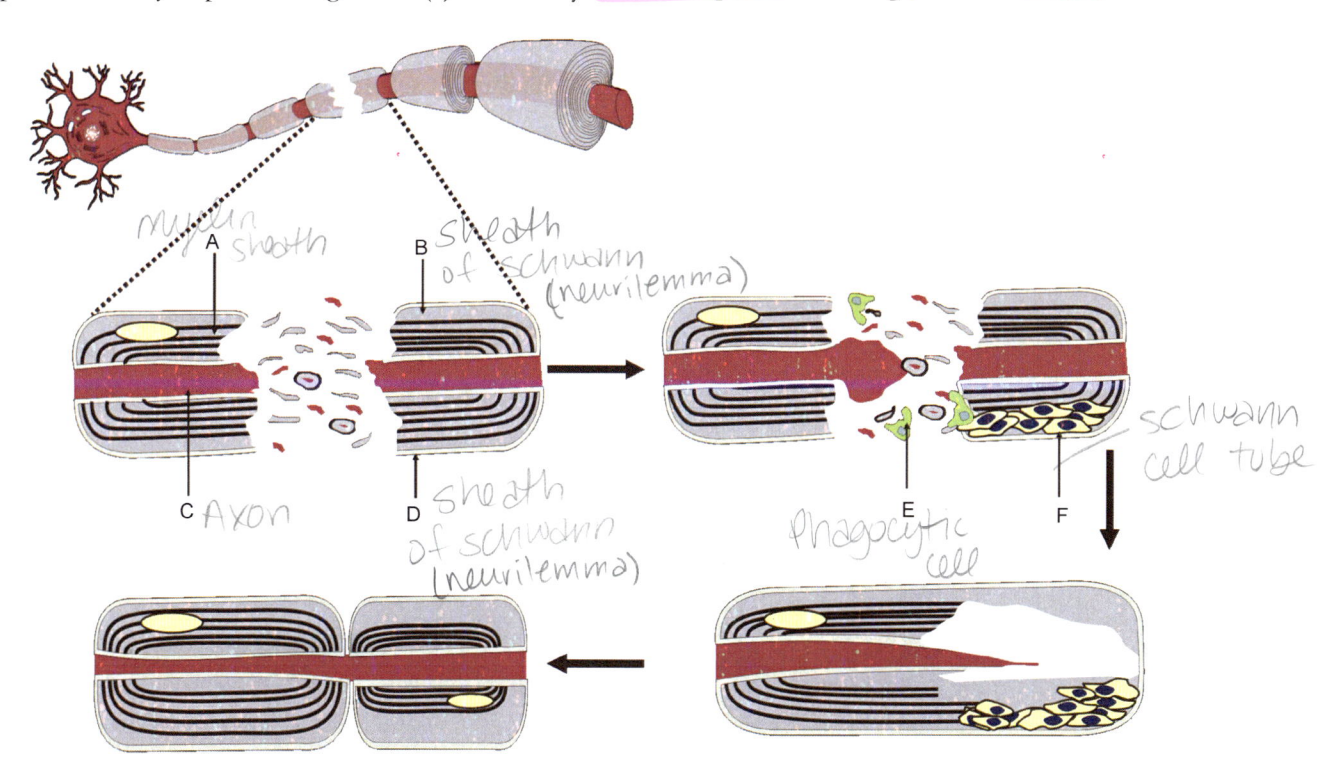

Figure 16-5. Repair of damaged axons

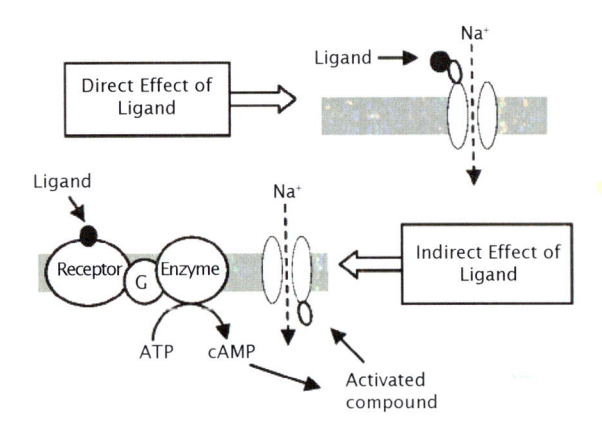

Figure 16-6. Action of neurotransmitters

case, the neurotransmitter will directly affect the plasma membrane's permeability to specific ions. For example, binding a neurotransmitter to a Na⁺ channel can open the channel and allow Na⁺ to diffuse into the cell, resulting in depolarization. Binding the neurotransmitter to a K⁺ channel can open the channel and allow K⁺ ions to diffuse out of the cell, resulting in hyperpolarization.

Indirect Effect of Neurotransmitters

A neurotransmitter can *indirectly* affect a cell by binding to a receptor that can initiate reactions inside the cell. In some cases, these cytosolic reactions may affect one or more aspects of the cell's metabolism and/or it may affect the plasma membrane's permeability. One example of a neurotransmitter's indirect effect is the formation of **cyclic AMP** (cAMP; *cyclic* refers to the ringed structure of the molecule). The cAMP functions as a *second messenger* for the neurotransmitter since the neurotransmitter (the *first* messenger) cannot enter the cell. The formation of cAMP occurs as follows:

1. The neurotransmitter attaches to the receptor on the postsynaptic cell's plasma membrane.
2. The membrane-bound receptor containing the neurotransmitter stimulates an adjacent chemical, called a *G protein*, also located in the plasma membrane.
3. The stimulated G protein activates a membrane-bound enzyme that dephosphorylates ATP twice,

by removing two phosphate groups from it, to form cAMP. The cAMP, in turn, initiates reactions in the cytoplasm.

The effect of a neurotransmitter persists as long as the neurotransmitter remains on the receptor. However, the neurotransmitter remains attached to the receptor only a short time and then it detaches. After detaching from the receptor, the neurotransmitter may diffuse out of the synapse, be broken down by enzymes in the synapse, or be actively transported back into the presynaptic neuron's axon terminal.

Depending on how they affect the postsynaptic cell, neurotransmitters (or ligands) are either *excitatory* or *inhibitory*. When the postsynaptic cell is another neuron, these words relate to electrical changes in the neuron's plasma membrane.

Excitatory neurotransmitters cause the postsynaptic cell to become more active. On neurons and muscle cells, these neurotransmitters open ligand-gated Na⁺ or Ca²⁺ channels, causing the membrane to *depolarize* (the inside border becomes less negative). Depolarization of a postsynaptic membrane by a neurotransmitter is an **excitatory postsynaptic potential (EPSP)**. It is a graded potential because it weakens as it spreads across the cell.

Inhibitory neurotransmitters cause the postsynaptic cell to become less active. On neurons and muscle cells, these neurotransmitters normally open ligand-gated K⁺ or Cl⁻ channels, causing the membrane to *hyperpolarize* (the inside border becomes more negative). Hyperpolarization caused by a neurotransmitter is a graded potential known as an **inhibitory postsynaptic potential (IPSP)**.

A particular neurotransmitter may cause an EPSP on one type of cell, but may cause an IPSP on another cell. For example, acetylcholine (Ach) is excitatory when it attaches to skeletal myofibers, but it is inhibitory when it attaches to cardiac myofibers.

ACTION POTENTIALS IN NEURONS

Neurons follow the **all-or-none principle** with regard to action potentials (AP), meaning that an AP will occur on an axon or it will not occur; i.e., there are no partial APs on axons. Furthermore, an AP occurring at one location on the axon will initiate an AP at an adjacent

INTRODUCTION TO THE NERVOUS SYSTEM

site, and so on. The resulting series of APs occurring one after another at adjacent sites appear to move along the axon as a "wave" known as an **impulse**.

Once it begins, an impulse travels the entire length of the axon. The initiation of APs and the resulting impulse depends on the opening of voltage-gated channels in the axolemma. Normally, the site where the first AP for an impulse occurs is at the axon hillock, but adequate stimulation of another site on the axon can also initiate an AP; thus, an impulse can originate at that location as well. The events associated with an AP at any particular site on an axon are as follows (Figure 16-7):

1. Resting membrane potential (RMP): The axon's voltage-gated channels are closed and the membrane potential is relatively stable. The leakage of Na$^+$ into the cell and K$^+$ ions out of the cell is equalized by the action of the cell's Na$^+$/K$^+$ pumps. Most neurons have a RMP of about -70 mV.

2. Depolarization: Any decrease in membrane potential away from the resting potential is called **depolarization**. Depolarization on the axon begins when a stimulus decreases the voltage in the region to threshold (usually around -55 mV), causing voltage-gated Na$^+$ channels to open. In a multipolar neuron, the first voltage-gated Na$^+$ channels to open are usually at the axon hillock, and are in response to a graded potential spreading across the neuron's cell body. In unipolar and bipolar neurons, the first channels to open are where a dendrite and axon meet. At other sites along an axon, the stimulus is simply a change in electrical voltage spreading into the region from an adjacent site. A massive influx of Na$^+$ through the voltage-gated channels causes the membrane potential to reverse—become positive.

The depolarization phase of the action potential occurs through positive feedback. Initially, the opening of only a few voltage-gated Na$^+$ channels at a particular site on the axon increases the membrane's permeability for Na$^+$ at that site. The resulting influx of Na$^+$ at that site causes threshold to be reached at other voltage-gated Na$^+$ channels in the same region. Influx of Na$^+$ through those channels causes threshold to be reached at still other voltage-gated Na$^+$ channels in the area, and so on. As a result of the influx of Na$^+$ through so many channels, the membrane potential at that site reverses. The time required for this reversal of polarity is about 1 msec.

Normally, while a section of an axon is experiencing an action potential it will not respond to another stimulus; this is called the *refractory period*. More specifically, when a section of the axon is

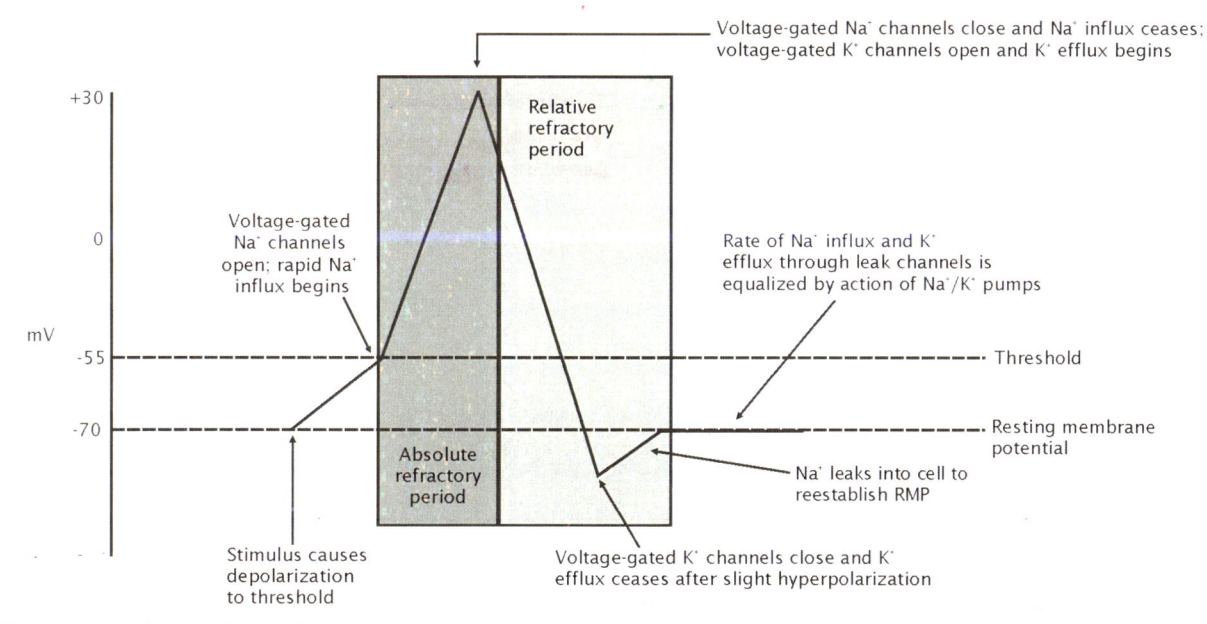

Figure 16-7. Graph of an action potential

depolarizing due to an influx of Na⁺ through voltage-gated Na⁺ channels, that section cannot respond to another stimulus; this is the **absolute refractory period**. However, shortly after the membrane begins to repolarize, a very strong stimulus may reopen the voltage-gated Na⁺ channels and initiate another depolarization; this is the **relative refractory period**. Keep in mind, the only way to initiate another stimulus during the relative refractory period is to apply a stronger-than-normal stimulus.

3. Repolarization: After being open for about 1 msec during the depolarization phase of the AP, the voltage-gated Na⁺ channels in the region close and depolarization stops. At the same time, *slow* voltage-gated K⁺ channels begin to open allowing an efflux (outflow) of K⁺ from the cell. The stimulus for the opening of these channels occurs during depolarization; however, since there is a delay before they open, they are called "slow" channels. The efflux of K⁺ causes the membrane potential to reverse again, returning to the negative inside condition. The return to a negative membrane potential from a positive potential is called **repolarization**.

4. Hyperpolarization: Usually during the repolarization phase, the voltage-gated K⁺ channels remain open slightly longer than is needed to reestablish the resting membrane potential. Consequently, enough K⁺ flows out of the cell to make the membrane potential slightly more negative than the RMP; this is called **hyperpolarization**. Finally, all of the voltage-gated K⁺ channels close and efflux of K⁺ ceases. The more negative inside border of the membrane has a stronger-than-normal pull on Na⁺ ions in the ECF, causing more of them to leak into the axon. This depolarizes the membrane back to the RMP. At this point, the diffusion of Na⁺ and K⁺ through the membrane is equalized by the transport of these ions by the Na⁺/K⁺ pumps.

SIGNAL SUMMATION

Unlike skeletal muscle cells, which receive impulses from a single neuron, a single neuron may receive impulses from hundreds of other neurons simultaneously. Some of the presynaptic neurons may generate EPSPs while others generate IPSPs. The effects of these incoming signals are additive, which means their individual effects reinforce one another, or summate. There are two types of summation: *temporal* and *spatial*.

Temporal summation (TEM-por-al; "time") occurs when a presynaptic neuron transmits a series of impulses to a postsynaptic membrane in a short period. The effect of neurotransmitter molecules released during one impulse on the presynaptic neuron may add to the effect remaining from a previous impulse. If enough neurotransmitter accumulates to make the membrane potential reach threshold, an impulse on the postsynaptic neuron will result.

Spatial summation (SPĀ-shul; "space") occurs when several neurons transmit impulses simultaneously to the same postsynaptic cell. In some cases, a single impulse from one neuron may not cause the release of enough neurotransmitter molecules to initiate an impulse. However, several neurons releasing excitatory neurotransmitter simultaneously can create an EPSP that can initiate an impulse.

SIGNAL INTEGRATION

Spatial summation and temporal summation may occur simultaneously or separately, and the effect on the postsynaptic neuron depends on a phenomenon called **signal integration**. What happens if an excitatory and an inhibitory neuron release neurotransmitters onto the same postsynaptic membrane at the same time? If the EPSP reaching the axon hillock is greater than the IPSP, an impulse occurs. If the IPSP is greater than the EPSP, no impulse occurs. Moreover, presynaptic neurons with axon terminals near the postsynaptic neuron's axon hillock have a greater effect than those with axon terminals farther away from the hillock. A single EPSP generated near the axon hillock may override several IPSPs created farther away. In contrast, a single IPSP near the axon hillock may override several EPSPs created farther away.

METHODS OF IMPULSE CONDUCTION

There are two methods of impulse conduction along axons in the nervous system: *continuous* and *saltatory*.

INTRODUCTION TO THE NERVOUS SYSTEM

Continuous conduction is the slowest type of conduction and is the method used by *unmyelinated* axons. The word "continuous" means that ion exchange between the axoplasm and ECF occurs along every part of the axolemma (Figure 16-8). The reason that impulses move slower along unmyelinated axons is that these axons are not well insulated from the ECF. Without an insulating cover, there can be considerable diffusion of ions through the axon's leak channels. Due to the leakiness of the unmyelinated axon, it takes longer for a voltage change on one segment of the axon to depolarize an adjacent segment to threshold.

To visualize continuous conduction, consider a line of people standing shoulder to shoulder along the entire length of a football field. You hand a football to the first person in line and tell each person to take the ball and hand it to the next person in line. Think about how long it would take to move the football from person to person from one end of the field to the other. Remember this analogy to contrast the relatively slow continuous conduction to the much faster saltatory method.

Saltatory impulse conduction (SOL-ta-tor-ē; *salta*, to leap) is the fastest type of conduction and occurs only in *myelinated* axons. It is so-named because ion exchange between the axoplasm and ECF occurs only at nodes of Ranvier; thus, impulses appear to "jump" from one node to the next (Figure 16-9).

The insulated part of an axon beneath a myelin sheath cannot exchange ions with the ECF. Depolarizing one node changes the electrical condition of the ECF around a second node, causing voltage-gated channels in the second node to open. Consequently, the impulse appears to "jump" from the first node to the second. When the second node depolarizes, the electrical condition of the ECF around the next node changes sufficiently so that the impulse jumps again, and the process continues.

In our football field analogy, saltatory conduction is analogous to having a person stand on each goal line and one at the 50-yard line. The person at the goal passes the ball to the person at the 50-yard line, who then passes the ball to the person at the other goal line. As you can see, the ball will move 100 yards much quicker than during the "continuous" method described earlier. Not only is saltatory conduction much faster than continuous conduction, it allows the

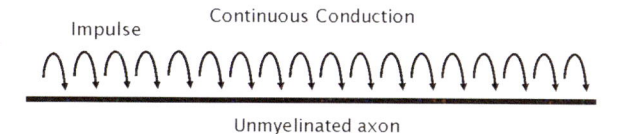

Figure 16-8. Continuous conduction

neuron to conserve ions and energy. The influx of Na^+ ions during depolarization, and the loss of K^+ ions from the axon during repolarization, occurs only at the nodes; therefore, ATP-driven Na/K pumps exist only at the nodes and not beneath the myelin sheaths. Consequently, with fewer Na/K pumps, the cell expends less ATP energy to maintain its ion balance with the ECF.

FACTORS AFFECTING IMPULSE CONDUCTION

The rate of impulse conduction along an axon correlates *positively* with temperature, axon diameter, and the axon's degree of myelination (Figure 16-10). When the body temperature rises, axons can conduct impulses at a faster rate. This is because at a higher temperature the ions, enzymes, and membrane channels operate faster.

Large-diameter axons conduct impulses faster than smaller-diameter axons. This is similar to large metal wires conducting electricity faster than small diameter wires, because large wires offer less resistance than small wires. Think about how traffic slows when moving from an 8-lane highway down to a 2-lane highway.

One reason why small children lack the coordination seen in adults is that they lack adequate myelination in their nervous system. Infants and toddlers have more of their impulses traveling by continuous conduction. As children grow, more myelination occurs, thereby allowing more rapid saltatory conduction. Patients with *multiple sclerosis* experience deterioration of myelin sheaths accompanied by a decrease in saltatory conduction.

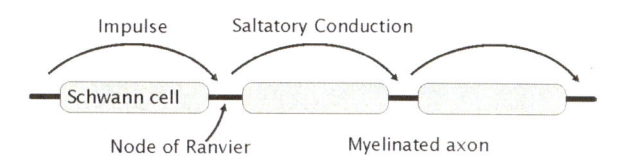

Figure 16-9. Saltatory conduction

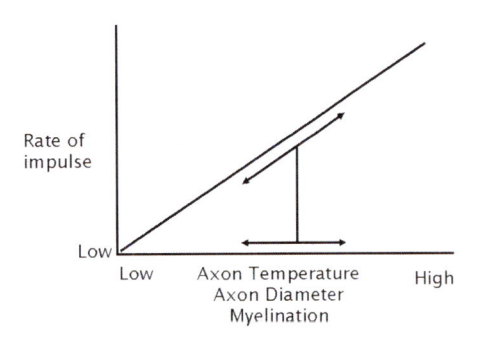

Figure 16-10. Factors affecting impulse conduction

CLASSIFICATION OF AXONS

Neurologists classify axons (neuron fibers) based on their diameter and speed of impulse conduction.

- **Class A fibers** have a large diameter with myelination and perform rapid, saltatory impulse conduction (~150 meters/sec or 300 mph). Class A fibers conduct sensory impulses from stretch receptors, tactile receptors, pressure receptors, and thermoreceptors. In addition, they conduct motor impulses to skeletal muscles.

- **Class B fibers** have a medium diameter with myelination and perform saltatory impulse conduction. However, the smaller diameter of class B fibers causes their speed of impulse conduction to be only about 15 m/sec (~40 mph). Class B fibers conduct sensory impulses from visceral organs, and they conduct motor impulses through special neurons, called *preganglionic neurons*, in the autonomic nervous system.

- **Class C fibers** have a small diameter and lack myelination, so they perform slow, continuous impulse conduction (about 1 m/sec or 2 mph). Class C fibers conduct sensory impulses from pain receptors, certain tactile and pressure receptors, and thermoreceptors. They also conduct motor impulses on *postganglionic neurons* in the autonomic nervous system.

TOPICS TO KNOW FOR CHAPTER 16 (NERVOUS TISSUE)

absolute refractory period
action potentials in neurons
afferent impulses
all-or-none principle
amitotic
association neurons
astrocytes
autonomic nervous system
axolemma
axon
axon collaterals
axon hillock
axon terminal
axoplasm
bipolar neurons
cell body
central nervous system
cerebral cortex
class A fibers
class B fibers
class C fibers
classification of axons
classification of neurons

columns
connector neurons
continuous conduction
dendrites
depolarization
direct effect of neurotransmitters
effectors
efferent impulses
ependymal cells
EPSP
excitatory neurotransmitter
excitatory postsynaptic potential
factors affecting impulse
    conduction
ganglion
glial cells
gliomas
graded potentials
gray matter
horn
hyperpolarization
impulse
indirect effect of

neurotransmitters
inhibitory neurotransmitter
inhibitory postsynaptic potential
integration center
interneurons
internuncial neurons
involuntary nervous system
IPSP
ligand
methods of impulse conduction
microglial cells
motor (efferent) division
motor (efferent) neurons
multipolar neurons
myelin sheath
myelination in the CNS
myelination in the PNS
myelination of axons
Na+/K+ pumps
nerve fiber
nerves
neurilemma
neurofibril nodes

INTRODUCTION TO THE NERVOUS SYSTEM

neurofibrils
neurofilaments
neurolemmocytes
neurology
neurons
neurotransmitters
neurotubules
Nissl bodies
nodes of Ranvier
nucleus
oligodendrocytes
parasympathetic division
perikaryon
peripheral nervous system
postsynaptic cell
presynaptic cell

receptors
refractory period
regulatory systems
relative refractory period
repair of damaged axons
repolarization
saltatory impulse conduction
satellite cells
Schwann cells
sensory (afferent) division
sensory (afferent) neurons
sheath of Schwann
signal integration
signal summation
soma
somatic nervous system

somatic sensory division
spatial summation
stimulus
sympathetic division
synapse
synaptic cleft
synaptic knob
telodendria
temporal summation
tracts
unipolar neurons
unmyelinated axons
visceral sensory division
voluntary motor division
white matter

CHAPTER 17

Central Nervous System

OVERVIEW OF THE CNS

While we might compare our nervous system to a computer, the nervous system is much more complex. Even so, a computer makes a good analogy. What would you say is most like the computer's keyboard—maybe sensory receptors? What would be most like the wires leading from the keyboard to the computer—maybe the nerves? Then we have the computer's hard drive, which integrates the information sent to it from the keyboard and sends out information to a monitor screen to show us what's going on inside the computer. The computer's hard drive would be most like our nervous system's integration center, or the *central nervous system*.

The central nervous system (CNS) includes the *brain* and *spinal cord*. The brain is the primary integrating organ for the CNS and the spinal cord is a tubular structure that courses through the vertebral column and conducts impulses between the brain and other parts of the body.

OVERVIEW OF THE BRAIN

Your brain, the part of the nervous system enabling you to understand what you are reading now, occupies your *cranial vault* (the cavity surrounded by the cranium). The adult brain, in males and females, weighs about 1500 grams (3-4 lbs) and includes four major regions: The *cerebrum* is responsible for most of a person's perception of stimuli and all of a person's thoughts. The *diencephalon* contains several functional areas, and is the major control center for the autonomic nervous system. The *brain stem* conducts impulses between the brain and spinal cord and is the site of many important "centers" that control various involuntary activities, such as breathing, heart rate, etc. The *cerebellum* helps a person maintain balance and equilibrium. See the parts of the brain in Figure 17-1.

THE CEREBRUM

The **cerebrum** (se-RĒ-brum; "brain") is the largest part of the brain, making up approximately 80% of its total weight. Several noticeable grooves separate different regions of the cerebrum. The **longitudinal fissure** (FISH-ur; groove) divides the cerebrum into right and left *cerebral hemispheres*. The **transverse cerebral fissure** separates the cerebrum from the cerebellum.

The surface of each cerebral hemisphere displays numerous ridges called **gyri** (JI-rī), and each ridge is

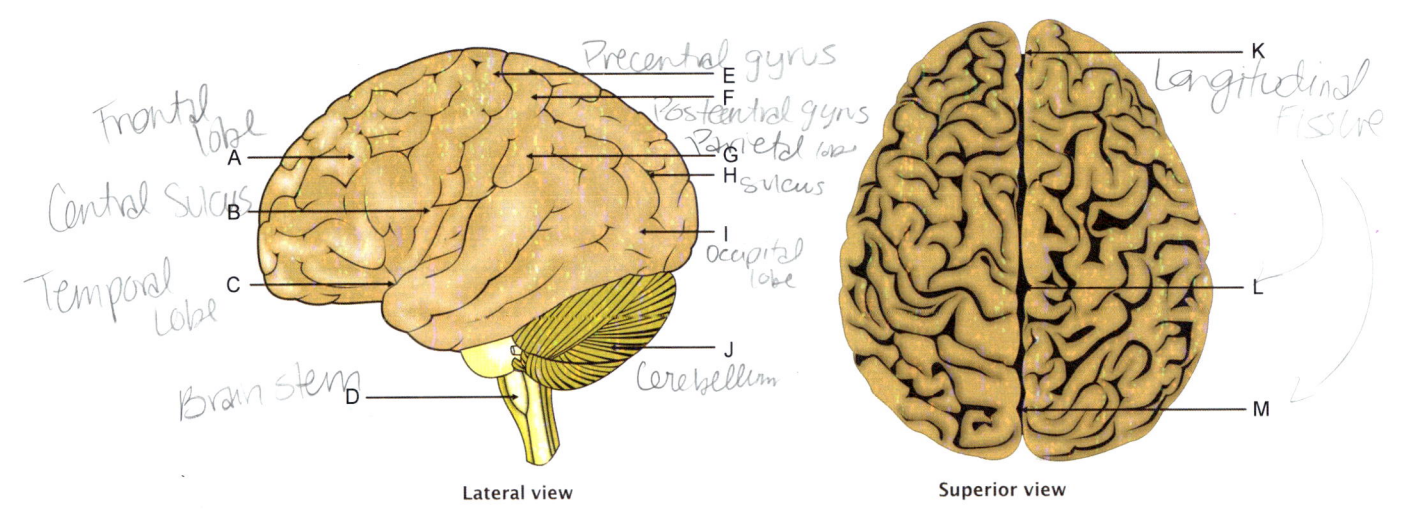

Figure 17-1. The brain

a **gyrus** (JI-rus; *gyros*, circle). The grooves separating the gyri are called **sulci** (SUL-sī), and each groove is a **sulcus** (SUL-kus, "ditch"). The gyri greatly increase the brain's surface area. As a result, more cerebral tissue can exist in the cranial cavity than would be possible if the brain's surface were not rippled. Think about how much farther you would run around a track if you weave back and forth (making gyri patterns) as opposed to running a straight path on the inside lane. There are six major sulci (one on each side cerebral hemisphere), and they separate the cerebrum into ten *cerebral lobes* (five on each side):

- **Central sulcus**: separates the *frontal lobe* from the *parietal lobe*. Immediately anterior to this is the *precentral gyrus*, which is part of the frontal lobe. Immediately posterior to the central sulcus is the *postcentral gyrus*, which is part of the parietal lobe.

- **Parieto-occipital sulcus**: separates the *parietal lobe* from the *occipital lobe*.

- **Lateral sulcus**: separates the frontal and parietal lobes from the *temporal lobe*. The *insula* (IN-sū-la; "island") is a cerebral lobe lying deep to the frontal, parietal, and temporal lobes, and is visible in the lateral sulcus when the temporal lobe is pulled inferiorly.

The outer few millimeters (~1/8 inch) of the cerebrum consist of gray matter called the **cerebral cortex** (*cortex*, bark), and it has sensory, association, motor, and integrative areas (Figure 17-2).

Sensory Areas of the Cortex

The *sensory* areas of the cerebrum interpret afferent information sent in from sensory receptors in the PNS (sense literally means, "to feel"), and include:

- **Gustatory cortex** (GUS-ta-tor-ē; *gusta*, taste): located in the insula, it is responsible for perception of taste.

- **Olfactory cortex** (OL-fak-tor-ē; *olfact*, to smell): located partly in the temporal lobes and partly in the frontal lobes, it is responsible for perception of smell.

- **Primary auditory cortex** (AW-di-tor-ē; *audio*, to hear): located in the temporal lobes, it is responsible for hearing sounds and its different aspects, such as its loudness, pitch (bass, treble, etc.), and location.

- **Primary somatosensory cortex**: located in the postcentral gyrus, it is responsible for the sense of touch, and perception of temperature and pressure. It is also responsible for *spatial discrimination*, the ability to know which region of the body is being stimulated.

- **Primary visual cortex**: located in the occipital lobe, it is responsible for perception of light, color, and the shape and movement of objects viewed.

- **Vestibular cortex**: located in the insula, it is responsible for giving a person a sense of balance and equilibrium.

CENTRAL NERVOUS SYSTEM

- **Visceral sensory area** (VIS-ser-al; *viscera*, internal organ): located in the insula, it is responsible for perception of various sensations originating in the internal organs of the thorax and abdomen.

Association Areas of the Cortex

The *association* areas receive impulses from the sensory areas and determine actions to take in response.

- **Auditory association area**: in the temporal lobes; interprets sounds, such as recognizing a gunshot.
- **Somatosensory association area**: in the postcentral gyrus; interprets touch; allows a person to determine the size and texture of an object by touch; e.g., distinguishing an apple from an orange inside a bag.

- **Visual association area**: located in the occipital lobe; interprets visual stimuli; e.g., recognizing an apple as an apple when you see it.

Motor Areas of the Cortex

The *motor* areas (*motor* means "to move") initiate efferent information that eventually reaches skeletal muscles to control voluntary muscle movement.

- **Premotor area**: located immediately anterior to the precentral gyrus in the frontal lobe; responsible for storing memory for skilled motor movement such as finger movements used when playing a piano. One region in this area, called the *frontal eye field*, controls learned eye movements, such as reading the words of a sentence in the proper order.

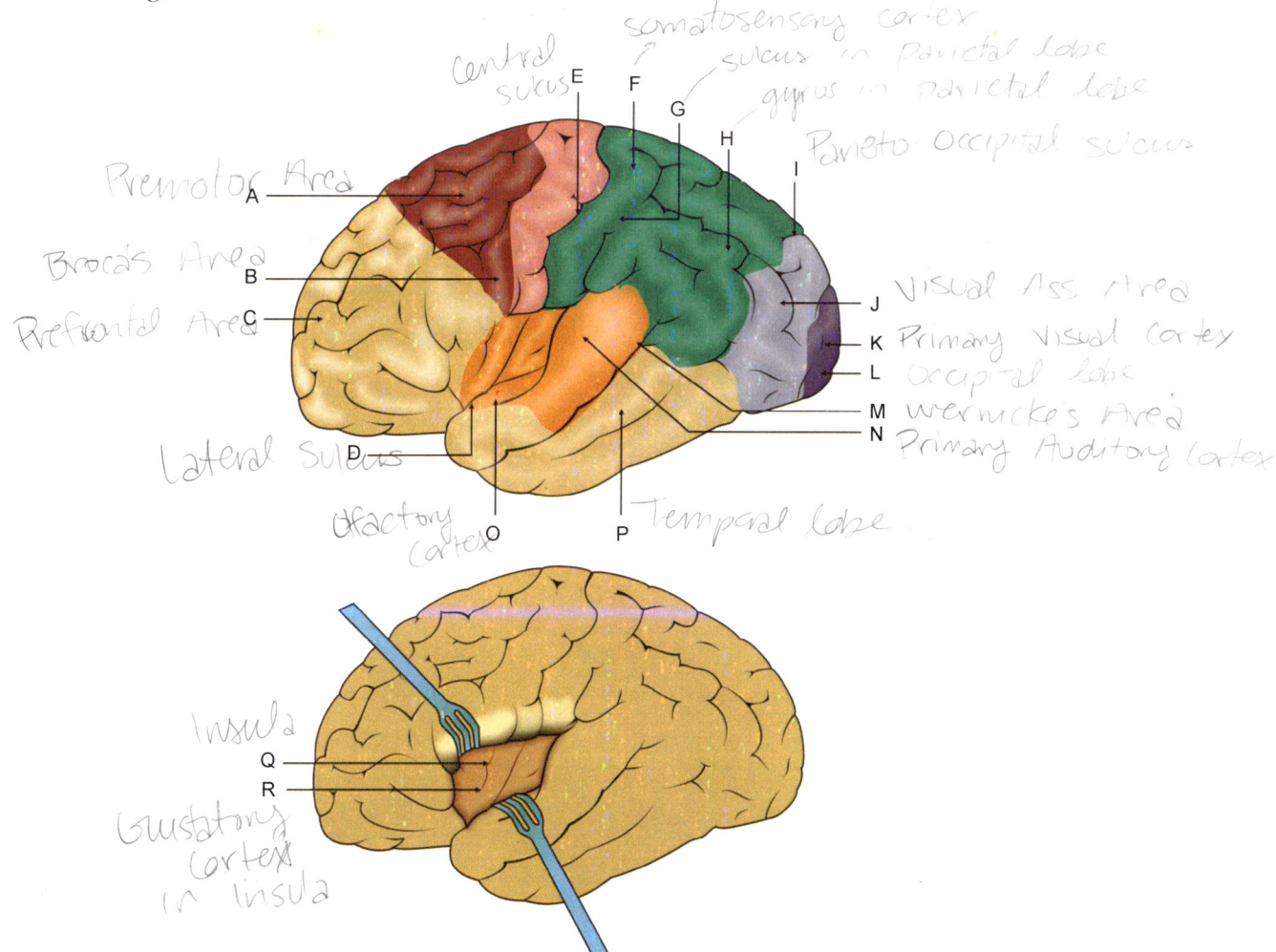

Figure 17-2. Functional aspects of the cerebrum

- **Primary motor cortex**: located in the precentral gyrus; controls voluntary muscle movements. The neurons residing in this region are called *pyramidal cells*, so-named because of their pyramid-like cell bodies.

Integrative Areas of the Cortex

The *integrative* areas receive impulses from association areas, evaluate it, and send out impulses to other areas of the brain for normal functioning in everyday life, including analyzing and solving problems.

- **Motor speech area** (also called the **speech center** or **Broca's area**; BRŌ-kahz): located most often in the left frontal lobe, it controls tongue, lip, and throat movements for speech. This is an integrative area because it receives input from auditory areas to allow a person to know how loud to speak and how to put words together appropriately in conversation.

- **General Interpretative Area** (also called **Wernicke's area** or the **gnostic area**—NOS-tik; "knowledge"): located only on one side of the brain; in most people, it is in the parietal and temporal lobes on the left side near the posterior end of the lateral sulcus. It receives input from the visual and auditory association areas, allowing a person to respond to visual and audible stimuli. For example, it enables a person to understand language and know how to respond appropriately when asked questions or given commands.

- **Prefrontal cortex**: located in the frontal lobes anterior to the premotor area, it is responsible for intellectual thoughts. In most people, the *right* prefrontal cortex is responsible for imagination, insight, forming images of sensations, artistic ability, and appreciation, whereas the *left* prefrontal cortex is responsible for science and math skills, analysis, reasoning, reading, writing, etc.

Impulse Pathways in the Cerebrum

White matter in the cerebrum consists primarily of myelinated axons that conduct millions of impulses through the CNS. Neurologists classify these cerebral axons (fibers) based on where they conduct impulses:

- **Association fibers** conduct impulses within a single hemisphere.

- **Commissural fibers** (kom-I-shur-al; "united") conduct impulses from one hemisphere to the other. Most of these fibers pass through a structure called the *corpus callosum* (KOR-pus ka-LŌ-sum, meaning "thick body"). Commissural fibers enable the left and right cerebral hemispheres to communicate and work together as a single unit.

- **Projection fibers** conduct impulses from the cerebral hemispheres to other parts of the brain and spinal cord.

Nuclei in the Cerebrum

Several gray matter regions, called **basal nuclei** (formerly called *basal ganglia*), are found deep within each cerebral hemisphere (Figure 17-3). They constantly monitor and influence impulses sent out from the primary motor cortex and prefrontal areas, thereby preventing unnecessary muscle movements. For example, they help coordinate the semivoluntary swinging motion of the arms when a person is walking. The basal nuclei include the **caudate nucleus** (KAW-dāt; *cauda*, tail), **putamen** (pū-TĀ-men; "pod"), and **globus pallidus** (GLŌ-bus PAL-i-dus; *glob*, sphere; *pallid*, pale). The putamen and globus pallidus together form the **lentiform nucleus** (LEN-ti-form; *lenti*, bean).

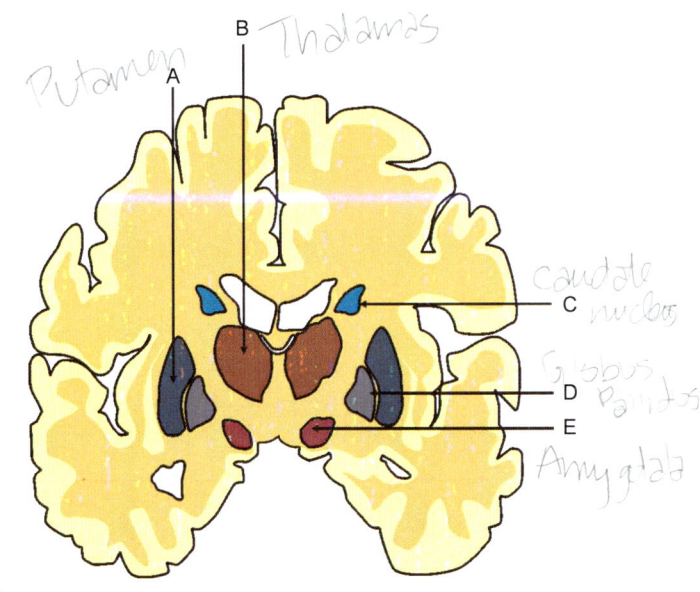

Figure 17-3. Basal nuclei

CENTRAL NERVOUS SYSTEM

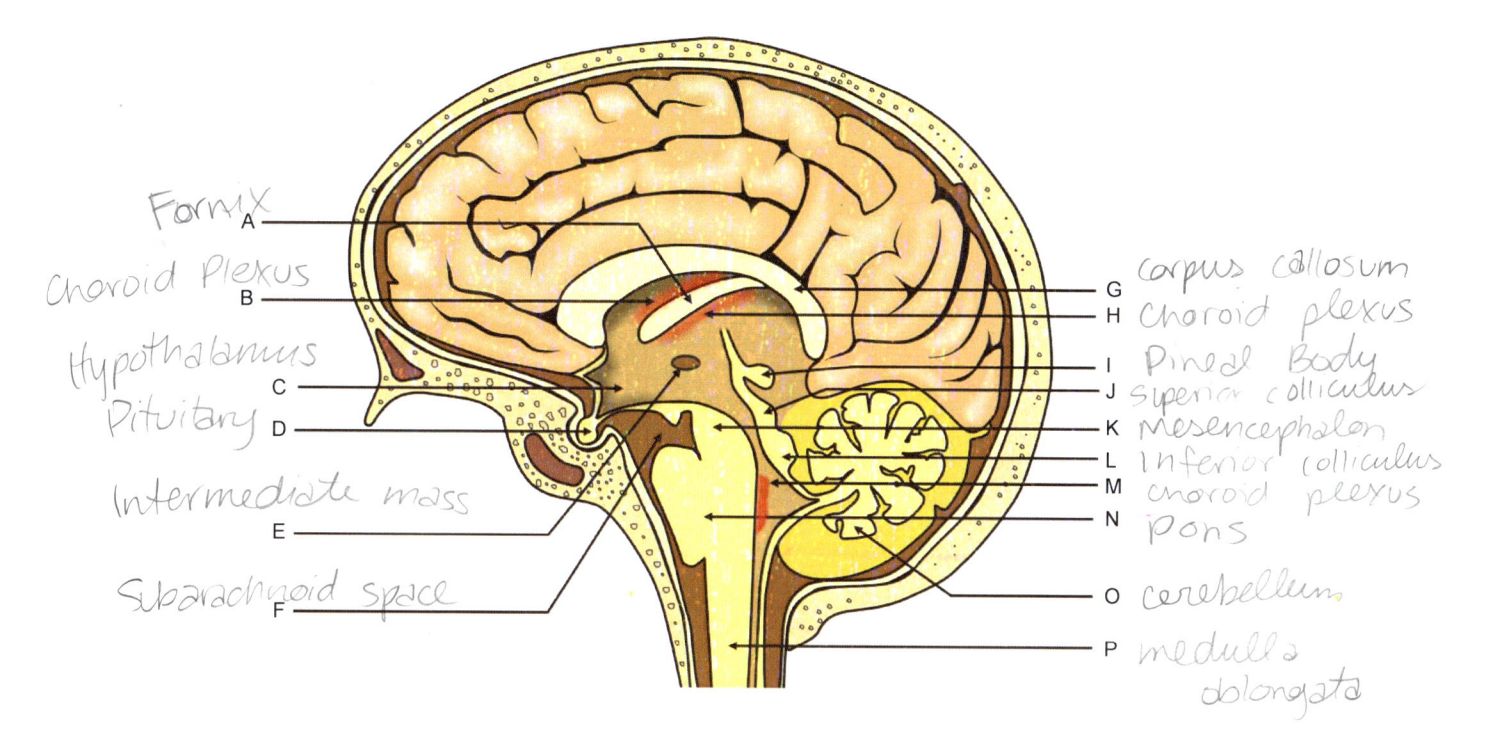

Figure 17-4. View of the diencephalon and brain stem

Labels (handwritten):
- A: Fornix
- B: Choroid Plexus
- C: Hypothalamus
- D: Pituitary
- E: Intermediate mass
- F: Subarachnoid space
- G: Corpus callosum
- H: Choroid plexus
- I: Pineal Body
- J: Superior colliculus
- K: Mesencephalon
- L: Inferior colliculus
- M: Choroid plexus
- N: Pons
- O: Cerebellum
- P: Medulla oblongata

The lentiform nucleus and caudate nucleus together form the **corpus striatum** (stri-Ā-tum; *stria*, striped).

THE DIENCEPHALON

The **diencephalon** (dī-en-SEF-a-lon; *die*, through; *encephalon*, brain) is located superior to the mesencephalon and inferior to the corpus callosum, and includes three major regions: the *epithalamus, thalamus,* and *hypothalamus* (Figure 17-4).

Epithalamus

The **epithalamus** (ep-i-THAL-a-mus; *epi*, upon; *thalamus*, inner room), located inferior to the corpus callosum, forms the superior rim of the diencephalon. The pinecone shaped **pineal body** (PIN-e-al) projects from the posterior end of the epithalamus and is important in a person's *circadian rhythm* (daily sleep-wake cycles; ser KĀ-dē-an; *circa*, around, *dia*, day). The pineal body secretes a hormone called **melatonin** (mel-a-TŌ-nin) that promotes drowsiness. The rate of melatonin secretion correlates positively with exposure to dim light or darkness. Prolonged exposure to low-light conditions causes excessive secretion of melatonin. The result may be *seasonal affective disorder (SAD)*, characterized by mood swings. Treatment of SAD may involve periodic exposure to bright light for regulated periods. Prolonged exposure to light, such as when a person stays awake for extended periods during a long trip, causes less melatonin secretion. This may upset the biological clock and may cause insomnia, fatigue, etc. *Jet lag* is a feeling of fatigue resulting from a lack of melatonin.

Thalamus

The **thalamus** (THAL-a-mus; "inner room") is the largest part of the diencephalon, and is located inferior to the epithalamus. It consists of two oval shaped halves held together by an **intermediate mass.** Each half of the thalamus includes clusters of nuclei that serve as relay centers for all sensory impulses passing from the spinal cord to the cerebrum. Additionally, regions called geniculate bodies (je-NIK-ū-lāt; *genu*, bent) serve as relay centers for visual and auditory signals. It also plays a role in learning and memory.

Hypothalamus

The **hypothalamus** (hī-pō-THAL-a-mus) is the lower, anterior portion of the diencephalon and it performs numerous functions related to homeostasis. Anatomically, the hypothalamus displays several distinct structures. Two pea-shaped structures called **mammillary bodies** (MAM-mil-ar-e; *mamma*, breast) project from the inferior surface of the hypothalamus. These bodies receive and evaluate impulses involved in smell, and they control certain muscle movements in the mouth involved in eating. Anterior to the mammillary bodies is a funnel-shaped tube, the **infundibulum** (in-fun-DIB-u-lum; funnel), projects anteriorly from the hypothalamus and suspends the bean-shaped *pituitary gland*. Physiologically, the hypothalamus has eight major functions:

- Controls the Autonomic Nervous System (ANS): The hypothalamus controls the ANS by regulating the activity of various centers in the brain stem, which in turn, regulate the activity of smooth muscle, cardiac muscle, and various glands. As a result, the hypothalamus can help regulate heart and breathing rates, blood pressure, activities of digestive organs, etc.

- Regulates Limbic System Output: The hypothalamus is a major component of the *limbic system*, or emotional part of the brain described under the heading "Functional Systems of the Brain". In short, the hypothalamus influences motor output to skeletal muscles responsible for performing movements associated with feelings of pleasure, fear, rage, hunger, satisfaction, and libido (li-BĒ-do; "sex drive").

- Major Coordinator of the Endocrine System: One of the most important functions of the hypothalamus is its influence on the endocrine system. The pituitary gland has been deemed the endocrine system's "master gland," because its numerous hormones influence the activities of most of the other endocrine glands. The hypothalamus controls the production and release of all hormones from the pituitary gland.

- Produces Hormones: The hypothalamus produces two hormones: ADH and oxytocin. **ADH** (antidiuretic hormone) causes the kidneys to conserve water and produce less urine; thus, more water stays in the blood preventing a decrease in blood pressure. **Oxytocin (OT**; ok sē-TŌ-sin, "swift birth") stimulates contraction of smooth muscle tissue in the uterus and mammary glands (promotes childbirth and milk secretion, respectively). ADH and OT are made in cell bodies of neurons in the hypothalamus, but then travel through axons that have axon terminals in the pituitary gland; thus, while these hormones enter the blood from the pituitary gland, they are actually produced in the hypothalamus.

- Controls Food Intake: The hypothalamus contains the **feeding center**, which responds to changes in blood glucose levels. When blood glucose levels drop below normal, the feeding center makes the person feel hungry. Taking in food counteracts this feeling by raising the blood glucose levels. When the blood glucose rises above normal, the hunger center makes the person feel satiated (no longer hungry).

- Controls Fluid Intake: The hypothalamus contains the **thirst center**, which responds to changes in blood osmotic pressure. The hypothalamus helps maintain blood osmotic (OP) pressure through the action of its *osmoreceptors*. When the blood OP rises above normal, the thirst center makes the person feel thirsty. In addition, the hypothalamus releases more ADH through the pituitary gland (mentioned earlier). By drinking more fluids and producing less urine, more water remains in the blood and lowers the blood's OP.

- Controls Circadian Rhythm: The hypothalamus contains a person's "biological clock," or more accurately, the **suprachiasmatic nucleus** (SŪ-pra-kī-az-MA-tik), which regulates sleep-wake cycles (i.e., one's circadian rhythm). This nucleus receives sensory input from the eyes and sets the cycle period according to the lengths of daylight and darkness in a 24-hour period. In addition,

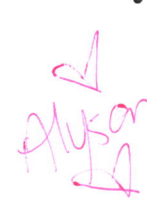

CENTRAL NERVOUS SYSTEM

the nucleus sends impulses to the pineal gland to regulate its release of melatonin.

- **Controls Body Temperature**: The hypothalamus contains the body's "thermostat," which influences activities affecting a person's body temperature. Setting the thermostat to a higher value promotes activities that increase body temperature, such as shivering, increased metabolism, and constriction of blood vessels in the skin to prevent heat loss. Setting the thermostat to a lower value promotes activities that decrease body temperature; e.g., sweating, decreased metabolism, and dilation of vessels in the skin allowing more heat loss.

THE BRAIN STEM

The brain stem serves as a connection between the other parts of the brain and the spinal cord. From most superior to most inferior, the **brain stem** includes the *mesencephalon*, *pons*, and *medulla oblongata*.

Mesencephalon

The **mesencephalon** (mez-en-SEF-a-lon; *mes*, between), or **midbrain**, is the most superior portion of the brain stem. Its ventral (anterior) surface displays bulges called **cerebral peduncles** (pe-DUNG-klz; "little feet"), which contain *motor tracts* that relay impulses passing between the cerebrum and spinal cord.

The dorsal (posterior) surface of the mesencephalon displays four knoblike structures, known collectively as the **corpora quadrigemina** (KOR-por-a, "bodies"; kwod-ri-JEM-i-na, "four twins"); each knob is a *colliculus* (ko-LIK-ū-lus; "mound"). The **superior colliculi** (ko-LIK-ū-lī; plural for colliculus) contain nuclei responsible for movements of the eyes and head in response to visual stimuli; e.g., flinching when you detect something out of the corner of your eye. The **inferior colliculi** contain nuclei responsible for reflexive movement of the head in response to *sound*; e.g., flinching in response to a gunshot. Since the corpora quadrigemina covers the dorsal surface of the midbrain, it is referred to as the *tectum* ("roof").

The basal nuclei in the cerebrum connect with a mesencephalic nucleus called the **substantia nigra** (sub-STAN-shē-a NĪ-gra; "black substance"), so named for its melanin content. Because of its interaction with the basal nuclei, some neurologists consider the substantia nigra as part of the basal nuclei. Neurons in the substantia nigra release the neurotransmitter *dopamine*, which inhibits unnecessary muscle movements. A deficiency in dopamine secretion from the substantia nigra is primarily responsible for the uncontrollable muscle movements associated with *Parkinson's disease*.

The **red nucleus** is gray matter lying near the substantia nigra and named for its reddish appearance, which is due to iron-containing pigments. The red nucleus relays *motor* impulses passing from the cerebrum to the spinal cord and affect movements of the limbs. This nucleus is also part of the *reticular formation*, described shortly.

Pons

The **pons** ("bridge") is a large bulge located immediately superior to the medulla. It contains mostly white matter and functions as a relay center for *sensory* and *motor* impulses traveling between the brain stem and cerebellum and between the brain and spinal cord. It contains the *salivation center* (stimulates salivary glands to release saliva) and parts of the *respiratory center* and *reticular formation*. In addition, the pons is the origin of three pairs of cranial nerves: the *trigeminal*, *abducens*, and *facial*, which we will describe in the next chapter.

Medulla Oblongata

The **medulla oblongata** (me-DŪ-la, "marrow"; ob-lon-GOT-a, "long") is the most inferior part of the brain stem and houses nuclei responsible for various involuntary activities related to homeostasis. It is located at the level of the skull's foramen magnum, and connects the brain stem directly to the spinal cord. Axons connecting higher brain centers with the spinal cord "cross over" in the medulla; neurologists call this anatomical feature *decussation* (dē-ku-SĀ-shun; "crossing"). Consequently, each side of the brain monitors and controls the opposite side of the body.

Two parallel ridges called **pyramids** run longitudinally along the anterior portion of the medulla and contain *motor tracts* passing between the cerebrum and spinal cord. Inferior and lateral to the pyramids are two oval-shaped mounds called **olives**, which contain *sensory tracts* that relay impulses from stretch receptors in skeletal muscles and joints to the cerebellum. This enables the cerebellum to monitor and control motor impulses sent to skeletal muscles from the precentral gyrus.

The medulla oblongata contains part of the *reticular formation* and includes a number of nuclei that serve as important regulatory *centers*:

- **Cardiovascular center:** regulates blood flow and blood pressure in the cardiovascular center. This center is subdivided into two centers: the *cardiac center* controls heart rate (how fast the heart beats) and stroke volume (how much blood the heart pumps out with each beat). The *vasomotor center* (vā-zō-MŌ-ter; *vaso*, vessel) helps control blood vessel diameter by regulating vasoconstriction and vasodilation.
- **Respiratory center:** regulates the rate and depth of breathing. Part of the respiratory center is in the pons.
- **Deglutition center:** (dē-glū-TISH-un; *deglut*, swallow) controls involuntary muscle movements associated with swallowing, coughing, sneezing, and hiccupping.
- **Emetic center:** (ē-ME-tik) controls muscle actions associated with vomiting.

CEREBELLUM

Located inferior to the occipital lobe of the cerebrum, the **cerebellum** (ser-e-BEL-um; "small brain") is the second largest part of the brain. It includes right and left *cerebellar hemispheres* divided by a central region called the **vermis** (VER-mis; "worm"), so named because of its worm-like appearance. The outer surface of the cerebellum displays thin convolutions called **folia** (FŌ-lē-a; "leaves"), so named because of their leaf-like (foliage) appearance. These convolutions greatly increase the cerebellum's surface area in the same way that gyri increase the surface area of the cerebrum. The **primary fissure** splits the cerebellum into a smaller *anterior lobe* and a larger *posterior lobe*.

Like the cerebrum, the cerebellum contains gray matter in its cortex and white matter in its inner region. Large neurons called **Purkinje cells** (pur-KIN-jē) reside in the cerebellar cortex. The white matter of the cerebellum exists in a branch-like pattern called **arbor vitae** (AR-bor; "tree"; VĒ-tā; "life"). The white matter surrounds the **cerebellar nuclei**, located more centrally. The cerebellum communicates with other parts of the brain through tracts located in pairs of cerebellar peduncles (one peduncle on each side). The **superior cerebellar peduncles** transmit impulses between the cerebellum and mesencephalon; the **middle cerebellar peduncles** transmit impulses between the cerebellum and pons, and the **inferior cerebellar peduncles** transmit impulses between the cerebellum and medulla oblongata.

The cerebellum constantly receives and translates sensory information from joints, muscles, eyes and the inner ear (which contains organs for equilibrium), and sends out impulses that help coordinate muscle movements to maintain balance and equilibrium. Depending on body position, the cerebellum sends impulses to the brain stem nuclei, which in turn modify motor impulses sent from the precentral gyrus to skeletal muscles. This constant monitoring and evaluation of sensory input and signaling to the cerebrum and brain stem makes the cerebellum crucial for maintaining coordination, posture, and balance.

BRAIN VENTRICLES

Different regions of the brain contain cavities, called *ventricles*, which contain a liquid called *cerebrospinal fluid (CSF)* (Figure 17-5). The two largest and most superior ventricles are **lateral ventricles**; one is located in each cerebral hemisphere. A thin clear membrane, called the **septum pellucidum** (SEP-tum; "partition"; pe-LŪ-si-dum; "clear") separates the lateral ventricles from one another. The **third ventricle** is in the diencephalon and connects to the lateral ventricles via the **interventricular foramen** (or *foramen of Monro*). The **fourth ventricle** is immediately anterior to the cerebellum and connects to the third ventricle through the **mesencephalic aqueduct**.

CENTRAL NERVOUS SYSTEM

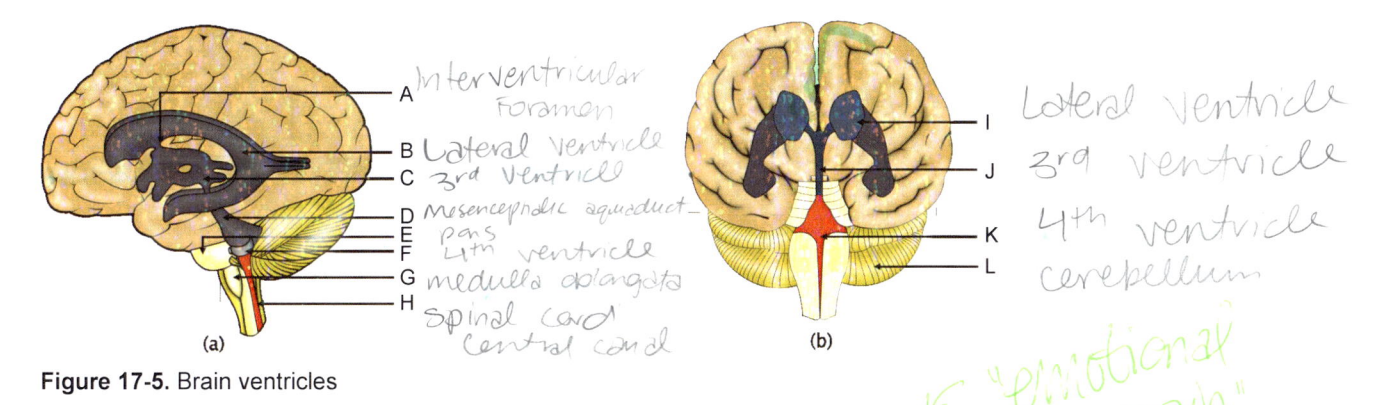

Figure 17-5. Brain ventricles

FUNCTIONAL SYSTEMS OF THE BRAIN

A *functional system* in the brain is one that performs specific functions but has neurons that extend through multiple regions of the brain. The brain's functional systems are the *reticular formation* and the *limbic system*.

The Reticular Formation

The **reticular formation** is a group of neurons that have axons extending through the entire brain stem and into the diencephalon, cerebellum, and spinal cord. The **red nucleus**, located in the mesencephalon, is part of the reticular formation that helps coordinate skeletal muscle movements in the limbs. The nuclei for the various centers described for the medulla oblongata are also in the reticular formation.

Part of the reticular formation in the brain stem functions in maintaining consciousness and is called the **reticular activating system (RAS)**. The RAS monitors sensory impulses reaching the brain and sends impulses to the thalamus, which in turn relays the impulses to the cerebral cortex to maintain consciousness and alertness. The RAS filters out most of the sensory input so that we are not consciously aware of every little stimulus. However, a person can become aware of these stimuli if reminded of them. For example, you were probably not aware of the shoe pressing on your foot until you were reminded of it just now. The RAS is important in sleep-wake cycles, where it is responsible for arousal from sleep. Sudden trauma to the RAS, which can happen in boxing when the brain stem twists due to a hard punch to the side of the jaw, can cause unconsciousness (the person gets "knocked out").

The Limbic System

The **limbic system** is a collection of nuclei located between the cerebrum and diencephalon and is responsible for one's emotions and the integration of emotions with thoughts. For this reason, the limbic system has the nickname "emotional brain." The word limbic means "ring," and refers to the way in which the nuclei in the cerebrum surround the superior portion of the brain stem. Major structures of the limbic system and their functions include the following (Figure 17-6):

- **Amygdala** (a-MIG-da-la; "almond"), or **amydaloid nucleus**: region responsible for a person's expressions of fear and recognizing fear and anger in other people. It also plays a role in a person's emotional reactions to remembered thoughts.

- **Cingulate gyrus** (SIN-gū-lāt; "belt"): Important in helping a person display emotions, such as making a "yucky" face when smelling soured milk.

- **Fornix** (FOR-niks; "arch"): contains tracts connecting the upper and lower regions of the limbic system.

- **Hippocampus** (hip-ō-KAM-pus; "seahorse"): plays a role in a person's emotional reactions to remembered thoughts.

- **Hypothalamus**: responsible for a person's perception of pleasure, anger, and fear, and it plays a role in the sex drive and regulating sleep-wake cycles.

BRAIN WAVES

Billions of impulses pass through the brain continuously and show up on monitoring equipment as **brain** waves. The graphical display of brain waves is an *electroencephalogram* (e-LEK-trō-en-SEF-a-lō-gram), or EEG. Reading an EEG allows evaluation of brain health and state of mind. There are four types of brain waves:

- **Alpha waves** are the most common when a person is awake but in a relaxed state with eyes closed. As soon as the person falls asleep or opens the eyes to focus on various tasks, the alpha waves disappear.
- **Beta waves** are typical in a person who is conscious, alert, thinking, and receiving sensory input.
- **Theta waves** are common in children but their appearance in adults suggests emotional stress or certain brain abnormalities.
- **Delta waves** are normally seen only when the person is asleep. The presence of delta waves in a person who is awake suggests some sort of brain abnormality.

SLEEP

Sleep is a state of *unconsciousness* in which adequate stimulation can bring about consciousness. In order to understand sleep, we must first understand what it means to be awake. When a person is *conscious* (awake), a variety of synonyms may describe that person: alert, aware, attentive, cognizant, mindful of surroundings, etc. *Coma* is also a state of unconsciousness, but unlike sleep, even intense stimulation will not arouse a person from a coma. While we might think the brain is not doing much during sleep, it is still active and processing information. There are two major types of sleep: *non-rapid eye movement sleep* and *rapid eye movement sleep*.

Non-rapid eye movement (NREM) sleep occurs with the first hour of unconsciousness and has four stages:

- **Stage 1 NREM**: eyes are closed and the person has sporadic thoughts; the EEG is dominated by alpha waves, and immediate arousal is possible.
- **Stage 2 NREM**: irregular brain waves intermingled with sporadic short bursts of specific brain waves; arousal is more difficult than in stage 1.
- **Stage 3 NREM**: vital signs diminish; decrease in body temperature and blood pressure; some dreaming (nightmares); EEG is dominated by theta and delta waves; arousal is difficult.
- **Stage 4 NREM**: deep sleep; delta waves common; awakening causes slow responses due to minimal vital sign activity; bedwetting or sleepwalking may occur.

Rapid eye movement (REM) sleep, so named because the eyes experience a fluttering movement, occurs after stage 4 of NREM sleep. REM sleep begins about 90 minutes after NREM sleep begins. During REM sleep, almost complete paralysis of skeletal muscles occurs. With the exceptions of nightmares, most dreaming occurs during REM sleep.

A person's normal sleep pattern exhibits **sleep cycles**, in which periods of NREM and REM sleep alternate with one another. After about the first 90

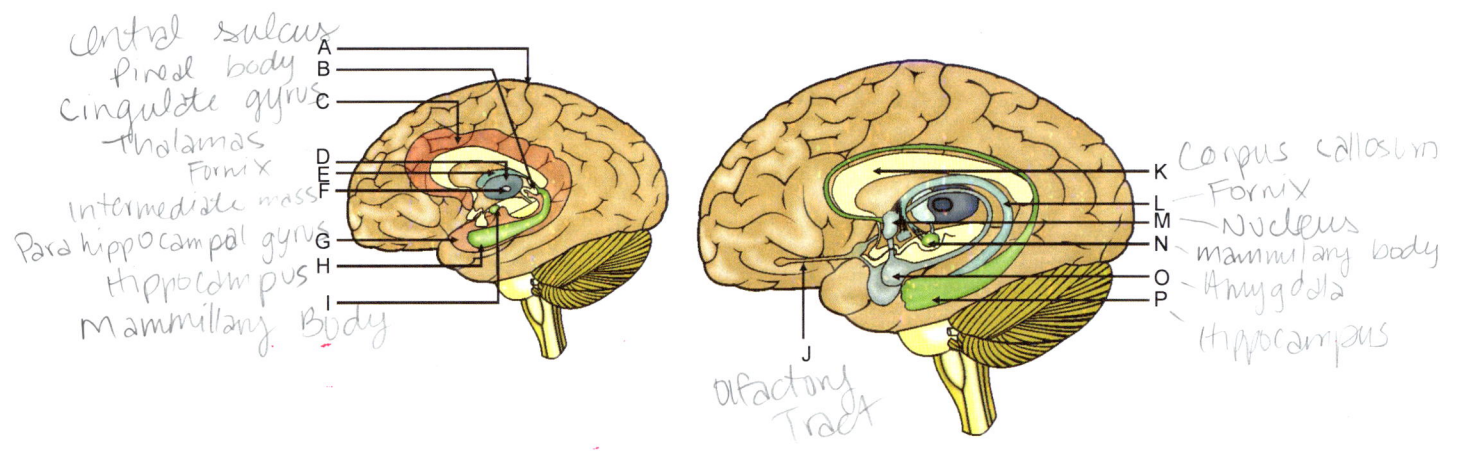

Figure 17-6. The limbic system

CENTRAL NERVOUS SYSTEM

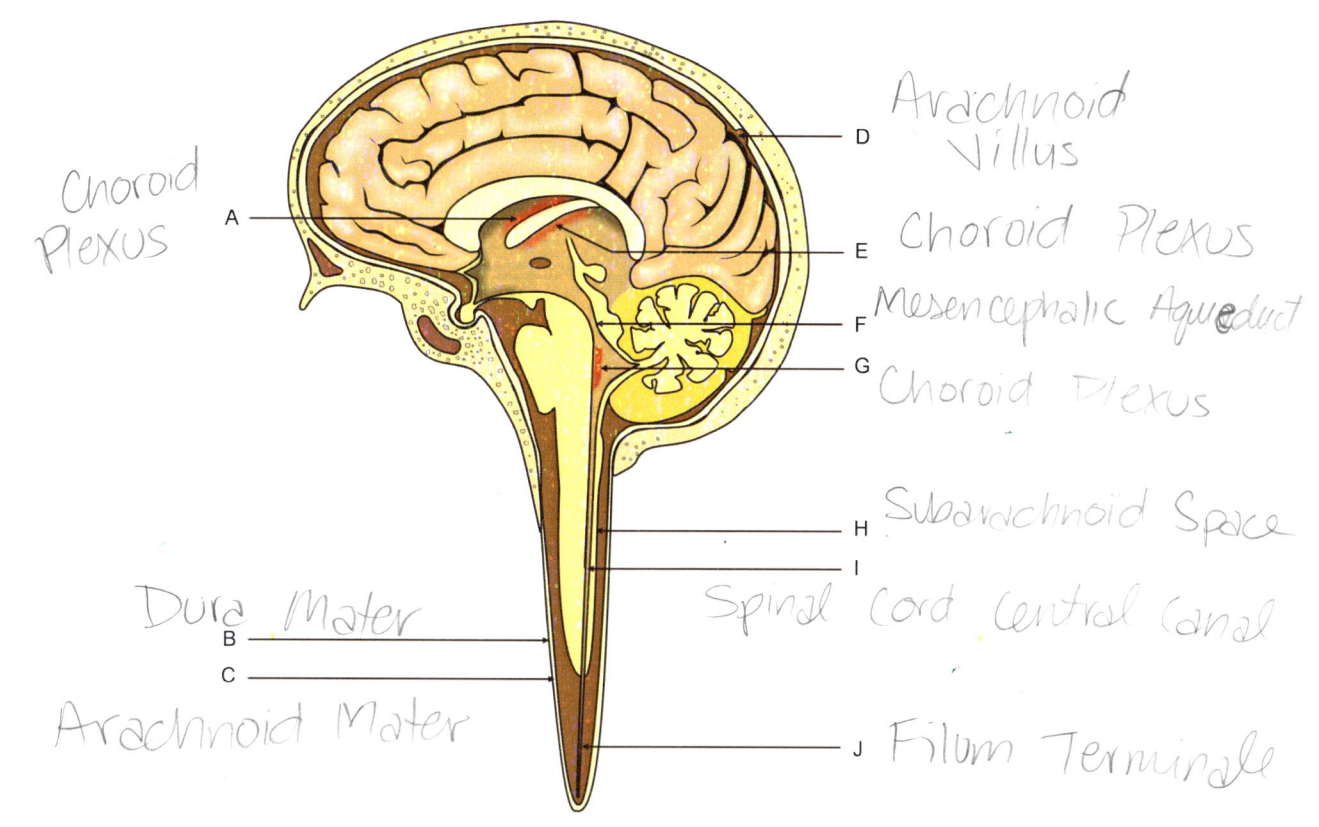

Figure 17-7. Circulation of CSF

Labels (handwritten annotations):
- A: Choroid Plexus
- B: Dura Mater
- C: Arachnoid Mater
- D: Arachnoid Villus
- E: Choroid Plexus
- F: Mesencephalic Aqueduct
- G: Choroid Plexus
- H: Subarachnoid Space
- I: Spinal Cord Central Canal
- J: Filum Terminale

minutes of sleep, a person has experienced all stages of NREM then experiences REM for 5-10 minutes. The person then reverts to the early stages of NREM and the cycle repeats with REM occurring about 90 minutes later. While each NREM episode lasts about 90 minutes, each successive REM episode lasts longer, so that near morning, REM episodes may last an hour or so. For this reason, long dreams occur near morning.

PROTECTION OF THE BRAIN

As important as the brain is to maintaining homeostasis, it is not surprising that it is protected by a number of items, including the skull, *meninges, cerebrospinal fluid,* and the *blood-brain-barrier*.

Meninges

Protective connective tissue membranes called **meninges** (me-NIN-jēz; *meninx*, membrane) lie between the skull and the brain's surface, and include the *dura mater, arachnoid mater,* and *pia mater* (Figure 17-7).

Dura mater (DUR-a, "tough"; MA-ter, "mother"), the most superficial and thickest meninx, is an opaque, dense connective tissue covering that resembles a leather cap. Around the brain, the dura mater exists as two layers that enclose the *dural sinuses*, which drain blood from the brain. Anteriorly, the dura mater lies in the longitudinal fissure where it forms the **falx cerebri** (FALKS, "sickle"; SER-e-brē). Anteriorly, the falx cerebri attaches firmly to the crista galli of the ethmoid bone. Posteriorly, the falx cerebri becomes the **falx cerebelli** (ser-e-BEL-ī), which separates the two cerebellar hemispheres. The **tentorium cerebelli** (ten-TOR-ē-um; "tent") is dura mater that separates the cerebrum from the cerebellum. Dura mater does not extend into sulci.

Arachnoid mater (a-RAK-noyd; *arach*, spider; *noid*, resembles), the middle meninx, lies deep to the dura mater and is named for its spider web-like appearance. The arachnoid mater is thinner and more transparent than the dura mater and supports the large blood vessels around the brain. The **subarachnoid space** lies deep to the arachnoid and contains CSF. Fingerlike projections called **arachnoid villi** (VIL-ī;

331

"shaggy hair") extend into the dural sinus and drain cerebrospinal fluid into the blood.

Pia mater (PĒ-a; "gentle"), the deepest meninx, is a thin, transparent membrane that adheres to the brain's surface. It dips into the sulci and supports small vessels and capillaries on the surface of the brain. The pia cannot be removed easily without damaging the cerebral cortex.

Cerebrospinal Fluid

A clear, watery fluid called **cerebrospinal fluid (CSF)** flows around the brain and through its ventricles and canals. It originates as blood plasma (the liquid part of blood around the blood cells) and then squeezes out of a cluster of blood capillaries called **choroid plexuses** (KOR-oyd PLEK-sus-ez; *chor*, membrane; *plexus*, braid). Each brain ventricle contains a choroid plexus. CSF circulates through the CNS with the help of beating cilia on ependymal cells that cover the choroid plexuses.

CSF has several important functions: (1) reduces the weight of the brain and spinal cord; (2) acts as a shock absorber; (3) prevents dramatic temperature changes in the CNS; and (4) delivers nutrients and removes waste materials from nervous tissue. CSF returns to the blood through *arachnoid villi*, which penetrate into a blood-filled *superior sagittal sinus* along the longitudinal fissure.

Blood-Brain-Barrier

The **blood-brain-barrier (BBB)** is the protective barrier between blood capillaries and the brain's tissues. Part of the BBB is attributable to tight junctions between endothelial cells that form the inner lining of the brain's capillaries. In addition, the basement membrane on which the endothelial cells rest is thicker than that in most other capillaries; consequently, materials leaving the blood must pass through the cytoplasm of the endothelial cells. This pathway allows the endothelial cells to detoxify potentially harmful substances before they enter the brain's tissues.

Part of the BBB includes microglial cells surrounding the vessels and neurons. They help regulate the types of materials that pass between the blood and brain tissue. The BBB does not exist in the hypothalamus or the emetic center in the medulla oblongata; therefore, these parts of the brain can monitor various blood-borne chemicals and make adjustments in the body's metabolic activity in order to maintain homeostasis. The BBB of an infant is not well developed.

THE SPINAL CORD

The spinal cord relays impulses between the brain and most of the rest of the body. It courses through the vertebral foramina and extends from the medulla oblongata into the lumbar region of the vertebral column (Figure 17-8).

The most inferior portion of the cord is a cone-shaped region, the **conus medullaris** (KŌ-nus, "cone"; med-u-LAR-is). The cord stops growing at about age 5, but the vertebral column continues to lengthen; thus, the conus exists at about the second lumbar vertebra (L2) in the adult and at about L3 in an infant.

The spinal cord is nearly divided into two halves by a **posterior median sulcus** and an **anterior medial sulcus**. The posterior sulcus is the deeper of the two sulci. Centrally located within the cord and running the entire length of the cord is a narrow tube, the **central canal**, through which CSF flows.

Support of the Spinal Cord

The same meninges that cover the brain cover the spinal cord. The pia mater covers the cord's surface and attaches to the arachnoid and dura mater by **denticulate ligaments** (den-TIK-ū-lāt; "tooth-like"), which are slender extensions of the pia. CSF circulates within the subarachnoid space. The arachnoid and dura extend inferiorly from the conus medullaris to the level of the second sacral vertebra (S2). The pia mater anchors inferiorly to the coccyx by a fibrous cord called the **filum terminale** (FĪ-lum, "filament"; ter-mi-NA-lē, "end").

> **Note**: During a *spinal tap* in an adult, the physician removes CSF from the subarachnoid space inferior to L2, reducing the chance of puncturing the spinal cord. Analysis of CSF can often reveal information about the health of the individual.

CENTRAL NERVOUS SYSTEM

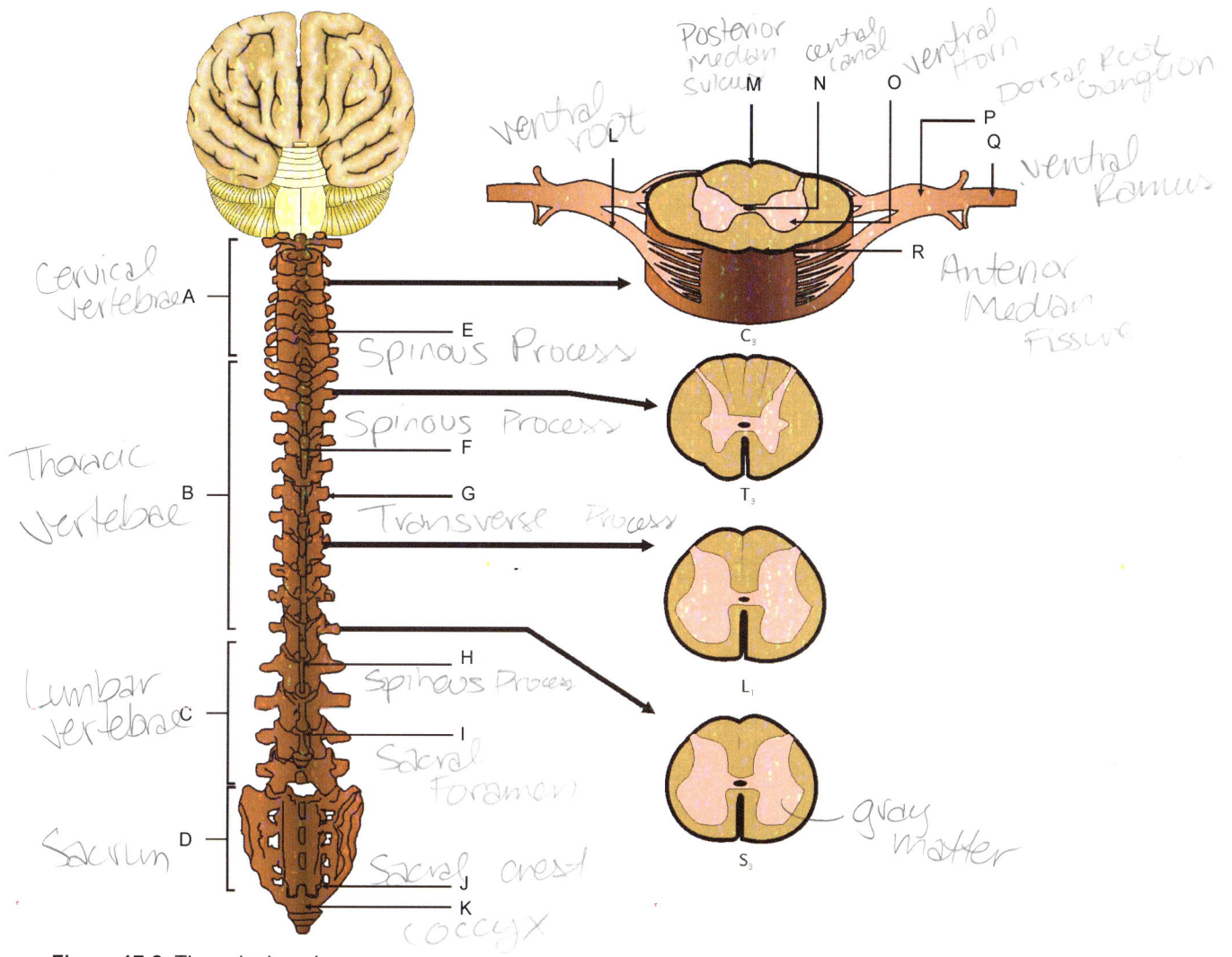

Figure 17-8. The spinal cord

Gray Matter of the Spinal Cord

Gray matter exists in the entire spinal cord as two parallel tubes extending from the medulla oblongata to the conus medullaris. These tubes of gray matter (nuclei) are connected to one another along their entire length by the **gray commissures** (KOM-i-shūrz; "combine"), which contain interneurons that conduct impulses from one side of the spinal cord to the other. Along most of their length, these two tubes of gray matter have projections called *horns*. When viewed in cross section, the cord's gray matter resembles a butterfly, with the "wings" connected in the middle (at the gray commissures) and displaying three projections (horns). The gray matter is organized according to the functions of its neurons as follows:

- **Posterior (dorsal) horns**: contain cell bodies of *interneurons* that receive sensory input from somatic sensory neurons with receptors in the skin, skeletal muscles, and joints, and visceral sensory neurons with receptors in visceral organs. Specific interneurons may relay the impulses to the brain and/or other neurons in the spinal cord.

- **Anterior (ventral) horns**: contain cell bodies of *somatic motor neurons*, which receive impulses from other neurons in the spinal cord and send impulses to skeletal muscles.

- **Lateral horns**: contain cell bodies of *visceral motor neurons*, which receive impulses from other neurons in the spinal cord and send impulses to

Table 17-1. Major tracts in the spinal cord

Sensory Tracts in the Spinal Cord		
Tract Name	Pathway for Tracts	Conducts sensory impulses for
Fasciculus	Posterior columns→Thalamus→Postcentral gyrus	Stretch, touch, vibration in neck, trunk, limbs
Spinothalamic	Anterolateral columns→Thalamus→postcentral gyrus	Touch, pressure, pain, temperature in skin
Spinocerebellar	Lateral columns →Cerebellum	Muscle stretch in trunk/lower limbs
Motor Tracts in the Spinal Cord		
Tract Name	Pathway for Tracts	Conducts motor impulses for
Corticobulbar	Precentral gyrus→Brain stem	Movements involving head, eye, face, chewing, swallowing
Corticospinal	Precentral gyrus→Pyramids→anterolateral columns	Movements of trunk/limbs
Vestibulospinal	Inner ear→Anterior columns	Movements for balance and equilibrium
Tectospinal	Corpora quadrigemina (tectum)→Anterior columns	Head/upper limb reflexes in response to visual/audible stimuli
Reticulospinal	Reticular formation→Lateral columns	Muscle tone and reflexes
Rubrospinal	Red nucleus→Lateral columns	Muscle tone and precise movements of hands and fingers

involuntary muscle tissue and glands. There are no lateral horns in the cervical region of spinal cord.

White Matter of the Spinal Cord

The nervous tissue surrounding the spinal cord's gray matter consists of white matter arranged in regions called *columns*. There are three pairs of columns named according to location: **posterior (dorsal) columns, anterior (ventral) columns,** and **lateral columns**.

Spinal cord columns contain tracts, or *fasciculi* (fa-SIK-ū-lī; *fascicle,* bundle), which are bundles of axons belonging to interneurons. Sensory impulses relayed to interneurons in a posterior horn then travel to the brain through **ascending tracts**; whereas, impulses traveling from the brain to motor neurons in the anterior horns move along **descending tracts**. At some point along the way, most tracts decussate (cross over) to the opposite side of the cord. Many tracts decussate in the medulla oblongata, but others decussate within the spinal cord. This explains why the *right* side of the brain receives impulses from and sends impulses to the *left* side of the body, and why the *left* side of the brain receives impulses from and sends impulses to the *right* side of the body. Major tracts in the spinal cord are shown in Table 17-1."

Ascending (Sensory) Tracts

Ascending tracts conduct impulses superiorly through the spinal cord's white matter (columns) and into the brain. These impulses originate at sensory receptors in the peripheral nervous system. The neurons that conduct the impulses into the spinal cord are **first-order neurons**. In turn, first-order neurons transfer impulses to second-order neurons, located inside the spinal cord. The **second-order neurons** conduct impulses superiorly within the cord and transfer them to either the thalamus or cerebellum. **Third-order neurons**, located in the thalamus but not in the cerebellum, transmit impulses to the primary

CENTRAL NERVOUS SYSTEM

somatosensory cortex. Second and third-order neurons are *interneurons*; whereas, first-order neurons are *sensory* neurons.

Descending (Motor) Tracts

Descending tracts conduct impulses inferiorly through the spinal cord's columns and into ventral horns, where they synapse with motor neurons. Both the somatic and autonomic nervous systems utilize descending tracts, but we will only consider those for the somatic nervous system (which innervate skeletal muscles). Motor impulses for the somatic nervous system always pass through two neurons within the CNS. The first neurons are located in the cerebrum and are called **upper motor neurons**. The second neurons are located within nuclei of the brain stem or spinal cord and are called **lower motor neurons**. Descending tracts utilized by upper motor neurons are located within anterior and lateral columns of the spinal cord.

TOPICS TO KNOW FOR CHAPTER 17 (CENTRAL NERVOUS SYSTEM)

- alpha waves
- amygdala
- anterior columns
- anterior horns
- anterior medial sulcus
- arachnoid mater
- arachnoid villi
- arbor vitae
- ascending tracts
- association areas
- association fibers
- auditory association area
- basal nuclei
- BBB
- beta waves
- blood-brain-barrier
- brain stem
- brain waves
- Broca's area
- cardiac center
- cardiovascular center
- caudate nucleus
- central canal
- central nervous system
- central sulcus
- cerebellar hemispheres
- cerebellar nuclei
- cerebellum
- cerebral cortex
- cerebral hemispheres
- cerebral pathways
- cerebral peduncles
- cerebrospinal fluid
- cerebrum
- choroid plexuses
- cingulate gyrus
- circadian rhythm
- coma
- commissural fibers
- conus medullaris
- corpora quadrigemina
- corpus callosum
- corpus striatum
- corticobulbar tracts
- corticospinal pathways
- crista galli
- CSF
- decussation
- deglutition center
- delta waves
- denticulate ligaments
- descending tracts
- diencephalon
- dopamine
- dorsal (posterior) horns
- dura mater
- dural sinuses
- electroencephalogram
- emetic center
- epithalamus
- falx cerebelli
- falx cerebri
- fasciculus
- filum terminale
- first-order neuron
- folia
- foramen of Monro
- fornix
- fourth ventricle
- frontal eye field
- functions of brain parts
- general interpretative area
- geniculate bodies
- globus pallidus
- gnostic area
- gray commissures
- gustatory cortex
- gyri
- hippocampus
- horns
- hypothalamus
- inferior cerebellar peduncles
- inferior colliculi
- infundibulum
- insula
- integrative areas
- intermediate mass
- interventricular foramen
- jet lag
- lateral columns
- lateral horns
- lateral sulcus
- lateral ventricles
- lemniscal pathway
- lentiform nucleus
- limbic system
- longitudinal fissure
- lower motor neurons
- mammillary bodies
- medial pathway
- medulla oblongata
- melatonin
- meninges
- mesencephalic aqueduct
- mesencephalon
- midbrain
- middle cerebellar peduncles
- motor areas of cortex
- motor speech area
- non-rapid eye movement sleep
- NREM
- nuclei in cerebrum
- olfactory cortex
- olives
- parieto-occipital sulcus
- Parkinson's disease
- pia mater
- pineal body
- pituitary gland
- pons
- postcentral gyrus
- posterior (dorsal) columns
- posterior median sulcus

precentral gyrus
prefrontal cortex
premotor area
primary auditory cortex
primary fissure
primary motor cortex
primary somatosensory cortex
primary visual cortex
projection fibers
protection of the brain
Purkinje cells
putamen
pyramidal cells
pyramids
rapid eye movement sleep
red nucleus
REM
respiratory center
reticular activating system (RAS)
reticular formation
reticulospinal tracts
rubrospinal tracts
salivation center

seasonal affective disorder (SAD)
second-order neuron
sensory areas of cortex
septum pellucidum
sleep
sleep cycles
somatosensory association area
spatial discrimination
speech center
spinal cord
spinal cord gray matter
spinal cord support
spinal cord white matter
spinal tap
spinocerebellar pathways
spinocerebellar tracts
spinothalamic tracts
stage 1 NREM
stage 2 NREM
stage 3 NREM
stage 4 NREM
subarachnoid space
substantia nigra

sulci
superior cerebellar peduncles
superior colliculi
tectospinal tracts
tectum
tentorium cerebelli
thalamus
theta waves
third ventricle
third-order neuron
tracts
transverse fissure
unconsciousness
upper motor neurons
vasomotor center
ventral columns
ventral horns
vermis
vestibular cortex
vestibulospinal tracts
visceral sensory area
visual association area
Wernicke's area

CHAPTER 18

Peripheral Nervous System (Part 1): Nerves and Somatic Reflexes

PERIPHERAL NERVOUS SYSTEM

The peripheral nervous system (PNS) includes all nervous system structures not located within the brain or spinal cord. In a way, the PNS is related to the CNS in the same way that the appendicular skeleton is related to the axial skeleton. In both cases, there is a centrally located "main frame" (the CNS and axial skeleton) and a set of more peripherally located structures (the PNS and appendicular skeleton, respectively). In general, the major anatomical features of the PNS include *nerves, nerve roots, rami, plexuses, ganglia, sensory receptors,* and *axon terminals.*

The PNS contains sensory and motor neurons, and a few interneurons, and it is divided into the *somatic* and *autonomic* divisions. In this chapter, we will describe nerves, nerve roots, rami, and plexuses, and their roles in the somatic nervous system. In the next chapter, we will describe details of the autonomic nervous system. Let's begin with a description of a typical nerve.

OVERVIEW OF NERVES

A **nerve** is a collection of axons and blood vessels bundled together within connective tissue outside the central nervous system (Figure 18-1).

The outermost connective tissue covering of a nerve is the **epineurium** (ep-i-NŪ-rē-um) which consists of dense, irregular connective tissue. The epineurium is continuous with the dura mater of the spinal cord and brain. Axons within a nerve exist within bundles called **fascicles** (FAS-i-klz, "bundles"). An extension of the epineurium, called the **perineurium** (per-i-NŪ-rē-um), surrounds each fascicle. Blood vessels course between the fascicles and supply nutrients to and remove wastes from the cellular components of the nerve. The perineurium extends within each fascicle as the **endoneurium** (en-dō-NŪ-rē-um), which surrounds individual axons.

Innervation (e-ner-VĀ-shun) refers to the connection between the CNS and either a sensory

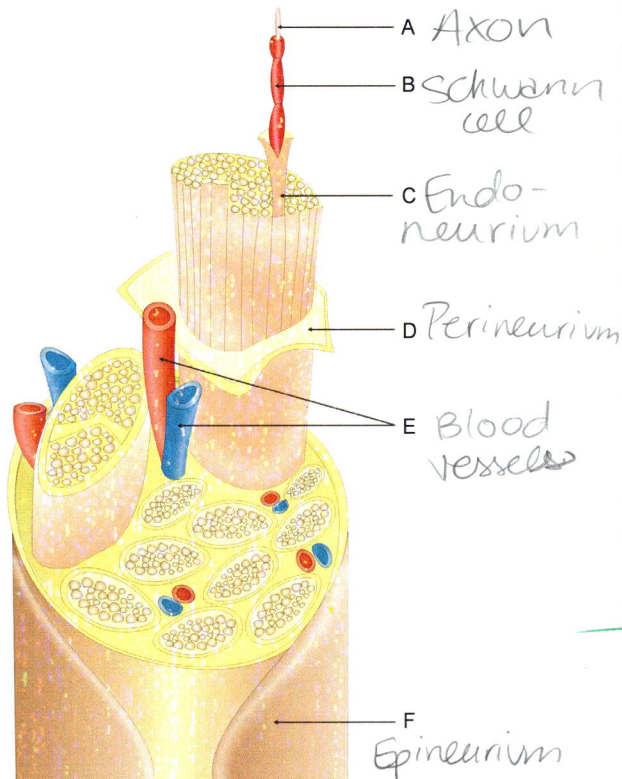

Figure 18-1. Structure of a nerve

- A — Axon
- B — Schwann cell
- C — Endoneurium
- D — Perineurium
- E — Blood vessels
- F — Epineurium

structure or an effector in the PNS by way of a nerve. Nerves are classified based on (1) the function of the axons within them, and (2) their origin, the site where the nerve connects to the CNS.

Classification based on function

Based on the function of the axons within them, nerves may be *sensory*, *motor*, or *mixed*.

- **Sensory nerves** contain only axons of sensory neurons; thus, sensory nerves conduct impulses only from the PNS to the CNS.

- **Motor nerves** contain mostly axons of motor neurons, and therefore conduct impulses mainly to effectors (muscles or glands).

- **Mixed nerves** contain abundant axons of sensory and motor neurons. These nerves are the most common and function like two-lane highways. Keep in mind that a single axon will conduct impulses in only one direction, so the impulses that are traveling in opposite directions within a mixed nerve are traveling along different axons.

Classification based on origin

Based on their origin along the CNS, nerves are either *cranial nerves* or *spinal nerves*. Cranial nerves connect to the brain, while spinal nerves attach to the spinal cord by way of spinal roots (described shortly).

CRANIAL NERVES

Cranial nerves are nerves that arise from the inferior surface of the brain, and include twelve pairs (one nerve on each side of the brain's midline). All of these nerves, except one pair, the vagus nerves, innervate structures in the head and neck. Most cranial nerves are mixed nerves, and some conduct both somatic and autonomic impulses. Some cranial nerves contain mostly motor axons but also contain a few sensory axons that conduct impulses from *proprioceptors* (stretch receptors in muscles). Since sensory axons are so few in these particular "mixed" nerves, we will say the nerves are *primarily* motor nerves.

Neurologists use Roman numerals to number the cranial nerves, with the lower numbers being more anterior and superior to the others. The cranial nerves are as follows:

I: **Olfactory** (ŌL-fak-to-rē; *olfact*, smell): the first pair of cranial nerves is actually a number of very short nerves that pass through the *olfactory foramina* of the ethmoid bone on either side of the nasal septum. These are sensory nerves, which conduct impulses for smell from sensory receptors in the olfactory epithelium to the olfactory bulbs of the brain. The olfactory epithelium is a mucous membrane located in the superior portion of the nasal cavity. The olfactory bulbs are two knob-like structures that rest on the cribriform plate of the ethmoid bone, just on either side of the crista galli.

II: **Optic** (OP-tik; "eye"): the second pair of cranial nerves arises from the posterior surface of the eyeballs and passes through the *optic canals*. They are sensory nerves that conduct impulses from the light-sensitive regions of the eyeball to the optic chiasma, which is an X-shaped structure on the inferior surface of the brain. Impulses traveling through the optic nerves are necessary for vision.

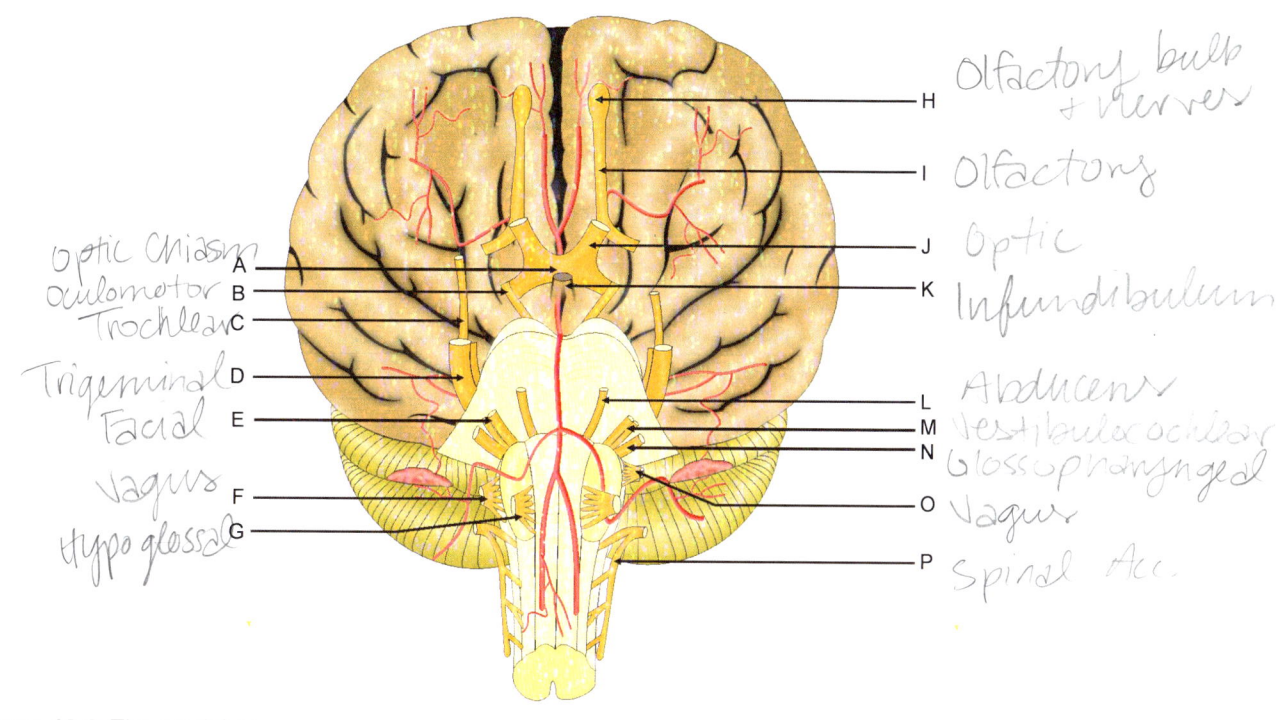

PERIPHERAL NERVOUS SYSTEM (PART 1) NERVES AND SOMATIC REFLEXES

Figure 18-2. The cranial nerves

Labels (handwritten):
- A: Optic Chiasm
- B: Oculomotor
- C: Trochlear
- D: Trigeminal
- E: Facial
- F: Vagus
- G: Hypoglossal
- H: Olfactory bulb + nerves
- I: Olfactory
- J: Optic
- K: Infundibulum
- L: Abducens
- M: Vestibulocochlear
- N: Glossopharyngeal
- O: Vagus
- P: Spinal Acc.

III: Oculomotor (ok-ū-lō-MŌ-tor; *oculo*, eye; *motor*, movement): the third pair of cranial nerves arises from the midbrain and passes through the superior orbital fissure. They are primarily motor nerves that conduct impulses to most of the *extrinsic* eye muscles, which attach to the outside of the eyeballs, and all *intrinsic* eye muscles, which are located inside the eyeball. The extrinsic eye muscles move the eyeball so that a person can look at different objects without moving the head. The intrinsic eye muscles control the diameter of the pupil and change the shape of the eye's internal lens so that a person can focus clearly on objects at different distances.

IV: Trochlear (TRŌK-lē-ar; *trochea*, pulley): the fourth pair of cranial nerves arises from the midbrain and passes through the *superior orbital fissure*. These are primarily motor nerves that stimulate the superior oblique eye muscle, causing the eyeball to point inferiorly and laterally. The nerve gets its name because the muscle it innervates passes through a trochlea (pulley-like structure) on the medial side of the orbit.

V: Trigeminal (trī-JEM-i-nal; "threefold"): the fifth pair of cranial nerves arises from the pons, and it is named for its three major branches. *[superior orbital fissure]* The **ophthalmic branches** (of-THAL-mik; *ophthal*, eye) are sensory nerves that pass through the *superior orbital fissure* and conduct impulses from the upper eyelids, upper part of the nose, lacrimal (tear) glands in the orbit, and anterior part of the scalp. The *[foramen rotundum]* **maxillary branches** (MAKS-i-lar-ē; *maxilla*, jaw) are sensory nerves that pass through the *foramen rotundum* and conduct impulses from the lining of the nasal cavity, palate (roof of mouth), upper teeth, and skin of the lower eyelid, cheek, and upper lip. The **mandibular branches** (man-DIB-ū-lar; *mandib*, jaw) are *[foramen ovale]* mixed nerves that pass through the *foramen ovale*. They conduct sensory impulses from the tongue (but not its taste buds), the lower teeth, scalp in the temple regions and skin of the chin. They conduct motor impulses to muscles involved in moving the lower jaw for chewing.

VI: **Abducens** (ab-DŪ-senz; *abduct*, take away): the sixth pair of cranial nerves arises from the pons and passes through the *superior orbital fissure*. They are primarily motor nerves that conduct impulses to the *lateral rectus* eye muscle, which causes the eyeball to look laterally.

VII: **Facial**: the seventh pair of cranial nerves arises from the pons and passes through the *stylomastoid foramen*. The facial nerves are *mixed*. They conduct sensory impulses from taste buds on the anterior two-thirds of the tongue, and conduct motor impulses to muscles of the face, lacrimal glands, most salivary glands (except the largest), and mucous glands in the lining of the nasal cavity.

VIII: **Vestibulocochlear** (ves-TIB-ū-lō-KOK-lē-ar): the eighth pair of cranial nerves, formerly called the *acoustic* or *auditory* nerves, arises from the junction between the pons and medulla oblongata and passes through the *internal auditory meatus*. These are sensory nerves, which conduct impulses from the inner ear. The inner ear includes two parts: (1) the vestibule, which contains receptors to detecting body position so that the brain can make adjustments in skeletal muscle tension to maintain balance and equilibrium for maintaining balance; and (2) the cochlea, which contains receptors for hearing.

IX: **Glossopharyngeal** (glos-sō-fa-RIN-jē-al; *gloss*, tongue; *pharynx*, throat): the ninth pair of cranial nerves is *mixed* and arises from the medulla oblongata and passes through the *jugular foramen*. These nerves conduct sensory impulses from taste buds on the posterior one-third of the tongue, and from chemoreceptors and baroreceptors in the neck's carotid arteries. Chemoreceptors respond to different chemicals in the blood, while baroreceptors respond to vessel stretch due to blood pressure. These nerves conduct motor impulses to skeletal muscles in the pharynx for swallowing movements and to the largest salivary glands (parotid glands).

X: **Vagus** (VĀ-gus; "vagabond" or "wanderer"): the tenth pair of cranial nerves arises from the medulla oblongata and passes through the *jugular foramen*. These are *mixed* nerves and the only cranial nerves that extend below the neck. They conduct sensory impulses from external ear, throat, esophagus, heart, lungs, abdominal visceral organs, baroreceptors in the aorta (large artery exiting the heart), and chemoreceptors in the aorta and carotid arteries. They conduct motor impulses to the heart and lungs for regulating breathing and heart rates, and to the abdominal visceral organs to regulate digestive and urinary system activity.

XI: **Accessory**: the eleventh pair of cranial nerves, also called the *spinal accessory* nerves, is the only cranial nerve pair that arises partly from the spinal cord; it also connects to the medulla oblongata and passes through the *jugular foramen*. These nerves are primarily motor nerves that conduct impulses to muscles of the throat, neck, and upper back.

XII: **Hypoglossal** (hī-pō-GLOS-al): the twelfth pair of cranial nerves arises from the medulla oblongata and passes through the *hypoglossal canal*. They are motor nerves that conduct impulses to the tongue to change its shape and position during chewing and talking.

> **Note**: Use the following to remember the order of the cranial nerves: "**O**n **O**ld **O**lympus **T**owering **T**ops, **A** **F**inn **V**ery **G**ladly **V**iewed **S**ome **H**ops." Use the following to remember the primary function of each pair of cranial nerves in their proper order; S=sensory; M=motor; B=both (mixed): **S**ister **S**ays **M**arry **M**oney **B**ut **M**y **B**rother **S**ays **B**ad **B**oys **M**arry **M**oney.

SPINAL ROOTS

The **spinal roots** connect the spinal cord to a spinal nerve and include *dorsal* and *ventral* roots (Figure 18-3).

The **dorsal (posterior) roots** connect to the posterior-lateral sides of the spinal cord and contain

PERIPHERAL NERVOUS SYSTEM (PART 1) NERVES AND SOMATIC REFLEXES

Figure 18-3. Spinal roots, spinal nerves, and rami

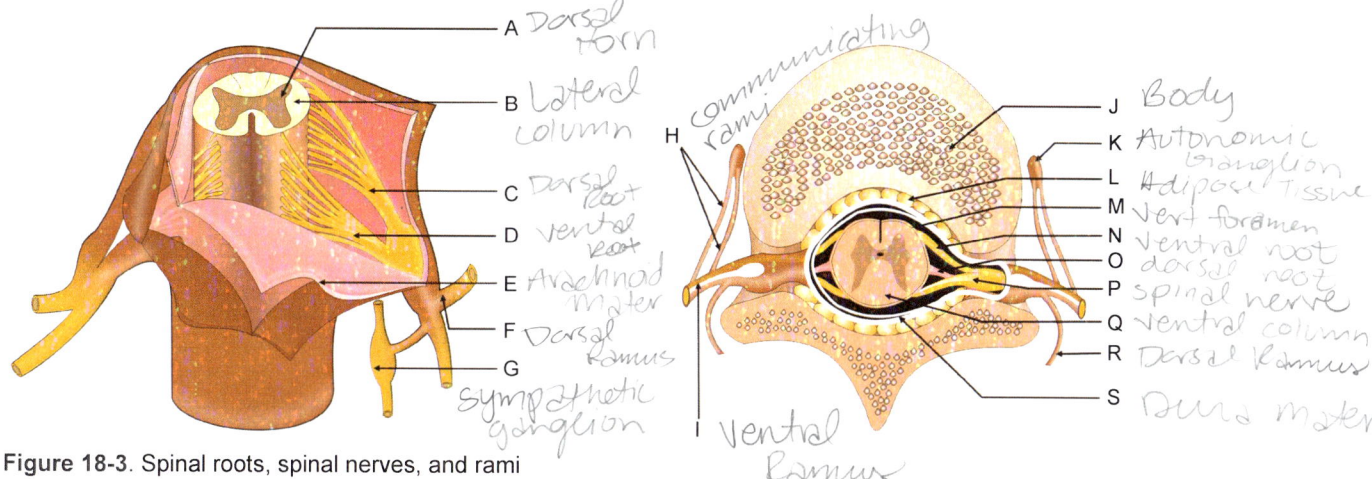

only *axons of sensory neurons*. The cell bodies of sensory neurons exist within a swollen region called the **dorsal root ganglion**, located on the dorsal root. The **ventral (anterior) roots** connect to the anterior-lateral sides of the cord and contain only *axons of motor neurons*. There are no neuron cell bodies in the ventral root. Most spinal roots are very short, extending no farther out than the lateral end of a vertebra's transverse process. However, roots that attach to the spinal cord in the lumbar region are extremely long, some of which extend inferiorly through the vertebral foramina all the way to the coccyx. This mass of long spinal roots in the section of the vertebral column below the conus medullaris (inferior end of the spinal cord) is called the **cauda equina** (KAW-da, "tail"; ē-KWĪ-na; "horse"), so named for its horse tail appearance. Nerve roots give rise to spinal nerves at different levels of the vertebral column and exit the column through *intervertebral foramina*.

SPINAL NERVES

The dorsal and ventral roots unite laterally to form a very short **spinal nerve**, which is only about 2 cm long. The spinal nerve then extends peripherally from the spinal cord and divides into a dorsal and ventral ramus (described below). There are 31 pairs of spinal nerves, and neurologists group them based on the region of the spine to which they attach. All spinal nerves are mixed nerves and include eight **cervical** pairs (C_1–C_8), twelve **thoracic** pairs (T_1–T_{12}), five **lumbar** pairs (L_1–L_5), five **sacral** pairs (S_1–S_5), and one **coccygeal** pair (C_0).

RAMI, PLEXUSES, and PERIPHERAL NERVES

A few centimeters lateral to the vertebral column, a spinal nerve branches into a **dorsal ramus** (RĀ-mus; "branch") and **ventral ramus**. Along most of the vertebral column (but not in the thoracic region), ventral rami (RĀ mī) arising from several levels along the spinal cord come together to form braid-like networks called plexuses (PLEK-sus-ez; "braids"). In turn, plexuses give rise to **peripheral nerves**, which innervate muscles, glands, skin, and other structures. There are four pairs of plexuses (one plexus of each pair is on opposite sides of the body) (Figure 18-4).

Cervical plexuses

The cervical plexuses arise from spinal segments C_1–C_5, and give rise to five major pairs of nerves:

- **Auricular nerves** (aw-RIK-ū-lar; *auricle*, ear) innervate the external ear.
- **Occipital nerves** (ok-SIP-i-tul; *occip*, back of head) innervate the scalp on back of head.
- **Phrenic nerves** (FRE-nik; *phren*, diaphragm) innervate the diaphragm, the skeletal muscle separating the thoracic and abdominopelvic cavities.
- **Cervical nerves** innervate muscles of neck and upper back.
- **Suprascapular nerves** innervate muscles of upper back, shoulder, and chest.

Table 18-1. Summary of the cranial nerves

Name of Nerve Pair	Type*	Major Associated Functions	Problems with Nerve
I: Olfactory	Sensory	Smell	Inability to smell or identify odors
II: Optic	Sensory	Vision	Blindness, blurred vision, decreased field of vision
III: Oculomotor	Motor	Most eye movements, pupil and lens changes for image focusing; raising eyelids	Blurred vision; pupil problems; inability to direct eyes; droopy eyelid
IV: Trochlear	Motor	Looking down and to side	Can't direct eyes; causes double vision
V: Trigeminal	Mixed		
Ophthalmic branch	Sensory	Sensing touch, pain, temperature in regions listed	Loss of sensitivity in regions listed
Maxillary branch	Sensory	Sensing touch, pain, temperature in regions listed	Loss of sensitivity in regions listed
Mandibular branch	Motor	Sensing touch, pain, temperature in regions listed; chewing motions	Loss of sensitivity in regions listed; can't move jaw adequately
VI: Abducens	Motor	Looking laterally	Can't look laterally
VII: Facial	Mixed	Taste (except bitter) Facial expressions, producing tears and saliva	Loss of certain tastes, decreased saliva secretion; can't close eyes; *Bell's Palsy* produces facial paralysis
VIII: Vestibulocochlear	Sensory	Hearing & equilibrium	Impaired hearing; loss of balance
IX: Glossopharyngeal	Mixed	Bitter taste; sensing touch, pain, temperature in regions listed; monitoring blood pressure and blood chemistry Swallowing; saliva secretion	Loss of bitter taste; impaired ability to regulate blood pressure and chemistry; difficulty swallowing; decreased saliva secretion
X: Vagus	Mixed	Sensing touch, pain, temperature in regions listed; monitoring blood pressure and chemistry; monitoring activity of visceral organs; regulation of muscle contractions in pharynx, neck, and visceral organs of thorax and abdomen; secretion of enzymes, hormones, and other substances from visceral organs	Loss of sensitivity in regions listed; impaired ability to control digestion and heart rate
XI: Accessory	Motor	Turning head and raising shoulders	Trouble turning head or shoulders
XII: Hypoglossal	Motor	Moves tongue	Can't move tongue properly; affects chewing, talking, and swallowing

Brachial plexuses

The brachial plexuses arise from spinal segments C_4-T_1, and give rise to five major pairs of nerves (Figure 18-5):

- **Axillary nerves** (AKS-i-lar-ē; "armpit") innervate the deltoid and teres minor muscles.

- **Median nerves** innervate the flexor muscles in the forearm and skin of the palm; inflammation of this nerve is responsible for *carpal tunnel syndrome*.

- **Musculocutaneous nerves** (MUS-kū-lō-kū-TĀN-ē-us; *musculo*, muscle; *cutan*, skin) innervate

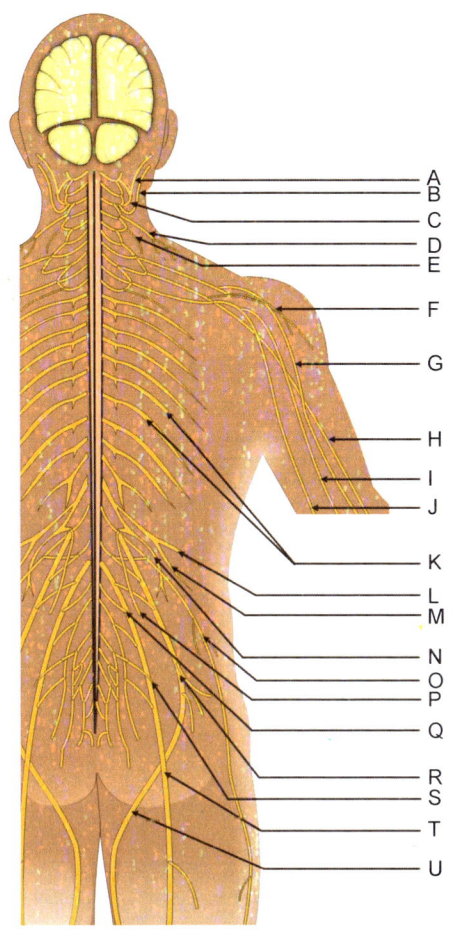

PERIPHERAL NERVOUS SYSTEM (PART 1) NERVES AND SOMATIC REFLEXES

343

Figure 18-4. Spinal plexuses and selected nerves

the flexor muscles in arm and the skin of the lateral forearm.

- **Radial nerves** innervate the extensor muscles and skin of the arm and forearm.
- **Ulnar nerves** innervate the skin of the medial forearm; called the "funny bone" because of the tingling arm sensation one gets after hitting it.

Lumbar plexuses

The lumbar plexuses arise from spinal segments T_{12}-L_4, and gives rise to two major pairs of nerves (Figure 18-6):

- **Femoral nerves** innervate the quadriceps muscles of the thigh and the skin on medial aspect of the leg.
- **Obturator nerves** innervate the adductors in the thigh and the skin on medial aspect of the thigh.

Sacral plexuses

The sacral plexuses arise from spinal segments L4-S4, and gives rise to several nerves:

- **Sciatic nerves** (sī-AT-ik; "hip") are the largest nerves in the body. Each sciatic nerve is actually two nerves: the *tibial* nerve innervates muscles and skin along the medial portion of the leg, and the *fibular nerve* innervates muscles and skin along the lateral portion of the leg.
- **Gluteal nerves** (GLŪ-tē-al; "buttock") innervate the buttocks muscles.
- **Pudendal nerves** (pū-DEN-dal; "feel ashamed") innervate the external genitalia (sex organs) and the muscles and skin of the lower pelvis.

There are no plexuses in the thoracic region. Instead, ventral rami in this region become *intercostals nerves* that innervate skin of the thorax and intercostal muscles between the ribs.

REFLEXES

A **reflex** is a rapid, involuntary response to a stimulus. Some reflexes are **somatic reflexes** that involve "voluntary" skeletal muscles. Reflexes involving cardiac and smooth muscle are **visceral (autonomic) reflexes.** You will learn about somatic reflexes in this chapter and visceral reflexes in the next chapter. An example of a somatic reflex is the *knee-jerk reflex* that occurs when a physician taps your knee with a percussion hammer. Jerking your hand away from a hot stove is another example. The pathway of impulses in a basic reflex occurs in a **reflex arc**, and it includes a receptor, sensory (afferent) neuron, integration center (brain or spinal cord), motor (efferent) neuron, and effector (muscle) (Figure 18-7).

Reflexes that use the spinal cord as the integration center are called **spinal reflexes**. A spinal reflex that does not utilize an association neuron within the spinal cord is a *monosynaptic reflex arc*; that is, the sensory neuron synapses directly with the motor neuron in the spinal cord. In a *polysynaptic reflex arc*, the impulses pass through at least one association neuron in the spinal cord.

CHAPTER 18

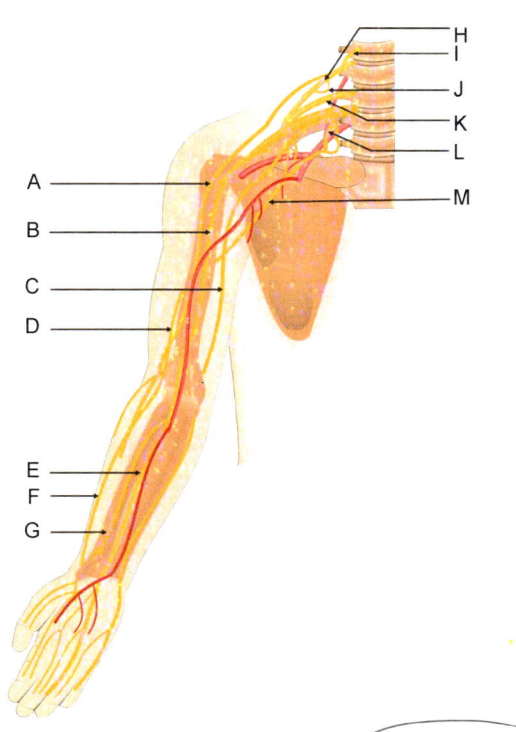

Figure 18-5: Nerves from the brachial plexus

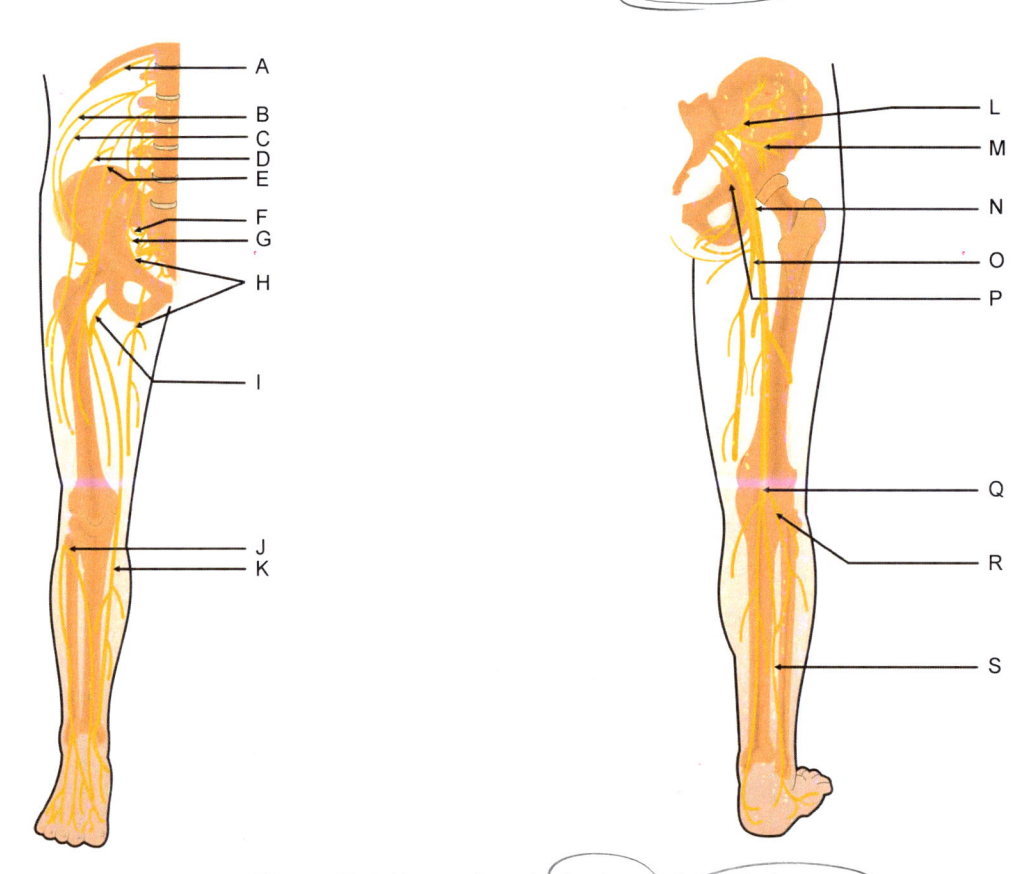

Figure 18-6. Nerves from the lumbar and sacral plexuses

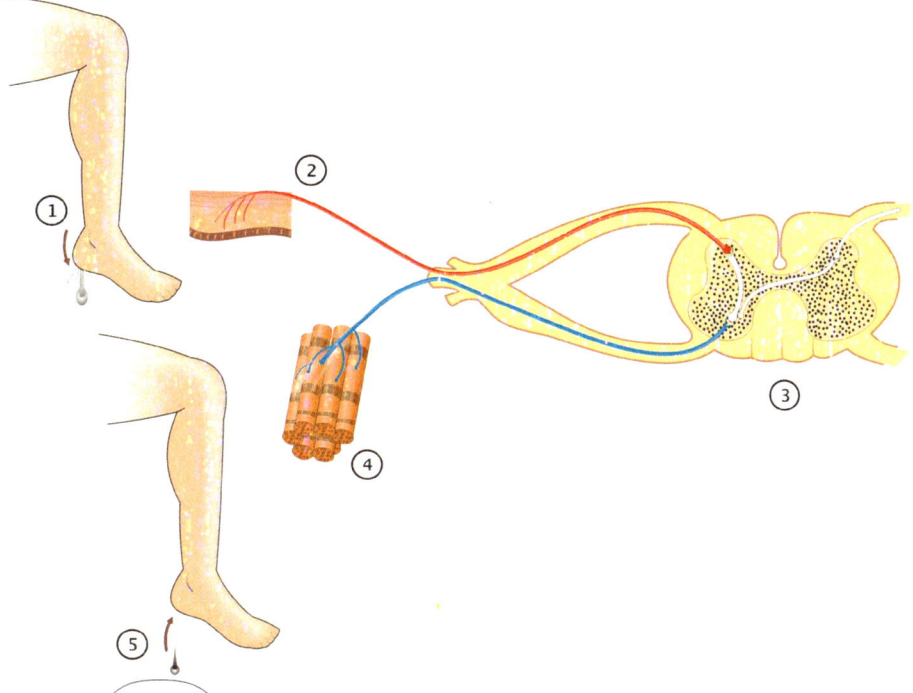

PERIPHERAL NERVOUS SYSTEM (PART 1) NERVES AND SOMATIC REFLEXES

Figure 18-7. Parts of a reflex arc

SOMATIC REFLEXES

There are three types of somatic reflexes: *stretch*, *tendon*, and *flexor* (withdrawal) reflexes.

Stretch Reflex

A stretch reflex is a monosynaptic reflex in which a *stretched muscle contracts* to help prevent overstretching of the muscle (Figure 18-8). This often works to help a person maintain balance. Modified skeletal myofibers called **muscle spindles** act as the receptors for a stretch reflex. When a muscle stretches, its muscle spindles depolarize and initiate action potentials on sensory neurons wrapped around the spindle. The sensory neuron, in turn, conducts the impulse into the spinal cord and transmits it to motor neurons that innervate the stretched muscle. In response, the motor neurons send efferent impulses to the stretched muscle, causing it to contract.

At the same time the stretched muscle contracts as part of the stretch reflex, its antagonistic muscle relaxes. While this action is not necessary for the stretch reflex, it ensures that the stretched muscle will be able to contract and not have to work against a contraction from the antagonistic muscle. During the stretch reflex,

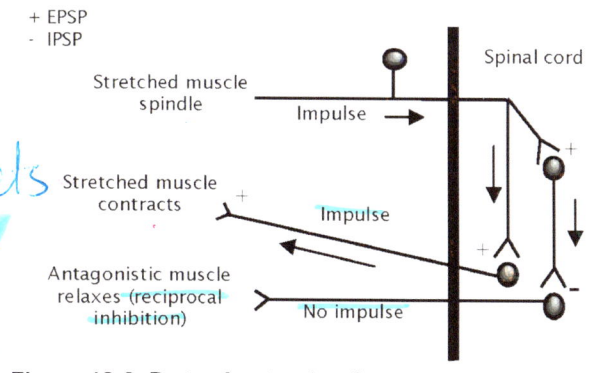

Figure 18-8. Parts of a stretch reflex

the sensory neuron transmitting the impulse from the muscle spindles to the spinal cord stimulates association neurons that inhibit motor neurons of the antagonistic muscles; consequently, the antagonistic muscle relaxes. The phenomenon is **reciprocal inhibition** of the antagonistic muscle and increases the efficiency of the stretch reflex.

Tendon Reflex

The **tendon reflex** is a polysynaptic reflex in which a *contracted muscle relaxes* in response to excessive stretch in its tendon (Figure 18-9). The excessive stretch of the tendon could be the result of muscle contraction. The tendon reflex is important in preventing damage to a muscle or its tendons. The receptor for this reflex is a **Golgi tendon organ**, which is a group of specialized neuron endings located within the tendon.

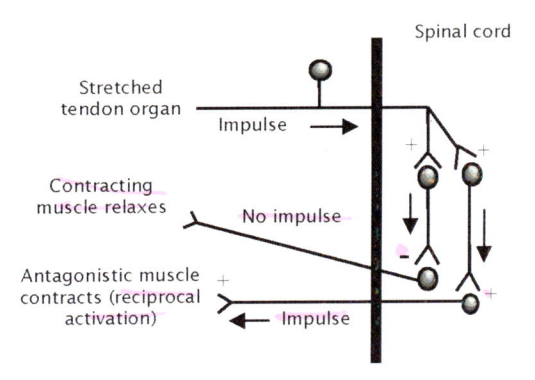

Figure 18-9. Parts of a tendon reflex

When excessive stretch of the tendon occurs, the tendon organs initiate sensory neuron impulses that travel to the spinal cord. In the cord, the sensory neuron stimulates an association neuron that hyperpolarizes (inhibits) motor neurons of the contracted muscle. As a result, impulses to the contracted muscle cease and the muscle relaxes. To ensure the efficiency of the tendon reflex, impulses from the sensory neurons stimulate association neurons that, in turn, stimulate motor neurons of the antagonistic muscle, causing this muscle to contract. This is **reciprocal activation** of the antagonist muscle.

Flexor (Withdrawal) Reflex

The **flexor (withdrawal) reflex** is a polysynaptic reflex in which a flexor typically contracts in response to a pain

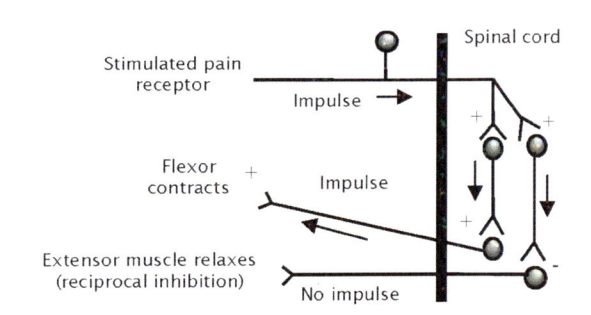

Figure 18-10. Parts of a withdrawal reflex

stimulus. An example is the reflex you might expect if you step on a tack. Suppose you step on a tack with the left foot. A pain receptor in the left foot depolarizes and initiates impulses that move along sensory axons into the spinal cord. In the cord, the sensory neuron stimulates association neurons that, in turn, stimulate motor neurons for flexor muscles of the left thigh. As a result, the left leg flexes, which pulls the left foot away from the pain stimulus. During this time, reciprocal inhibition occurs in the extensor muscles of the left thigh.

During a flexor reflex, impulses can pass across the spinal cord and stimulate *extensor* muscles on the opposite side of the body; this is a **crossed-extensor reflex**. In our example, sensory impulses entering the spinal cord on the left side will stimulate motor neurons for extensor muscles in the right thigh, causing them to contract. Therefore, when the person lifts the left foot off the tack, the right leg extends to prevent the person from falling. At the same time, the sensory neuron stimulates an association neuron that inhibits the motor neurons leading to the flexor muscles on the right side. In this way, reciprocal inhibition of flexor muscles in the right thigh prevents the right leg from flexing.

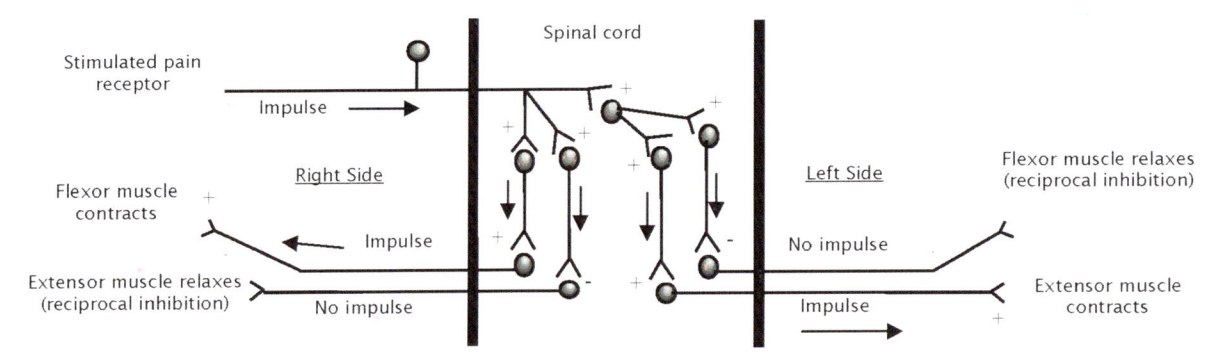

Figure 18-11. Parts of a crossed-extensor reflex

TOPICS TO KNOW FOR CHAPTER 18 (PERIPHERAL NERVOUS SYSTEM (PART 1): NERVES AND SOMATIC REFLEXES)

- auricular nerves
- axillary nerves
- baroreceptors
- brachial plexuses
- carpal tunnel syndrome
- cauda equine
- cervical nerves (C1 C8)
- cervical plexuses
- chemoreceptors
- classification of nerves
- CN I: olfactory
- CN II: optic
- CN III: oculomotor
- CN IV: trochlear
- CN V: trigeminal
- CN VI: abducens
- CN VII: facial
- CN VIII: vestibulocochlear
- CN IX: glossopharyngeal
- CN X: vagus
- CN XI: accessory
- CN XII: hypoglossal
- coccygeal nerve (C0)
- cochlea
- cranial nerves
- crossed-extensor reflex
- dorsal (posterior) roots
- dorsal ramus
- dorsal root ganglion
- endoneurium
- epineurium
- extrinsic eye muscles
- fascicles
- femoral nerves
- fibular nerve
- flexor (withdrawal) reflex
- foramen ovale
- foramen rotundum
- gluteal nerves
- Golgi tendon organ
- hypoglossal canal
- innervation
- intercostals nerves
- internal auditory meatus
- intervertebral foramina
- intrinsic eye muscles
- IV: trochlear
- IX: glossopharyngeal
- jugular foramen
- knee-jerk reflex
- lumbar nerves (L1–L5)
- lumbar plexuses
- mandibular branches
- maxillary branches
- median nerves
- mixed nerves
- motor nerves
- muscle spindles
- musculocutaneous nerves
- nerve
- obturator nerves
- occipital nerves
- olfactory foramina
- ophthalmic branches
- optic canals
- perineurium
- peripheral nerves
- peripheral nervous system
- phrenic nerves
- plexuses
- polysynaptic reflex arc
- pudendal nerves
- radial nerves
- reciprocal activation
- reciprocal inhibition
- reflex
- reflex arc
- sacral nerves (S1–S5)
- sacral plexuses
- sciatic nerves
- sensory nerves
- somatic reflexes
- spinal nerve
- spinal reflexes
- spinal roots
- stretch reflex
- stylomastoid foramen
- superior orbital fissure
- suprascapular nerves
- tendon reflex
- thoracic nerves (T1–T12)
- tibial nerves
- ulnar nerves
- ventral (anterior) roots
- ventral ramus
- vestibule
- visceral (autonomic) reflex

CHAPTER 19

Peripheral Nervous System (Part 2): The Autonomic Nervous System

AUTONOMIC NERVOUS SYSTEM

The **autonomic nervous system (ANS)** is a subdivision of the efferent (motor) division of the peripheral nervous system (PNS), and includes the **sympathetic** (sim-pa-THET-ik; *sympatho*, feel suffering with) and **parasympathetic** (par-a-sim-pa-THET-ik; *para*, alongside) divisions. The effectors stimulated by the ANS are glands, smooth muscle, and cardiac muscle. Motor impulses from the ANS travel through ganglia in the PNS on their way to these effectors (Figure 19-1).

In all cases except one, the ANS impulse passes through two motor neurons before reaching the effector. The **preganglionic neuron** (prē-gang-lē-ON-ik; *pre*, before) is the motor neuron that conducts the impulse out of the CNS (Figure 19-2). It has a class B axon (thin diameter, but myelinated). The preganglionic neuron synapses with a **postganglionic neuron** (post-gang-lē-ON-ik; *post*, after) inside a ganglion in the PNS. The postganglionic neuron conducts the impulse along a class C axon (thin diameter and unmyelinated) to the effector. The one exception to the "two motor neuron" rule is the stimulation of the adrenal gland. In this case, the adrenal gland receives stimulation from only a "preganglionic" neuron in the sympathetic division.

In some cases, an effector receives impulses from only one division of the ANS, but other effectors receive dual innervation; that is, they receive impulses from the sympathetic and parasympathetic divisions. When an effector is dually innervated, if the effect of one division is *excitation*, the effect of the other division is *inhibition*. Under normal conditions, both divisions of the ANS are active but at different levels. During fight-or-flight situations, the sympathetic division is highly active while the parasympathetic division is less active. In contrast, when the parasympathetic division is most active, the sympathetic division is less active.

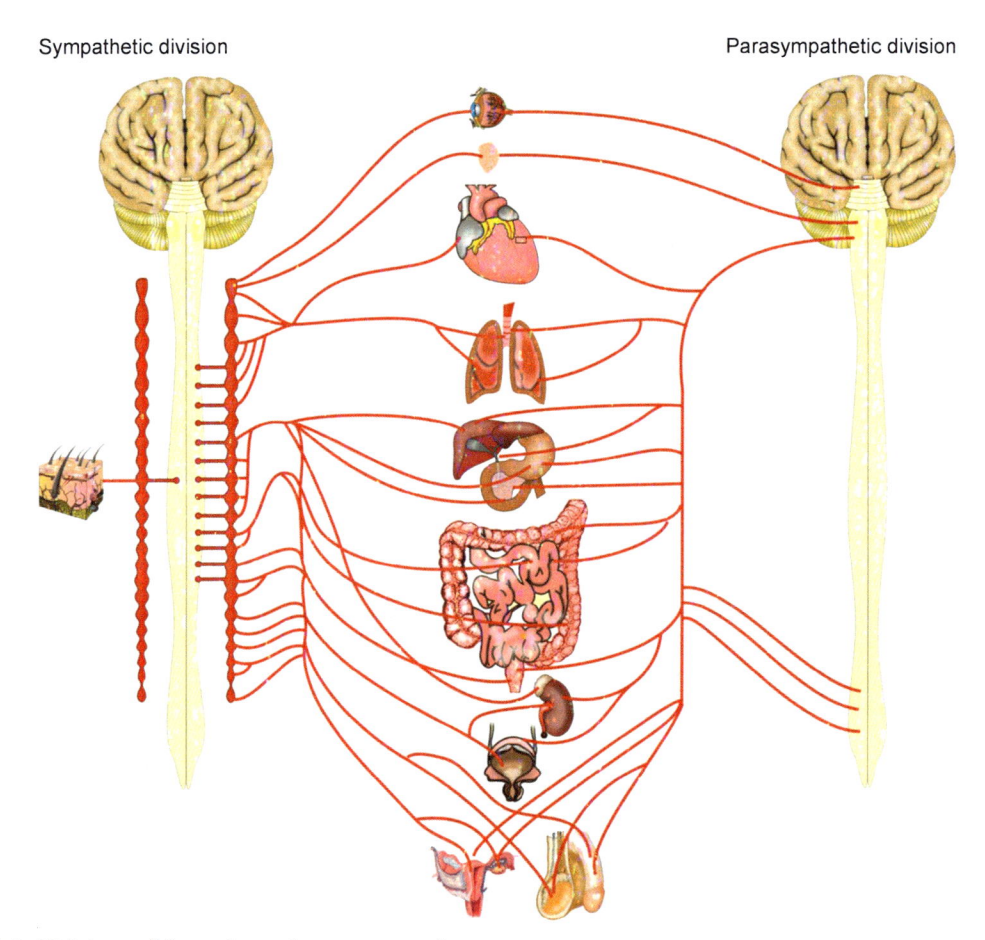

Figure 19-1. Divisions of the autonomic nervous system

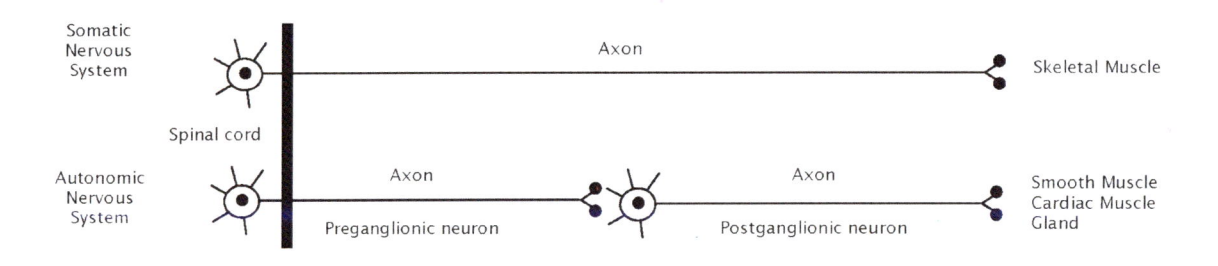

Figure 19-2. Comparison of somatic and autonomic innervation

SYMPATHETIC DIVISION

The **sympathetic division** has two other names based on its major associated functions and the location where its preganglionic neurons exit the dorsal cavity. Functionally, the sympathetic system is the nervous system's *fight-or-flight division* because its activity increases during times of physical and emotional stress, including exercise, anxiety, trauma, etc. It is also the *thoracolumbar division* (thor-ak-ō-LUM-bar) because its impulses exit the dorsal cavity only in the thoracic and lumbar regions (Figure 19 3).

The cell bodies of sympathetic, preganglionic neurons reside in the anterior (ventral) horns of the spinal cord. The axons of these neurons exit the cord

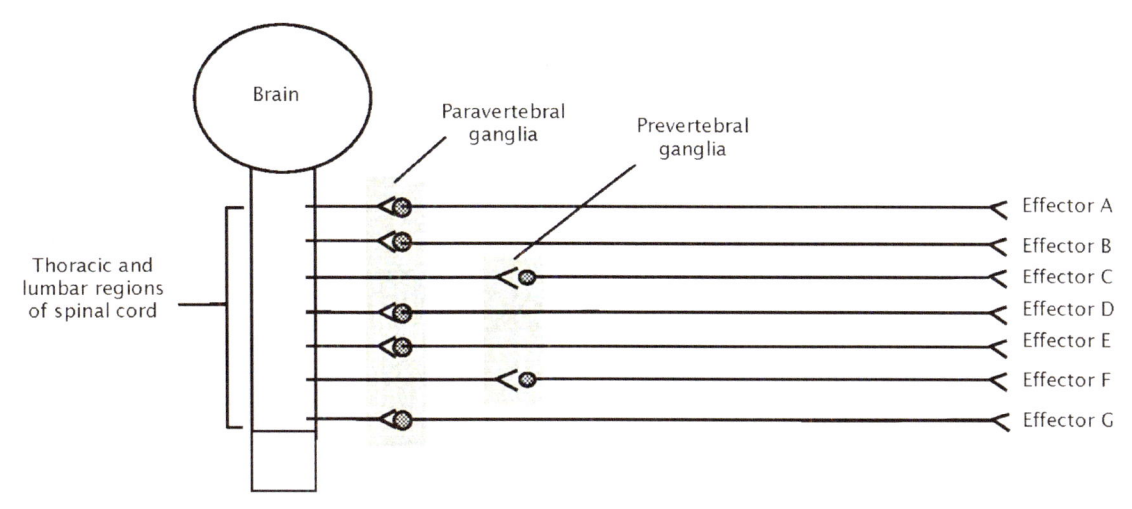

Figure 19-3. Pathways for sympathetic impulses

through thoracic or lumbar spinal nerves and pass through **paravertebral ganglia** (para-VER-te-bral), so-named because they are located alongside the vertebrae. There are 23 paravertebral ganglia aligned like a "chain of beads" on each side of the vertebral column. A preganglionic axon may synapse with a postganglionic neuron in a paravertebral ganglion, or it may pass through the paravertebral ganglia and synapse in a **prevertebral ganglion** (prē-VER-te-bral), so-named because it is anterior to (*pre-*, before) the vertebrae. Whether or not a sympathetic impulse passes through more than one paravertebral or prevertebral ganglion, it will pass along no more than two axons before reaching its effector.

The axons of preganglionic neurons in the sympathetic system are relatively short, while the postganglionic fibers are long. All preganglionic neurons in the sympathetic division release the neurotransmitter **acetylcholine** (**Ach**; as-e-til-KŌ-lēn) from their axon terminals. *Most* postganglionic neurons in this division release the neurotransmitter **norepinephrine** (**NE**; nōr-ep-i-NEF-rin), which is a catecholamine chemical described in chapter 3. On the other hand, a few postganglionic neurons in the sympathetic division release Ach onto their effectors. Effectors stimulated by Ach from sympathetic neurons include the *sweat glands*, *some blood vessels* coursing through skeletal muscles, and the *adrenal medulla* (the inner core part of the adrenal gland). However, the adrenal gland receives Ach stimulation directly from a preganglionic neuron. In response, the adrenal gland secretes the hormones epinephrine and norepinephrine; thus, the adrenal gland functions much like a typical postganglionic neuron in the sympathetic division. Epinephrine and norepinephrine usually promote similar effects on the same target organs.

It is often important for autonomic signals to reach a great number of effectors in a short amount of time. To facilitate this, one preganglionic neuron may synapse with more than one postganglionic neuron within a ganglion; this pattern of impulse flow is called **divergence** (dī-VER-jens) (Figure 19-4). While divergence is a part of both divisions of the ANS, it is more extensive and common in the sympathetic division. Divergence allows sympathetic impulses to "spread out" to numerous effectors more rapidly, which is an obvious advantage when one considers certain fight-or-flight responses.

PARASYMPATHETIC DIVISION

Like the sympathetic division, the **parasympathetic division** has two other names based on its major associated functions and the location where its preganglionic neurons exit the dorsal cavity. Functionally, the parasympathetic system is the nervous system's *rest-and-digest division* because its activity increases during times of rest, relaxation, and digestion. It is also the *craniosacral division* (krā-nē-ō-SĀ-kral) because its impulses exit the dorsal cavity only in the cranium (which houses the brain) and the sacral regions (Figure 19-5).

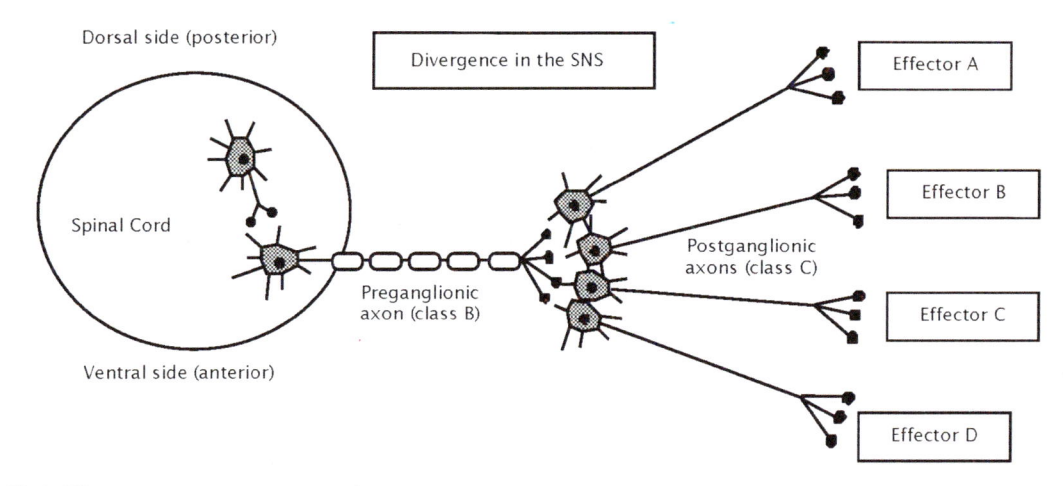

Figure 19-4. Divergence among autonomic neurons

The cell bodies of parasympathetic preganglionic neurons reside in gray matter of the brain and anterior horns of the spinal cord. Preganglionic fibers exit the dorsal cavity and pass through ganglia located close to the target organ (effector). Compared to the sympathetic division, the axons of the preganglionic neurons in the parasympathetic division are relatively long, while the postganglionic axons are short. All neurons (preganglionic and postganglionic) in the parasympathetic division release **acetylcholine** from their axon terminals.

RECEPTORS FOR ANS NEUROTRANSMITTERS

To be stimulated by the ANS, an effector must display receptors to which the ANS neurotransmitter can attach. Two major groups of receptors respond to ANS neurotransmitters: cholinergic and adrenergic receptors.

Cholinergic Receptors

Membrane receptors that bind Ach are called **cholinergic receptors** (kō-lin-ER-jik). There are two major classes of cholinergic receptors: *nicotinic* and *muscarinic*.

- **Nicotinic receptors** (nik-o-TIN-ik) bind Ach and nicotine (a chemical found in cigarette smoke). Nicotinic receptors are displayed on (1) all postganglionic neurons in the sympathetic and parasympathetic divisions, (2) cells in the adrenal medulla (bind Ach released from sympathetic "preganglionic" neurons), and (3) skeletal muscle

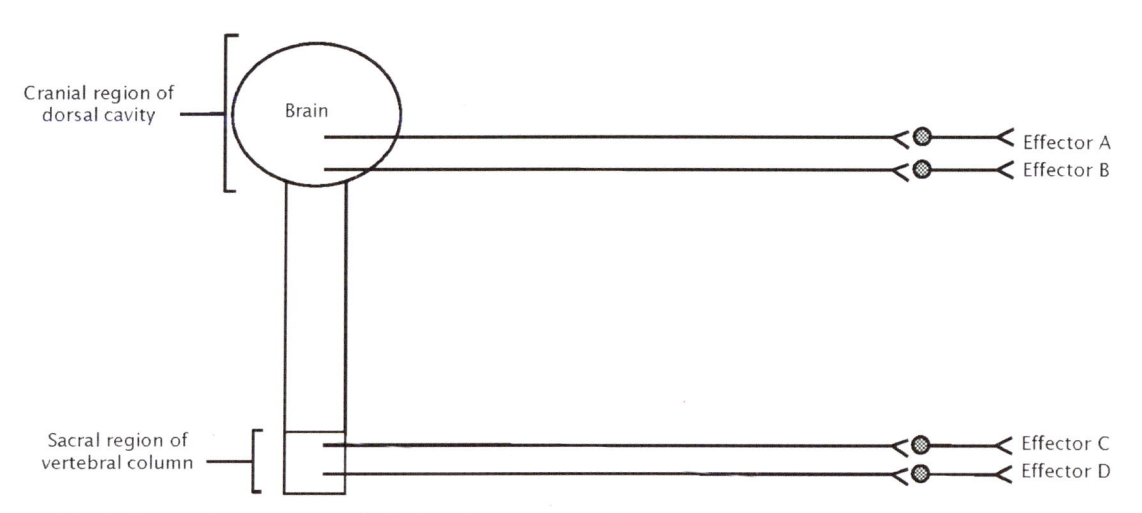

Figure 19-5. Pathways for parasympathetic impulses

cells, which bind Ach released from *somatic* motor neurons, not from autonomic neurons.

- **Muscarinic receptors** (mus-ka-RIN-ik) bind Ach and *muscarine* (MUS-ka-rēn), a chemical produced in a certain species of mushroom. Muscarinic receptors are displayed on all muscles and glands stimulated by the parasympathetic division. In addition, sweat glands and some blood vessels in skeletal muscles display muscarinic receptors that bind Ach released from postganglionic neurons of the sympathetic division.

While Ach can bind to both nicotinic and muscarinic receptors, nicotine cannot bind to muscarinic receptors, and muscarine cannot bind to nicotinic receptors. Certain drugs may bind to only one type of cholinergic receptor, or it may bind to both types. In this way, specific drugs can have either local effects or affect structures throughout the body. Nicotine at low doses is excitatory to postganglionic neurons and neuromuscular junctions of muscle fibers that bind Ach; however, at high doses, nicotine can inhibit these structures.

Adrenergic Receptors

The membrane-bound receptors that bind norepinephrine and epinephrine are called **adrenergic receptors** (ad-re-NER-jik), so named for *adrenaline* (a-DREN-a-lin, the former name for epinephrine). There are two major classes of adrenergic receptors: *alpha* (α) and *beta* (β). Norepinephrine (NE) normally binds more often to α receptors than to β receptors, while epinephrine (E) binds to α and β receptors.

- **Alpha (α) receptors** are the most common adrenergic receptor and are displayed on most cells in the body except cardiac muscle cells. There are two subclasses of alpha receptors: $α_1$ and $α_2$. Binding of NE to $α_1$ receptors usually results in *excitation* of the effector, whereas binding of NE to $α_2$ receptors usually results in *inhibition* of the effector.
- **Beta (β) receptors** are displayed on cardiac, smooth, and skeletal muscle cells and cells in the liver, kidneys, and adipose tissue. There are three classes of beta receptors:
  - $β_1$ **receptors** are found on the cardiac muscle cells, liver cells, and kidney cells. The binding of epinephrine to $β_1$ receptors usually results in *excitation*. $β_1$ receptors are also found on skeletal muscle cells but binding of E on these cells does not cause depolarization; instead, it causes an increase in cellular metabolism.
  - $β_2$ **receptors** are found on smooth muscle cells located in (1) blood vessels of the heart and skeletal muscles, (2) walls of bronchioles—air passageways in the lungs, and (3) walls of the intestine. Binding of E with $β_2$ receptors causes *inhibition*, or relaxation of smooth muscle in the locations listed. As a result, E causes vasodilation in the heart and skeletal muscles, dilation of bronchioles, and relaxation of intestines.
  - $β_3$ **receptors** are found on adipocytes (fat cells) in adipose tissue. Binding of E to these receptors results in *excitation*, whereby the adipocytes break down their stored lipids (a process called *lipolysis*) and release fatty acids into the blood.

> **Note**: To associate $α_1$ and $β_1$ receptors with excitation, and to associate $α_2$ and $β_2$ receptors with inhibition, remember that numerically, 1 comes before 2, and alphabetically excitation comes before inhibition.

The effects of different neurotransmitters on selected effectors are summarized in Table 19-1.

CONTROL OF THE ANS

The diencephalon and brain stem control various aspects of the ANS. Involuntary control centers involving heart regulation, urination, defecation, pupil diameter, and breathing exist in the medulla and pons. The hypothalamus regulates aspects of the sympathetic and parasympathetic divisions. About three-fourths of all parasympathetic activities involve the paired vagus nerves (cranial nerve X), which exit from the medulla oblongata.

VISCERAL (AUTONOMIC) REFLEXES

Visceral reflexes involve smooth and cardiac muscle tissues. Moreover, the impulse pathway in a visceral reflex arc follows the same general pattern as that in somatic arcs with one major exception: a visceral reflex arc always involves two motor neurons (a preganglionic neuron and a postganglionic neuron).

Table 19-1. Effects of sympathetic and parasympathetic neurotransmitters on selected effectors

SYMPATHETIC stimulation			
Target Organ	**Neurotransmitter**	**Receptor**	**Effect**
Adipose tissue	NE	Beta	Lipolysis (lipid breakdown)
Adrenal medulla	**Ach***	**Nicotinic**	Release of epinephrine and NE
Arrector pili muscles	NE	Alpha	Contraction (causes "goosebumps")
Blood vessels in the digestive system	NE	Alpha	Vasoconstriction
Blood vessels in the heart	NE	Beta	Vasodilation
Blood vessels in the kidneys	NE	Beta	Vasoconstriction
Blood vessels in the sex organs	NE	Alpha	Vasoconstriction (loss of erection)
Blood vessels in the skeletal muscles	**Ach****	**Muscarinic**	Vasodilation
Blood vessels in the skin	NE	Alpha	Vasoconstriction
Bronchiole tubes in lungs	NE	Beta	Dilation (increased air flow)
Cardiac muscle	NE	Beta	Increased heart rate
Digestive system	NE	Beta	Inhibits activity
Internal urethral sphincter	NE	Alpha	Constricts sphincter (prevents urination)
Iris radial muscle	NE	Alpha	Contraction (causes dilation of pupil)
Sweat glands	**Ach****	**Muscarinic**	Sweat secretion
Urinary bladder	NE	Beta	Relaxes bladder (prevents urination)
PARASYMPATHETIC Stimulation			
Target Organ	**Neurotransmitter**	**Receptor**	**Effect**
Blood vessels in sex organs	Ach	Muscarinic	Vasodilation (causes erection in penis and clitoris)
Bronchiole tubes in lungs	Ach	Muscarinic	Constriction
Cardiac Muscle	Ach	Muscarinic	Decreases heart rate
Digestive system	Ach	Muscarinic	Increases activity
Internal urethral sphincter	Ach	Muscarinic	Relaxation (allows urination)
Iris sphincter muscle	Ach	Muscarinic	Contraction (cause constriction of pupil)
Sex organs	Ach	Muscarinic	Causes erection in penis and clitoris
Tear glands	Ach	Muscarinic	Secretion of tears
Urinary bladder	Ach	Muscarinic	Constriction (promotes urination)

*Released from a "preganglionic" neuron.

**Released from a postganglionic neuron.

TOPICS TO KNOW FOR CHAPTER 19 (AUTONOMIC NERVOUS SYSTEM)

acetylcholine (Ach)
adrenergic receptors
alpha receptors
autonomic nervous system
beta receptors
cholinergic receptors
control of the ANS
craniosacral division
divergence
dual innervation
epinephrine (E)
fight-or-flight division

muscarinic receptors
nicotinic receptors
norepinephrine (NE)
parasympathetic division
parasympathetic stimulation on selected target organs (tables)
paravertebral ganglia
postganglionic neuron
preganglionic neuron
prevertebral ganglion
receptors for ANS neurotransmitters
rest-and-digest division

sympathetic division
sympathetic stimulation on selected target organs (tables)
thoracolumbar division
visceral (autonomic) reflexes
α_1 receptors
α_2 receptors
β_1 receptors
β_2 receptors
β_3 receptors

CHAPTER 20

The Senses

SENSATION AND PERCEPTION

A **sensation** (sin-SĀ-shun; *sense*, to feel) is the body's awareness of a change in its internal or external environment. The environment could be external (i.e., light, room temperature, touch of the skin, etc.), or it could be internal (tension in a muscle, pressure in the stomach, blood pH, levels of glucose in the blood, etc.). Sensations allow the body to maintain homeostasis by making appropriate behavioral and/or physiological modifications when environmental conditions change.

A sensation may be either conscious (one that you are aware of) or subconscious (one that you are not aware of). A *conscious* awareness of a sensation is called **perception**. Conscious sensations include touch, taste, smell, sight, hearing, pain, equilibrium, pressure, and temperature. Every sensation requires four things: (1) stimulus, (2) receptor, (3) afferent impulses traveling from a sensory receptor to the brain, and (4) interpretation of the afferent impulses in the brain.

Perceiving particular sensations fall into two major categories: *general senses* and *special senses*. **General senses** are those that correspond to stimulation of receptors widespread over the body, and include feelings of touch, pain, temperature, pressure, stretch, and vibration. **Special senses** are those that correspond to stimulation of receptors in a localized region, and include vision, hearing, smell, taste, and equilibrium.

SENSORY RECEPTORS

In order to detect stimuli, the body uses specialized structures called *sensory receptors*. A **sensory receptor** is a specialized cell or neuron ending that responds (depolarizes) when there is a change in its surrounding environment. The environmental change generates a graded potential on the receptor that can initiate an impulse. When a graded potential begins on a sensory receptor, it is called a **receptor potential**. The ability of a receptor to convert a stimulus into a nerve impulse is **transduction** (trans-DUK-shun, "lead across").

RECEPTOR ADAPTATION

Adaptation (or **accommodation**) is a phenomenon in which a receptor becomes less responsive to a stimulus, even if the stimulus is still present. For example, touch receptors in the skin adapt very quickly so that you do not feel clothes rubbing constantly on your skin. Adaptation may be due to the receptor's membrane becoming less permeable to ions during constant stimulation. Depending on its speed of adaptation, a receptor is either *phasic* or *tonic*.

Phasic receptors (FĀ-sik) adapt *rapidly*. The term *phasic* means that the receptor's sensitivity goes through phases; i.e., sometimes it is very sensitive, but at other times, it is less sensitive. Examples of phasic receptors include receptors for *touch, pressure, temperature,* and *smell*. Since olfactory receptors are phasic, you may "get used to" the smell of preserved specimens in an anatomy lab. The general role of phasic receptors is to make you aware of a change that occurs, but not to remind you constantly that the stimulus is present.

Tonic receptors adapt either very slowly or not at all. Examples include *nociceptors, chemoreceptors,* and *proprioceptors* (discussed below). The general role of tonic receptors is to provide a constant reminder of tissue damage or body position. Tonic proprioceptors in the inner ear make the brain aware of head position so that it can make muscle adjustments to maintain balance.

An **afterimage** is the perception of a stimulus after the stimulus no longer exists; i.e., an afterimage is the opposite of accommodation. Continuing to see a picture or scene after closing your eyes is an example. Afterimages may be due to the brain's continued processing of the sensory input and/or continued firing of the sensory receptors even after the stimulus no longer exists.

CLASSIFICATION OF RECEPTORS

Sensory receptors are classified based on (1) the location of the stimulus and (2) the type of stimulus to which they respond.

Classification by Location

Depending on the location of the stimulus to which they respond, sensory receptors are *exteroceptors, interoceptors,* or *proprioceptors*.

- **Exteroceptors** (eks-TER-ō-sep-terz) respond to stimuli from outside of the body; therefore, they exist near the body's surface. Most exteroceptors are in the skin or in mucous membranes, but photoreceptors in the eyes that respond to light are also exteroceptors. Examples of cutaneous exteroceptors are thermoreceptors, tactile (touch) receptors, pressure receptors (more forceful touch), and pain receptors.

- **Interoceptors** (IN-ter-ō-sep-terz) respond to stimuli inside the dorsal or ventral cavities. They include *chemoreceptors* and *baroreceptors* in blood vessels and in the CNS, *osmoreceptors* in the brain, and *nociceptors* (pain receptors) in visceral organs.

- **Proprioceptors** (PRŌ-prē-ō-sep-terz) respond to stretch, and exist in tendons, muscles, joints, and the inner ear. Specific examples include *joint kinesthetic receptors* in the capsules of synovial joints, *muscle spindles* in skeletal muscle, *Golgi tendon organs* in muscle tendons, and special receptors inside the inner ear. Proprioceptors allow the brain to determine the body's position and then make adjustments to maintain balance. Proprioceptors are tonic receptors.

Classification by Stimulus

Depending on the type of stimulus to which they respond, sensory receptors are generally *chemoreceptors, mechanoreceptors, nociceptors, osmoreceptors, photoreceptors,* or *thermoreceptors*.

- **Chemoreceptors** (KĒ-mō-rē-sep-terz) respond to chemicals, such as CO_2, O_2, and H^+ ions in blood and cerebrospinal fluid. They are tonic receptors and exist in large arteries of the thorax, neck and brain. Chemoreceptors are important in regulating blood chemistry.

- **Mechanoreceptors** (me-KAN-ō-rē-sep-terz) respond to mechanical forces such as stretch or pressure, and include *tactile receptors, baroreceptors,* and *proprioceptors*.

  □ **Tactile receptors** (TAK-til; "touch") respond to tension and pressure in the skin. Specific examples include *Meissner's corpuscles, Merkel's discs, Ruffini's organs, Krause corpuscles, Pacinian corpuscles,* and *hair root plexuses*. All tactile receptors are phasic.

  □ **Baroreceptors** (BAR-ō-rē-sep-terz; *baro,* pressure) exist in the walls of large blood vessels in the mediastinum and neck and respond to stretch in the blood vessel walls.

This allows the brain to utilize the vasomotor center to make adjustments in blood vessel diameter in order to maintain optimum blood pressure. Baroreceptors are tonic.

- **Proprioceptors** (described earlier)
- **Nociceptors** (NŌ-sē-sep-terz; *noci*, pain) are free nerve endings that generate impulses that the brain interprets as pain. A variety of stimuli can stimulate nociceptors, including chemicals released from or formed in damaged tissues. Nociceptors are tonic receptors.
- **Osmoreceptors** (OZ-mō-rē-sep-terz) are tonic receptors in the hypothalamus that respond to osmotic pressure (OP) changes in the blood or cerebrospinal fluid.
- **Photoreceptors** (FŌ-tō-rē-sep-terz; *photo*, light) are tonic receptors that respond to light, and include rods and cones in the retina of the eye.
- **Thermoreceptors** (THER-mō-rē-sep-terz; *therm*, heat) are free nerve ending receptors that respond to changes in temperature. Cold receptors are more abundant than warm receptors, and respond to temperatures between 54° and 95°, but also above 117° F. Warm receptors respond to temperatures between 95° and 117° F. Nociceptors respond to temperatures between 0° and 54° F, and above 117° F.

SPATIAL DISCRIMINATION

The ability of the brain to pinpoint the location of a stimulus is **projection** (or **spatial discrimination**). For example, stimulating pain receptors in the fingertip causes the brain's somatosensory regions to perceive that the pain is in the fingertip, not in the big toe. If a neurosurgeon stimulates the same parts of the brain's somatosensory region directly, the person perceives touch on the fingertip, even though there is no stimulus at the fingertip. Projection allows a person to take action to compensate for disruptions in homeostasis. If you cut your right hand, you know to treat the right hand, not the left one.

PAIN SENSATIONS

Nociceptors (pain receptors) are present in all tissues except the brain; however, the brain is the site of pain perception. More specifically, the diencephalon perceives most types of pain, which neurologists classify by intensity, duration, and location.

Photoreceptors	Exteroceptors	Mechanoreceptors
Cones in retina	Gustatory cells	Baroreceptors
Rods in retina	Hair root plexus	Crista ampullaris in ear
	Krause corpuscles	Golgi tendon organs
Proprioceptors	Meissner's corpuscles	Hair root plexus
Crista ampullaris	Merkel's disks	Joint kinesthetic receptors
Golgi tendon organs	Nociceptors	Krause corpuscles
Joint kinesthetic receptors	Olfactory cells	Meissner's corpuscles
Muscle spindles	Pacinian corpuscles	Merkel's disks
Saccule macula	Photoreceptors in eye	Muscle spindles
Utricle macula	Ruffini's corpuscles	Pacinian corpuscles
	Spiral organ (of Corti)	Ruffini's corpuscles
Visceroceptors	Thermoreceptors	Maculae in inner ear
Aortic baroreceptors		Spiral organ in inner ear
Aortic chemoreceptors	**Thermoreceptors**	
Carotid baroreceptors	Free nerve endings	**Chemoreceptors**
Carotid chemoreceptors		Aortic chemoreceptors
Chemosensitive area (brain)		Carotid chemoreceptors
Osmoreceptors	**Nociceptors**	Chemosensitive area (brain)
Visceral nociceptors	Free nerve endings	Gustatory cells
		Olfactory cells

Pain Classified Based on Duration

There are two types of pain classified by intensity and duration: *acute* and *chronic*:

- **Acute pain** (a-KŪT; "sharp") is sudden and sharp, such as when a needle penetrates the skin. Its duration is usually short, and afferent impulses perceived as acute pain travel along fast-conducting class A axons.

- **Chronic pain** (KRON-ik; *chron*, time) is more of a throbbing and recurring pain, such as a headache or arthritis pain. Afferent impulses perceived as chronic pain travel along slow-conducting class C axons.

Pain Classified Based on Origin

Based on the site of origin, pain is either *somatic* or *visceral*.

- **Somatic pain** (sō-MA-tik; *soma*, body) originates in the skin, muscles, or joints, and includes *superficial* and *deep* pain.

  □ **Superficial pain** is somatic pain that originates in the epidermis or in a mucous membrane. Most superficial pain is acute.

  □ **Deep pain** is somatic pain that originates in the dermis, hypodermis, skeletal muscles or joints. It usually has a long duration and suggests damage in deep tissues.

- **Visceral pain** occurs when stimulation of nociceptors in the thorax and abdomen occurs. Some of the impulses from these nociceptors may share common ascending tracts with impulses originating in certain somatic nociceptors; consequently, the brain is unable to project the exact source of the pain. An example is when a person experiencing a heart attack feels pain in the left arm. The pain impulse originates in the heart, but afferent impulses from the heart and regions of the left arm synapse with the same association neurons in the spinal cord. When the brain receives the impulses, it erroneously projects the pain to the arm. This erroneous projection is **referred pain**. Most people experience a form of referred pain when they hit their ulnar nerve ("funny bone"). When this happens, the person feels pain in the fingers, even though the fingers were not the site of nociceptor stimulation. Knowledge of referred pain can help medical personnel make better evaluations of various ailments.

Phantom pain is the perception of pain in a structure that no longer exists; e.g., an amputated limb. In this case the cut axons that earlier had connections with nociceptors in the lost limb discharge spontaneously. The brain, in turn, perceives these impulses as pain in the lost limb. Some amputees may have various sensations in the phantom limb when other regions (e.g., the face) are stimulated.

TASTE

A person perceives taste in the gustatory cortex of the brain's insula. Taste receptors exist within **taste buds**, groups of cells embedded in *tongue papillae* (bumps on the tongue's surface). A taste bud consists mostly of **sustenacular cells** (sus-ten-AK-ū-lar; "support"; also called **supporting cells**), which arise from nearby **basal cells**. Over time, the supporting cells develop into **gustatory cells** (GUS-ta-tor-ē; *gusta*, taste) which function as taste receptors (Figure 20-1).

Gustatory cells contain hair-like microvilli that make contact with saliva on the tongue's surface. These microvilli depolarize in response to various chemicals dissolved in saliva. Gustatory cells then stimulate dendrites of sensory neurons, which surround the gustatory cells. The dendrites initiate impulses that travel along the sensory neuron axons and then pass to association neurons in the brain. The association neurons then conduct the impulses to the gustatory cortex. Due to the wear-and-tear that occurs during eating, sustenacular cells replace gustatory cells about once every week.

Impulses leaving taste buds travel along one of two nerves. Impulses from the anterior two-thirds of the tongue travel to the brain through the *facial nerves*, which are the 7th pair of cranial nerves (CN 7). Impulses from the posterior one-third of the tongue travel through the *glossopharyngeal nerves* (CN 9).

THE SENSES

361

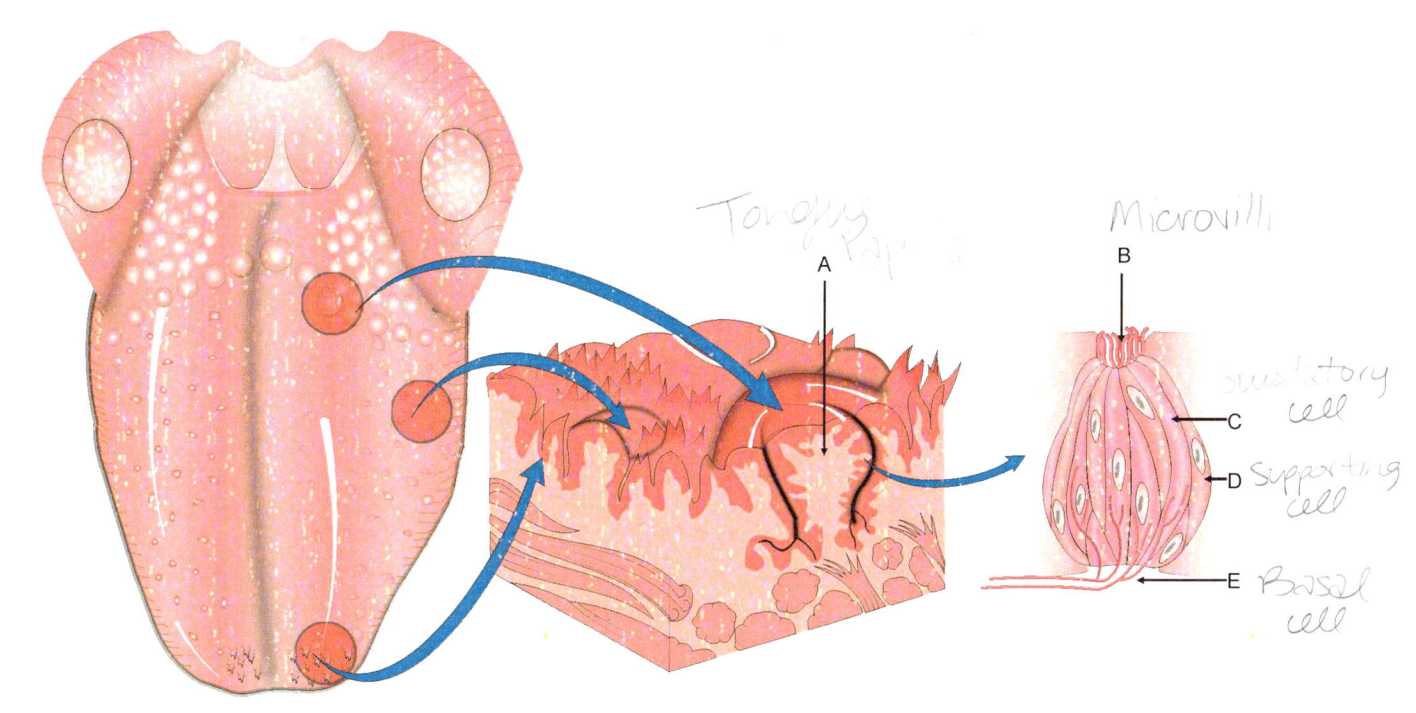

Figure 20-1. *Taste buds*

Gustatory cells in different parts of the tongue initiate impulses on sensory neurons in response to different chemicals, and the result is perception of different tastes:

- **Sweetness**: perceived when sugars, artificial sweeteners, alcohol, or certain lead salts stimulate taste buds at the *tip* of the tongue.
- **Sourness**: perceived when acidic substances stimulate taste buds along the *sides* of the tongue.
- **Saltiness**: perceived when metal ions from inorganic salts stimulate taste buds at the *tip of the tongue*.
- **Bitterness**: perceived when alkaline materials or other substances stimulate taste buds at the *back of the tongue*. Since many toxic plant materials contain alkaloid (base) materials, they have a bitter taste. It is ironic that detection of these bitter toxins occurs at the back of the mouth, since that is where swallowing begins.
- **Umami** (ū-MOM-ē): perceived as a "meaty" or "cheesy" taste in response to exposure to various amino acids, peptides, and polypeptides.

SMELL

Olfaction is the sense of smell and the brain perceives it in the olfactory cortex, which is part of the frontal and temporal lobes. The mammillary bodies, which are part of the limbic system, control flinching and grimacing reflexes in response to strong odors.

The receptors for smell reside in the **olfactory epithelium**, located in the superior regions of both nasal cavities (one cavity on each side of the nasal septum). This epithelium contains columnar-shaped **sustenacular (supporting) cells** that appear bright yellow. **Olfactory (Bowman's) glands**, which exist in the lamina propria beneath the membrane, secrete mucus onto the surface of the epithelium (Figure 20-2).

Sustenacular cells arise from nearby **basal cells** (similar to what happens in taste buds). Basal cells also develop into **olfactory neurons**, which are the only neurons to have direct contact with the outside environment. Moreover, olfactory neurons are the only neurons known that we replace throughout one's lifetime. A basal cell replaces an olfactory neuron about every two months. Olfactory neurons are bipolar and contain long cilia that extend into the mucus covering.

CHAPTER 20

Before a person can smell something, volatile (gaseous) chemicals must dissolve in the mucus of the olfactory epithelium and bind to the olfactory "hairs" (cilia) of the olfactory neurons. In response to this binding, Na^+ channels open in the olfactory neuron and create a receptor potential. The receptor potential then initiates an impulse on the axons of the olfactory neurons. The axons of **olfactory neurons** form the olfactory nerves (CN 1).

The olfactory nerves extend through the cribriform plate of the ethmoid bone to synapse with *mitral cells* in the **olfactory bulb**, which rests on the superior surface of the cribriform plate. **Mitral cells** (MĪ-tral; *miter*, bishop's hat) are neurons that conduct impulses to the olfactory cortex, which perceives the impulses as smell. As mitral cells become more active, so do nearby *granule cells* located in the olfactory bulb. **Granule cells** inhibit the activity of mitral cells, which may explain why a strong odor becomes less noticeable as time passes.

THE EYE AND VISION

Approximately three-fourths of all receptors in the body are inside the eye. These receptors are **photoreceptors**, which respond to light energy. Impulses conducted through the optic nerves (CN 2) pass to tracts that lead to the occipital lobes where perception of light occurs.

ANATOMY OF THE EYE

The eye consists of three layers (or tunics), a lens, and two major fluid-filled chambers. The three tunics of the eye include the *fibrous, vascular,* and *nervous* tunics (Figure 20-3).

FIBROUS TUNIC

The **fibrous tunic** is the outer layer of the eye and consists of dense, fibrous connective tissue. The **sclera** (SKLE-ra; "hard") is the white part of the eye that covers all but the anterior surface of the eye. It is avascular and provides a tough protective layer for the eye's internal components. It also serves as an attachment site for extrinsic eye muscles that move the eye within the skull's orbits.

At its posterior surface, the sclera is continuous with the dura mater that encloses the brain. The transparent anterior portion of the eye is the **cornea** (KOR-nē-a). It is continuous with the sclera, but its transparent nature is due to an ordered arrangement of very fine collagen fibers. The cornea allows light to enter the eye.

VASCULAR TUNIC

The **vascular tunic** (or **uvea**; Ū-vē-a; "grape") is deep to the sclera and has a rich supply of blood vessels

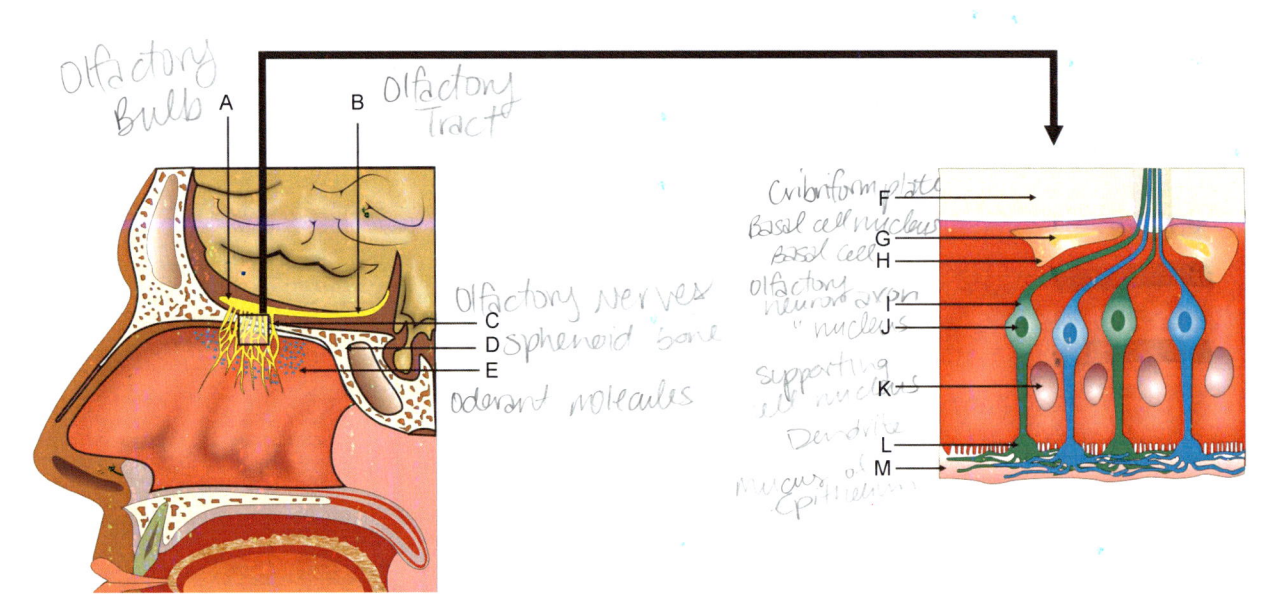

Figure 20-2. Olfactory epithelium

THE SENSES

Figure 20-3. Anatomy of the eye

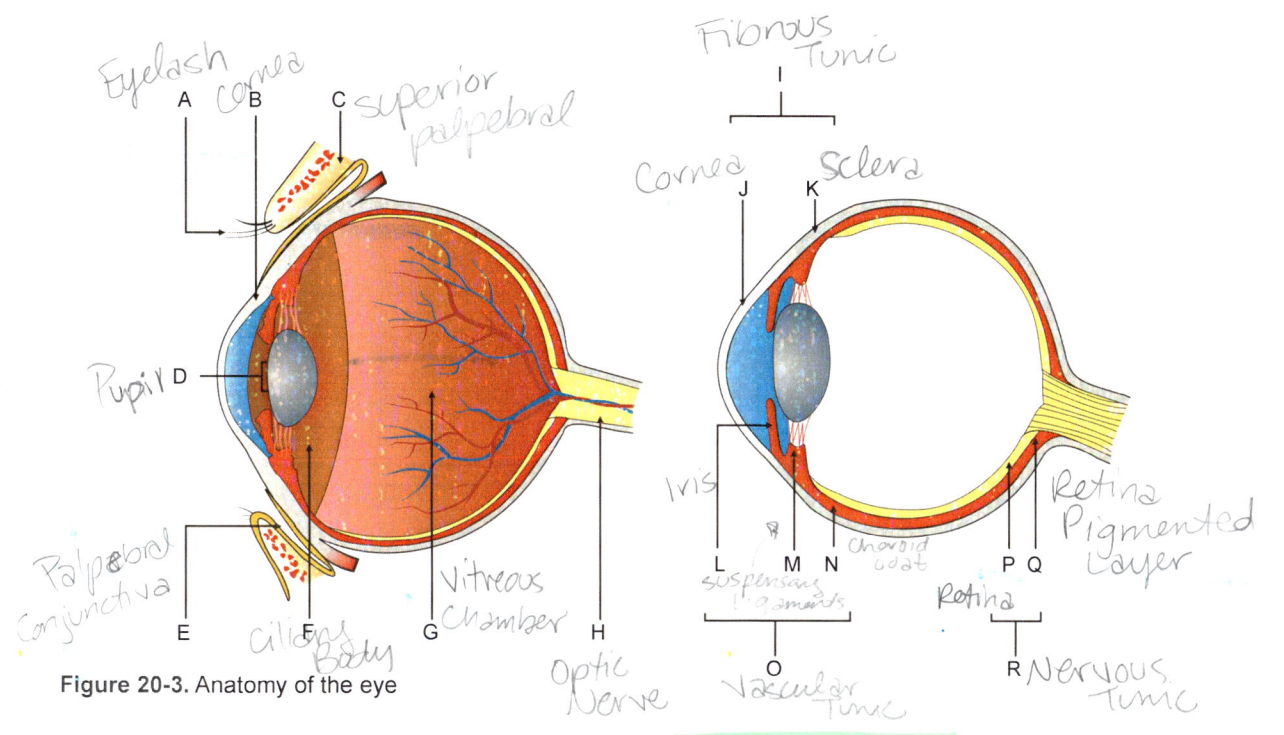

that supplies oxygen and nutrients to the fibrous and nervous tunics. Most of the vascular tunic consists of the **choroid coat** (KOR-oyd; *chor*, membrane) containing melanocytes. The melanin absorbs some of the light that enters the eye and prevents excessive light scattering within the eye.

Anterior to the choroid coat is the **ciliary body** (SIL-ē-ar-ē), which is a smooth muscular ring that alters the shape of the lens. The posterior, jagged boundary of the ciliary body is the **ora serrata** (ō-ra se-RA-ta; *ora*, mouth; *serrat*, jagged).

Anterior to the ciliary body is the **iris** (Ī-ris; "rainbow"), consisting of two groups of smooth muscle. It regulates the amount of light reaching the posterior part of the eye by controlling the diameter of an opening called the **pupil** (PŪ-pil; "doll"), so named because one's reflection seen in it resembles a doll. The *sphincter (circular) muscle* of the iris encircles the pupil. Contracting the sphincter muscle causes the pupil to constrict (its diameter decreases). The *dilator (or radial) muscle* has fibers that radiate outward from the sphincter muscle. When the radial muscle contracts, the pupil dilates (its diameter increases). The sphincter muscle receives impulses from parasympathetic axons in the oculomotor nerve. The radial muscle receives sympathetic fibers in thoracic nerves. Since the ciliary muscle and iris muscles are within the eye, they are *intrinsic* eye muscles.

NERVOUS TUNIC

The **nervous tunic** (or **retina**) is the inner coat of the eye. It is really part of the nervous system because it contains sensory receptors for sight. However, an outer, nonsensory portion of the retina, called the *pigmented layer*, exists next to the choroid. It contains melanocytes and extends anteriorly to cover the posterior surface of the iris. Melanin produced in the retina, along with that in the choroid, reduces light scattering within the eye. The inner portion of the retina is the *neural layer* and contains specialized neurons. It extends anteriorly to the ora serrata, but does not cover the posterior surface of the iris.

The **optic disc** is a hole in the posterior portion of the retina, where the optic nerve connects to the eye. Through this opening, a **central retinal artery** brings blood into the large vitreous chamber and a **central retinal vein** removes blood. These vessels have branches that spread out across the retina's surface providing nourishment and removing wastes from the retinal cells. An ophthalmologist (eye doctor) can view these vessels with an ophthalmoscope, which shines light through the pupil. The choroid coat also supplies blood to the retina. If the retina "detaches" from the choroid, it quickly atrophies due to a lack of nourishment.

The optic disc does not contain photoreceptors; therefore, a person is unaware of light striking this region of the eye's inner surface. For this reason, the optic disc is functionally a *blind spot*. Just lateral to the optic disc is a yellow oval region called the **macula lutea** (MAK-ū-la lū-TĒ-a; *macula*, spot; *lutea*, yellow). In the center of the macula is a tiny pit called the **fovea centralis** (FŌ-vē-a sen-TRAL-is; *fovea*, pit), which has a diameter of about 0.5 mm. The fovea is at the posterior end of eye's *visual axis* (representing a line drawn through the eye perpendicular to the cornea). When a person stares directly at an object, light from that object converges at the fovea.

PHOTORECEPTORS

There are two types of photoreceptor cells, rods and cones, so-named according to their general shape. There are about 120 million **rods** in each eye, and this accounts for 95% of all photoreceptors in the eye; however, there are no rods within the fovea centralis. Rods are most useful for non-color vision, peripheral vision, and vision in dim light. The remaining 6-7 million photoreceptors in each eye (5% of all photoreceptors present) are **cones**, and they are most abundant in the fovea centralis.

Each photoreceptor contains within its cytoplasm hundreds of membranous, disc-like organelles stacked together like coins. The phospholipid membrane of these discs contains special chemicals called **photopigments**, which change shape when certain wavelengths of light strike them.

The photopigment in rods is **rhodopsin** (rō-DOP-sin; "visual purple"). It consists of a glycoprotein called **scotopsin** (skō-TOP-sin; *scoto*, darkness) and a pigment called **retinal** (re-tin-AL), which the cell synthesizes from vitamin A. The liver can convert compounds called *carotene*, abundant in carrots and green vegetables, into vitamin A. Rhodopsin is extremely sensitive to light; i.e., even very dim light can activate rhodopsin. Since there are no rods in the fovea, a person staring directly at a dimly lit star may not see the star. The reason is that there is not enough light energy emitted from the star to activate the photopigments in cones, which are the only photoreceptors present in the fovea. However, looking to the side of the star causes light to move off the fovea and onto regions that contain rods. As a result, the star becomes visible in the peripheral vision.

The photopigment in cones is **iodopsin** (ī-ō-DOP-sin; "visual violet"), which is the pigment used for visual acuity and color vision. Cones are the only photoreceptors located in the fovea, but their numbers gradually decrease farther away from the fovea. Each iodopsin contains one of three varieties of opsin proteins called **photopsins** (fō-TOP-senz), and each cone contains only one type of iodopsin. Since all cones contain retinal, the color of light to which a particular cone responds depends on the type of photopsin present in a cone's iodopsin. Approximately 75% of the cones contain the iodopsin called **erythrolabe** (ē-RITH-rō-lāb; *erytho*, red), which responds to red light; 15% contain **cyanolabe** (sī-AN-ō-lāb; *cyan*, blue), which responds to blue light; and 10% contain **chlorolabe** (KLOR-ō-lāb; *chlor*, green), which responds to green light. The wide variety of colors that a person can perceive depends on the relative number of different cones stimulated.

OTHER CELLS IN THE RETINA

Other cells in the retina include *bipolar cells, ganglion cells, amacrine cells,* and *horizontal cells* (Figure 20-4).

- **Bipolar cells** are bipolar neurons that synapse with photoreceptors. They transmit graded potentials to neurons called *ganglion cells* that have axons in the optic nerve. More than one rod may synapse with a single bipolar cell, and several bipolar cells may synapse with a single ganglion cell. This increases *spatial summation* on the ganglion cell so that even very dim light can initiate an impulse. In contrast, usually only one cone synapses with only one bipolar cell, and the bipolar cell synapses with only one ganglion cell; consequently, light must be brighter to cause enough *temporal summation* on a ganglion cell to initiate an impulse.

- **Ganglion cells** are neurons that receive impulses from bipolar cells and conduct them to the brain. The axons of ganglion cells lie on the inner surface of the retina, but not over the fovea, and come together at the optic disc. The axons then course

THE SENSES

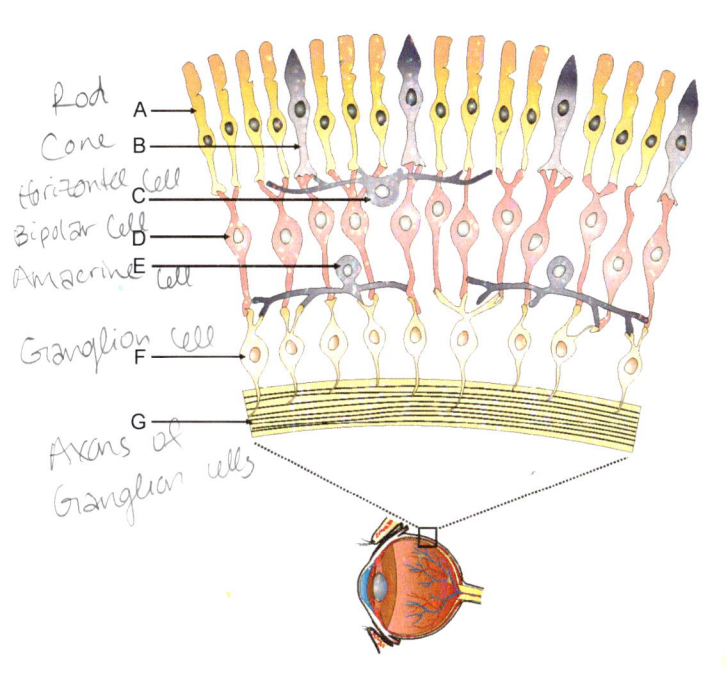

365

Figure 20-4. Cells of the retina

(handwritten labels: A - Rod, B - Cone, C - Horizontal Cell, D - Bipolar Cell, E - Amacrine Cell, F - Ganglion Cell, G - Axons of Ganglion cells)

through the optic nerves where they conduct impulses to the brain.

- **Horizontal cells** exist where photoreceptors synapse with bipolar cells, and modify the way in which these cells interact.

- **Amacrine cells** (Ā-ma-krin; "without long fibers") are positioned where bipolar cells synapse with ganglion cells, and modify the way in which these cells interact.

Horizontal cells and amacrine cells help the eye adjust to various light intensities. When light is too bright, these cells can inhibit the rate of depolarization of bipolar cells. When light is dim, these cells can help facilitate the depolarization of bipolar cells.

LENS

The **lens**, so named for its resemblance to a lentil bean, is a flexible clear structure located immediately posterior to the pupil. It consists of many layers of a globular protein called **crystallins** (KRIS-ta-lenz), arranged in layers like those of an onion. It connects to the ciliary body by thin strands of connective tissue called **suspensory ligaments**. When the ciliary muscle contracts, it moves anteriorly and reduces the tension on the suspensory ligaments, allowing the lens to become more round. When the ciliary muscle relaxes, it moves posteriorly and increases the tension on the suspensory ligaments. As a result, the lens flattens.

CHAMBERS OF THE EYE

The **aqueous chamber** (OK-wē-us; "watery") is anterior to the lens and posterior to the cornea and it contains a watery fluid called **aqueous humor** (HŪ-mor; "fluid"). The *posterior aqueous chamber* is posterior to the iris, while the *anterior aqueous chamber* is anterior to the iris. The ciliary body secretes aqueous fluid into the posterior aqueous chamber throughout one's life. It flows anteriorly through the pupil and into the anterior aqueous chamber. The aqueous humor drains into the blood through the **scleral venous sinus** (or **canal of Schlemm**), located at the junction between the iris and cornea. Aqueous humor supplies nutrients to and removes wastes from the lens. The ciliary body replaces all the aqueous humor about every 90 minutes.

The **vitreous chamber** (VIT-trē-us; "glassy") is the largest chamber in the eye and is posterior to the lens. It contains a viscous fluid called **vitreous humor**, which consists of very fine collagenous fibers embedded in a jelly-like matrix. The transparent nature of vitreous humor allows light to pass from the lens to the retina. It also maintains intraocular pressure, which prevents the eyeball from distorting when extrinsic, skeletal muscles contract and pull on the sclera. In addition, the vitreous humor keeps the retina pressed gently against the choroid coat, allowing the retina to receive nourishment from blood vessels in the choroid coat. The vitreous humor forms during embryological development.

ACCESSORY STRUCTURES OF THE EYE

Accessory structures are structures that help the eye function more efficiently and include the *eyebrows*, *eyelids*, various *glands*, and *extrinsic muscles* (Figure 20-5).

Eyebrows are short, bristly hairs located on the supraorbital ridges, superior to the eyes. They shade the eyes from light coming into the eye from above.

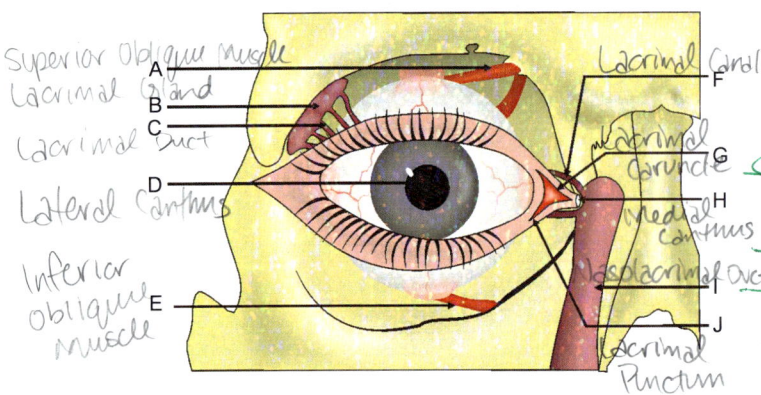

Figure 20-5. Accessory structures of the eye

Eyelids (or **palpebrae**; PAL-pe-brē) are fleshy flaps that come together over the anterior surface of the eye, protecting the eye from foreign particles and dehydration. They contain areolar connective tissue and a tarsal plate, consisting of dense connective tissue. The tarsal plate provides a firm structure to which two skeletal muscles can pull. Contraction of the *orbicularis oculi* muscle closes the eyelid, and contraction of the *levator palpebrae* elevates the upper eyelid. Blinking the eyelids helps keep the surface of the eye moist.

The upper and lower eyelids come together medially at the **medial canthus** (KAN-thus; "corner of eye") and laterally at the **lateral canthus**. The **lacrimal caruncle** (KAR-ung-kl; "small fleshy mass") is a protuberance in the medial canthus that contains sebaceous glands and sweat glands. These glands secrete a viscous white fluid that may accumulate in the medial canthus during sleep. In people of Asian descent, a vertical *epicanthic fold* (ep-ē-KAN-thik) may cover the medial canthus and obscure the lacrimal caruncle.

Eyelashes are hairs located at the margin of the eyelids. They shade the eye and help keep dust and debris away from the eye. **Ciliary glands** are modified sweat glands that secrete a lubricating fluid into the eyelash follicle. Large sebaceous glands, called **tarsal (meibomian**; mī-BŌ-mē-an) **glands**, exist along the inner margins of the eyelids, just posterior to the eyelashes. Their sebum prevents the eyelids from sticking together when blinking or sleeping.

The **conjunctiva** (kon-junk-TĪ-va; "bind together") is a mucous membrane that covers the anterior surface of the eye and the inner lining of the eyelids. It consists of very thin stratified squamous epithelium. The *bulbar conjunctiva* covers the anterior surface of the sclera but not the cornea, while the *palpebral conjunctiva* lines the inner surface of the eyelids. Both conjunctivae form a continuous membrane that prevents foreign objects, such as contact lenses, from moving behind the eye.

Lacrimal glands (LAK-ri-mal; "tears"), or **tear glands**, are located in the superior-lateral corner of each orbit. They secrete tears, a watery fluid that lubricates the eye and flushes foreign material from its surface. Tears contain antibodies and a chemical called *lysozyme*, which functions as an anti-bacterial agent. Lacrimal glands secrete tears continually in response to stimulation from parasympathetic axons in the facial nerves (CN 7). Tears pass over the eye's surface and drain into tiny openings, called **lacrimal puncta** (PUNGK-ta; *punctum*, a prick), located on upper and lower eyelid margins near the medial canthus. Tears pass through tiny **lacrimal canals** and into the **nasolacrimal duct** (NĀ-zō-LAK-ri-mal), which connects the orbit to the nasal cavity. The duct is a channel located between the lacrimal and maxillary bones. When a person cries, excess tears can spill out of the eye and out of the nose.

The *extrinsic* eye muscles attach to the sclera and move the eye within the orbit (see Table 20-1 and Figure 20-6). The lateral rectus receives stimulation from the *abducens nerve* (CN 6), whereas, the superior oblique receives stimulation from the *trochlear nerve* (CN 4). All other extrinsic eye muscles receive stimulation from the *oculomotor nerve* (CN 3).

Muscle	Actions on the eyeball
Medial rectus	Medial rotation
Lateral rectus	Lateral rotation
Superior rectus	Superior rotation/elevation
Inferior rectus	Inferior rotation/depression
Inferior oblique	Lateral rotation/elevation
Superior oblique	Lateral rotation/depression

THE SENSES

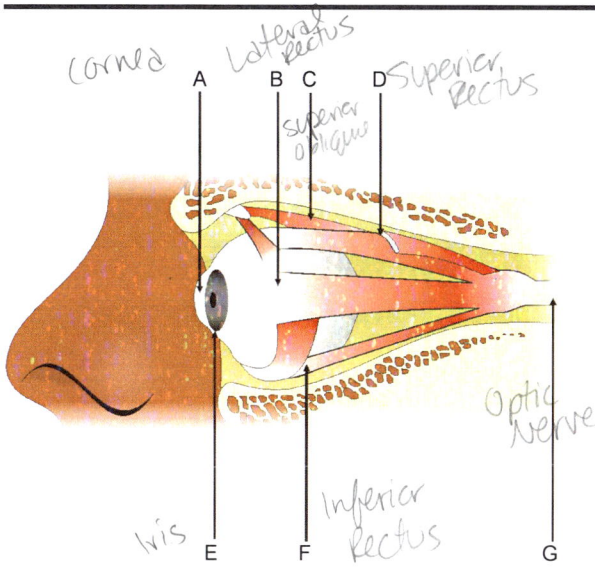

Figure 20-6. Extrinsic eye muscles

LIGHT REFRACTION IN THE EYE

To see an object clearly, the eye must focus the image precisely on the fovea centralis. As light first passes through the cornea, its waves bend in a process called **refraction** (rē-FRAK-shun; "to bend"). Light experiences refraction again as it passes through the lens. Normally, the cornea's refraction ability cannot change; however, contraction and relaxation of the ciliary muscle can change the shape of the lens, causing light refraction and precise focusing of an image on the fovea (Figure 20-7).

Making the lens more rounded due to contraction of the ciliary muscle is **lens accommodation**. When viewing objects closer than 20 feet, light enters the pupil at a greater angle and the eye must refract it more in order to pinpoint it on the fovea. For close-up vision, the ciliary muscle contracts and moves anteriorly, which reduces tension on the suspensory ligaments and allows the lens to become more rounded. The **near point of vision** is the closest distance that a person can focus an object clearly. In most people, this distance is about 4 inches.

Light rays from objects far away from the eye reach the eye in a more parallel fashion and need less refraction to focus on the fovea. In this situation, the ciliary muscle relaxes and moves posteriorly, causing the suspensory ligaments to become taut; thus, the lens becomes flatter. When viewing objects farther away than 20 feet, the eye needs no lens accommodation to focus the image on the fovea. The minimum distance away from the eye in which the lens does not need to accommodate is the **far point of vision**, which is usually about 20 feet. Viewing objects within 20 feet of the eye require varying degrees of accommodation.

The diameter of the pupil decreases as a viewed object moves closer to the eye. This prevents diverging light rays from entering the eye and blurring vision. The brain causes pupil constriction through *parasympathetic* stimulation of the iris's circular muscle. Also, when light gets brighter, the iris constricts. Excess light would stimulate more photoreceptors outside the fovea and generate too many impulses that would blur the vision.

EYE MOVEMENT

When a person stares at an object, both eyes focus simultaneously on that object. If the object moves

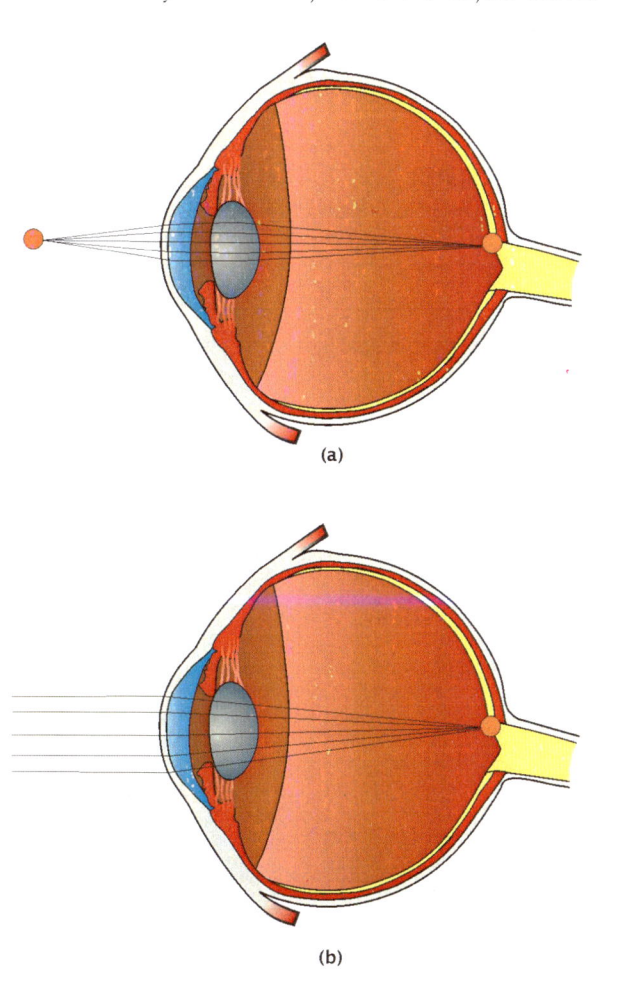

Figure 20-7. Effect of lens shape on focusing

closer, the eyes rotate medially in an action called **convergence**. Maximum convergence occurs when focusing both eyes at the tip of the nose and results in a "cross-eyed" condition. Without convergence, only one eye could view an object directly as it moves closer to the face. The other eye would focus on a different point and would force the brain to evaluate two different images simultaneously; consequently, the brain could not form a clear single image.

When a person is viewing his or her surroundings, the eyes usually move in a jerky manner known as **saccades** (sa-KADZ; *saccade*, sudden jerk of a horse). The frontal eye field, located in the frontal lobe, controls saccades and allows a person to see the entire field of vision in a short time. When turning the head, or when the eyes suddenly shift from one object to another, the eyelids often blink subconsciously, which prevents blurred vision.

STIMULATION OF PHOTORECEPTORS

Photoreceptors respond to light, which is kinetic energy that travels in waves. Also called **electromagnetic (radiant) energy**, physicists describe light as tiny packets of energy, called **photons**, which travel through space in a wave pattern. This energy can vary in intensity (brightness), which refers to the number of photons passing a given point in a given time. Light can also vary in *wavelength*, which is the distance between the wave peaks.

Different cones in the retina respond to different wavelengths and the brain perceives the different wavelengths as different colors. The **electromagnetic spectrum** includes all energy wavelengths. *Visible light* is that part of the electromagnetic spectrum that stimulates photoreceptors in the eyes. It includes wavelengths of about 380 nanometers (nm) to 750 nm. The visual cortex perceives the longest visible wavelengths as red, and the shortest wavelengths as violet. You can remember the visible wavelengths, from longest to shortest, by the acronym *ROY-G-BIV* (red, orange, yellow, green, blue, indigo, and violet). Each color has a specific range of wavelengths.

Before the brain can perceive it, light must pass through the cornea, aqueous humor, lens, vitreous humor, and a layer of ganglion cells, amacrine cells, bipolar cells, horizontal cells, and most of the cytoplasm of the photoreceptors. Finally, the light reaches the photopigment located in the rod or cone portion of the photoreceptor. This portion of the photoreceptor is adjacent to the pigmented layer of the retina.

Photoreceptors are unusual, compared to other receptors in the body, in that they *depolarize* when the stimulus is **not** present. In the dark, photoreceptors depolarize due to open sodium channels in the cell membrane. In response to depolarization, the photoreceptor releases an *inhibitory* neurotransmitter onto the bipolar cells. In contrast, when light of adequate intensity strikes a photopigment, the pigment undergoes a structural change in which the retinal and opsin separate. This process, called **bleaching**, initiates chemical reactions inside the photoreceptor that causes *hyperpolarization* of the photoreceptor (Figure 20-8).

Hyperpolarization of a photoreceptor in the light prevents the photoreceptor from releasing inhibitory neurotransmitter onto a bipolar cell. In response, the bipolar cell *depolarizes* spontaneously and releases an *excitatory* neurotransmitter onto a ganglion cell. The ganglion, in turn, depolarizes and conducts an impulse along its axon through the optic nerve. Bleaching cannot occur again until the photopigment regenerates (retinal and opsin reunite).

RETINAL PROCESSING

While ganglion cells can be stimulated by bipolar cells, not all ganglion cells respond to stimulation in exactly the same way. Bipolar cells are interconnected with more than one rod or cone, and ganglion cells receive input from more than one bipolar cell. All of the rods or cones that are functionally linked to a ganglion cell via bipolar cells are referred to as the ganglion cell's **receptive field**. Some ganglion cells depolarize more frequently when light strikes the center of their receptive field; these ganglion cells are said to have **on-center fields**. Other ganglion cells depolarize more frequently when light strikes the peripheral regions of the receptive field; these ganglion cells are said to have **off-center fields**. Having ganglion cells with receptive fields of different sensitivity allows the retina to send to the brain more precise messages about specific regions of the retina that are receiving light. In turn, the brain is better able to distinguish shapes and form accurate images of the objects being viewed.

THE SENSES

PERCEPTION OF COLOR

How can the brain perceive a multitude of colors if there are only three types of iodopsin in the retina? Perception of different colors (hues) depends on the ratio of different cones stimulated (see chart). When light stimulates all cones stimulated equally, the brain perceives white light.

Color	% red cones	% green cones	% blue cones
Red	60	0	0
Orange	97	42	0
Yellow	83	83	0
Green	31	67	36
Blue	0	0	97
Violet	0	0	65

LIGHT ADAPTATION

Adaptation to light refers to the ability of the retina to adjust its sensitivity to different intensities of light. Rhodopsin in rods is much more sensitive to light than is iodopsin in cones. Although rhodopsin bleaches very rapidly, it regenerates very slowly. In bright light, most rhodopsin molecules exist in a bleached condition, which makes the rods less responsive. In contrast, when iodopsin bleaches in bright light, it regenerates very quickly; i.e., there are always some iodopsin molecules available for bleaching. Due to the differences in bleaching and regeneration rates of their photopigments, cones are more important for vision under bright light conditions.

Light adaptation is the ability of the eyes to adjust to bright light. Being in the dark for about 30 minutes allows regeneration of virtually all photopigments molecules in the retina. However, moving into bright light causes bleaching of these photopigments, resulting

---

Rod's Rhodopsin

Scotopsin ↔ Retinal
↑ ↑
Amino Acids   Vitamin A
↑
Carotene

Cone's Iodopsin

Photopsin ↔ Retinal
↑ ↑
Amino Acids   Vitamin A
↑
Carotene

Photopigment
↗ ↖
Opsin   Retinal
↓
Photoreceptor cell depolarizes spontaneously
↓
Photoreceptor releases inhibitory neurotransmitter onto bipolar cell
↓
Bipolar cell remains at resting potential
↓
Bipolar cell do not release excitatory neurotrasmitter onto ganglion cell
↓
Ganglion cell remains at resting potential
↓
No impulse sent through optic nerve

Light → Photopigment
↗ ↖
Opsin   Retinal
↓
Photoreceptor cell hyperpolarizes
↓
No inhibitory neurotransmitter onto bipolar cell
↓
Bipolar cell depolarizes spontaneously
↓
Bipolar cell releases excitatory neurotrasmitter onto ganglion cell
↓
Ganglion cell depolarizes
↓
Impulse sent through optic nerve

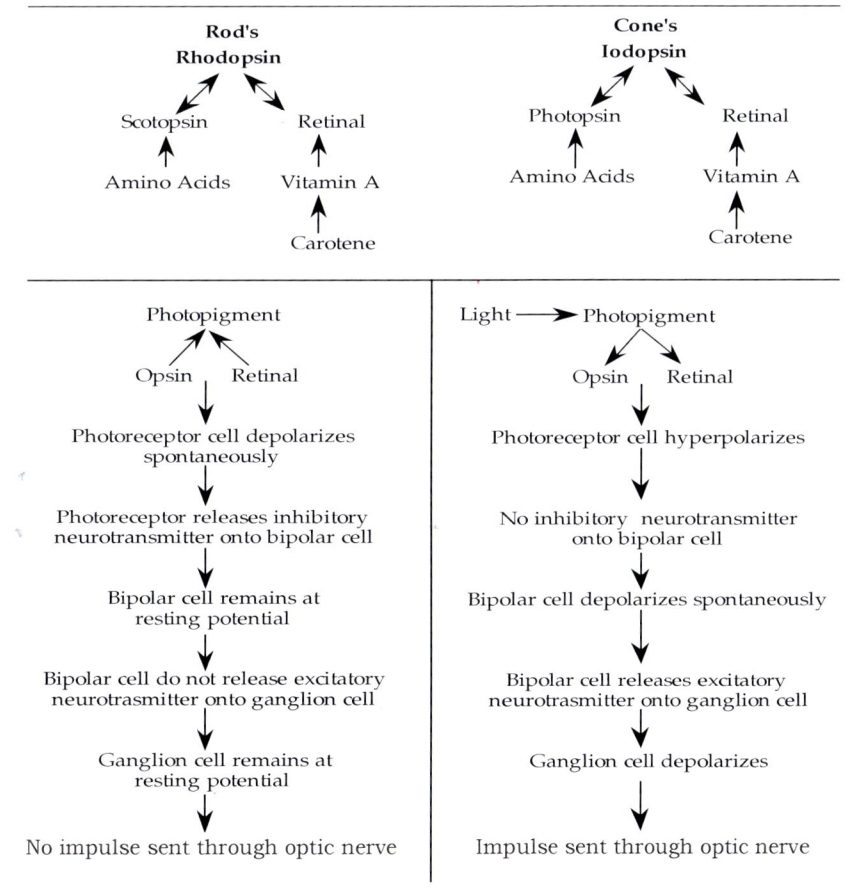

Figure 20-8. Stimulation of photoreceptors

in numerous impulses traveling to the visual cortex; consequently, the person sees a blinding glare. When most rhodopsin molecules have been bleached in bright light, the rods become much less active and the eyes are *light adapted*. On the other hand, the rate at which molecules of iodopsin bleach equals the rate at which they regenerate; therefore, cones are the main photoreceptors used in bright light. Light adaptation also involves pupil constriction that reduces the amount of light entering the eye. Light adaptation is relatively fast, requiring only 5-10 minutes.

Dark adaptation is the ability of the eyes to adjust to dim light. When entering a dark room, a person experiences temporary "blindness" for two reasons: (1) rhodopsin in rods is in the bleached condition, and (2) the dim light is unable to bleach iodopsin in cones. However, over the next few minutes more molecules of rhodopsin regenerate and allow the rods to respond to the dim light. Dark adaptation is much slower than light adaptation due to the slow rate at which rhodopsin regenerates. Complete dark adaptation may require 20-30 minutes.

VISUAL PATHWAY

Impulses generated through the optic nerve "cross over" in a region called the **optic chiasma** (kī-AS-ma; "crossing"). Here, impulses from the *medial* region of an eye cross over to the opposite side of the brain. Impulses from the *lateral* aspect of each eye do not cross over at the chiasma; instead, they synapse with neurons that conduct the impulses to the occipital lobe on the same side of the head as the eye where they originate. All impulses originating from bipolar cells in the retina eventually reach the primary visual cortex in the occipital lobe of the brain.

VISUAL FIELD AND 3-D VISION

An eye's **visual field** is the area that it can view at one time and it spans about 170°. The visual fields of both eyes overlap, allowing each eye to see the same object from a slightly different angle. The brain's visual cortex superimposes both images into one 3-dimensional image in a process called **depth perception**.

Since impulses passing from the retina do not reach the visual cortex immediately, we see an image for a fraction of a second longer than it actually appears; this is an example of an afterimage. This is similar to seeing a star from which light left it thousands or millions of light-years in the past, since it takes thousands or millions of light-years for that light to reach Earth. Taking advantage of afterimages made early motion pictures possible. A person will perceive a moving image whenever still-frame photographs pass in front of the eyes at a rate of about 24 frames per second.

VISUAL ACUITY

Visual acuity (a-KŪ-i-tē; "sharpness") is the ability to see objects clearly, and is attributable to cones in the fovea centralis. The average visual acuity for the human population receives a rating of 20/20. The numbers refer to distances in feet. **Near-sightedness** (**myopia**; mī-Ō-pē-a; *myo*, to shut; *opia*, eye) results in visual ratings with the bottom number being greater than the top number. If you have 20/200 vision, you would need to be 20 feet away from an object to see it clearly, whereas, a person with average vision could see it clearly from 200 feet away. If the bottom number is less than the top number, the person has better than average vision. For example, if you have 20/10 vision, you would be able to see an object clearly from 20 feet away, but the average person would need to be 10 feet closer to see it as clearly. **Far-sightedness** (**hyperopia**; hī-per-ŌP-ē-a) means that a person may be able to see objects far away clearly, but they need special lenses to see nearby objects clearly.

THE EAR AND HEARING

Sound refers to air vibrations the ear can convert to nerve impulses that the brain can perceive. When a person speaks, air molecules moving through the larynx (voice box) vibrate the vocal cords. Eventually, vibrating air molecules vibrate specialized structures in the ear. *Transduction* (conversion of a stimulus to an impulse) allows the brain to perceive the vibrations as sound. The brain perceives sound in the **auditory cortex** of the *temporal lobe*. Unlike light and electronic signals, sound cannot travel through a vacuum (e.g., outer space) because no air molecules are present.

THE SENSES

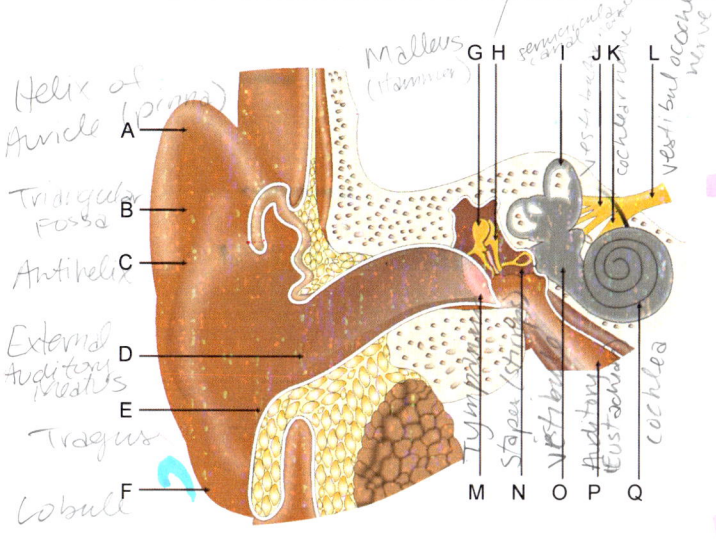

Figure 20-9. Parts of the ear

The anatomical structures involved in hearing include three major groups: *external ear, middle ear,* and *internal ear* (Figure 20-9).

EXTERNAL EAR

The **external ear** includes the *pinna, external auditory meatus,* and *tympanum.* The **pinna** (PIN-a), or **auricle** (AW-ri-kl), is a fleshy appendage on the side of the head that reflects sound vibrations into a tube called the **external auditory meatus**. The pinna is flexible due to the presence of elastic cartilage. The pinna consists of the **helix**, an outer curved portion, and the **antihelix**, an inner curved portion. The **tragus** (TRA-gus; "goat"), so named for its resemblance to a goatee, is an anterior projection of the pinna at the opening of the external auditory meatus, while the **antitragus** (AN-ti-trā-gus) is a posterior projection. The pinna has a **lobule** (**earlobe**) at the inferior end that lacks cartilage. Curved depressions between the helix, antihelix, and meatus are **conchae** (KONG-kē; "shells"), named for their resemblance to the inner curves of a seashell.

Sound vibrations travel through the external auditory meatus to the lateral surface of a membranous structure called the **tympanum** (tim-PAN-um; or **eardrum**). *Air conduction* of sound occurs as sound waves move through the external ear. The tympanum vibrates at the same frequency as the vibrating air molecules. *Ceruminous glands* lining the meatus secrete wax, which helps waterproof the meatus and repel small insects.

MIDDLE EAR

The **middle ear** (or **tympanic cavity**) exists between the tympanum and inner ear. Three tiny ear bones, called **ear ossicles** (OS-i-klz; "little bones") connect the tympanum to the inner ear. The **malleus** (MAL-ē-us; **hammer**) is the most lateral ear ossicle. It transmits vibrations from the tympanum to the middle ossicle, or **incus** (IN-kus; **anvil**). The incus, in turn, transmits the vibration to the medial ossicle, or **stapes** (STĀ-pēz; **stirrup**), which causes vibrations in the inner ear. The ear ossicles are responsible for *bone conduction of sound*.

The tympanum can vibrate freely only if the pressure on either side of it is equal. To equalize pressure, air can pass through the **auditory** (or **Eustachian**; ū-STĀ-shun) **tube** connecting the pharynx to the middle ear. Divers learn how to fill these tubes with air to compensate for water pressure on the outside of the tympanum. They close the nose and mouth and exhale gently so that the auditory tubes fill with air from the lungs, thus, pushing the tympanum outward to its normal resting position. On the other hand, when a person travels to a higher altitude, the tympanum bulges outward because the middle ear pressure is higher than the surrounding atmospheric pressure. Swallowing or opening the mouth while protruding the lower jaw may open the auditory tubes and allow air pressure on either side of the tympanum to equalize.

A tiny skeletal muscle, the **tensor tympani** (TEN-sor tim-PAN-nē), connects the wall of the auditory tube to the malleus. The **stapedius muscle** (sta-PĒ-dē-us) is the smallest skeletal muscle in the body and connects the stapes to the wall of the middle ear cavity. Both muscles contract reflexively, preventing excessive ossicle movement when exposed to loud sounds.

INNER EAR (LABYRINTH)

The **inner ear** (or **labyrinth**; LAB-e-rinth; maze) is a fluid-filled compartment consisting of a "maze" of tubes (Figure 20-10). The **bony labyrinth** is a series of cave-like compartments and tubes within the petrous portion of the temporal bone. The **membranous labyrinth** is a membrane-bound series of tubes and sacs located within the bony labyrinth. A watery fluid called **perilymph** (PER-i-limf) fills the space between the two labyrinths. Watery **endolymph** (EN-dō-limf) fills the membranous labyrinth. The components of the bony labyrinth include three *semicircular canals*, the *vestibule* and *cochlea*. The components of the membranous labyrinth include the *semicircular ducts*, *utricle* and *saccule*, and *cochlear duct*.

Semicircular Canals and Their Contents

The **semicircular canals** are ring-like tubes connected to the vestibule. The position of each canal is in a different anatomical plane: *sagittal*, *coronal*, and *transverse*. Inside each canal is a membranous **semicircular duct** filled with endolymph. Perilymph surrounds each duct. At the base of each duct is a saclike structure, called an **ampulla** (am-PUL-a; "two-handed bottle"), which also contains endolymph. Each ampulla contains a sensory structure called a **crista ampullaris** (KRIS-ta; am-pu-LAR-is; *crista*, crest). The cristae contain specialized epithelial cells called *supporting cells* that surround other cells called *hair cells*. The "hairs" consists of short microvilli called **stereocilia** (ster-ē-ō-SIL-ē-a; *stereo*, solid) and a single cilium called a **kinocilium** (kī-nō SIL ē-um; *kino*, to move). The stereocilia and kinocilium project into a gelatinous, ridge-shaped mass called the **cupula** (KU-pū la; "tub"). Dendrites of sensory neurons wrap around the base of the hair cells.

The Vestibule and Its Contents

The **vestibule** (VES-ti-būl; "entrance court") is the region of the bony labyrinth between the cochlea and semicircular canals. Two sac-like structures, the **utricle** (Ū-tri-kl; "leather bag") and **saccule** (SAK-ūl; "sac"), exist within the membranous labyrinth of the vestibule. Each sac contains a sensory structure called a **macula** (MAK-ū-la; spot). The macula in the saccule orients more *vertically* and responds to up or down movements, such as when a person is in an elevator. The macula in the utricle orients more *horizontally* and responds more to forward, backward, and side-to-side movements. The maculae consist of a layer of *supporting cells* surrounding *hair cells*. Like the cristae inside the semicircular ducts, the hair cells of the maculae have **stereocilia** and a **kinocilium**. Overlying the macula is a thick, flat gelatinous membrane embedded with tiny calcium carbonate ($CaCO_3$) crystals called **otoliths** (Ō-tō-liths; *oto*, ear; *lith*, stones). The gelatinous material and otoliths together make up the **otolithic membrane**.

The Cochlea

The **cochlea** (KOK-lē-a; "snail") is a snail-shaped structure that contains sensory receptors for hearing. A membranous tube called the **cochlear duct** (or **scala media**; SKA-la; "ladder"; *media*, middle) is inside the cochlea and divides the cochlea into three chambers. The cochlear duct is the middle chamber and contains endolymph. The superior canal is the **scala vestibuli** (ves-TIB-ū-lē). The **vestibular membrane** separates the scala vestibuli from the cochlear duct. The inferior canal is the **scala tympani** (TIM-pa-nē). The **basilar membrane** separates the scala tympani from the cochlear duct. The scala vestibuli and scala tympani contain *perilymph* and connect to one another at the distal end of the cochlear duct through a passageway called the **helicotrema** (hē-li-kō-TRĒ-ma; *helic*, spiral; *trema*, hole).

Sensory receptors for hearing are in the **organ of Corti** (KOR-tē, or **spiral organ**), located within the cochlear duct and resting on the basilar membrane. The spiral organ contains *supporting cells* and *hair cells*. The hair cells contain stereocilia embedded in an overlying

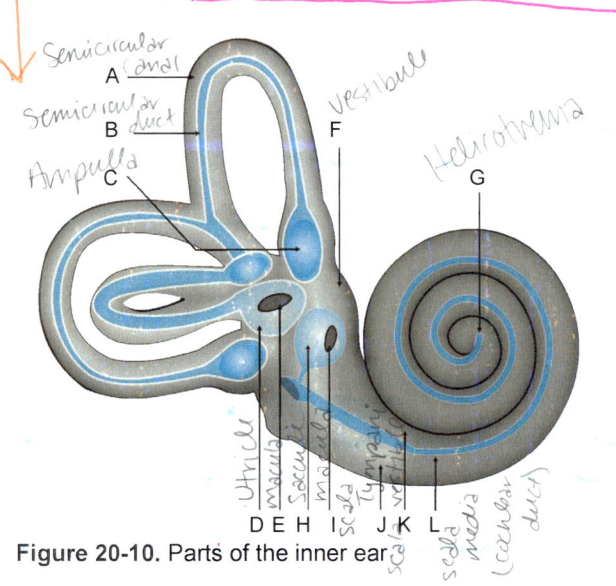

Figure 20-10. Parts of the inner ear

gelatinous structure called the **tectorial membrane** (tek-TOR-ē-al; "to cover"). The hair cells of the spiral organ do not contain a kinocilium.

The stapes connect directly to the scala vestibuli at a membrane-covered opening called the **oval window**. When the stapes vibrates in response to sound waves, it vibrates the oval window, causing waves to develop in the perilymph of the scala vestibuli. The waves travel through the three cochlear chambers and finally reach the end of the scala tympani at a membrane-covered opening called the **round window**. The round window pulsates at the same frequency as the oval window, thus, relieving pressure built up in the cochlea from waves initiated at the oval window. This is like the opposite of a drum vibrating when a drumstick strikes the other side. Liquid conduction of sound occurs inside the cochlea.

PERCEPTION OF SOUND

Sound waves vary in frequency and amplitude. **Sound frequency,** measured in *hertz* (Hz), refers to the number of wave peaks that pass a given point in a given amount of time. **Sound wavelength** refers to the distance between successive peaks. Short sound waves have a higher frequency than long sound waves. The average human can hear sounds with frequencies between 20 and 20,000 Hz, but are most sensitive to frequencies between 1500 and 4000 Hz. A **sound's pitch** relates to frequency. The brain perceives long sound waves (low frequency) as *bass* sounds (low pitch), and short wavelengths (high frequency) as *treble* (high pitch).

The energy in sound, measured in logarithmic units called *decibels* (dB), refers to the pressure difference created by the sound waves, and is a measure of the wave's height, called **amplitude (intensity** or **volume).** Two sounds with the same pitch can have different intensities. A sound at 50 dB is 10 times louder than 40 dB, and 100 times louder than 30 dB. Humans can detect sound as "soft" as 0.1 dB, or as "loud" as 130 dB or greater. Sounds of 130 dB or greater usually cause pain.

PHYSIOLOGY OF HEARING

Sound waves enter the external auditory meatus and vibrate the tympanum and ear ossicles. The vibrating stapes transmits vibrations into the cochlea via the oval window. The perilymph is set in motion in the scala vestibuli. Waves in the perilymph travel through the scala vestibuli and pass into the scala tympani through the helicotrema. As waves pass through the top chamber, they cause the vestibular membrane to vibrate. The vibrating vestibular membrane creates waves in the endolymph of the cochlear duct. The vibrating endolymph causes the basilar membrane to vibrate. The organ of Corti resting atop the basilar membrane vibrates against the gelatinous tectorial membrane. The vibration causes the hair cells' microvilli to bend and create a graded potential. This graded potential initiates an impulse in the sensory neurons connected to the hair cells. The impulses travel through the **cochlear nerve** and pass on through association neurons in the brain to reach the **auditory cortex** in temporal lobe.

Cochlear Sensitivity to Different Sounds

The basilar membrane is more flexible near the helicotrema than it is near the oval window. As a result, high frequency (treble) sounds are better able to stimulate hair cells near the proximal end of the spiral organ, while low frequency (bass) sounds stimulate hair cells nearer the helicotrema (Figure 20-11). Therefore, the brain perceives different pitches of sound depending on where the impulses originate along the spiral organ.

High intensity vibrations stimulate a larger number of hair cells within a given region of the spiral organ and the brain perceives this as louder sounds. Extremely high intensity sounds can damage hair cells in a certain region of the spiral organ resulting in a loss of ability to hear certain frequencies of sound. Listening to very loud music for prolonged periods may "fatigue" the hair cells, resulting in a temporary impairment of hearing ability. The cells may recover, or they may not.

EQUILIBRIUM

Equilibrium refers to a person's ability to determine body position and maintain balance, and includes *static* and *dynamic* equilibrium.

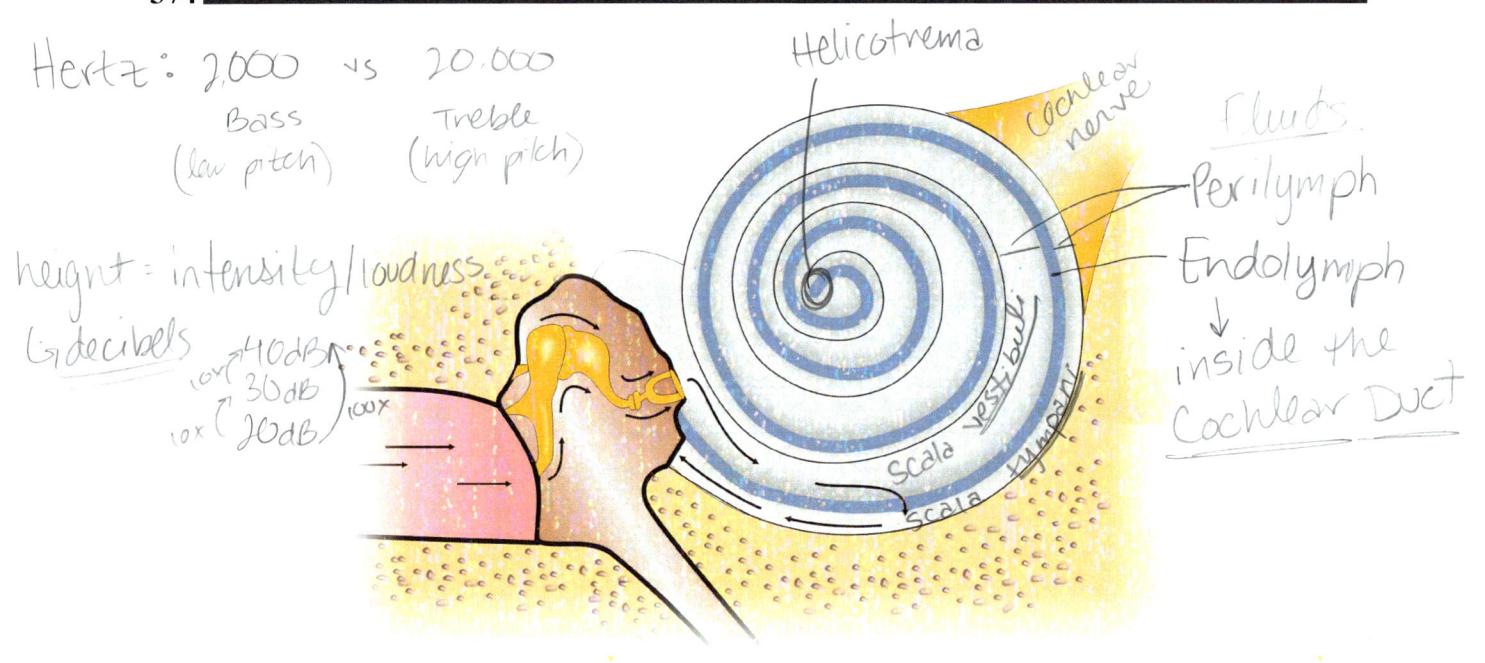

Figure 20-11. Sound conduction through the ear

Static Equilibrium

Static equilibrium relates to the head's position relative to the ground, and when the body moves in a "straight-line," such as during acceleration or deceleration (forward, backward, and side-to-side movements). The maculae within the saccule and utricle of the vestibule are important in helping the body maintain static equilibrium.

The hair cells of the maculae depolarize and repolarize constantly, but the frequency of impulses sent to the brain depends on the position of the stereocilia and kinocilium. When head position changes in response to acceleration or deceleration, the otolithic membrane shifts in the opposite direction and causes the stereocilia and kinocilium to bend. When these "hairs" bend in one direction, depolarization occurs more frequently; when they bend in the opposite direction, depolarization occurs less frequently. Impulses leave the maculae and travel to the cerebellum and higher brain centers by way of the **vestibular nerve**.

The brain can cause various skeletal muscles to contract or relax in order to compensate for changes in body position. The hair cells in the saccule respond more to up-and-down motions, such as when bending over or riding in an elevator. Hair cells in the utricle respond more to acceleration and deceleration.

Dynamic Equilibrium

Dynamic equilibrium relates to angular movements, such as spinning, turning, flipping, etc., but the sensory receptors involved also respond to static movements. Dynamic movement causes endolymph to move within the semicircular ducts. Depending on the type of movement, the fluid in one particular semicircular duct may move more than the fluid in another; therefore, its cupula (located on the crista within the ampulla) will bend to a greater degree in the endolymph's current. The swaying cupula bends the stereocilia and kinocilium of the hair cells located on the crista.

When the head is spinning, the endolymph within the *transverse duct* flows in the opposite direction of the spinning and presses on the cupula. In response to impulses arising from the crista within this duct, the brain can stimulate certain skeletal muscles and relax others to maintain balance. Impulses initiated in the ampullae travel to the cerebellum through the vestibular nerve. Consuming excessive amounts of alcohol can affect the specific gravity of the endolymph and perilymph. Consequently, the stereocilia and kinocilia of the cristae and maculae may sway more easily due to a lack of resistance. This, in turn, can contribute to difficulty in maintaining balance and equilibrium.

THE SENSES

TOPICS TO KNOW FOR CHAPTER 20 (SENSES)

accessory structures of the eye
accommodation
acute pain
afterimage
air conduction of sound
amacrine cells
ampulla
anatomy of the eye
anterior aqueous chamber
antihelix
antitragus
aqueous chamber
aqueous humor
auditory (Eustachian) tube
auditory cortex
auricle
baroreceptors
basal cells
basilar membrane
bass sounds
bipolar cells
bitterness
blind spot
bone conduction of sound
bony labyrinth
bulbar conjunctiva
canal of Schlemm
central retinal artery
central retinal vein
ceruminous glands
chambers of the eye
chemoreceptors
chlorolabe
choroid coat
chronic pain
ciliary body
ciliary glands
classification of pain
classification of receptors
classification of specific receptors (table)
cochlea
cochlear duct
cochlear nerve
cochlear sensitivity to different sounds
cones
conjunctiva
convergence
cornea
coronal semicircular duct
crista ampullaris
crystallins
cupula
cyanolabe
dark adaptation

decibels (dB)
deep pain
depth perception
dilator (or radial) muscle
dynamic equilibrium
ear conchae
ear ossicles
eardrum
electromagnetic (radiant) energy
electromagnetic spectrum
endolymph
endolymph
epicanthic fold
equilibrium
erythrolabe
external auditory meatus
external ear
exteroceptors
extrinsic eye muscles
eye movement
eyebrows
eyelashes
eyelids
facial nerves
far point of vision
far-sightedness (hyperopia)
fibrous tunic
fovea centralis
ganglion cells
general senses
glossopharyngeal nerves
granule cells
gustatory cells
hair cells in cochlea
helicotrema
helix
hertz (Hz)
horizontal cells
incus
inferior oblique
inferior rectus
inner ear (labyrinth)
interoceptors
intrinsic eye muscles
iodopsin
iris
kinocilium
kinocilium
lacrimal canals
lacrimal caruncle
lacrimal glands
lacrimal puncta
lateral canthus
lateral rectus

lens
lens accommodation
levator palpebrae
light adaptation
light intensity (brightness)
light refraction in the eye
light wavelength
liquid conduction of sound
lobule (earlobe)
lysozyme
macula
macula lutea
malleus
mechanoreceptors
medial canthus
medial rectus
membranous labyrinth
middle ear
mitral cells
nasolacrimal duct
near point of vision
near-sightedness (myopia)
nervous tunic
neural layer
nociceptors
off-center field
olfaction
olfactory (Bowman's) glands
olfactory bulb
olfactory epithelium
olfactory nerves
olfactory neurons
on-center field
ophthalmoscope
optic chiasma
optic disc
ora serrata
orbicularis oculi
organ of Corti
osmoreceptors
otolithic membrane
otoliths
oval window
pain sensations
palpebrae
palpebral conjunctiva
perception
perception of color
perception of sound
perilymph
phantom pain
phasic receptors
photons
photopigment bleaching

photopigments
photopsins
photoreceptors
physiology of hearing
pigmented layer
pinna
posterior aqueous chamber
projection
proprioceptors
pupil
receptive field
receptor adaptation
receptor potential
referred pain
retina
retinal (retinene)
retinal processing
rhodopsin
rods
round window
ROY-G-BIV
saccades
saccule
sagittal semicircular duct
saltiness
scala media
scala tympani
scala vestibuli
sclera
scleral venous sinus
scotopsin
semicircular canals
semicircular ducts

sensation
senses
sensory receptor
smell
somatic pain
sound
sound amplitude (intensity or volume)
sound frequency
sound pitch
sound wavelength
sourness
spatial discrimination
special senses
sphincter (circular) muscle
stapedius muscle
stapes
static equilibrium
stereocilia
stimulation of photoreceptors
superficial pain
superior oblique
superior rectus
supporting cells
supporting cells in cochlea
suspensory ligaments
sustenacular cells
sweetness
tactile receptors
tarsal (Meibomian) glands
tarsal plate
taste
taste buds
tear gland

tectorial membrane
tensor tympani
the ear and hearing
the eye and vision
thermoreceptors
tongue papillae
tonic receptors
tragus
transduction
transverse semicircular duct
treble sounds
tympanic cavity
tympanum
umami
utricle
uvea
vascular tunic
vestibular membrane
vestibular nerve
vestibule
visceral pain
visible light
visual acuity
visual axis
visual field
visual field and 3-D vision
visual pathway
visual ratings
vitamin A
vitreous chamber
vitreous humor

Appendix 1: Keys for Chapter Figures

CHAPTER 1

1-1
A. Chemical (atoms)
B. Chemical (molecules)
C. Cellular (organelles)
D. Cellular (muscle cells)
E. Tissue (muscle tissue)
F. Organ (heart)

1-2
A. Integumentary system
B. Cardiovascular system
C. Digestive system
D. Endocrine system
E. Muscular system
F. Urinary system
G. Reproductive system
H. Skeletal system
I. Respiratory system
J. Nervous system
K. Lymphatic system

1-4
A. Sweating, skin vasodilation
B. Shivering, vasoconstriction

CHAPTER 2

2-1 (a)
A. Frontal (forehead)
B. Cranial
C. Facial
D. Oral (mouth)
E. Mental (chin)
F. Axillary (armpit)
G. Brachial (arm)
H. Cubital (elbow) or Antecubital (front of)
I. Antebrachial (forearm)
J. Coxal (hip)
K. Carpal (wrist)
L. Pollex (thumb)
M. Digital (fingers) or Phalangeal
N. Palmar
O. Patellar (knee)
P. Crural (leg)
Q. Tarsal (ankle)
R. Digital (toes) or Phalangeal
S. Hallux (big toe)
T. Pedal (foot)
U. Fibular (Peroneal)
V. Femoral (thigh)
W. Genital
X. Inguinal
Y. Pelvic
Z. Umbilical (navel)
AA. Abdominal
BB. Pectoral (chest)
CC. Sternal (breastbone)
DD. Cervical (neck)
EE. Nasal (nose)
FF. Otic (ear)
GG. Buccal (cheek)
FF. Ocular (eye) or Orbital

2-1 (b)
A. Acromial (shoulder)
B. Vertebral or Spinal
C. Lumbar (lower back)
D. Natal cleft
E. Manual (hand)
F. Gluteal (buttock)
G. Gluteal fold
H. Popliteal (back of knee)
I. Sural
J. Calcaneal
K. Digital or Phalangeal
L. Volar or Plantar
M. Lower appendage
N. Upper appendage
O. Scapular
P. Cervical
Q. Cranial or Cephalic

2-2
A. Superior or Cephalic
B. Posterior or Dorsal
C. Inferior or Caudal
D. Anterior or Ventral
E. Proximal and Superior
F. Distal and Inferior
G. Distal and Inferior
H. Proximal and Superior

2-3
A. Frontal or Coronal
B. Sagittal
C. Transverse or Cross

2-4

A. Cranial
B. Spinal or Vertebral
C. Pleural
D. Pericardial
E. Thoracic
F. Diaphragm
G. Abdominal
H. Pelvic
I. Abdominopelvic
J. Cranial
K. Spinal or Vertebral
L. Dorsal
M. Pleural
N. Pericardial
O. Diaphragm
P. Abdominal
Q. Pelvic
R. Pleural
S. Spinal
T. Pericardial
U. Mediastinum

2-5

A. Upper right quadrant
B. Upper left quadrant
C. Lower right quadrant
D. Lower left quadrant
E. Epigastric
F. Right hypochondriac
G. Right lumbar
H. Right inguinal (Iliac)
I. Umbilical
J. Left hypochondriac
K. Left lumbar
L. Left inguinal (Iliac)
M. Hypogastric (Pubic)
N. Liver
O. Gallbladder
P. Large intestine (Colon)
Q. Small intestine
R. Appendix
S. Stomach
T. Spleen
U. Urinary bladder

CHAPTER 3

3-1

A. First (lowest) shell
B. Second energy shell
C. First energy shell
D. Third energy shell

3-2

A. Anion (e.g., chloride)
B. Cation (e.g., sodium)

3-5

A. Hydration shell
B. Hydration shells

3-7

A. Unsaturated fatty acid
B. Hydrogenated fatty acid
C. Trans fatty acid

CHAPTER 4

4-1

A. Cytoskeletal component
B. Cytoskeletal component
C. Centriole
D. Centrosome
E. Mitochondrion
F. Peroxisome
G. Transport vesicle
H. Bound ribosome
I. Lysosome
J. Cilium
K. Rough ER
L. Microvillus
M. Cytosol
N. Peroxisome
O. Nucleolus
P. Nuclear membrane
Q. Nuclear pore

4-2

A. Mitochondrion
B. Microfilament
C. Microtubule
D. Vesicle
E. Microtubule
F. Intermediate filament
G. Endoplasmic reticulum

4-5

A. Microtubule in cilium
B. Basal body

4-6

A. Large ribosomal subunit
B. Small ribosomal subunit

4-7

A. Matrix (inner compartment)
B. Inner membrane
C. Outer membrane
D. Intermembrane space (outer compartment)

4-9

A. Rough ER
B. Bound ribosome

4-10

A. Golgi complex
B. Vesicle
C. Trans face

CHAPTER 5

5-1

A. Nucleoplasm
B. Chromatin

APPENDIX 1: KEYS FOR CHAPTER FIGURES

C. Nucleolus
D. Nuclear membrane
E. Nuclear pore

5-2
A. Plasma membrane
B. Chromatid
C. Centromere
D. Nucleosome
E. DNA

5-4
A. DNA
B. Phosphate-Sugar backbone
C. RNA polymerase
D. Nucleotide
E. RNA transcript
F. Released RNA molecule

5-7
A. Amino acid (methionine)
B. tRNA
C. Large ribosomal subunit
D. mRNA
E. Amino acid
F. Small ribosomal subunit
G. Amino acid
H. Large ribosomal subunit

5-8
A. Centrosome
B. Nuclear membrane
C. Nucleolus
D. Plasma membrane
E. Chromatin in nucleoplasm
F. Centriole
G. Centromere
H. Chromatid
I. Spindle fiber
J. Replicated chromosome
K. Spindle fiber
L. Metaphase plate

M. Centriole
N. Sister chromosome
O. Uncoiling chromosome
P. Cleavage furrow
Q. RNA polymerase

5-9
A. Original DNA molecule
B. Original DNA side
C. New DNA side

CHAPTER 6

6-1
A. Integral protein
B. Cholesterol
C. Phospholipid bilayer
D. Carbohydrates
E. Transmembrane proteins
F. Fatty acid tails
G. Phospholipid bilayer
H. Glycerol heads
I. Cytoskeletal components

6-12
A. Bacterium
B. Forming phagosome
C. Phagosome
D. Lysosome
E. Enzymes
F. Vesicle

CHAPTER 7

7-4
A. Basal lamina of basement membrane
B. Reticular lamina
C. Connective tissue
D. Basal cell (squamous)
E. Basal cell (cuboidal)
F. Basal cell nucleus
G. Basement membrane

H. Connective tissue
I. Basal cell (columnar)
J. Basal cell nucleus
K. Basement membrane
L. Apical cells (squamous)
M. Epithelial cell
N. Basement membrane
O. Connective tissue
P. Apical cell (cuboidal)
Q. Epithelial cell
R. Basement membrane
S. Connective tissue
T. Apical cell (columnar)
U. Basal cell (columnar)
V. Apical cell (transitional)
W. Epithelial cell
X. Basal epithelial cell

7-5
A. Fibroblast
B. Adipocyte
C. Basophil
D. Eosinophil
E. Monocyte
F. White blood cell Neutrophil
G. Erythrocyte
H. Adipocyte
I. Fibroblast
J. Fibroblast

7-6
A. Collagenous fiber
B. Fibroblast
C. Collagenous fiber
D. Fibroblast
E. Collagenous fiber

7-7
A. Chondrocyte in lacuna
B. Chondrocyte in lacuna
C. Elastic fiber

D. Collagenous fiber
E. Chondrocyte in a lacuna

7-8
A. Canaliculus
B. Central (Haversian) canal
C. Osteocyte in lacuna
D. Canaliculus
E. Central canal
F. Osteocyte in lacuna

CHAPTER 8

8-1
A. Dermis
B. Epidermis
C. Papillary dermis
D. Reticular dermis
E. Hypodermis
F. Hair shaft
G. Free nerve ending
H. Tactile receptor
I. Sweat gland duct
J. Papillary plexus vessel
K. Arrector pili muscle
L. Tactile receptor
M. Reticular plexus artery
N. Reticular plexus vein
O. Reticular plexus

8-3
A. Stratum corneum
B. Stratum lucidum
C. Stratum granulosum
D. Stratum spinosum
E. Stratum basale
F. Stratum corneum
G. Stratum lucidum
H. Stratum granulosum
I. Stratum spinosum
J. Stratum basale

8-4
A. Melanin in melanosome of melanocyte
B. Melanin granule in keratinocyte

8-5
A. Hair shaft
B. Opening of hair follicle
C. Sebaceous gland
D. Arrector pili muscle
E. Hair medulla
F. Hair cortex
G. Dermal sheat
H. Hair bulb
I. Hair cortex (white)
J. Dermal sheath
K. External epithelial sheath
L. Internal epithelial sheath
M. Hair cuticle (gray)
N. Hair cortex (white)
O. Hair medulla (pink)

8-6
A. Nail fee edge
B. Nail body
C. Lunula
D. Nail fold
E. Edge of eponychium
F. Edge of eponychium
G. Nail fold
H. Nail body
I. Phalanx (bone)
J. Epidermis
K. Hyponychium
L. Nail body
M. Eponychium
N. Nail root
O. Stratum basale
P. Middle phalanx
Q. Distal phalanx
R. Epidermis

8-7
A. Red blood cell
B. Platelet
C. Epidermis
D. Dermis
E. Granulation tissue
F. Open wound
G. Fibroblast
H. Collagenous fiber
I. Fibroblast
J. Fibrocyte

CHAPTER 9

9-1
A. Flat bone
B. Short bone (sesamoid)
C. Irregular bone
D. Long bone
E. Short bone

9-2
A. Head of long bone
B. Compact bone
C. Medullary cavity (pink)
D. Proximal epiphysis
E. Proximal metaphysis
F. Diaphysis
G. Distal metaphysis
H. Distal epiphysis

9-3
A. Sspongy bone trabecula
B. Lymphatic vessel
C. Nutrient artery
D. Compact bone
E. Lamella of osteon
F. Compact bone lamella
G. Lymphatic vessel

APPENDIX 1: KEYS FOR CHAPTER FIGURES

H. Perforating (Volkmann's) canal
I. Artery
J. Central (Haversian) canal
K. Osteocyte in lacuna

9-5

A. Bony collar
B. Medullary cavity
C. Secondary ossification center
D. Articular cartilage
E. Compact bone below epiphyseal disc (blue)
F. Medullary cavity
G. Blood vessel
H. Compact bone
I. Epiphysis

CHAPTER 10

10-1

A. Skull
B. Cervical vertebrae
C. Ribs/thoracic vertebrae
D. Lumbar vertebrae
E. Sacrum
F. Coccyx
G. Sternum

10-2

A. Lacrimal
B. Sphenoid's greater wing
C. Superior orbital fissure
D. Temporal
E. Nasal bones
F. Infraorbital foramen
G. Inferior nasal concha
H. Vomer
I. Squamous suture
J. Temporal (squamous part)
K. Zygomatic process
L. Lambdoid suture
M. External auditory meatus
N. Mastoid process
O. Styloid process
P. Parietal
Q. Coronal suture
R. Frontal
S. Supraorbital foramen
T. Temporal
U. Sphenoid
V. Sphenoid
W. Inferior orbital fissure
X. Zygomatic
Y. Middle nasal concha
Z. Perpendicular plate of ethmoid
AA. Mandible
BB. Mental foramen
CC. Coronal suture
DD. Frontal
EE. Sphenoid's greater wing
FF. Nasal
GG. Ethmoid
HH. Maxilla
II. Maxilla
JJ. Zygomatic
KK. Mental foramen
LL. Mandible
MM. Temporal process

10-2 (continued)

A. Maxilla
B. Zygomatic
C. Sphenoid
D. Vomer
E. Foramen ovale
F. External auditory meatus
G. Jugular foramen
H. Condylar foramen
I. Lambdoid suture
J. Occipital
K. Superior nuchal line
L. Anterior cranial fossa
M. Crista galli
N. Cribriform plate
O. Sphenoid's greater wing
P. Occipitomastoid suture
Q. Posterior cranial fossa
R. Hard palate of maxilla
S. Maxilla
T. Palatine
U. Zygomatic arch
V. Pterygoid process
W. Pterygoid process
X. Foramen lacerum
Y. Carotid canal
Z. Occipital condyle
AA. Foramen magnum
BB. External occipital protuberance
CC. Sella turcica
DD. Foramen rotundum
EE. Foramen ovale
FF. Foramen spinosum
GG. Temporal (petrous part)
HH. Internal auditory meatus
II. Hypoglossal canal
JJ. Occipital

10-3

A. Sphenoid
B. Superior orbital fissure
C. Inferior orbital fissure
D. Maxilla
E. Zygomatic
F. Supraorbital margin
G. Frontal
H. Optic canal

381

I. Ethmoid
J. Lacrimal (red)
K. Nasal (pink)
L. Nasolacrimal duct
M. Maxilla
N. Infraorbital foramen

10-4
A. Frontal
B. Frontal sinus
C. Perpendicular plate of ethmoid
D. Nasal
E. Nasal septum cartilage
F. Palatine
G. Maxilla
H. Sella turcica above sphenoid sinus
I. Vomer
J. Pterygoid process

10-5
A. Nasal
B. Maxilla
C. Mandible
D. Frontal
E. Coronal suture forming
F. Sphenoid fontanel
G. Squamous suture forming
H. Lambdoid suture forming
I. Mastoid fontanel
J. Occipital
K. Temporal
L. Frontal suture
M. Coronal suture (lateral to anterior fontanel)
N. Posterior fontanel (blue)
O. Sagittal suture

10-6
A. Cervical curvature
B. Thoracic curvature
C. Lumbar curvature
D. Sacral curvature
E. Cervical vertebrae
F. Thoracic vertebrae
G. Lumbar vertebrae
H. Sacrum
I. Coccyx

10-7
A. Superior articular process
B. Transverse process
C. Spinous process
D. Inferior articular process
E. Pedicel
F. Vertebra body (centrum)
G. Inferior articular facet
H. Superior articular facet
I. Pedicle
J. Lamina
K. Intervertebral disc
L. Body of vertebra
M. Spinous process
N. Inferior articular process
O. Transverse process
P. Articular facet
Q. Body of vertebra
R. Vertebral foramen
S. Spinous process
T. Lamina
U. Pedicle
V. Superior articular facet
W. Lamina
X. Spinous process
Y. Intervertebral foramen
Z. Pedicle
AA. Superior articular process
BB. Body of vertebra
CC. Inferior articular facet

10-8
A. Posterior arch of atlas
B. Lateral mass
C. Dens (odontoid process)
D. Anterior arch of atlas
E. Lamina of axis

10-9
A. Sacral canal
B. Articular facet
C. Ala
D. Lateral sacral crest
E. Median sacral crest
F. Median sacral crest
G. Sacral hiatus
H. Coccyx
I. Sacral promontory
J. Median sacral crest
K. Lateral sacral crest
L. Median sacral crest
M. Median sacral crest
N. Median sacral crest
O. Ala
P. Sacral promontory
Q. Sacral foramen
R. Transverse ridge

10-10
A. Jugular notch
B. Manubrium
C. Costal notch
D. True ribs (1-7)
E. False ribs (8-12)
F. Superior thoracic aperture
G. 1st thoracic vertebra
H. 2nd thoracic vertebra
I. Vertebrocostal joint
J. Sternal body (gladiolus)
K. Xiphoid process
L. Costal cartilages

APPENDIX 1: KEYS FOR CHAPTER FIGURES

M. Floating ribs (11-12)
N. Inferior thoracic aperture

CHAPTER 11

11-1
A. Cranium of skull
B. Mandible
C. Cervical vertebra
D. Clavicle
E. Scapula
F. Sternum
G. Humerus
H. Rib
I. Lumbar vertebra
J. Ulna
K. Radius
L. Sacrum
M. Carpal
N. Proximal phalanx
O. Distal phalanx
P. Femur
Q. Patella
R. Tibia
S. Fibula
T. Tarsal
U. Metatarsal
V. Phalanx

11-2
A. Scapula
B. Clavicle
C. Manubrium
D. Sternoclavicular joint
E. Sternal end of clavicle
F. Acromial end of clavicle
G. Body of clavicle

11-3
A. Acromion process
B. Coracoid process
C. Superior border
D. Superior angle
E. Lateral angle
F. Subscapular fossa
G. Axillary (lateral) border
H. Inferior angle
I. Vertebral (medial) border
J. Acromion process
K. Lip of glenoid cavity
L. Coracoid process
M. Acromion process
N. Lip of glenoid cavity
O. Axillary border
P. Inferior border
Q. Supraspinous fossa
R. Coracoid process
S. Acromion process
T. Spine of scapula
U. Lip of glenoid cavity
V. Infraspinous fossa
W. Axillary border
X. Vertebral border
Y. Inferior border

11-4
A. Head of humerus
B. Neck of humerus
C. Lesser tubercle
D. Intertubercular groove
E. Greater tubercle
F. Neck of humerus
G. Diaphysis
H. Coronoid fossa
I. Radial fossa
J. Lateral epicondyle
K. Capitulum
L. Trochlea
M. Medial epicondyle
N. Greater tubercle
O. Diaphysis
P. Trochlea
Q. Olecranon fossa

11-5
A. Ulnar trochlear notch
B. Ulnar coronoid process
C. Head of radius
D. Radial neck
E. Radial tuberosity
F. Diaphysis
G. Radius distal epiphysis
H. Head of ulna
I. Styloid process of radius
J. Ulnar olecranon process
K. Ulnar coronoid process
L. Head of radius
M. Radial neck
N. Diaphysis of ulna
O. Diaphysis of radius
P. Interosseous membrane
Q. Head of ulna
R. Ulnar notch
S. Styloid process of radius
T. Styloid process of ulna

11-6
A. Triquetral
B. Lunate
C. Scaphoid
D. Trapezium
E. Trapezoid
F. Capitate
G. Metacarpal #1
H. Hamate
I. Proximal phalanx
J. Distal phalanx
K. Trapezoid
L. Lunate
M. Scaphoid
N. Pisiform

O. Trapezium
P. Trapezoid
Q. Capitate
R. Hamate
S. Metacarpophalangeal joint
T. Head of metacarpal #2
U. Proximal phalanx
V. Middle phalanx
W. Distal phalanx

11-7
A. Iliac crest
B. Anterior superior iliac spine
C. Ala
D. Anterior inferior iliac spine
E. Gluteal line
F. Sciatic notch
G. Posterior inferior iliac spine
H. Lip of acetabulum
I. Lip of acetabulum
J. Superior ramus of pubis
K. Pubic crest
L. Inferior ramus of pubis
M. Ischial tuberosity
N. Ischial ramus
O. Iliac fossa
P. Iliac fossa
Q. Posterior superior iliac spine
R. Articular surface
S. Posterior inferior iliac spine
T. Sciatic notch
U. Ischial spine
V. Ischial ramus
W. Ischium
X. Ischial tuberosity
Y. Articular surface
Z. Pubic crest

11-9
A. Head of femur
B. Greater trochanter
C. Neck of femur
D. Lesser trochanter
E. *Adductor tubercle*
F. Lateral epicondyle
G. Lateral condyle
H. Medial condyle
I. Medial epicondyle
J. Greater trochanter
K. Intertrochanteric crest
L. Gluteal tuberosity
M. Gluteal tuberosity
N. Linea aspera
O. Diaphysis
P. Intercondylar line
Q. Lateral epicondyle
R. Intercondylar notch
S. Lateral condyle
T. Medial condyle

11-10
A. Medial condyle
B. Lateral condyle
C. Head of fibula
D. Tibial tuberosity
E. Diaphysis of tibia
F. Tibia
G. Fibula
H. Medial malleolus
I. Distal tibiofibular joint
J. Lateral malleolus
K. Medial condyle
L. Intercondylar eminence
M. Proximal tibiofibular joint
N. Head of fibula
O. Tibial tuberosity
P. Fibula
Q. Tibia
R. Medial malleolus
S. Lateral malleolus

11-11
A. Calcaneus
B. Trochlea of talus
C. Talus
D. Navicular
E. Cuboid
F. Lateral cuneiform
G. Metatarsal #2
H. Proximal phalanx-digit 5
I. Middle phalanx
J. Distal phalanx
K. Proximal phalanx-digit 1
L. Distal phalanx
M. Phalanges
N. Metatarsal
O. Lateral cuneiform
P. Navicular
Q. Talus
R. Calcaneus

CHAPTER 12

12-1
A. Medullary cavity
B. Compact bone
C. Periosteum
D. Articular cartilage
E. Synovial cavity
F. Synovial membrane
G. Periosteum

12-2
A. Hand (wrist) extension
B. Hand (wrist) flexion
C. Arm lateral rotation
D. Arm medial rotation
E. Head (neck) flexion
F. Head (neck) extension
G. Thigh (hip) flexion
H. Thigh (hip) extension
I. Arm abduction

APPENDIX 1: KEYS FOR CHAPTER FIGURES

J. Arm adduction
K. Thigh (hip) abduction
L. Thigh (hip) adduction
M. Hand (wrist) adduction
N. Hand (wrist) abduction
O. Arm circumduction

12-2 (continued)

A. Head neck rotation
B. Arm lateral rotation
C. Arm medial rotation
D. Supination of palm
E. Pronation of palm
F. Eversion of foot (ankle)
G. Inversion of foot (ankle)
H. Dorsiflexion
I. Plantar flexion
J. Opposition
K. Depression of mandible
L. Elevation of mandible
M. Head (neck) lateral flexion

12-3

A. Acromion process
B. Coracoacromial ligament
C. Subacromial bursa
D. Head of humerus
E. Synovial cavity
F. Muscle tendon
G. Clavicle
H. Acromioclavicular ligament
I. Scapula
J. Glenoid fossa of scapula
K. Edge of glenoid labrum
L. Fibrous capsule
M. Medullary cavity

12-4

A. Humerus
B. Radial annular ligament
C. Ulnar olecranon process
D. Humeral lateral epicondyle
E. Radial collateral ligament
F. Humerus
G. Radial annular ligament
H. Ulnar collateral ligament
I. Ulnar olecranon process

12-5

A. Greater trochanter
B. Muscle tendon
C. Pubofemoral ligament
D. Iliofemoral ligament
E. Obturator foramen
F. Obturator membrane
G. Lesser trochanter
H. Ischium
I. Femur
J. Muscle tendon
K. Iliofemoral ligament
L. Greater trochanter
M. Ischiofemoral ligament
N. Synovial capsule
O. Lesser trochanter
P. Femur
Q. Greater trochanter
R. Synovial capsule
S. Coxal (hip) bone
T. Synovial membrane
U. Ligamentum teres
V. Articular cartilage
W. Acetabular labrum
X. Synovial capsule
Y. Medullary cavity

12-6

A. Fibular collateral ligament
B. Tibial collateral ligament
C. Medial condyle of femur
D. *Meniscofemoral ligament*
E. Medial meniscus
F. Posterior cruciate ligament
G. Head of fibula
H. Fibular collateral ligament
I. Lateral condyle of femur
J. Posterior cruciate ligament
K. Medial condyle of femur
L. Medial meniscus
M. Anterior cruciate ligament
N. Lateral meniscus
O. Fibular collateral ligament
P. Head of fibula

CHAPTER 14

14-2

A. Skeletal muscle
B. Tendon fibers
C. Epimysium
D. Fascicles
E. Muscle cell (myofiber)
F. Nuclei
G. Cytoplasm
H. Sarcolemma
I. Sarcoplasmic reticulum
J. Mitochondrion
K. Myofibrils
L. Z discs
M. Thin myofilament
N. Thick myofilament
O. Thick myofilament
P. Thin myofilament
Q. Titin

14-3

A. Myofilament
B. Myofibril
C. Sarcolemma of myofiber
D. Nucleus
E. Myofibril
F. Myofilaments

G. A band
H. I band
I. Z disc
J. Thin myofilament
K. Thick myofilament within myofibril
L. Mitochondria
M. Terminal cisternae of SR
N. SR
O. T tubule

14-4
A. Myofilament
B. Myofibrils
C. Sarcolemma of myofiber
D. Nucleus
E. Myofibril
F. Myofilament
G. Z disc
H. H zone of A band
I. Z disc
J. I band
K. A band
L. I band
M. M line

14-5
A. I band
B. H zone
C. Thin myofilament
D. M line
E. Thick myofilament
F. Z disc
G. A band

14-6
A. I band
B. A band
C. I band
D. Z disc
E. H zone

F. Z disc

14-15
A. Contractile unit between dense bodies
B. Dense body
C. Thick myofilament
D. Thin myofilament

14-16
A. Axon of motor neuron

CHAPTER 15

15-1
A. Epicranial aponeurosis
B. Temporalis
C. Scalenus muscle
D. Clavicle
E. Deltoid
F. Pectoralis major
G. Biceps brachii (short head)
H. Biceps brachii (long head)
I. Brachialis
J. Triceps brachii
K. Palmaris longus
L. Brachioradialis
M. Tensor fasciae latae
N. Rectus femoris
O. Vastus lateralis
P. Iliotibial tract
Q. Patella
R. Tibia
S. Tibialis anterior
T. Extensor digitorum
U. Extensor retinaculum
V. Extensor retinaculum
W. Frontalis
X. Sternocleidomastoid
Y. Scalenus
Z. Sternum
AA. Serratus anterior

BB. Latissimus dorsi
CC. External oblique
DD. Rectus abdominis
EE. Linea alba
FF. Brachioradialis
GG. Flexor carpi radialis
HH. Brachioradialis tendon
II. Tensor fasciae latae
JJ. Flexor retinaculum
KK. Aductor longus
LL. Adductor magnus
MM. Gracilis
NN. Sartorius
OO. Vastus medialis
PP. Gastrocnemius
QQ. Soleus
RR. Medial malleolus
SS. Lateral malleolus

15-1 (continued)
A. Occipitalis
B. Nuchal ligament
C. Sternocleidomastoid
D. Latissimus dorsi
E. Lumbodorsal fascia
F. Gluteus maximus
G. Gracilis
H. Gastrocnemius
I. Gastrocnemius
J. Calcaneal (Achilles') tendon
K. Extensor digitorum
L. Nuchal ligament
M. Trapezius
N. Deltoid
O. Triceps brachii
P. Triceps brachii
Q. Flexor carpi ulnaris
R. Extensor retinaculum
S. Intrinsic hand muscle

APPENDIX 1: KEYS FOR CHAPTER FIGURES

T. Semitendinosus
U. Vastus lateralis
V. Gastrocnemius
W. Extensor retinaculum
X. Intrinsic foot muscle

15-2

A. Orbicularis oculi
B. Nasalis
C. Levator labii superioris
D. Zygomaticus muscles
E. Oribicularis oris
F. Mentalis
G. Depressor labii
H. Depressor anguli oris
I. Frontalis
J. Temporalis
K. Corrugator supercilii
L. Procerus
M. Nasalis
N. Orbicularis oris
O. Risorius
P. Platysma (cut)
Q. Mentalis
R. Epicranial aponeurosis
S. Temporoparietalis
T. Occipitalis
U. Masseter
V. Buccinators
W. Sternocleidomastoid
X. Trapezius
Y. Temporoparietalis
Z. Temporalis
AA. Levator labii superioris alaeque nasi
BB. Levator labii superioris
CC. Zygomaticus muscles
DD. Masseter
EE. Orbicularis oris
FF. Mentalis
GG. Trapezius
HH. Strenocleidomastoid
II. Platysma

15-3

A. Longissimus (cut)
B. Spinalis cervicis
C. Middle scalenus
D. Posterior scalenus
E. Semispinalis cervicis
F. Longissimus cervicis
G. Semispinalis thoracis
H. Longissimus thoracis
I. Multifidus
J. Quadratus lumborum
K. Semispinalis capitis (cut)
L. Splenius
M. Longissimus capitis
N. Longissimus cervicis
O. Iliocostalis cervicis
P. Iliocostalis thoracis
Q. Spinalis thoracis
R. Iliocostalis lumborum
S. Erector spinae

15-4

A. Platysma
B. Clavicle
C. Deltoid
D. Pectoralis major
E. Serratus anterior
F. Latissimus dorsi
G. Rectus abdominis
H. External oblique
I. Tendinous sheath
J. Transversus abdominis
K. Inguinal canal
L. Sternocleidomastoid
M. Nuchal ligament
N. Trapezius
O. Spine of scapula
P. Infraspinatus
Q. Deltoid
R. Teres minor
S. Triceps brachii
T. Latissimus dorsi
U. Erector spinae
V. External oblique
W. Iliac crest
X. Gluteus medius
Y. Sternocleidomastoid
Z. Trapezius
AA. Subclavius
BB. Deltoid (cut)
CC. Pectoralis minor
DD. Subscapularis
EE. Pectoralis major (cut)
FF. Biceps brachii
GG. Serratus anterior
HH. External intercostal
II. Internal intercostal
JJ. Internal oblique (cut)
KK. External oblique (cut)
LL. Tensor fasciae latae
MM. Spinalis
NN. Splenius
OO. Levator scapulae
PP. Rhomboid minor (cut)
QQ. Superior serratus posterior
RR. Rhomboid major (cut)
SS. Serratus anterior
TT. Inferior serratus posterior
UU. Latissimus dorsi (cut)
VV. External oblique
WW. Latissimus dorsi (cut)

15-5

A. Trapezius

B. Infraspinatus
C. Deltoid
D. Teres minor
E. Teres major
F. Serratus anterior
G. Levator scapulae
H. Rhomboid minor
I. Rhomboid major
J. Triceps brachii

15-6

A. Spine of scapula
B. Deltoid
C. Deltoid
D. Triceps brachii
E. Brachialis
F. Brachioradialis
G. Flexor carpi radialis
H. Flexor carpi ulnaris
I. Palmaris longus tendon
J. Flexor retinaculum
K. Spine of scapula
L. Deltoid
M. Triceps brachii
N. Triceps brachii
O. Brachioradialis
P. External carpi radialis
Q. Humeral medial epicondyle
R. Anconeus
S. Flexor carpi ulnaris
T. Extensor carpi ulnaris
U. Abductor pollicis
V. Extensor digitorum tendon
W. Extensor retinaculum

15-7

A. Flexor digitorum superficialis
B. Flexor pollicis
C. Supinator
D. Flexor digitorum profundus
E. Flexor pollicis
F. Pronator quadratus
G. Lumbricals
H. Anconeus
I. Supinator
J. Abductor pollicis
K. Extensor pollicis longus
L. Extensor indicis
M. Anconeus
N. Extensor carpi radialis
O. Extensor carpi ulnaris
P. Extensor digitorum
Q. Abductor pollicis brevis
R. Extensor pollicis brevis
S. Extensor digitorum tendon
T. Dorsal interossei

15-8

A. Abductor pollicis
B. Opponens pollicis
C. Flexor pollicis
D. Adductor pollicis
E. Adductor pollicis tendon
F. Dorsal interossei
G. Tendon sheath
H. Tendon sheath
I. Extensor carpi ulnaris
J. Palmaris longus tendon
K. *Palmaris brevis (cut)*
L. Abductor digiti minimi
M. Flexor digiti minimi
N. Opponens digiti minimi
O. Lumbricals
P. Flexor digitorum tendons
Q. Tendon sheaths
R. Extensor indicis tendon
S. Extensor pollicis tendon
T. Extensor digiti minimi
U. Extensor digitorum tendon
V. Dorsal interossei

15-9

A. Psoas major
B. Ilacus
C. Obturator
D. Adductor magnus
E. Gluteus maximus
F. Piriformis
G. Gemellus superior
H. Obturator externus
I. Gemellus inferior
J. Nerve ending
K. Semitendinosus
L. Piriformis
M. Obturator
N. Pectineus
O. Adductor brevis
P. Adductor longus
Q. Gracilis
R. Sartorius
S. External oblique (cut)
T. Gluteus medius (cut)
U. Gluteus minimus
V. Gluteus medius (cut)
W. Quadratus femoris
X. Gluteus maximus (cut)
Y. Femur
Z. Adductor magnus (part)
AA. Biceps femoris

15-10

A. Gluteus medius
B. Tensor fasciae latae
C. Vastus lateralis
D. Patella
E. Inguinal ligament
F. Iliacus
G. Psoas major
H. Psoas minor
I. Pectineus

APPENDIX 1: KEYS FOR CHAPTER FIGURES

J. Adductor longus
K. Sartorius
L. Rectus femoris
M. Vastus medialis
N. Iliac crest
O. Semitendinosus
P. Adductor magnus
Q. Biceps femoris
R. Gracilis
S. Semimembranosus
T. Vastus medialis
U. Gluteus medius
V. Gluteus maximus
W. Iliotibial tract
X. Vastus lateralis
Y. Plantaris

15-11 (top of page)
A. Plantaris
B. Gastrocnemius
C. Gastrocnemius
D. Soleus
E. Calcaneal tendon
F. Popliteus
G. Soleus
H. Gastrocnemius
I. Calcaneal tendon
J. Lateral condyle of tibia
K. Gastrocnemius
L. Tibialis anterior
M. Fibularis (Peroneus) longus
N. Extensor digitorum
O. Flexor digitorum
P. Calcaneal tendon
Q. Lateral malleolus
R. Extensor retinaculum
S. Extensor retinaculum

15-11 (bottom of page)
A. Tibialis posterior
B. Flexor digitorum
C. Flexor halluces
D. Fibularis (peroneus) brevis
E. Medial malleolus
F. Calcaneus
G. Tibialis posterior
H. Flexor digitorum
I. Quadriceps tendon
J. Patella and tibia
K. Patellar ligament
L. Gastrocnemius
M. Soleus
N. Retinaculum
O. Medial malleolus
P. Flexor digitorum tendon
Q. Tibialis anterior tendon
R. Calcaneal tendon
S. Flexor hallucis tendon

15-12
A. Extensor hallucis tendon
B. Extensor retinaculum
C. Medial malleolus
D. Extensor retinaculum
E. Extensor digitorum longus tendons
F. Extensor digitorum brevis
G. Lumbrical tendons
H. Lumbrical
I. Extensor hallucis tendon
J. Lumbrical tendon
K. Lumbricals
L. Flexor digitorum brevis
M. Flexor digitorum brevis
N. Flexor digiti minimi
O. Abductor digiti minimi
P. Tendon sheaths
Q. Abductor hallucis
R. Calcaneal tendon
S. Calcaneus

CHAPTER 16

16-2
A. Nucleus
B. Cell body
C. Axon
D. Telodendron
E. Mitochondrion
F. Golgi complex
G. Axon terminal
H. Dendrite
I. Neurofilament
J. Golgi complex
K. Presynaptic cell axon
L. Telodendron
M. Postsynaptic cell body

16-3
A. Schwann cells
B. Sheath of Schwann
C. Node of Ranvier
D. Myelin sheath
E. Myelinated axon in CNS
F. Oligodendrocyte

16-4
A. Neuron cell body
B. Node of Ranvier
C. Schwann cell
D. Axon
E. Schwann cell cytoplasm
F. Schwann cell nucleus
G. Sheath of Schwann
H. Myelin sheath
I. Cell body
J. Unmyelinated axon

16-5
A. Myelin sheath
B. Sheath of Schwann
C. Axon
D. Sheath of Schwann

APPENDIX 1: KEYS FOR CHAPTER FIGURES

E. Phagocytic cell
F. Schwann cell tube

CHAPTER 17

17-1
A. Frontal lobe
B. Central sulcus
C. Temporal lobe
D. Brainstem
E. Precentral gyrus
F. Postcentral gyrus
G. Parietal lobe
H. Sulcus
I. Occipital lobe
J. Cerebellum
K. Longitudinal fissure
L. Longitudinal fissure
M. Longitudinal fissure

17-2
A. Premotor area
B. Broca's area
C. Prefrontal area
D. Lateral sulcus
E. Central sulcus posterior to motor cortex (pink)
F. Somatosensory cortex
G. Sulcus in parietal lobe
H. Gyrus in parietal lobe
I. Parieto-occipital sulcus
J. Visual association area
K. Primary visual cortex
L. Occipital lobe
M. Wernicke's area
N. Primary auditory cortex
O. Olfactory cortex
P. Temporal lobe
Q. Insula
R. Gustatory cortex in insula

17-3
A. Putamen
B. Thalamus (not a basal nucleus)
C. Caudate nucleus
D. Globus pallidus
E. Amygdala (not a basal nucleus)

17-4
A. Fornix
B. Choroid plexus
C. Hypothalamus
D. Pituitary gland
E. Intermediate mass
F. Subarachnoid space
G. Corpus callosum
H. Choroid plexus
I. Pineal body
J. Superior colliculus
K. Mesencephalon
L. Inferior colliculus
M. Choroid plexus
N. Pons
O. Cerebellum
P. Medulla oblongata

17-5
A. Interventricular foramen
B. Lateral ventricle
C. Third ventricle
D. Mesencephalic aqueduct
E. Pons
F. Fourth ventricle
G. Medulla oblongata
H. Spinal cord central canal
I. Lateral ventricle
J. Third ventricle
K. Fourth ventricle
L. Cerebellum

17-6
A. Central sulcus
B. Pineal body
C. Cingulate gyrus (pink)
D. Thalamus
E. Fornix
F. Intermediate mass
G. Parahippocampal gyrus
H. Hippocampus
I. Mammillary body
J. Olfactory tract
K. Corpus callosum
L. Fornix
M. Nucleus
N. Mammillary body
O. Amygdala
P. Hippocampus

17-7
A. Choroid plexus
B. Dura mater
C. Arachnoid mater
D. Arachnoid villus
E. Choroid plexus
F. Mesencephalic aqueduct
G. Choroid plexus
H. Subarachoid space
I. Spinal cord central canal
J. Filum terminale

17-8
A. Cervical vertebrae
B. Thoracic vertebrae
C. vertebrae
D. Sacrum
E. Spinous process
F. Spinous process
G. Transverse process
H. Spinous process
I. Sacral foramen

APPENDIX 1: KEYS FOR CHAPTER FIGURES

J. Sacral crest
K. Coccyx
L. Ventral root
M. Posterior median sulcus
N. Central canal
O. Ventral horn
P. Dorsal root ganglion
Q. Ventral ramus
R. Anterior median fissure

CHAPTER 18

18-1

A. Axon
B. Schwann cell
C. Endoneurium
D. Perineurium
E. Blood vessels
F. Epineurium

18-2

A. Optic chiasm
B. Oculomotor nerve
C. Trochlear nerve
D. Trigeminal nerve
E. Facial nerve
F. Vagus nerve
G. Hypoglossal nerve
H. Olfactory bulb and nerves
I. Olfactory tract
J. Optic nerve
K. Infundibulum
L. Abducens nerve
M. Vestibulocochlear nerve
N. Glossopharyngeal nerve
O. Vagus nerve
P. Spinal accessory nerve

18-3

A. Dorsal horn
B. Lateral column
C. Dorsal root
D. Ventral root
E. Arachnoid mater
F. Dorsal ramus
G. Sympathetic ganglion
H. Communicating rami
I. Ventral ramus
J. Body of vertebra
K. Autonomic ganglion
L. Adipose tissue
M. Vertebral foramen
N. ventral root
O. Dorsal root
P. Spinal nerve
Q. Ventral column
R. Dorsal ramus
S. Dura matter

18-4

A. Superficial cervical
B. Auricular
C. Occipital
D. Supraclavicular
E. Phrenic
F. Axillary
G. Musculocutaneous
H. Radial
I. Median
J. Ulnar
K. Intercostals
L. *Iliohypogastric*
M. *Ilioinguinal*
N. *Genitofemoral*
O. *Lateral femoral*
P. Obturator
Q. *Gluteal (superior)*
R. Femoral
S. *Gluteal (inferior)*
T. Sciatic
U. Saphenous

18-5

A. Musculocutaneous
B. Median
C. Ulnar
D. Radial
E. Radial (deep)
F. Radial (superficial)
G. *Palmar interosseous*

18-6

A. Intercostal
B. *Iliohypogastric*
C. *Ilioinguinal*
D. *Femoral cutqneous*
E. *Genitofemoral*
F. *Gluteal (superior)*
G. *Gluteal (inferior)*
H. Obturator
I. Sciatic
J. Common fibular
K. Saphenous
L. *Gluteal (superior)*
M. *Gluteal (inferior)*
N. Sciatic
O. *Femoral cutaneous*
P. Pudendal
Q. Tibial
R. Common fibular
S. Sural

CHAPTER 20

20-1

A. Tongue papilla
B. Microvilli
C. Gustatory cell
D. Supporting cell
E. Basal cell

20-2
A. Olfactory bulb
B. Olfactory tract
C. Olfactory nerves
D. Sphenoid bone
E. Odorant molecules
F. Cribriform plate
G. Basal cell nucleus
H. Basal cell
I. Olfactory neuron axon
J. Olfactory neuron nucleus
K. Supporting cell nucleus
L. Dendrite
M. Mucus of epithelium

20-3
A. Eyelash
B. Cornea
C. Superior palpebral
D. Pupul
E. Palpebral conjunctiva
F. Ciliary body
G. Vitreous chamber
H. Optic nerve
I. Fibrous tunic
J. Cornea
K. Sclera
L. Iris
M. Suspensory ligaments
N. Choroid coat
O. Vascular tunic
P. Retina
Q. Retina pigmented layer
R. Nervous tunic

20-4
A. Rod
B. Cone
C. Horizontal cell
D. Bipolar cell
E. Amacrine cell
F. Ganglion cell
G. Axons of ganglion cells

20-5
A. Superior oblique muscle
B. Lacrimal gland
C. Lacrimal duct
D. Lateral canthus
E. Inferior oblique muscle
F. Lacrimal canal
G. Lacrimal caruncle
H. Medial canthus
I. Nasolacrimal duct
J. Lacrimal punctum

20-6
A. Cornea
B. Lateral rectus
C. Superior oblique
D. Superior rectus
E. Iris
F. Inferior rectus
G. Optic nerve

20-9
A. Helix of auricle (pinna)
B. Triangular fossa
C. Antihelix
D. External auditory meatus
E. Tragus
F. Lobule
G. Malleus (hammer)
H. Incus (anvil)
I. Semicircular canal
J. Vestibular nerve
K. Cochlear nerve
L. Vestibulocochlear nerve
M. Tympanum (eardrum)
N. Stapes (stirrup)
O. Vestibule
P. Auditory (Eustachian) tube
Q. Cochlea

20-10
A. Semicircular canal
B. Semicircular duct
C. Ampulla
D. Utricle
E. Macula
F. Vestibule
G. Helicotrema
H. Saccule
I. Macula
J. Scala tympani
K. Scala vestibule
L. Scala media (cochlear duct)

Appendix 2: Eponyms in Anatomy & Physiology

Achilles: Achilleus in Greek mythology; Achille's (calcaneal) tendon

Adam: first man; Adam's apple (thyroid cartilage)

Addison: Thomas Addison, English physiologist, 1793-1860; Addison's disease

Alzheimer: Alois Alzheimer, German neurologist, 1864-1915; Alzheimer's disease

Apgar: Virginia Apgar, U.S. anesthesiologist, 1909-1974; APGAR score for newborns

Auerbach: Leopold Auerbach, German anatomist, 1828-1897; Auerbach (myenteric) plexus

Bainbridge: Francis Arthur Bainbridge, English physiologist, 1874-1921; Bainbridge (right heart--atrial) reflex

Barr: Yvonne M. Barr, English virologist, 20th century; Epstein-Barr virus

Bartholin: Caspar Thomeson Bartholin, Danish anatomist, 1655-1738; Bartholin's (vestibular) glands

Bell: Sir Charles Bell, Scottish physiologist, 1774-1842; Bell's palsy

Bohr: Christian Bohr, Danish physiologist, 1855-1911; Bohr effect

Bowman: Sir William Bowman, English physician, 1816-1892; Bowman's (glomerular) capsule

Boyle: Robert Boyle, English physicist, 1627-1691; Boyle's Law

Breuer: Josef Robert Breuer, Austrian physician, 1842-1925; Hering-Breuer reflex

Broca: Pierre Paul Broca, French anatomist, anthropologist, and surgeon, 1824-1880; Broca's (motor speech) area

Brunner: Johann Conrad Brunner, Swiss anatomist, 1653-1727; Brunner's (duodenal) glands

Corti: Alfonso Corti, Italian anatomist, 1822-1888; Organ of Corti (spiral organ)

Cowper: William Cowper, English surgeon, 1666-1709; Cowper's (bulbourethral) glands

Cushing: Harvey Williams Cushing, American surgeon, 1869-1939; Cushing's disease

Dalton: John Dalton, English chemist and physicist, 1766-1844; Dalton's Law

Duchenne: Louis Theophile Joseph Duchenne, French physiologist, 1845-1917; Duchenne muscular dystrophy

Epstein: Albert Anthony Epstein, English physician, 1921- ; Epstein-Barr virus

Eustachian: Bartolommeo Eustachio, Italian anatomist, 1524-1574; Eustachian (auditory) tubes

Fallopio: Gabriele Fallopio, Italian anatomist, 1523-1562; Fallopian (uterine) tubes

Frank: Oto Frank, German physiologist, 1865-1944; Frank-Starling principle

Golgi: Camillo Golgi, Italian neurologist and histologist; 1843-1926; Golgi body, Golgi (tendon) organ

Graaf: Reijer de Graaf, Dutch physician and anatomist, 1641-1673; Graafian (mature) follicle

Haldane: John Scott Haldane, Scottish physiologist, 1860-1936; Haldane effect

Haversian: Cloptin Havers, English physician and anatomist, 1650-1702; Haversian (central) canal

Heimlich: Henry Jay Heimlich, American surgeon, 1920- ; Heimlich (abdominal thrust) maneuver

Henle: Friedrich Gustav Jakob Henle, German anatomist, 1809-1885; Loop of Henle (nephron loop)

Henry: William Henry, English chemist, 1774-1836; Henry's Law

Hering: Heinrich Ewald Hering, German physiologist, 1866-1948; Hering-Breuer reflex

His: Wilhelm His, Swiss physician, 1863-1934; Bundle of His (atrioventricular bundle)

Hodgkin: Thomas Hodgkin, English physician, 1798-1866; Hodgkin's disease

Huntington: George Sumner Huntington, American physician, 1850-1916; Huntington's disease

Korotkoff: Nicolai Sergeevich Korotkoff, Russian physician, 1874-1920; Korotkoff's sounds

Krause: Johann Friedrich Krause, German anatomist, 1833-1910; Krause end organs (tactile corpuscle)

Kreb: Sir Hans Adolf Kreb, German-born British biochemist, 1900-1981; Kreb's (citric acid) cycle

Kupffer: Karl Wilhelm von Kupffer, German anatomist, 1829-1902; Kupffer (stellate reticuloendothelial) cells

Langerhans: Paul Langerhans, German pathologist, 1847-1888; Islets of Langerhans (pancreatic islets)

Leydig: Franz von Leydig, German anatomist, 1821-1908; Leydig cells (interstitial endocrinocytes)

Lieberkuhn: Johann Nathaniel Lieberkuhn, German anatomis, 1711-1756; Crypts of Lieberkuhn (intesinal crypts)

Malpighian: Marcello Malpighi, Italian anatomist, 1628-1694; Malpighian cells (keratinocytes)

Marfan: Antonin Bernard Jean Marfan, French pediatrician, 1858-1942; Marfan's syndrome

Meissner: Georg Meissner, German physiologist, 1829-1905; Meissner's (tactile) corpuscle, Meissners' (submucosal) plexus

Merkel: Friedrich Sigmund Merkel, German anatomist, 1845-1919; Merkel's disc (tactile disc)

Oddi: Ruggero Oddi, Italian physician, 1864-1913; Sphincter of Oddi (hepatopancreatic sphincter)

Pacinian: Filippo Pacini, Italian anatomist, 1812-1883; Pacinian (lamellated) corpuscles

Paget: Sir James Paget, English surgeon, 1814-1899; Paget's disease

Parkinson: James Parkinson, English physician, 1755-1824; Parkinson's disease

Peyer: Johann Conrad Peyer, Swiss anatomist, 1653-1712; Peyer's (aggregated lymphatic) patches

Punnett: Reginald Crundall Punnett, English geneticist, 1875-1967; Punnett square

Purkinje: Johannes Evangelista Purkinje, Czech physiologist, 1787-1869; Purkinje fibers (conduction myofibers)

Pylorus: In Greek mythology - "gatekeeper"; pyloric sphincter

Ranvier: Louis Antoine Ranvier, French pathologist, 1835-1922; Nodes of Ranvier (neurofibril node)

Reye: Ralph Douglas Reye, Australian physician, 20th century; Reye's syndrome

Rivinus: Augustus Quirinus Rivinus, German anatomist and botanist, 1652-1723; Rivinus (sublingual) ducts

Ruffini: Angelo Ruffini, Italian anatomist, 1864-1929; Ruffini's (tactile) corpuscle

Sachs: Bernard Parney Sachs, New York physician, 1858-1944; Tay-Sachs disease

Schlemm: Friedrich Schlemm, German anatomist, 1795-1858; Canal of Schlemm (scleral venous sinus)

Schwann: Theodor Schwann, German anatomist and physiologist, 1810-1882; Schwann cells (neurolemmocytes)

Sertoli: Enrico Sertoli, Italian histologist, 1842-1910; Sertoli's (sustenacular) cells

Sharpey: William Sharpey, Scottish anatomist and physiologist, 1802-1880; Sharpey's (perforating) fibers

Skene: Alexander Johnston Chalmers Skene, American gynecologist, 1838-1900; Skene's (paraurethral) glands

Starling: Ernest Henry Starling, English physiologist, 1866-1927; Frank-Starling's principle

Stensen: Niels Stensen, Danish physician, anatomist in Italy, 1638-1686; Stenson's (parotid) duct

Tay: Warren Tay, English physician, 1843-1927; Tay-Sachs disease

Valsalva: Antonio Valsalva, Italian anatomist, 1666-1723; Valsalva maneuver

Vater: Abraham Vater, German anatomist, 1684-1751; Ampulla of Vater (hepatopancreatic ampulla)

Volkmann: Richard von Volkmann, German surgeon, 1830-1889; Volkmann's (perforating) canals

APPENDIX 2: EPONYMS IN ANATOMY & PHYSIOLOGY

Wernicke: Karl Wernicke, German neurologist, 1848-1905; Wernicke's (audiotory association) area

Wharton: Thomas Wharton, English physician and anatomist, 1614-1673; Wharton's jelly (mucous connective tissue)

Willis: Thomas Willis, English anatomist and physician, 1621-1675; Circle of Willis (cerebral arterial circle)

Worm: Olaus Worm, Danish anatomist, 17th century; Wormian (sutural) bones

INDEX

A

abdomen 16, 109, 192, 285, 288-9, 323, 342, 360
abdominopelvic quadrants 23-4
abduction 210, 212-13, 216, 220-3
abductor hallucis 302-3
abducts 212, 277, 288, 293, 295, 297-8, 301-3, 340
accessory structures 206-7, 365-6, 375
acetabula 194
acetabulum 191-2, 195, 200, 207-8, 216-17
Ach 247, 249-50, 273, 314, 351-5
Achilles 238, 299, 377
acids 33-5, 43, 45, 149, 156
    strong 34, 46
    weak 34-5, 46
ACL (anterior cruciate ligament) 218, 223
actin 42, 45, 242-6, 249-52, 254, 268-9, 272-3
actin molecules 49, 243
action of neurotransmitters 314
action potentials 228, 305, 314, 345
active transport 87-8, 94-7, 101
    secondary 97-8, 101
adduction 210, 212-13, 216, 220, 222-3, 298, 301
adductor 295, 301, 303
adductor hallucis 302-3
adducts 212, 287-9, 293, 295, 299, 301, 303
adenine 43-4, 66, 68-9, 79
adipocytes 48, 109, 114, 129, 145, 205, 207, 353
adipose tissue 109, 114, 116, 126, 140, 145, 173, 207, 237, 353-4
aerobic respiration 254-6, 258-60, 265-6
aggregation of keratin fibrils 123
amacrine cell 365
amino acid sequence 72, 78-9
amino acids 41, 48, 60, 66, 68-70, 72, 78-9, 86-7, 89, 113, 154, 242, 256, 361, 369
amphiarthrosis 202, 219, 221-2
anabolism 6, 13, 31-2
analysis of CSF 332
anaphase 75-6, 81
anatomical position 15, 18, 188, 191, 195-6, 198, 207, 210-13, 215, 217, 220
anatomy 2-3, 7, 13, 15, 18-19, 143, 158-9, 165, 173, 202, 233, 236, 239, 258, 266, 362-3
    developmental 3, 13
    gross 2-3, 13, 15, 146
    microscopic 2-3

ankle 17, 141, 143, 153, 194, 198, 207, 210, 213, 218, 220, 222-3, 299, 303
ANS (Autonomic Nervous System) 130, 306, 312, 318, 321, 326, 335, 337, 349-53, 355
ANS neurotransmitters 352
antagonistic muscle 345
anterior 19-20, 23, 140, 167-72, 174, 180, 186, 188-9, 191-3, 322-3, 326-8, 333-5, 340-1, 350-2, 363, 365
    serratus 285, 288
    tibialis 299, 301
anterior aqueous chamber 365, 375
anterior cruciate ligament see ACL
antibodies 41-2, 100, 366
anticodon 70, 81
AP (action potential) 228-31, 247-52, 271, 305, 314-16, 318, 345, 369
apical cells 105-6, 114
apical surface 106, 114, 120-2, 128
apocrine glands 104, 129-30
aponeuroses 238, 262, 287, 289, 303
    epicranial 238, 280, 282
    palmar 291
appendicular skeleton 140, 143, 159, 161, 175, 182, 185-7, 189, 191, 193, 195, 197, 199-200, 337
APs 234-5, 238, 240, 247-50, 268, 315
    generating 235
    partial 314
    transmit 267
arachnoid mater 331
arches 120, 178, 194, 199-200, 215, 329
    vertebral 176-7, 184
arm 2, 9, 15-17, 127, 131-2, 141, 153, 175, 182, 185-9, 212-14, 262, 276-7, 285, 287-91, 343
arm muscles 187, 257, 276
arrangement of epithelial cells 106
arteries 125, 145, 166, 170, 174, 217, 238
arterioles 125
articular capsule 205, 214, 216, 218, 223
articular cartilages 143, 152, 158, 205-7, 214, 216, 223
articular facets 178-81
    superior 179-80, 184
articular processes 177-8, 180
articular surfaces 188, 202-3, 207-10
    free 202
    superior 179
articulating bones 202-11, 213-14, 218, 220, 235

INDEX

ascending tracts 334
astrocytes 306-7
atoms 3, 13, 27-32, 39, 45
    neutral 29
ATP 39, 43-5, 50, 55-6, 86-7, 94-8, 240, 242, 245-6, 254-60, 265-7, 269, 273, 314
    deficiency of 258
    dephosphorylates 314
    extra 255
    generating 255
    muscle fiber's 256
    producing 56, 259
    stored 254-5, 258
    surplus 256
ATP 39, 44-5, 50, 55, 86-7, 94, 97-8, 242, 245-6, 254-60, 265-7, 269, 273
    muscle fiber's 256
    stored 254-5, 258
ATP molecules 43, 56, 96, 255-6
ATP synthesis 55-6, 240, 254, 256, 259, 266
ATPase site 244-5, 269, 273
    myosin's 245, 269
ATPase site hydrolyzes ATP 243
attachment sites 112, 144, 161, 166-71, 175, 178, 181-2, 185-8, 192, 196-7, 277, 283, 362
    muscle's 275
auditory ossicles 161-2, 166
autonomic nervous system 130, 306, 312, 318, 321, 326, 335, 337, 349-51, 353, 355
autophagia 60, 122, 137
autorhythmicity 272
autosomes 64-5, 81
axial regions 15-16, 20
axial skeleton 140, 143, 145, 158-61, 163, 165, 167, 169, 171, 173, 175, 181-3, 185-6, 191, 194, 337
axial, antecubital region anterior appendicular regions 24
axon hillock 309, 315-16, 318
axons 52, 246, 263, 267-8, 273, 307-18, 326-7, 329, 337-8, 349-52, 360, 362, 364, 368
    myelinated 309-11, 317, 324
    postganglionic 352
    preganglionic 351-2
    unmyelinated 311, 317
axoplasm 309, 317-18

B

bacteria 5, 38, 42, 55, 85, 98-9, 109, 118, 122-3, 131, 136, 144, 157, 206
ball-and-socket 209, 214, 216, 219, 221-2
bands 50, 103, 110, 126, 135, 140, 206, 238, 241, 243-4, 273, 293, 299
baroreceptors 340, 358-9, 375
Basal 53, 121, 324, 361
    basal cell 121

basal cells 105, 113-14, 121-2, 360-1, 375
basal nuclei 324, 327
basement membrane 105-6, 108, 114, 121-2, 124-6, 132, 135, 332
basioccipital process 170
BBB (blood-brain-barrier) 331-2, 335
Bell's Palsy 342
biaxial 209, 221-2
biceps brachii 277, 290-1
biceps femoris 298-9, 301
biceps muscles 254, 262, 266, 290
biceps, skeletal muscle names biceps brachii 303
bilayer 40, 45, 83-4, 86, 89
binding of ATP to atpase 269
binding of LDL 100
binding of NE 353
binding of tonofilaments 123
bipolar cells 364-5, 368-70, 375
birth 3, 16, 131, 150-1, 159, 173, 175-6, 178, 185, 193, 203
blood 1, 15, 27, 47-9, 63, 103-4, 112-15, 118, 123-5, 139, 148-9, 156-7, 159, 233-6, 258-60, 357-9
    movement of 1, 15, 27, 47, 63, 103, 115, 139, 159, 185, 201, 225, 233, 235, 275, 305
    warm 10, 118
blood capillaries 332
blood cell 94, 109, 145, 150, 332
    specialized white 109, 157
    traps 113, 136
blood cells form 141
    trapped 136
blood chemistry 305, 342
blood clot 11, 113-14, 157-8
blood clotting 10-11, 112-13, 156
blood flows 113, 136, 256, 328
blood formation 141
blood loss 113, 136, 157
blood pH 257, 357
blood plasma 129, 332
blood pressure 129, 326, 328, 330, 340, 342
blood supply 1, 15, 27, 47, 63, 103, 115, 139, 159, 185, 201, 225, 233, 238, 273, 275
    brain's 167
    skin's 118
blood transports 8, 118
blood type 39, 85
blood vessels 1-2, 7-8, 10, 85, 105-6, 108-10, 113, 132, 143-5, 147, 150-2, 168-72, 205-6, 233-8, 267-9, 353-4
    dense network of 118
    large 268, 331, 358
    nourishing 147, 152
    skin's 125
blood vessels coursing 109, 351
Blood-Brain-Barrier 332
bloodstream 104, 112
body 1-12, 15, 18-22, 27-30, 35-7, 41-2, 47-9, 103-6, 115-19, 125-31, 139-42, 178-83, 200-1, 233-5, 275-7, 305

INDEX

basal 53, 61
ciliary 363, 365, 375
dense 268-9, 272-3
ischial 192
living 169, 176
mammillary 326, 361
mandible's 171-2
pineal 325, 335
sphenoid's 168
sternal 183-4
sternum 221
body cavities 20-1, 53, 105-6
body cells 47-53, 56, 58, 98
    damaged 109
    dead 99
    typical 47, 55, 63-4, 239
body movements 141, 143, 209
    coordinated 275-6
body organization 15, 17, 19, 21, 23-5
body temperature 7, 9-12, 31, 118, 130, 317, 327, 330
    person's 31, 327
    regulating 118, 125, 129
body weight 155, 199, 218
body's 185
    broken 146, 155, 157
    cancellous 145, 158
    compact 143-8, 150-1, 153, 158, 182
    cortical 144, 158
    cuneiform 143, 198
    forearm 187-8, 210, 291
    funny 159, 343, 360
body's blood vessels 1, 15, 27, 47, 63, 103, 115, 139, 159, 185, 201, 225, 233, 275, 305, 321
body's surface 10, 19, 358
body's weight 7, 153, 176, 178, 180, 191, 197-9, 297
bonds 29, 32, 39, 41, 44, 49, 69-70, 77, 84
    chemical 28-31, 45, 56, 255
    covalent 29-30, 33, 37, 41, 43, 45, 68
    peptide 46, 70, 72
bone cells 139, 144, 146-8=group of 139
bone density 155, 158
bone deposition 148, 154-5, 158
bone marrow 110, 145, 147, 153, 158
bone matrix 109, 146, 148-51, 153-8
bone models 149-50, 158
bone movement 202, 205, 207-8, 220, 234
    skeletal muscles cause 234
bone remodeling 155-6, 158, 193
bone resorption 147, 149, 155, 158
bone surface 149, 180
bones 108-12, 139-62, 165-6, 168-9, 173-6, 181-2, 185, 187, 189-91, 193-4, 196-9, 201-4, 206-14, 218-20, 234-5, 275-6
    adjacent 141, 178, 201, 204
bones function 139, 275
bones move 207, 210

bony labyrinth 371-2, 375
Bowman 361, 375, 377
brachial 17, 342
brachialis 276, 290-1, 303
brachioradialis 291, 303
brain 3-4, 9-10, 20-1, 126-7, 141, 161-2, 165-70, 305-7, 312, 321-2, 324-34, 337-8, 351-2, 357-62, 367-70, 373-4
brain abnormalities 330
brain cells 50
brain stem 167, 170, 325-9, 335
brain ventricles 328, 332
brain waves 329-30
brain's somatosensory regions 359
buttocks 16-17, 109, 295, 343

C

calcaneal tendon 299
calcaneus 198-9, 218, 238, 299, 301-3
calcification 148-9, 154, 156, 158
calcified cartilage 151-2, 157
calcitonin 156, 158
calcium 7, 27, 119, 142, 149, 154, 156, 226
    body's 142, 156
calmodulin 269, 271, 273
calvaria 165
canaliculi 147-9, 155, 158
canals 147-8, 153-4, 160, 167-8, 332, 372, 377, 379
    central 147-8, 158, 332, 335
    nasolacrimal 172, 174, 184
    optic 168, 170, 184, 338
    sacral 181, 184
    semicircular 372
capillaries 106, 113, 124-5, 238-9, 256, 260-1, 266, 332
carbohydrates 6-7, 13, 35, 38-40, 52, 57-8, 85, 261
carbon chain 39-40
carbon dioxide 6, 30-2, 35, 48, 89, 118
cardiac muscle cells 266-7, 353
cardiac muscle squeeze blood 234
carpal bones 189-90, 215, 293
carpals 17, 188-91, 200, 209, 216, 222, 291, 295
carriers 86-7, 94-8, 100-1
cartilage 4, 23, 108-9, 111-12, 114, 139-41, 149-52, 154, 158-9, 182, 201-6, 275, 371
    skeletal 140-1
cartilage matrix 109, 150, 152
cartilage model 150-2, 155
cartilaginous 202-3, 221-2
cartilaginous joints 202-5, 208, 219
catabolic reaction 32
catabolism 6, 13, 32, 45
catalase 43, 45, 61
catalysts 33, 36, 45
cavities 20-2, 104, 111, 141, 145, 147, 151, 160, 162, 165-6, 174, 205, 214, 216, 235, 307

abdominal 20-2, 182, 289-90
abdominopelvic 20-3, 235, 341
major 20-2
oral 21, 162, 169, 171
pelvic 20-2, 181, 192
pericardial 20, 22
vertebral 20-1, 306
cell biologists 49, 51, 53-5, 57-60, 74, 79, 86, 239
cell bodies 266, 308-9, 312, 318, 324, 333, 341, 350, 352
cell connections 103, 114
cell cortex 49-50, 52-3
cell crawling 49-50, 52
cell cycle 63, 65, 67, 69, 71, 73-7, 79-81
cell division 52, 64, 73-4, 77, 79-81, 121, 266, 312
cell junctions 52
cell membrane 40, 42, 44, 47, 72, 83, 101, 105, 228-9, 235, 239-40, 308, 368
cell types 47, 85, 109
cells 3-8, 30-1, 39-40, 47-64, 66-8, 72-6, 79-80, 83-100, 103-9, 120-7, 133-6, 147-9, 226-9, 308-10, 313-17, 352-3
adjacent 87, 103-4, 121, 309
adjoining 104
amacrine 364-5, 368, 375
body's 8, 38
cancer 79
connected 104
cuticle 133
damaged 40, 61, 113
dead 50, 113
ependymal 306-7, 318, 332
ethmoid air 169-70, 173, 183
fat 109, 353
fat-storing 48, 141
few types of 63, 73
formed 6-7, 239
generalized 48, 50
glandular 104, 130
glial 306-7, 309, 311, 318
groups of 3, 63, 80, 103, 133, 360
gustatory 360-1
hemopoietic 145, 151
horizontal 364-5, 368, 375
human 47, 68, 80, 83, 91-2
layers of 106, 122
liver 4, 57, 74, 85, 94, 353
longest muscles 234
mast 109, 124, 136, 205
mesenchyme 109, 157
mitral 362, 375
multinucleated 149
myoepithelial 130
nerve 52
nervous system 246
nucleated 73
organized 63
osteogenic 148, 150-1, 157-8

pacemaker 234, 268, 273
parent 74-5, 77-9
person's 87
photoreceptor 364
plant 39
postsynaptic 309, 313-14, 316
pyramidal 324, 336
satellite 239, 260-1, 273, 306, 319
sex 47, 64, 234
single 6, 73
somatic 47
special 6, 118, 309
specialized 57, 145, 305, 308, 357
sperm 53, 85
spiny 122, 138
stimulates 154
stratum corneum 123, 131
supporting 360, 372, 376
transitional 106, 114
typical 47, 63, 73-5, 78, 88
uninucleate 63
cell's plasma membrane 83, 85
cellular differentiation 73, 81, 133
cellularity 6-7, 13
cellulose 39, 45
centrioles 51-4, 61, 74
centromere 51, 75-6
centrosomes 51, 61, 74, 76
cerebellum 165, 321, 327-9, 331, 334, 374
cerebrospinal fluid 328, 331-2, 358-9
cerebrum 312, 321-5, 327-9, 331, 335
ceruminous 130, 371
cervical 16, 176-81
cervical nerves 341
cervical vertebra 167, 170, 178-9, 209
cervical vertebrae 167, 176-81, 283-4, 287
change shape 21, 30, 38, 44, 84, 86, 95-7, 106, 243, 249, 364
channels 86-7, 89-90, 94, 98, 100-1, 104, 227-9, 247-50, 271, 273-4, 308, 313-16, 362, 366
ligand-gated 89, 101, 228, 231, 247
voltage-gated calcium 271, 274
characteristics of life 5
chemical reactions 6-7, 28, 31-3, 36, 43, 45, 47, 53-4, 56, 59, 86, 136, 157, 235, 255-6, 271
chemicals 3-4, 6-7, 9, 11, 27-8, 32, 35, 41, 47, 73, 79, 112-13, 126, 154, 234-5, 358-62
chemistry 27, 45, 342
chemistry overview 27, 29, 31, 33, 35, 37, 39, 41, 43, 45
chemoreceptors 9, 340, 358, 375
chest 2, 16, 141, 176, 182-3, 186, 212, 234, 236, 262, 276, 282-3, 286-8, 295, 341
chew 233-4, 282-3
chin 16, 172, 174, 254, 282-3, 339
cholesterol 41, 45, 57, 61, 83, 85, 99-101, 124
cholinergic receptors .352-3
chondroblasts 109, 111, 150, 157

INDEX

chondrocytes 109, 111, 114, 140, 150-2, 154, 205
choroid coat 363, 365, 375
chromatids 51, 75-6
    sister 75-6, 81
chromatin 64, 67, 74-6, 81
    strands of 74-5
chromosome Number 64
chromosomes 51, 64-6, 68, 73, 75-6, 80, 239, 309
    replicated 75-6, 81
    sex 64-5, 81
ciliary 53, 366
cilium 53
cingulate 329
circuit 1, 15, 27, 47, 63, 103, 115, 139, 159, 185, 201, 225, 233, 275, 305, 321
circumduction 210, 212-13, 216, 220-2
circumducts 288
circumferential 147
Cl 28-9, 34
    chloride pumps transport 96
Cl- ions 271
    charged 227
classification 31, 41, 45, 86, 101, 105-6, 114, 142-3, 146, 202, 208, 219, 221-3, 338, 358, 375
classifying Joints 201
clathrin 100
clavicle 153, 183, 185-7, 200, 209, 221, 283-5, 287-8
clot 112, 136-7
CNS (central nervous system) 305-7, 309-10, 312-13, 321, 323-5, 327, 329, 331-3, 335, 337-8, 349, 358
CO_2 30-2, 35, 48, 88-9, 219, 358
coccyx 19, 176, 180-1, 191, 193-4, 332, 341
cochlea 340, 372-3
code 66, 68-9, 78, 80
codons 68-70, 72, 78, 81
coenzyme 36
collagen 41, 43, 45, 108, 125, 127, 146, 154
collagen fibers 105, 110-11, 119, 124-5, 127, 132, 137, 139-40, 144, 146-7, 149-50, 154, 157-8, 202-6, 267, 362
collarbones 150, 183, 185
colloids 28-9, 45, 47
columnar cells 106, 114
    single layer of 107
commissural fibers 324
compounds 27-8, 32-7, 40, 43-4, 59-61, 72, 206, 255, 364
concentration gradient 88-90, 93-7, 226-7, 231=steep 97, 248
concentration of catalysts 33
concentration of reactants 33
concentration of transported particles 95
condyle 160, 188, 196, 200, 209, 218
    tibial 196, 217-18
connective tissue bands 143, 203, 275, 289, 293, 298-9
connective tissues 4, 13, 23, 58, 105, 108-14, 117, 126, 140-1, 202-3, 205, 234, 236, 238, 289, 365-6
    dense 108-11, 114, 140, 203, 331, 366

dense regular 144, 162, 178, 206-7, 238, 289
    most 108-9
    sheath of dense irregular 237-8
contact inhibition 79, 81, 113-14
continuous conduction 317
contractile components, skeletal muscle's 262
contractility 235-6, 273
    muscle fiber's 240
contraction
    concentric 262, 276
    eccentric 262, 276
    isometric 261-2, 266, 273
    isotonic 261-2, 273
contraction bulges 252
contraction cycles 269, 271
contraction periods 250-1
conus medullaris 332-3, 341
core temperature, body's 8, 85
cornea 362, 364-8, 375
coronoid process 171, 174, 188-9, 200, 215, 283, 290
corpus callosum 324-5, 335
corpuscles 127, 378
corrugator 282
cortex 133, 144, 322-4, 328, 336
Corti organ of 372-3, 375
corticobulbar tracts 334
corticospinal tracts 334
costal cartilages 140-1, 182-3
CP (creatine phosphate) 255, 258, 266, 273
cranial 16, 21, 162, 165, 221, 338, 352
cranial bones 161-2, 165-6, 168-71, 173, 175, 183, 221
cranial cavity 20-1, 165-6, 168, 173, 183, 306, 322
cranial nerves 327, 338-40, 342, 353
cranium 20, 162, 165-6, 169, 183, 321, 351
crista 168, 372, 374
crista galli 168-70, 183, 331, 335, 338
cristae 55, 372, 374
crossbridge cycles 244, 246, 250, 258-9, 273
crossbridges 242-6, 249-52, 254, 269-70
crosses, skeletal muscle's tendon 235
cube-shaped cells 73, 106-7
cuboid 198, 301-2
cuboidal 105-6
cultures 119, 189
cupula 372, 374-5
curvatures, secondary 176
curve 159, 167-8, 194
cushions 20, 48, 204, 206-7, 218
cutaneous receptors 126
cycles of hair growth 133
cyclins 79-80
cytokinesis 74-7, 80-1, 121, 152, 260, 266
cytoplasm 47, 50, 52-3, 55-6, 58, 60-1, 64, 70, 76, 83, 85, 87-8, 97, 103-4, 109, 308-9
cytosine 43, 45; 66, 69

401

cytoskeleton 49-52, 54, 59-61, 98, 100, 103-4, 121, 268, 309
cytosol 47-55, 60-1, 64, 72, 83-4, 86-90, 95-101, 225-8, 240, 247-52, 254-5, 258-9, 268-71, 308

D

dehydration synthesis 37, 44
deltoid 288, 303, 342
dendrites 121, 308-9, 312, 315, 360
dendrites of sensory neurons 372
density of capillaries 261
density of mitochondria 261
depolarize 228-9, 249, 267-8, 314, 316-17, 357, 368
depression 100, 160, 166, 183, 187, 212, 220-1, 223, 366
dermal blood flow 125
dermal blood vessels 120, 125
dermal papillae 119-20, 124-5, 127, 132
dermal root sheath 132
dermal tension lines 125, 137
dermis 116-27, 129-32, 134-5, 236, 360
desmosomes 103-5, 114, 121, 123, 133, 266
detachment of myosin 245
development of lamellar bone 150
development of osteoblasts 148
development of osteoclasts 149
dialysis 92-3, 101
diaphragm 20-1, 341
diaphysis 143, 145-6, 150-2, 160, 189, 195, 204
diaphysis side 152, 204
diarthrosis 203, 219, 221-2
diencephalon 321, 325-6, 328-9, 353, 359
digestion 60-1, 351
dilation 327, 353-4
discs 189, 204, 240-3, 266, 268, 272, 274, 364
    intercalated 234, 266-7, 272-3
    intervertebral 111, 141, 177-8, 204
    optic 363-4, 375
diseases 1-3, 7, 12-13, 40, 119
distal 19, 24, 84, 143, 189, 194, 204, 210-11, 221-2, 291, 294, 299, 309, 313
distal epiphysis 188, 196-7
    tibia's 197
distal phalanges 293, 301
distal phalanx 143, 191, 199-200, 301
distal tarsals 198
distribution of muscle fibers 260
DNA 28, 38, 44-5, 51, 55, 63-4, 66-8, 70, 74-5, 77-81, 123
    nuclear 128
    replicating 74
DNA expression 65-7, 69, 71, 73, 75, 77, 79, 81
DNA molecule 55, 63, 66-8, 74-5, 77, 80
DNA nucleotides 77
    exposed 77
    free 77
DNA of living cells 44

DNA of living organisms 66
DNA polymer 77-8
DNA proofreading 78, 81
DNA replication 74, 77-9, 81
DNA sequence 79
DNA template 68, 77-8, 81
DNA triplets 68
dorsal cavity 20-1, 306, 350-2
dorsal interossei 295, 303
dorsiflexes 299, 301
dorsiflexion 213, 220, 222, 299
ducts 104, 107, 129-30, 135, 366, 372, 374, 378
    cochlear 372-3
    semicircular 372, 374
dyneins 52

E

ear ossicles 21, 277, 371, 373, 375
ECF 8, 13, 59-60, 83, 88, 95-7, 225-8, 247-8, 259-60, 268, 271, 307, 310-11, 316-17
EEG 330
efflux 316
elasticity 110, 236, 252
    muscle fibers eccentric isotonic contraction 273
elastin fibers 43, 124
elbow 17, 19, 140-1, 159, 187-9, 209-12, 214-17, 219, 221, 236, 243, 254, 276, 290
electrical condition 89, 225, 228, 240, 247, 317
electrochemical energy 30
electrodes 225
electrons 27-30, 32, 35, 61
EMG 247-8, 273
emotions 119, 189, 280, 329
endochondral 150-1
endocytosis 60-1, 98-101
    receptor-mediated 98-100
endolymph 372-4
endomembrane system 58-9, 61
endomysium 238, 262, 266-7, 272-3
endoplasmic reticulum 56-7, 61, 309
endosteum 143, 145-9, 153
Endosymbiotic theory 56
endothelial cells 332
end-plate 247
energy 7, 10, 29-32, 36, 39, 43, 48, 50, 54, 56, 60, 86, 94-7, 254-6, 258-9, 368
    cellular 87-8, 96, 207
    mechanical 30
energy shells 29
energy systems 254-5, 257, 273
enzyme activity 37, 258
enzymes 35-9, 41, 43-5, 57, 60-1, 63-4, 68, 70, 77-80, 86-7, 101, 148-9, 247, 254-5, 269, 314
ependymal 307

epicondyle, lateral 188, 196, 200, 214, 293, 299
epicranial 282
epidermal cells 120-1, 123-4, 126-7, 129, 131
    modified 133
    undamaged 135
epidermal nerve endings 126-7, 137
epidermal pegs 119-20, 124, 127, 137
epidermal ridges 119, 124, 137
epidermal tissue 132
epidermal wounds 135
epidermis 52, 105, 116-17, 119-29, 131-5, 137, 234, 360
epidermis functions 137
epimysium 238, 262, 272-3
epinephrine 351, 353-5
epineurium 337, 347
epiphyseal lines 143, 145, 152, 202, 219
epiphyseal plates 151-4, 158, 188, 201, 204, 223
epiphyses 143, 145-6, 151-2, 158, 160, 188, 195, 204
epithalamus 325
epithelial cells 74, 105-6
epithelial tissues 4, 13, 104-5, 108, 120
eponychium 135, 137
EPP (end-plate potential) 247-50, 273
EPSP 314, 316, 318, 345
    single 316
equilibrium 93, 166, 225, 321-2, 328, 334, 340, 342, 357, 373-5
    dynamic 373-4
    static 374, 376
erection 354
escalator 95-6
esophagus 4, 20-1, 106, 340
ethmoid 165, 168-9, 171, 173
ethmoid bone 162, 165, 168-70, 172-3, 183, 331, 338, 362
etymology 1-2, 13
eumelanin 127-8, 134, 137
excitation-contraction coupling 249
excitatory 268, 271, 314, 316, 353
exocytosis 98-101, 104, 130, 313
exposure 41, 43, 128, 325, 361
extensor digitorum 277, 291, 293, 299, 301, 303
extensor digitorum tendon 291, 293, 295, 303
extracellular fibers 108, 112
extracellular fluid 8, 13, 48, 53, 59, 72-3, 84-90, 96, 98, 100, 145, 225, 240, 267-8, 271-2
eye muscles
    extrinsic 339, 362, 366-7, 375
    intrinsic 339, 347, 363, 375
eyeballs 2, 21, 49, 166, 168, 173, 234, 250, 263, 268, 312, 338-40, 365
eyebrows 131, 133-4, 165-6, 280, 282, 365, 375
eyelashes 131, 133-4, 366, 375
eyelids 116, 131, 280, 282, 365-6, 368, 375
eyes 9, 18, 131, 162, 168, 173, 280, 282, 312, 326-8, 330, 334, 338-9, 358-9, 362-70, 375-6
    direct 342

F

Facial 169, 280, 340, 342
facial bones 141, 162, 165-6, 168-9, 171-4
    skull's 169
facial expressions 119, 161, 171, 234, 280, 283, 342
falx cerebri 331, 335
far-sightedness 370
fascia
    deep 237-8, 273, 298
    superficial 126, 138, 236-7, 280
    thoracolumbar 288-9
fascicles 238, 277, 280, 288-9, 337
fasciculi 334-5
fast glycolytic fibers 259-60, 263, 265-6, 273
fast oxidative fibers 259-60, 263, 265-6, 273
fatty acids 39-40, 46, 56, 60-1, 85, 87, 89, 131, 256, 258-9
    saturated 39-40, 46
    unsaturated 39-40
feedback 9, 11, 13
    negative 8-10, 12, 67, 79
    positive 10-13, 315
female pelvis 181, 193-4
femoral condyles 218
femoris, rectus 298, 301
femur 15, 143, 191, 194-7, 200, 205, 208, 216-18, 222, 276, 295, 297-9, 301
fibroblasts 109-10, 113, 124-5, 127, 132, 137, 150, 157, 203, 205-6
fibrocartilage 111, 140, 177-8, 189-90, 202-5, 207, 214, 216
fibrocartilage callus 157
fibrocartilage pads 140, 177-8, 190, 204
fibrosis 113-14, 137
fibrous 113, 132, 137, 150, 178, 202-3, 205, 207-8, 221-3, 234, 362-3
fibrous capsule 205-7, 223, 289
fibrous joints 202-4
fibrous layer 144-5
fibrous membrane 111, 150, 152, 175
fibrous periosteum 144, 158
fibrous tissue 203
fibula 15, 196-7, 202, 204, 217-18, 222, 298-9, 301
fibular 17
field, receptive 368, 376
filamentous proteins 41, 46, 103, 108, 120, 243
flexion 210, 212-18, 220-3
    lateral 213, 220, 223
flexor 291, 295, 301, 303, 346
flexor 291, 342, 345-7
flexor carpi ulnaris 291, 303
flexor digitorum 291, 301, 303
flexor pollicis 291, 294-5, 303
flexor retinaculum 293, 295, 301, 303
follicles 127, 131-4, 377
fontanels 150, 158, 173, 175, 183, 203
foot 17, 37, 153, 194, 196-9, 207, 213, 218, 222, 238, 297, 299, 301-4, 329

foot muscles, intrinsic 302-4
foramina 167-8, 172, 179, 181
forearm 17, 141, 145, 153, 159, 185, 187-91, 201-2, 204, 210-12, 214-15, 220, 262, 277, 290-3, 342-3
forehead 16, 18, 165-6, 203, 282
fossa 160, 165, 171, 183, 186, 209
    anterior cranial 165, 168, 173
    posterior cranial 165-7
fovea 160, 183, 364, 367
fovea centralis 364, 367, 370
gree nerve endings (FNEs) 122, 126, 135, 137, 359
frontal lobe 159, 165, 322-3, 368
frontal planes 19, 24
fructose 37-9, 46

G

G-actin 49, 52
GAGs 108
ganglia 312, 337, 349, 351-2, 368
    paravertebral 351, 355
ganglion cells 364-5, 368-9, 375
gap junctions 103-4, 114, 148-9, 155, 234, 267-8, 272
gastrocnemius 250, 299, 301
genes 66-8, 73, 78-9, 81
genetic material 63-4, 73-5, 79, 81
glabella 165, 170
glands 9, 104, 106-7, 114-15, 117, 120, 129-31, 166, 173, 305-6, 312, 326, 338-9, 353-4, 365-6, 376-8
    adrenal 22, 154, 349, 351
    eccrine 129-30
    holocrine 104, 131
    mammary 104, 130, 326
glandular epithelium 104
glossopharyngeal 340
glucose molecules 39, 43, 48, 91-2, 240, 255, 259
gluteal 16-17, 343
gluteal regions 24, 295-6
gluteus 298, 301
gluteus medius 295, 297-8, 301, 304
glycocalyx 85, 101
glycogen 39, 46, 48, 62, 240, 255-6, 259-60, 266
glycolysis 255-6, 258-60, 266, 273
glycoproteins 57, 60, 85, 99, 101, 103, 105, 124, 267, 364
goblet cells 104, 106-7
Golgi 54, 57-62, 72, 346-7, 358, 377
gomphoses 203-4, 219, 221
gracilis 298, 301, 304
gray matter 309, 311-12, 318, 322, 327-8, 333, 352
groin 16
ground substance of connective tissues 108
growth hormone (GH) 154, 158
guanine 43-4, 46, 66, 69

H

hair bulb 132-3, 137
hair cells 133, 372-5
hair follicles 125, 127, 129-34, 137, 234
hair growth 119, 133-4
hair growth cycle 133-4, 137
hair matrix 133-4, 137
hair papilla 132-4, 137
hair receptors 127, 132, 137
hair roots 49, 126, 133, 137
hair shaft 133, 137
Hair Texture and Color 134
hairs 4, 41, 43, 52-3, 115, 117, 119, 125, 127, 129-35, 137, 193, 362, 365-6, 372, 374
    club 134, 137
    dark 134
    vellus 131
    white 134
hamstring muscles 193, 233
H-bond 30, 77
    intermolecular 30
    intramolecular 30
hearing 2, 161, 166, 277, 340, 342, 357, 370-3, 376
heart 1-2, 15, 19-22, 27, 47, 63, 103, 115, 139, 159, 185, 201, 225, 233-4, 275, 305
heart beats 266, 328
heart rates 321, 340, 342
helix, double 44-5, 68, 77, 242
hemocytoblasts 109
hemoglobin 41-2, 46, 49, 79, 129, 256
Hemopoietic 145
hemopoietic tissue 145, 150
heterogeneous mixture 28-9
hinge 209, 215, 219, 221-3
hip 16-17, 161, 175, 180, 191-2, 195, 205, 207-9, 216-17, 219, 222-3, 297-8, 343
hipbones 112, 140, 191-4, 216
histamine 109, 136
HIV (human immunodeficiency virus) 44
Holocrine 104
homeostasis 6-9, 12-13, 33, 87, 94, 115, 119, 125, 129, 156, 158, 305, 307, 326-7, 332, 357
homeostatic control systems 8-9
homeostatic imbalance 12
homogeneous mixture 28
hormones 4, 79, 83, 87, 99, 104, 112, 128, 130, 154, 156, 158, 234, 271, 305, 325-6
    parathyroid 156, 158
Human Genome Project 66
human skeletal muscles 259
humeral head 200, 207, 213-14
humeroradial 215, 221, 223

INDEX

humeroulnar 215, 221
humerus 187-9, 202, 210-15, 221, 287-91, 293
hyaline cartilage 111, 140, 150, 154, 169, 178, 182, 202-5
hydration shells 33, 37, 91
hydrogen atoms 29-30, 32, 37, 39, 41
hydrogen bonds 29-30, 43-4, 66, 68, 70
hydrogen ions 29, 32, 34
hydrolysis 37-8, 44, 46, 60
hydrophobic 40, 83, 89
hyperextension 210-12, 215, 220
hyperosmotic 93
hyperpolarization 226, 228, 231, 247, 271, 314, 316, 318, 368
hyperthermia 31
hypochondriac 23
hypodermis 117, 124-7, 129-32, 135, 236, 273, 360
hypoglossal 170, 340, 342
hypothalamus 325-7, 329, 332, 335, 353, 359
hypothenar Group 295
hypothermia 31
hypotonic 91-2, 94, 101

I

iliac crest 192, 194-5, 200, 289, 298
iliac region 295
iliacus 276, 295, 298, 304
iliocostalis 284
iliotibial tract 298, 301, 304
ilium 192-4, 200, 209, 222, 284, 288, 298, 301
illness 12-13, 119
impulse pathways 324, 343, 353
impulses 118, 126-7, 228-9, 231, 308-9, 312-13, 315-18, 323-4, 326-9, 333-4, 338, 345-6, 349, 359-64, 367-70, 373-4
    afferent 305, 357, 360
    conducts 306-7, 321
    nerve 130, 357, 370
    sympathetic 351
indirect effect of neurotransmitters 314
inferior nasal conchae 172
inferior surface 177-8, 180, 197, 326, 338
inflammation 113, 135, 157-8, 342
infraorbital 174
infraspinatus 288-9
inner ear 166, 328, 340, 358, 371-2, 375
innervate 335, 339, 341-3, 345
insensible perspiration 123
insula 322-3, 335
integumentary system 115-19, 121, 123, 125, 127, 129, 131, 133, 135, 137
intercarpal 216, 219, 222
intermediate 19, 52, 261, 272
intermediate filaments 49, 51-2, 103-4, 121, 123, 268, 273
Intermolecular 30
Intermolecular hydrogen bonds 30
internal oblique 288-9, 304

internal organs 20-1, 192, 267, 323
internasal 174
interneurons 312, 333-5, 337
interphalangeal 222
interphase 74, 76, 79-80
interpretative area 324
intervertebral 178, 204, 219, 221
intramembranous 150
intramembranous ossification 150, 175, 203
intramolecular h-bonds 30
introns 69
inversion 213, 220, 222, 301
iodopsin 364, 369, 375
ion channels 89-90, 101, 313
IPSPs 314, 316, 345
iris 363, 365, 367, 375
irregular bones joints 158
irritability 6-7, 13, 235, 273
ischial spines 192-4, 297
ischial tuberosity 192-4, 200, 233, 297-9
ischium 192-3, 200, 298, 301
Isoosmotic 93
isotonic 90-2, 94, 101, 261, 266
isotopes 30, 46

J

jaw 141, 169, 171, 282-3, 329, 339
joint capsule 217
joint cavity 205-6, 214
joints 108, 112, 140-1, 162, 198, 201-11, 213, 215, 217, 219-21, 223, 235, 306, 328, 333, 360
    ball-and-socket 209
    hinge 209
    interphalangeal 209, 295, 302-3
    metacarpophalangeal 209, 295
    metatarsophalangeal 209, 302-3
    multiaxial 208
    synarthrotic 202-3
jugular 170

K

keratin fibrils 122-3
keratinocytes 120-4, 128-9, 132-4, 378
keratohyalin 122-3
keratohyalin granules 122
kidneys 4, 21-3, 93, 105-6, 111, 124, 256, 326, 353-4
    left 19, 23
kinesins 52
kinetic energy 30, 46, 88, 93, 97, 368
kinetochore 51, 62, 76
kinetochore fibers 76
kinocilium 372-5
kneecap 17, 143, 196

L

lactic acid   118, 255-8, 260, 273
lacunae   111, 114, 147-8, 151-2, 155, 158
lambdoid suture   162, 165-7, 175
lamella   147, 153=outer 147-8
lamellae   127, 147-8, 151, 158
    circumferential   147, 153-4
Lamellar   122, 147
lamellar bone   146-7, 150, 157-8
laminae   178-9
Langerhans cells   122, 132
large cells   52, 73, 131
large muscles   183, 189
lateral condyle   196-7, 200, 217-18, 293, 298-9
lateral cuneiform   198, 200, 302
lateral rotation   220, 223, 366
lateral side   162, 171, 177-8, 188-9, 191, 195, 197, 293
latissimus   288
latissimus dorsi   288-9, 304
LDL receptors   100
leak channels   227, 231
learning skeletal muscles   277
leg bones   155, 196-7
leg muscles   266, 299
lesser wing   168, 170
levator   282, 288
levator labii superioris   280, 282, 304
ligaments   4, 58, 110, 139-40, 144, 158-60, 186, 189, 192, 196, 199, 203-4, 206-9, 213-18, 223, 235
    capsular   207, 214, 216
    coracohumeral   213-14
    inguinal   288-9
ligand   86, 89, 101, 228, 231, 247, 271, 313-14
ligase   43
linea alba   288-9, 304
linea aspera   196, 200, 298
lipid-soluble   89
lipoproteins   100-1
liver   2, 4, 21, 23, 39, 48, 55, 63, 85, 110, 124, 154, 256, 258, 353, 364
long bones   15, 142-3, 145-7, 150, 152-4, 158, 160, 187-8, 191, 196, 204, 207
longissimus   284
longus, palmaris   291, 293
lower limbs   15-17, 24, 140, 143-5, 153, 176, 181, 185, 191, 193-4, 197, 199-201, 213, 297, 334
lumbar curvature   176, 180, 285
lumbar vertebra   179-80, 332
lumbar vertebrae   176-8, 180-1, 295
lunate   190, 200, 215-16
lungs   1-2, 4, 8, 15, 19-22, 27, 47, 49, 63, 103, 106-8, 110, 112, 182, 340, 353-4
lymphatic   4, 145
lysosomes   58, 60-2, 72, 99-100, 122

M

macromolecules   28, 30, 35, 54, 64, 83
macrophages   99, 101, 109, 112, 122, 158, 205-6
maculae   372, 374
malnutrition   150
mammary   16, 104, 130
mandible   174, 282-3
mandibular   171, 174, 342
manubriosternal   221
manubrium   182-3, 186, 204, 221
marrow
    red   141, 145-6, 150-1, 158
    yellow   141, 145, 158
mastoid process   167, 171, 175, 283
    air cells   183
mater, dura   170, 331-2, 337, 362
matrix   55, 108-9, 111, 133, 146, 149-50, 152-3, 155, 365
matter   3, 6, 27-30, 46, 123
    white   311-12, 319, 324, 327-8, 334, 336
maxillae   162, 168-9, 172-4, 183
maximum contraction   255, 260
mechanisms   8, 72, 88
mechanoreceptors   126-7, 358
medial canthus   366, 375
medial condyle   196, 217-18
medial cuneiform   198, 299
medial epicondyle   188-9, 196, 214, 291, 299
medial surface   172, 188, 192, 197, 289
mediastinum   20-1, 358
medulla oblongata   170, 327-9, 332-5, 340, 353
medullary cavity   143, 145-7, 151-3, 157-8
melanin   48-9, 62, 123, 127-8, 134, 363
melanocytes   49, 121, 127-8, 132, 134, 363
melatonin   325, 327, 335
membrane   22, 52-6, 59-60, 84-9, 93-8, 100, 105-6, 144, 149-50, 225-9, 231, 239-40, 247-9, 258, 271, 314-16
    basilar   372-3, 375
    epithelial   104-5
    glassy   132
    inner   55, 64
    interosseous   204, 293, 299
    nuclear   56, 70, 74
    outer   55-6, 64
    positive   248-9
    postsynaptic   314, 316
    ruffled   149, 158
    semipermeable   88, 90-1, 93
membrane channels   89, 94, 229-30, 247, 317
membrane phospholipids   84-5
membrane proteins   59, 86-7, 101
membrane receptors   100, 352
membrane structure   85, 87, 89, 91, 93, 95, 97, 99, 101
membranous epithelium   105-6, 113
membranous labyrinth   372
membranous organelles   53-4, 57-8, 61
meninges   170, 331-2, 335

INDEX

Merkel cells 121, 127
merocrine glands, mast cells membranous epithelium 114
mesencephalon 325, 327-9
mesenchyme 108
messenger RNA 68
metabolism 6-7, 13, 31, 239
    metacarpal 190-1
    metatarsal 197-8
    metacarpals 191, 198, 200, 209, 222, 291, 293, 295, 299
    adjacent 191, 294-5
metaphase 75-6
metaphysis 143
metatarsals 198-200, 209, 222, 299, 301-3
microfilaments 49-53, 62, 98, 100, 309
microglia 306-7
microscopic structures 2-3, 146, 234
microtubules 49-53, 56, 61-2, 76, 309
microvilli 52-3, 62, 360, 373
midbrain 327, 339
middle ear 21, 166, 171, 371
minimi
    abductor digiti 294, 302-3
    gluteus 276, 295, 297-8, 301, 304
mitochondria 54-6, 59, 61-2, 72, 88, 109, 240, 255-6, 258-9, 261, 266-7
mitosis 74-7, 79-81, 121, 152, 260, 266, 309
MLC (myosin light-chain) 269, 273
MLCK (myosin light-chain kinase) 269-70, 273
molecules 3, 8, 13, 27-30, 32, 35, 37, 40, 43-4, 50, 54-6, 59-61, 83, 86-8, 93, 370
    dynein 51
    large 60, 86
    lipid 57-8, 86, 109
    phosphate 40, 96
monosaccharides 38
motor molecules 50-2, 59-60, 76, 98-100
motor neurons 246, 249-50, 263, 267-8, 271, 273, 312, 334-5, 337-8, 343, 345-6, 349, 353
    upper 335
MPF (mitosis-promoting factor) 80-1
mRNA 68-70, 72, 79
multinucleate 63, 81, 239, 272-3
muscarinic receptors 353, 355
    skeletal muscles display 353
muscle cells 39, 48, 57, 228, 233, 266, 273, 314
    neighboring cardiac 267
    skeletal 63, 73, 266-7, 316, 353
muscle contractions 57, 125, 156, 246, 257, 261, 345
muscle contracts 207, 265
    ciliary 365, 367
    skeletal 208, 238
muscle fiber contracts 235, 243, 246
    skeletal 246, 251
muscle fibers 233-6, 238-40, 243, 246-52, 254-6, 258-69, 272-4, 353
    cardiac 234, 240, 243, 267-9, 271
    single 261, 263
muscle tissue 1, 15, 27, 47, 63, 103, 115-16, 139, 159, 185, 201, 225, 233-5, 271, 273, 275
    cardiac 234, 273, 353
    multicellular organism 13
    skeletal 234-6, 259, 273
    smooth 234, 236, 267, 269, 271-2, 274, 326
muscles 125-6, 141-3, 165-7, 175, 180-3, 206-8, 233-9, 250-2, 254, 257-8, 260-6, 275-7, 280-303, 338-40, 342-3, 345-6
    antagonistic 345-6
    arrector pili 125, 133, 234, 268, 354
    cardiac 234-6, 240, 272, 306, 326, 349, 354
    ciliary 363, 367
    circular 280, 282, 367
    stapedius 371, 376
musculocutaneous 342
myelination 309-10, 317-18
myoglobin 240, 256, 258-60, 266, 273
myosin 42, 52, 62, 241-5, 265, 272-3
myosin light-chain kinase (MLCK) 269-70, 273

N

nasal bones 162, 165, 169, 172, 174, 184, 282
    left 168, 172, 203
nasal cavity 4, 21, 105-7, 131, 162, 166, 168-9, 172-5, 184, 308, 338-40, 361, 366
nasal conchae 162, 168-70, 172-4, 184
nasal septum 21, 168-70, 172-4, 184, 338, 361
nerve fiber 105, 127, 309
nerves 2-4, 116, 121, 126-7, 142-5, 147, 153, 159-60, 165-9, 172-4, 180-1, 188, 236-8, 312-13, 337-45, 347
    optic 168, 170, 338, 362-5, 368-70
    peripheral 341
    vestibular 374
neurology 305
neurons 73, 122, 228, 246-7, 263, 271, 305-9, 311-12, 314, 316-18, 326-7, 329, 332-5, 343, 361-2, 364
    bipolar 312, 315, 318, 364
    multipolar 312, 315
    postganglionic 318, 349, 351-5
    postsynaptic 316
    presynaptic 316
    unipolar 312, 319
neurophysiology 3
neurotransmitter molecules 267, 316
nociceptors 126, 138, 358-60, 375
nose 16, 18, 111, 116, 141, 165, 172-3, 185, 276, 280, 282, 312, 339, 366, 368, 371
nozzle 229, 249
NREM (Non-rapid eye movement) 330-1, 336
nuclear membrane dismantles 75-6
nucleic acids 35, 38, 43-4, 66-7
    single-stranded 44
nucleoplasm 64, 68, 77

O

organic compounds 6, 35, 37, 41, 43, 48, 206
organic molecules 30, 37, 54, 59, 127
organs 1-4, 7, 9, 19-22, 103-5, 115-16, 118-19, 125-7, 139, 141-3, 159-60, 233-6, 305-6, 321, 372-3
    living 139
    sex 343, 354
    spiral 372-3
osmoreceptors 326, 358-9
osmosis 90-1, 101
osseous tissue 108-9, 112, 114, 139-41, 143-9, 151, 153, 155, 157-8, 202-3
ossification 149-50, 152, 158, 204
    endochondral 150-2, 157
    primary 151
osteocytes 109, 112, 114, 147-9, 155, 158
oxygen 3, 7-8, 27, 30-3, 38, 56, 61, 63, 79, 88-9, 113, 120, 124, 238-9, 255-6, 258-9

P

parathyroid 156
parietal bones 143, 146, 162, 165-7, 170, 184, 202, 280
    left 162, 166, 203
parietal lobe 322
parietal peritoneum 22, 289
patellar ligament 217, 223, 298
PCL (posterior cruciate ligament) 218, 223
PDGFs (platelet-derived growth factors) 113-14
pectoral girdle 185-7, 191-2, 285, 287-8, 295
pectoralis 276-7, 285, 287-8, 304
pelvic 16, 21, 153, 194
pericardial 21
perichondrium 111, 114, 140, 150-1, 205
perilymph 372-4
perimysium 238, 262, 272-3
periosteum 143-8, 150-1, 153, 158, 203, 205
peroxisomes 58, 60-2, 72
phagocytosis 98-9, 101, 122, 128, 136, 149
phalanges 190-1, 197-200, 209, 222, 291
phasic receptors 358, 375
pheomelanin 127-8, 134
phosphagen system 256, 258, 273
phospholipid molecules 83-6, 89
phospholipids 39-40, 53, 57, 83-7, 100-1, 309
photopigments 364, 368-9
physiology 2-3, 7, 27-8, 139, 159, 258, 266
pinocytosis 98-101
pituitary gland 168, 170, 326, 335
pivot 179, 209, 215, 219, 221
pivot joints 209
plantar flexion 213, 220, 223, 299, 301
plasma membrane 39, 47, 49-50, 52-4, 56-60, 73, 83-5, 87-90, 92-3, 96, 98-101, 103-4, 122, 225-9, 307-8, 313-14
platelet-derived growth factors (PDGFs) 113-14

platysma 282-3
pleura 20, 22
plexuses 337, 341, 343
PNS (peripheral nervous system) 305-10, 312-13, 322, 334, 337-9, 341, 343, 345, 347, 349, 351, 353, 355
polar molecules 29-30, 33, 37, 91
polymers 35, 39, 41, 43-4, 46, 48, 66, 68
    single-stranded 43-4
polypeptides 41, 66, 72-3, 78, 243, 361
    growing 70, 72
polyribosome 72, 81
polysaccharides 39, 108
posterior forearm 293
posterior muscles 283, 293
posterior side 156, 188-9, 196, 236, 250, 262, 285, 288, 290, 293
    ulnar head's 189
posterior surface 156, 162, 166, 179, 181, 186, 188, 196, 198, 214, 293, 295, 301, 338, 362-3
preganglionic neurons 318, 349-55
pressure receptors 126, 137, 318, 358
pronation 212, 215, 220-1
proprioceptors 338, 358-9
prostaglandins 40
protein fibers 108, 110, 124, 157
Protein synthesis 41, 56, 61, 66, 68, 72, 74-6, 154, 308
proteins 6-8, 35-6, 41-2, 44-9, 51-2, 55-9, 63-4, 66-70, 72-4, 78-80, 85-7, 100, 121-2, 154, 241-3, 307-9
    adhesion 86-7, 108
    cells secrete 124
    contractile 42, 45, 241
    histone 64, 74-5
    immunological 42
    integral 86-7, 89, 94, 101, 104
    peripheral 86, 101, 240
    secondary-level 41
    soluble blood 136
    structural 41, 241
    tertiary 79
    transmembrane 86, 101, 104
proteoglycans 62, 108, 124, 146
proximal epiphysis 187, 195-7
proximal phalanges 209, 222, 294-5, 303
pseudopodia 50, 62, 98-100, 307
pubic bones 193, 200, 205, 222=left 193, 204
pudendal 343
putamen, brain Purkinje cells 336
pyrimidines 43, 46
pyruvic acid 255-6, 258-9

Q

quickness 266

INDEX

R

radialis muscles 291, 293
radialis, flexor carpi 291, 293, 303
radioisotopes 30
radioulnar 202, 219, 221
radius 188-90, 200, 202, 204, 209-10, 212, 214-15, 221-2, 290-1, 293
rapid eye movement (REM) 330-1, 336
RAS (reticular activating system) 329, 336
RDS (respiratory distress syndrome) 12
reactants 31-3, 35-7, 46-7
reactions 6-7, 9, 11, 29, 31-7, 228, 254-5, 271, 314
    body's 9-10, 12
receptors 9, 59, 86-7, 95-6, 99-100, 105, 121-2, 126-7, 228, 247, 305-6, 312-14, 352-3, 355, 357-9, 361-2
    adrenergic 352-3
    membrane-bound 314, 353
    nicotinic 352-3, 355
    tactile 126, 138, 318, 358, 376
    tonic 358-9, 376
    warm 359
reciprocal activation 346-7
recognition, cellular 85, 101
recovery stroke 53, 245-6, 269, 273, 289
rectus abdominis 288-9
red blood cells (RBCs) 39, 41, 49, 63, 85, 91, 112, 114, 128-9, 141, 256
reflexes 334, 343, 345-7, 353, 355
regenerate 113, 129, 261, 308, 313, 369-70
regions 15-16, 23-4, 68, 70, 75-7, 88, 90, 104-5, 125-6, 165-6, 191-3, 225-7, 312, 315-16, 321-5, 341-3
    abdominopelvic 23
    antecubital 19
    appendicular 15, 17
    buccal 18=cephalic 18, 20
    charged 91, 227
    depolarized 229, 251
    epigastric 23
    inguinal 23-4
    lateral 23
    repolarized 251
    thoracic 19, 178, 180, 341, 343
    umbilical 16, 23, 25
REM (Rapid eye movement) 330-1, 336
repair of damaged axons 313
replication 74-5, 77-8, 80
repolarization 226, 231, 248, 252, 258, 316-17
RER (rough endoplasmic reticulum) 56, 62, 64, 309
resorption 149, 155-7
respiratory center 327-8, 336
resting conditions 227-8
resting membrane 225, 227, 231, 248-9, 315-16
reticular plexus 125
reticular region 124-5, 129, 131, 135
reticulospinal 334
retina 359, 363-5, 368-70

rhodopsin 364, 369-70
ribose 38, 43-4
ribosomal RNA 68
ribosomal subunits 55, 64, 70, 72
    large 70
    small 55, 64, 68, 70, 72
ribosomes 54-7, 61-2, 64, 66, 68-70, 72, 74, 108, 239, 308
    bound 55, 61, 72
    free 55, 62, 72
    functional 55, 64, 68, 70
RME (Receptor-mediated endocytosis) 98-101
RMP (resting membrane potential) 226-8, 231, 247-9, 315-16
RNA 38, 44, 46, 64, 66, 68, 70, 72, 76-8, 81, 308
    formed 74
    ribosomal 55, 62, 68, 81
    transfer 68-9, 81
rough endoplasmic reticulum (RER) 56, 62, 64, 309
rubrospinal 334

S

saccule 372, 374, 376
sacral hiatus 181, 184
sacral plexuses 343-4
sagittal 19, 210, 372
saltatory conduction 317
sarcolemma 239-40, 246-52, 256, 258, 267-8, 271-2
sarcomeres 240-3, 246, 249-52, 254, 258, 262, 265, 268-9, 272-3
sarcoplasm 239-40, 247, 250, 256, 259, 267-8, 273
sartorius 298, 301
scala tympani 372-3, 376
scala vestibuli 372-3, 376
scapula 153, 185-7, 200, 202, 207, 214, 221, 284-5, 287-91
scar tissue 137-8, 313
Schwann cells 306-7, 309-11, 313, 319
sciatic nerves 192, 343
sebaceous glands 117, 123, 125, 129-33, 366
secretory cells 59, 130
sella turcica 168, 170, 184
semimembranosus 299, 301
Semipermeability 87
Semispinalis 284
sensory impulses, fibers conduct 318
sensory neurons 309, 312, 335, 338, 341, 345-6, 360-1, 372-3
sensory receptors 116-18, 122, 124, 132, 136, 161, 309, 312, 321-2, 334, 337-8, 357-8, 363, 372, 374, 376
serous membranes 21-2, 106, 114
    body's 22
sex hormones 41, 130, 154
short bones 142-3, 146, 154, 158, 187, 190, 198
shoulder bones 140
shoulder girdle 185, 191, 200
shoulder muscles 214, 289

signal recognition particle (SRP) 72, 81
simple diffusion 88-9
sinuses, paranasal 173, 184
skeletal bones 140, 185
skeletal muscle anatomy 273
skeletal muscles 161, 166-7, 179, 182, 185-8, 190-2, 197-8,
    234-8, 246-7, 258, 260-5, 272-3, 275-7, 306, 328, 350-4
    adult 260
    flat 238
    large 180, 236
    outermost 237
    smallest 371
    typical 236
    voluntary 343
skin 4, 10, 19, 43, 48-9, 104-6, 108-9, 115-36, 138-9, 280,
    282-3, 327, 333-4, 339, 341-3, 357-8
    forehead 280
    human 127
    pale 128
    scalp 282
skin constrict 10, 118
skin derivatives 115, 117, 129, 138
skin glands 129, 138
skin pigments 129, 138
skin repair 135-6, 138
skin trichosiderin types 138
skull bones 140, 160, 162, 165-8, 173, 201, 203
slow oxidative fibers 259-60, 263, 273
smooth muscle 125, 132, 234-6, 267-73, 306, 326, 343,
    349, 353, 363
    single-unit 267, 273
smooth muscle cells 104, 353
smooth muscle contraction 269-70, 273
smooth muscle fibers 234, 236, 267-9, 271
smooth muscle tone 271, 274
spongy bone 143-8, 150-2, 158, 182
squame cells 122-3, 138
SR (sarcoplasmic reticulum) 240, 259, 267-8, 271-4
SRP (signal recognition particle) 72, 81
stereocilia 372, 374, 376
sternum 140, 153, 182-4, 186, 209, 221, 283-4, 287-8
steroids 39-40, 46, 89
switching 263
stimulus 9-13, 86, 89-90, 117, 126, 206, 228-9, 235, 248-9,
    252, 271, 305-6, 312, 315-16, 329, 357-9
stomach 2, 4, 21, 23, 43, 104-6, 234, 236, 268, 271, 357
strata 105, 117, 120-1, 135
    membranous epithelia squamous cells 114
stratum basale 120-3, 126-8, 132, 135
stratum corneum 120, 122-3, 135
stratum germinativum 121, 123-4, 135
stratum granulosum 120, 122-3
stratum lucidum 120, 122-3
stratum spinosum 120-3, 126, 128, 132, 135
stress 10, 12-13, 130, 144-6, 155, 157, 176, 270-1, 306
    physical 152, 155-6

stretch reflex 345
stretch, excessive 345-6
stretched muscle contracts 345
structural design 41, 201-3, 209
structures 1-3, 9, 15, 19, 63-5, 103-4, 115-16, 126, 139, 159,
    161-2, 175-6, 184-5, 201-2, 206-7, 338-9
    associated 23
    movable 262
    specialized 2, 4, 47, 104, 305, 309, 357, 370
    stratified 115
styloid process 167, 171, 175, 184, 189-90, 216, 291
    pointed 189
subclavius 285, 288
subscapularis 288-9
substances 7, 28, 31-5, 37, 42, 48, 53, 57-60, 79, 86-91, 93-5,
    97-8, 100, 104, 113, 123-4
    diffusing 88-9, 93
    water-soluble 84, 89
substitution mutation 78-9
substrate detaches 95
substrate molecules 95
sucrose molecules 37
sugar, simple 38-9, 46, 85
sulfanilamide 38
superior portion 168-9, 171-3, 182, 280, 327, 329, 338
supination 212, 215, 220-1
supraorbital 170
surface area to volume ratio 259-60
sutures 113, 143, 162, 165-6, 175, 184, 203-4, 219, 221, 223
    sagittal 162, 165-6, 175, 184, 202-3
sweat 6, 11, 115, 117-18, 129-30
    eccrine 129-30
sweat glands 10, 104, 117, 125, 132, 135, 351, 353-4, 366
    apocrine 130-2
symphyses 204, 219, 221-3
synapse 309, 313-14, 335, 351, 362, 364, 370
synaptic cleft 246-7, 249, 309, 319
synarthrosis 202, 219, 221, 223
synarthrotic 203-4, 221
synchondroses 204, 219, 221, 223
syndesmoses 203-4, 219, 222-3
synergists 276
synostosis 202-4, 223
synovial cavity 202-3, 205-6, 219, 223
synovial fluid 21, 205-7, 219, 223
synovial joints 202, 205-10, 218-20, 358
synovial membrane 205-7, 219, 223
synthesis 31-2, 66, 68, 72, 74, 77, 118, 123, 129, 255
synthesize 35, 43, 54, 61, 63-4, 72, 74, 78, 128, 258
    connective tissue cells 108
systems 2-5, 8-9, 13, 115, 139, 240, 254-5, 257, 305-6, 311,
    350
    digestive 2, 4, 7, 39, 161, 234-5, 354
    endocrine 4, 8-9, 235, 305, 326
    functional 329
    immune 85, 87

INDEX

limbic 326, 329-30, 335, 361
regulatory 305, 319
somatic nervous 306, 312, 319, 335, 337
urinary 234-5

T

tactile 126-7, 318, 358
talus 198-9, 209, 218, 222
tarsal bones 197-8
    largest 198, 218
tarsals 17, 198-200, 209, 222, 301, 303, 366, 376
tarsometatarsal 222
taut 207, 217-18, 262-3, 367
tectospinal 334
telogen 133-4, 138
telomeres 80
telophase 75-6
template 68, 77-8
temporal bone 21, 162, 165-6, 168, 171-2, 174-5, 184, 221, 282-4, 372
temporal lobes 165, 322-4, 361, 370, 373
temporalis 282-3
temporoparietalis 280, 282
tendon reflex 345-6
tendon sheaths 206-7, 214
tendons 4, 43, 58, 143-4, 159-60, 206-8, 213-14, 233-5, 238, 262, 289, 293, 298-9, 301-2, 345-6
tension 103, 108, 111, 146-7, 180, 208, 233-6, 243-4, 246, 249-52, 254, 260-6, 268-9, 274, 357-8, 365
    internal 90, 262-4, 273
    maximum 252, 254
tension of ligaments 208
tensor fasciae latae 297-8
teres 288-9, 342
    pronator 291, 293
terminal cisternae 240-1, 246, 249-52, 259
tetanus 252, 273
thalamus 325, 329, 334
thenar group 295
theory
    endosymbiotic 55-6
    sliding filament 243, 245, 273
thermoreceptors 9-10, 126, 318, 358-9
thermoregulation 10-11
thigh muscle tendon 196
thighbones 15, 145, 191
thin myofilaments 241-3, 245-6, 249-50, 252, 265, 268-9, 272, 274
thoracic 16, 21, 176-8, 181, 285, 306, 341, 350-1
thoracic cage 160, 182, 184-6, 191
thoracic cavity 20, 22, 182
thoracic vertebrae 176, 179-82, 184, 287
thorax 161, 182, 184, 220, 276, 285, 323, 342-3, 358, 360
threshold stimulus 249-50, 274

throat 4, 32, 167, 183, 283, 340
thymine 43-4, 46, 66, 68
thyroxine 154, 158
tibia 159, 194, 196-8, 200, 202, 204, 209, 217-18, 222, 298-9, 301
tibial tuberosity 196, 200, 217, 298
tilts 209, 283-5
tissue necrosis 113-14
tissues 3-4, 7, 35, 41, 49-50, 63, 80, 89, 99, 103-7, 109-15, 118, 123-4, 268, 306, 359-60
    areolar 109, 114, 124
    dense irregular 110-11, 114, 238
    dense regular 110-11, 114
    nervous 4, 185, 305-6, 318, 332, 334
    reticular 109-10, 114
    soft 141, 143, 149, 171, 199, 280
toes 17, 19, 117, 153, 198-200, 210-11, 213, 220, 222, 299, 301-3
tongue 4, 21, 162, 167, 175, 283, 339-40, 342, 360-1
torsion 146-7, 204
torso 179-80, 182, 265, 285, 290
torso muscles 288
trabecula 147
trabeculae 145-8, 150-1, 157-8
trachea 4, 20-1, 106-7, 111
transcribe 66-7, 73, 76, 79
transcription 66-8, 72, 77, 79, 81, 308
transcription factors 67, 81
translocation 70, 72, 81
transport blood 145
transport vesicles 57, 59-60, 62
transverse plane 19, 212
transverse processes 177-81, 184, 283, 285, 287, 295
trapezoid 190, 200
trigeminal nerve 170
    maxillary branch of 170, 174
triglycerides 40, 46, 48, 126, 131, 237, 256
triplets 53, 66, 68, 70, 78, 81
triquetrum 190, 200
trochlea 188-9, 200, 215, 339
tropomyosin 243-4, 246, 249-51, 268, 272, 274
troponin 243-4, 246, 249-51, 272
tubercles 160, 184, 188, 200, 214, 289
    lesser 188, 200, 214, 289
tubes 104, 106-7, 127, 130, 147, 152, 166, 181, 235, 309-10, 371-2, 375
    auditory 371
    tiny 104-6
tubules 57, 239-41, 247, 249-50, 267-8, 272
Tympanic 171
tympanum 166, 371, 373

U

ulnar head 189, 200

ulnar nerve 159, 188, 360
ultraviolet B (UVB) 124, 138
umbilical 16, 23
uniaxial 209-10, 215, 217-18, 221-2
uninucleate 63, 81, 272
upper limbs 15-16, 140, 185-91, 194, 197, 200, 214, 237
urinary bladder 4, 21-3, 106, 108, 193, 234, 236, 269, 354
urine 3, 6, 106, 234, 236, 326
utricle 372, 374, 376

V

vascular tunic 362-3, 376
vasoconstriction 125, 138, 354
vasodilation 113, 125, 328, 353-4
veins 2, 125, 145, 153, 167
ventral 19, 21, 327, 333-4, 341, 347, 350
ventricles 328, 332, 335-6
    lateral 328, 335
vertebrae 21, 111, 140, 146, 153, 176-81, 184, 204, 221, 283-5, 288, 298, 351
    adjacent 178, 180, 285
vertebral column 160, 175-81, 184-6, 204, 213, 220, 276, 283, 285, 289, 321, 332, 341, 351-2
vesicles 4, 50, 54, 57-62, 72, 76, 85, 98-101, 128, 268, 313
    endocytic 59-61, 98-9, 101
    secretory 59, 62
vesicular 59
vestibular membrane 372-3
vestibule 340, 372, 374
vestibulocochlear 340, 342
vestibulospinal 334
viruses 7, 42, 44, 60, 85, 98-9, 118
visceral organs 20-3, 105-6, 181, 235, 272, 318, 333, 342, 358
    abdominal 340
vitamins 7, 32, 34-6, 41, 46, 99, 118, 123-4, 129, 154, 158, 364, 369, 376
vitreous humor 365, 368, 376
voltage 225-6, 228, 231, 247-8, 315
voltage-gated channels 89, 101, 228-9, 231, 247-8, 309, 315, 317

W

water concentration 90
water molecules 30, 33, 37, 84, 89-91
water-resistant 131
wave summation 251-3
wavelengths 364, 368
waves 30, 53, 228, 248, 250-2, 315, 330, 335, 367-8, 373
    alpha 330, 335
    delta 330, 335
weight 28, 91, 116, 124, 141, 145, 152, 176-7, 181, 191, 199, 214, 263, 332
    molecular 28, 30, 100
    plasma membrane's 83, 86
white blood cells 40, 50, 60, 84-5, 99, 112, 114, 122, 141
Wormian bones 143, 158, 184
wrinkles 119, 125, 165, 280, 282

X

X-rays 30, 149

Z

zygomatic arch 166-7, 171-2, 184, 282-3
zygomatic bones 162, 165-6, 169-74, 184, 282
zygomaticus 280, 282